"The PEERS® program has been a gift to autistic and other neurodivergent teens and adults, their families and professionals who work with them by providing a fun, innovative way of building social skills and opportunities for interaction. This version for preschool children provides a modified version of its step by step, evidence-based, positive approach to how to support younger children in social relationships. It will bring joy, confidence and skills to many children, their parents (who are actively involved from the word go) and the providers who get to work with them."

Catherine Lord, PhD, *Distinguished Professor of Psychiatry, Semel Institute of Neuroscience and Human Behavior, UCLA David Geffen School of Medicine*

"A marvelous addition to our tools for developing social-communication skills in preschoolers this valuable, evidence based program teaches social skills using lessons, play based materials, and group activities. Designed to have materials that are readily taught and used, this book will be an invaluable guide to foster social skills in the preschool population."

Fred R. Volkmar, MD, *Irving B. Harris Professor Emeritus, Child Study Center, Yale University School of Medicine*

PEERS® for Preschoolers

This manual builds on the success of the Program for the Education and Enrichment of Relational Skills (PEERS®), an internationally renowned program used in over 150 countries and translated into numerous languages. PEERS® has now expanded to work with autistic and neurodivergent preschool-aged children, as well as those with other social challenges. Through this new manual, providers will learn about important skills to enhance positive peer interactions and friendship development for young children, how to structure sessions and encourage skill-building effectively, and how to educate and empower parents to be valuable social coaches for their children. Every chapter includes a therapist guide for each session and parent resources such as lessons, homework, handouts, worksheets, and social coaching play cards. This latest edition to the PEERS® program is ideal for professionals and educators who provide social-emotional therapeutic services and support to young children (between the ages of four and six years) diagnosed with autism or other social challenges.

Dr. Elizabeth Laugeson is a licensed clinical psychologist, Clinical Professor at the UCLA David Geffen School of Medicine, and Director of the UCLA PEERS® Clinic and UCLA Tarjan Center UCEDD.

Dr. Mina Park is a licensed clinical psychologist in private practice, a former Assistant Clinical Professor in the Department of Psychiatry at UCLA, and an Associate Clinical Professor in the Department of Psychiatry at UCSF.

Dr. Jennifer Sanderson is a licensed clinical psychologist in Miami, Florida. She currently directs the Autism Clinic within a private practice, providing psychological and consultative services across the lifespan.

PEERS® for Preschoolers

Friendship Skills for Autistic and Neurodivergent Children

Elizabeth Laugeson, Mina Park, and Jennifer Sanderson

Routledge
Taylor & Francis Group
NEW YORK AND LONDON

Designed cover image: Rawpixel © Getty Images

First published 2025
by Routledge
605 Third Avenue, New York, NY 10158

and by Routledge
4 Park Square, Milton Park, Abingdon, Oxon, OX14 4RN

Routledge is an imprint of the Taylor & Francis Group, an informa business

ISBN: 978-1-032-82106-1 (hbk)
ISBN: 978-1-032-80139-1 (pbk)
ISBN: 978-1-003-50296-8 (ebk)

DOI: 10.4324/9781003502968

Typeset in Times New Roman
by Deanta Global Publishing Services, Chennai, India

For Product Safety Concerns and Information please contact our EU representative:
GPSR@taylorandfrancis.com
Taylor & Francis Verlag GmbH, Kaufingerstraße 24, 80331 München, Germany

Dedicated to every child who dreams of making a new friend and to the parents, teachers, and therapists who guide them with love.

Contents

Tables

Preface

This manual builds on the success of the Program for the Education and Enrichment of Relational Skills (PEERS®), which is an internationally renowned program, used in over 150 countries and translated into numerous languages. *PEERS® for Preschoolers: Friendship Skills for Autistic and Neurodivergent Children* is the fourth in a series of *PEERS®* manuals published by Routledge. Other manuals include:

- *Social Skills for Teenagers with Developmental and Autism Spectrum Disorders: The PEERS Treatment Manual* (Laugeson & Frankel, 2010)
- *The PEERS® Curriculum for School-Based Professionals: Social Skills Training for Adolescents with Autism Spectrum Disorder* (Laugeson 2014)
- *PEERS for Young Adults: Social Skills Training for Adults with Autism Spectrum Disorder and Other Social Challenges* (Laugeson 2017).

Through this new manual, providers will learn about important skills to enhance positive peer interactions and friendship development for young children, how to structure sessions and encourage skill-building effectively, and how to educate and empower parents to be valuable social coaches for their children. Unlike other social skills programs, *PEERS® for Preschoolers* has a strong evidence base with numerous research studies supporting its efficacy in improving friendship skills for young children. With a strong emphasis on teaching ecologically valid social skills, children and parents will be taught strategies that have been shown to be effective in making and keeping friends according to research.

Like other *PEERS®* programs, *PEERS® for Preschoolers* uses a strengths-based approach with neuro-affirming principles. The focus will not be on exploring the challenges faced by the child, but rather on identifying their strengths, building upon their skills related to making and keeping friends, and identifying supportive and inclusive environments where they can thrive and feel accepted.

The purpose of any *PEERS®* program is not to change the person, but to enhance their social interactions so others can appreciate them for who they already are. This underscores the importance of intrinsic motivation and the desire to learn the skills taught in *PEERS®* for both children and parents, as the forcing of friendship skills upon unwilling participants would be unethical. But just as the imposing of social skills programs upon those who do not want to learn them is unethical, it is also unethical to withhold the learning of friendship skills for those who do want to learn more.

Essentially, the purpose of *PEERS®* is to help decode the social world in a way that is navigable to those who want to learn about the rules and steps that many use in making and keeping friends.

To some, these rules and steps come naturally and are learned over time and with practice. For others, more structured learning may be desired to learn to navigate the social world. This once again highlights the importance of providing ecologically valid friendship skills packaged in an empirically supported program to achieve desired goals.

PEERS® for Preschoolers is not only an empirically supported program, but incorporates several evidence-based methods of instruction, including parent social coaching, didactic lessons with concrete rules and steps of social etiquette related to making and keeping friends, and homework assignments to practice newly learned skills in more natural social settings. Aspects of the program that are unique to *PEERS® for Preschoolers* include child-focused puppet-facilitated didactic lessons and roleplay demonstrations to enhance attention and engagement, behavioral rehearsal activities that incorporate skills practice into familiar childhood games (i.e., Musical Chairs, Red Rover, Ring Around the Rosie), and in-session parent-coached play activities in which children and parents are placed into dyads with other group members during mock playdates to practice parent social coaching with the support of the program team. All skills are taught using a neuro-affirming approach, which celebrates neurodiversity and does not seek to change the child, but rather enhance social interactions so others can appreciate the children for who they already are.

The primary intended audience for this manual is professionals and educators who provide social-emotional supports and educational services to young children between the ages of four and six years. *PEERS® for Preschoolers* facilitators may include educators, speech-language pathologists, behavior therapists, occupational therapists, recreational therapists, ABA therapists, BCBAs, social workers, marriage and family therapists, psychologists, psychiatrists, and other mental health, medical, or school-based professionals. *PEERS® for Preschoolers* may be provided in various settings, such as schools, community-based clinics, hospital-based outpatient clinics, camps, afterschool programs, extracurricular activities, sports programs, and at home.

While *PEERS® for Preschoolers* has been more extensively studied for use with autistic children, the program is used clinically for children with other social difficulties. In addition, while this manual was originally developed as a group-based curriculum, providers may also choose to teach the skills individually if deemed clinically appropriate.

Acknowledgments

I would like to extend my heartfelt gratitude to the families who have participated in and supported our research. Your dedication, insights, and unwavering commitment to your children inspire us every day. To our exceptional clinical and research team at UCLA, thank you for your expertise, passion, and tireless efforts in making this manual a reality. Your dedication to improving the lives of young children is truly commendable. I also want to express my deepest appreciation to my family and friends for their unwavering support and encouragement throughout this journey. Your belief in me and this work has been a constant source of strength. Finally, to my co-authors, Mina Park and Jennifer Sanderson, I want to thank you for the persistence and dedication you have shown in bringing this work to life. Together, we strive to make a difference in the lives of young children, empowering them to build meaningful friendships with confidence and joy. – Elizabeth Laugeson, PsyD

I am incredibly grateful for the amazing families who have helped shape and give life to this work. My deepest appreciation to the parents and families who joined our research journey and partnered with us; your enthusiasm, hope, dedication, and feedback are the foundation and guiding light of this work. I also wish to thank my UCLA family of colleagues, mentors, and friends for their support and encouragement. And an extra special thanks to Liz Laugeson for the endless hours role playing puppet scripts with me and her unwavering support. Jenn, I am grateful for our new friendship that blossomed from this project. And finally, to my dear family and friends, a simple heartfelt thank you for everything that you do. – Mina Park, PhD

I am so excited to see this research project come to completion and I will be eternally grateful to the children, families, therapists, colleagues, and researchers at UCLA who made this work possible. To my mentor and friend, Liz Laugeson, thank you for the incredible opportunity during my internship year to begin developing a friendship training curriculum for young children on the autism spectrum with you. Your dedication to helping others through PEERS®, passion for clinical research, and tireless efforts to mentor and guide trainees and professionals is something truly special that I feel very lucky to have experienced. To my co-author Mina Park, I am thankful and awed at your phenomenal efforts to solidify this curriculum and create such an extensive research base. To my friends and family, I am forever grateful for your unwavering support and friendship. Lastly, words cannot adequately express how much of a privilege it has been to work with the many children, adults, and families navigating life on the autism spectrum. You have challenged, humbled, and inspired me, and shaped my life and career. Being an only child, my friendships have played such a critical role throughout my life in both my personal and professional development. Every child deserves the joy, love, and support of great friends, and it is my sincere hope that this project and friendship skills curriculum help to make this a reality. – Jennifer Sanderson, PsyD

Author Biographies

Dr. Elizabeth Laugeson is a licensed clinical psychologist and a Clinical Professor in the Department of Psychiatry and Biobehavioral Sciences at the University of California, Los Angeles (UCLA) David Geffen School of Medicine. She is the Founder and Director of the UCLA PEERS® Clinic, which is an outpatient hospital-based clinic providing evidence-based social skills programs for individuals from preschool to adulthood. She is also the Director of the UCLA Tarjan Center, which is a University Center for Excellence in Developmental Disabilities, and serves as the Program Director for the Predoctoral Psychology Internship Program in Autism and Neurodevelopmental Disabilities at UCLA. Dedicated to supporting those with neurodevelopmental disabilities and their families, Dr. Laugeson has also held positions as Founding Director of The Help Group – UCLA Autism Research Alliance (2007–2017), Training Director for the UCLA Tarjan Center (2014–2021), Director of the UCLA Early Childhood Clubhouse Program (2007–2010), and Associate Director for the UCLA Parenting and Children's Friendship Training Program (2007–2010).

Dr. Laugeson received her doctorate in clinical psychology from Pepperdine University in 2004 and completed a predoctoral psychology internship and postdoctoral fellowship at UCLA in 2004 and 2007, respectively. Considered one of the world's leading experts in evidence-based social skills programming, she was a two-time recipient of the Ruth L. Kirschstein National Research Service Award from the National Institutes of Health in 2004 and 2006, recipient of the Semel Scholar Award for Junior Faculty Career Development in 2008, and received the Distinguished Alumnus Award from Pepperdine University in 2010.

Dr. Laugeson has been a principal investigator and collaborator on numerous nationally funded studies investigating social skills programs from preschool to early adulthood and has authored four books related to social skills, including the critically acclaimed, *The Science of Making Friends*. As the developer of PEERS®, she has trained tens of thousands of mental health professionals, educators, and families worldwide and is dedicated to developing, testing, and disseminating evidence-based treatments to improve social skills for individuals across the lifespan and across the globe. As one of the only empirically supported and internationally recognized social skills programs for neurodivergent youth, her programs are currently used in over 150 countries and have been translated into over a dozen languages. Her work has been featured in numerous media outlets, including People Magazine, USA Today, the Washington Post, LA Times, New York Times, ABC, NBC, CBS, Fox, and the Emmy award-winning Netflix series, Love on the Spectrum. In this current work, Dr. Laugeson shares her research-supported strategies for teaching social skills to young autistic children and those with other social difficulties.

Dr. Mina Park is a licensed clinical psychologist who has dedicated her training and clinical practice to serving autistic and neurodivergent individuals, their families, and other mental health and service providers. She was an Associate Clinical Professor at the University of California, San Francisco (UCSF) Department of Psychiatry and Behavioral Sciences (2017–2022), working with families in the UCSF Center for Autism and Neurodevelopmental Disabilities. Prior to this, she was an Assistant Clinical Professor at the UCLA Department of Psychiatry and Biobehavioral Sciences (2015–2017) and provided care to families through the UCLA Child and Adult Neurodevelopmental Clinic, UCLA PEERS® Clinic, and the UCLA ABC Child Partial Hospitalization and Intensive Outpatient Programs.

Dr. Park received her doctorate in counseling/clinical/school psychology (clinical emphasis) from the University of California, Santa Barbara (UCSB) in 2012, where she trained and specialized in the delivery of naturalistic developmental behavioral interventions for autistic youth and their families. She continued her training at UCLA, completing her predoctoral psychology internship and postdoctoral fellowship. Currently, Dr. Park has transitioned from the clinical academic setting and continues to provide autistic and neurodivergent-affirming care through her private practice in California.

Dr. Jennifer Sanderson is a licensed clinical psychologist with experience in the diagnosis and treatment of autism and other developmental, behavioral, social-emotional, and learning challenges. She is passionate about improving the lives and long-term outcomes of autistic individuals and ameliorating mental health concerns through increased awareness and acceptance of neurodevelopmental differences and higher-quality services and supports. She currently serves as Director of the Autism Clinic, providing psychological services across the lifespan and clinical expertise at a private practice in Miami, Florida. Before transitioning into private practice full-time, she worked at Florida Atlantic University Center for Autism and Related Disabilities (2014–2016), providing support, clinical consultation, and training to autistic children and adults and their families. In this role, Dr. Sanderson also delivered training in autism screening and diagnosis, improving awareness and acceptance and the implementation of evidence-based clinical services to thousands of professionals, service providers, and university students/trainees working within schools, therapeutic settings, social services, hospitals, first responders, and the community at large.

Dr. Sanderson completed her undergraduate education at the University of Florida in 2003. She received both her master's and doctoral degrees in clinical psychology from Nova Southeastern University (2003–2012). Her graduate clinical training included working with children and families through The Children and Family Consortium at Easter Seals and the University of Miami Mailman Center for Child Development. She also worked with autistic children and those with other developmental disabilities through Achievement and Rehabilitation Centers, Inc. (ARC Broward). Dr. Sanderson completed a clinical psychology internship specializing in developmental disabilities at the UCLA Semel Institute for Neuroscience and Human Behavior (2007–2008), followed by a two-year postdoctoral psychology fellowship in the highly acclaimed UCLA PEERS® Clinic (2008-2010), providing and developing evidence-based social skills programs for autistic children, adolescents, young adults, and those with other social difficulties. She also completed a postdoctoral residency in autism at Nova Southeastern University's Mailman Segal Center (2012–2013), providing early intervention and school-based consultation, completing diagnostic evaluations, and supervising and training psychology doctoral students.

In addition to her work in private practice, Dr. Sanderson enjoys training, mentoring, and collaborating with other professionals. She taught and developed graduate coursework in developmental disabilities and applied behavior analysis as an Adjunct Professor at Nova Southeastern University (2012–2014) and Florida Atlantic University (2015–2016). She has participated in expert panels, presented at continuing education and research conferences, served on regional and legislative committees, worked as an independent clinical expert in legal proceedings involving autistic children, and has been featured in popular online and print media, including Parenting Plus Magazine of The Palm Beaches and The Treasure Coast, Well+Good Digital Publication, and several regional magazines from Best Version Media within Palm Beach, Florida.

Introduction

Purpose of the Manual

This manual builds on the success of the *Program for the Education and Enrichment of Relational Skills (PEERS®),* which is an internationally renowned program, used in over 150 countries, and culturally adapted and translated into numerous languages. *PEERS®* is widely regarded as one of the only evidence-based social skills programs for autistic youth in the world, but the programs can be used clinically with anyone interested in learning the skills taught. *PEERS® for Preschoolers: Friendship Skills for Autistic and Neurodivergent Children* is the fourth in a series of *PEERS®* manuals published by Routledge. Other manuals include:

- *Social Skills for Teenagers with Developmental and Autism Spectrum Disorders: The PEERS Treatment Manual* (Laugeson & Frankel, 2010)
- *The PEERS® Curriculum for School-Based Professionals: Social Skills Training for Adolescents with Autism Spectrum Disorder* (Laugeson 2014)
- *PEERS for Young Adults: Social Skills Training for Adults with Autism Spectrum Disorder and Other Social Challenges* (Laugeson 2017).

Through this new manual, providers will learn about important skills to enhance positive peer interactions and friendship development for young children, how to structure sessions and encourage skill-building using a neuroaffirming approach, and how to educate and empower parents to be valuable ***social coaches*** for their neurodivergent children in a way that honors neurodiversity.

The term neurodiversity essentially means that people have different ways of thinking. These differences do not make us less than or more than any other person. Arguably, there are great strengths in neurodiversity and PEERS® is a strengths-based approach. While the focus of PEERS® for Preschoolers is to help develop and enhance friendship skills for autistic and neurodivergent children, the PEERS® method is meant to be delivered using a neuroaffirming approach. Therefore, in teaching social strategies for making and keeping friends, it is important to respect the role of neurodiversity. Simply put, learning and/or using the strategies taught in PEERS® should NOT be about changing a person. Rather, learning and using these skills should be about enhancing social interactions so others can appreciate our children for who they already are. Ultimately, learning and/or using the skills taught in PEERS® will be the choice of every family.

To highlight the importance of choice and respect for neurodiversity, each session begins with a *Neuroaffirming Pledge*. This pledge is also used in updated practice guidelines for PEERS® programs for teens and young adults as well. The *PEERS® Neuroaffirming Pledge* states the following principles:

DOI: 10.4324/9781003502968-1

- We value neurodiversity, acceptance, and authenticity.
- We honor the diverse ways people experience the world.
- We respect each person's unique perspectives and communication styles.
- We recognize there is no one right way to connect with others.
- If using the strategies taught in PEERS® feels like camouflaging or masking and/or they don't align with your goals or the goals of your family, then you do not have to use them.
- Learning and using the skills taught in PEERS® is a PERSONAL CHOICE.

The primary intended audience for this treatment manual is professionals and educators who provide social-emotional therapeutic services and supports to young children between the ages of four and six years. These professionals may include teachers and other special education providers, speech-language pathologists, behavior therapists, occupational therapists, recreational therapists, ABA therapists, BCBAs, social workers, marriage and family therapists, psychologists, psychiatrists, and other mental health and/or medical professionals.

PEERS® for Preschoolers may be provided as a group-based program in various settings, such as schools, community-based clinics, hospital-based outpatient clinics, camps, afterschool programs, extracurricular activities, sports programs, and at home. Social skills groups are highly desirable in many of these community and public settings as they allow for the efficient delivery of care to several children and families at a single time. In addition, though this manual was originally developed as a group-based curriculum, providers may also choose to implement the strategies and skills to families individually if deemed clinically appropriate.

While the *PEERS® for Preschoolers* manual will commonly be used for neurodivergent youth, such as those diagnosed with autism spectrum disorder (ASD) and/or attention-deficit/hyperactivity disorder (ADHD), the program may be used with other youth who would benefit from learning the skills taught. The importance of providing support around friendship skills may be particularly helpful for autistic children who often struggle socially. Social communication differences may manifest in the first few years of life. These differences often persist throughout development and do not typically resolve on their own. Studies have identified numerous short- and long-term consequences of social difficulties, including increased feelings of loneliness, fewer friendships and poorer friendship quality, peer rejection and isolation, anxiety and mood problems, behavior problems, and lower academic and occupational achievement. Social skills programs have increased in popularity and utilization and are now commonplace in addressing these social differences. However, research reveals that most social skills programs for neurodivergent youth have focused on older-aged children and adolescents, with little support for those in early childhood. In addition, despite their popularity, most social skills programs available in the community lack sufficient empirical support, unlike *PEERS® for Preschoolers*.

Inclusion of Parents

A highly unique aspect of *PEERS® for Preschoolers* that differs from other social skills groups is the inclusion of parents as ***social coaches***. This model involves simultaneously occurring *social coaching groups* that meet in tandem with child groups. Essentially, while children are learning about friendship skills in their own group, parents attend a concurrent *social coaching group* to learn about how to assist children in the development and maintenance of friendships. The rationale behind including parents as ***social coaches*** is that the skills will more easily generalize to other settings and improvements will be more durable over time for the following reasons:

1. ***Social coaching in natural social settings.*** Greater generalization of skills is expected through ***social coaching*** because parents will be able to provide ***social coaching*** during *coachable moments* in natural social environments. Better durability of outcomes over time is expected because parents will be able to provide ***social coaching*** long after the program has ended.

2. ***Assistance with weekly socialization assignments.*** Generalization of skills will be promoted through the completion of weekly *socialization homework assignments*. Parents are integral to ensuring the completion of these practice assignments by enrolling their children in ***playgroups***, arranging ***playdates***, practicing newly learned skills, and helping troubleshoot any barriers to homework completion. The durability of outcomes is further enhanced by parents continuing to encourage the use of the *PEERS®* skills long after the program has ended and no formal assignments are given.

3. ***Assistance with finding a source of friends.*** The inclusion of parents is also useful in assisting children in finding a source of friends outside of the program setting. The purpose of *PEERS® for Preschoolers* is not to provide *friendship matching*, where group members become friends with other group members. Instead, parents are taught how to help children find ***playmates*** more independently in the real world. Parent involvement is critical throughout this process by identifying ***playgroups*** in the community where children might find accepting groups of peers with common interests. Moreover, parents not only enroll children in these activities, but they also ensure that children continue to attend ***playgroups*** long after the program has ended, thereby further enhancing the durability of gains.

Organization of the Manual

PEERS® for Preschoolers is conducted using a structured group format, focusing on teaching children the skills necessary to develop and maintain friendships. An overview of the 16 didactic sessions is presented in Table 0.1.

This manual is intended to serve as a step-by-step outline for each lesson and is meant to be used during each group. Memorization of the material in the manual is neither required nor encouraged. Children and parents seem comfortable with group leaders having the manual open in front of them as they guide the group through the skills. The rationale for following the manual closely is that program staff need to cover all the necessary elements being taught to maintain fidelity and enhance outcomes.

The current chapter provides an introduction to the curriculum and includes information about the organization of the manual, composition of groups, screening guidelines, required personnel, physical facilities, materials needed, teaching methods, and information about how to track progress, along with an overview of previous research outcomes. *Sessions 1–16* include therapist guides highlighting the 16-week *PEERS® for Preschoolers* curriculum. The material includes information about how to conduct *Homework Review* with parents, how to present *Didactic Lessons*, including puppet shows for children with role-play demonstrations, procedures for conducting *Behavioral Rehearsal* exercises for children, guidelines for conducting *Parent Coached Play* between children and their parents, as well as photocopiable material meant to be distributed to parents each week, including *Parent Handouts*, *Parent Coached Play Cards*, and *Parent Homework Worksheets*.

Table 0.1 Overview of Curriculum

Week	*Parent Didactic Lesson*	*Child Didactic Lesson*	*Homework Review*	*Child Behavioral Rehearsal 1*	*Child Behavioral Rehearsal 2*	*Homework Assignments*
1	Introduction	Listening and Following Directions	None	Simon Says	Head, Shoulders, Knees, and Toes	1. Practice listening and following directions. 2. Bring a turn-taking game.
2	Finding Playgroups	Meeting and Greeting Friends	1. Practice listening and following directions. 2. Bring a turn-taking game.	What Time Is It, Friend?	Red Light, Green Light	1. Find a playgroup for your child. 2. Practice meeting and greeting friends. 3. Provide social coaching on previously learned skills. 4. Bring a turn-taking game
3	Choosing Playgroups	Sharing and Giving a Turn	1. Find a playgroup for your child. 2. Practice meeting and greeting friends. 3. Provide social coaching on previously learned skills. 4. Bring a turn-taking game.	Sweet Potato Soup	Musical Share Chairs	1. Find a playgroup for your child. 2. Practice sharing and giving a turn. 3. Provide social coaching on previously learned skills. 4. Bring a turn-taking game
4	Preparing for Playgroups	Asking for a Turn	1. Find a playgroup for your child. 2. Practice sharing and giving a turn. 3. Provide social coaching on previously learned skills. 4. Bring a turn-taking game	Duck, Duck, Goose	Swap Draw	1. Find a playgroup for your child. 2. Practice asking for a turn. 3. Provide social coaching on previously learned skills. 4. Bring a turn-taking game

(*Continued*)

Table 0.1 Continued

5	Planning Playdates	Keeping Cool	1. Find a playgroup for your child. 2. Practice asking for a turn. 3. Provide social coaching on previously learned skills. 4. Bring a turn-taking game.	Mother, May I?	Musical Share Chairs	1. Identify playmates for playdates. 2. Playgroups. 3. Practice keeping cool. 4. Provide social coaching on previously learned skills. 5. Bring a turn-taking game.
6	Suggesting Playdates	Being a Good Sport	1. Identify playmates for playdates. 2. Playgroups. 3. Practice keeping cool. 4. Provide social coaching on previously learned skills. 5. Bring a turn-taking game.	Elbow to Elbow	Head, Shoulders, Knees, and Toes	1. Identify potential playmates. 2. Playgroups. 3. Practice being a good sport. 4. Provide social coaching on previously learned skills. 5. Bring a turn-taking game.
7	Preparing for Playdates	Show and Tell During Play	1. Identify potential playmates. 2. Playgroups. 3. Practice being a good sport. 4. Provide social coaching on previously learned skills. 5. Bring a turn-taking game.	Simon Says	Show Go Lego	1. Playdates. 2. Practice show and tell during play. 3. Provide social coaching on previously learned skills. 4. Bring a turn-taking game
8	Coaching During Playdates	Don't be Bossy	1. Playdates. 2. Practice show and tell during play. 3. Provide social coaching on previously learned skills. 4. Bring a turn-taking game.	Hot or Cold	Swap Draw	1. Playdates. 2. Practice not being bossy. 3. Provide social coaching on previously learned skills. 4. Bring a turn-taking game
9	Social Coaching Strategies	Asking a Friend to Play	1. Playdates. 2. Practice not being bossy. 3. Provide social coaching on previously learned skills. 4. Bring a turn-taking game.	Red Rover	Swap and Play	1. Playdates. 2. Practice asking a friend to play. 3. Provide social coaching on previously learned skills. 4. Bring a turn-taking game.

(*Continued*)

Table 0.1 Continued

Week	*Parent Didactic Lesson*	*Child Didactic Lesson*	*Homework Review*	*Child Behavioral Rehearsal 1*	*Child Behavioral Rehearsal 2*	*Homework Assignments*
10	Social Coaching Strategies for Joining a Game	Joining a Game	1. Playdates. 2. Practice asking a friend to play. 3. Provide social coaching on previously learned skills. 4. Bring a turn-taking game.	What Time Is It, Friend?	Ring Around the Rosie	1. Playdates. 2. Practice joining a game. 3. Provide social coaching on previously learned skills. 4. Bring a turn-taking game.
11	Social Coaching Strategies for Asking to Play Something Different	Asking to Play Something Different	1. Playdates. 2. Practice joining a game. 3. Provide social coaching on previously learned skills. 4. Bring a turn-taking game	Elbow to Elbow	Swap and Play	1. Playdates. 2. Practice asking to play something different. 3. Provide social coaching on previously learned skills. 4. Bring a turn-taking game.
12	Social Coaching Strategies for Asking and Giving Help	Asking and Giving Help	1. Playdates. 2. Practice asking to play something different. 3. Provide social coaching on previously learned skills. 4. Bring a turn-taking game.	Tinker Toy Town	Hot or Cold	1. Playdates. 2. Practice asking and giving help. 3. Provide social coaching on previously learned skills. 4. Bring a turn-taking game.
13	Social Coaching Strategies for Staying in Our Own Space	Staying in Our Own Space	1. Playdates. 2. Practice asking and giving help. 3. Provide social coaching on previously learned skills. 4. Bring a turn-taking game	Ring Around the Rosie	Simon Says	1. Playdates. 2. Practice staying in our own space. 3. Provide social coaching on previously learned skills. 4. Bring a turn-taking game.
14	Social Coaching Strategies for Using an Inside Voice	Using an Inside Voice	1. Playdates. 2. Practice staying in our own space. 3. Provide social coaching on previously learned skills. 4. Bring a turn-taking game.	Duck, Duck, Goose	Sweet Potato Soup	1. Playdates. 2. Practice using an inside voice. 3. Provide social coaching on previously learned skills. 4. Bring a turn-taking game.

(Continued)

Table 0.1 Continued

15	Disclosing a Diagnosis or Condition with Others	Final Review (Part 1)	1. Playdates. 2. Practice using an inside voice. 3. Provide social coaching on previously learned skills. 4. Bring a turn-taking game.	Red Rover	Swap Draw	1. Playdates. 2. Make a list of previously learned skills that still need refinement. 3. Practice a previously learned skill that needs refinement using the 4 Ps. 4. Practice disclosing a diagnosis or condition with others (optional assignment).
16	Sharing a Diagnosis or Condition with Your Child	Final Review (Part 2)	1. Playdates. 2. Make a list of previously learned skills that still need refinement. 3. Practice a previously learned skill that needs refinement using the 4 Ps. 4. Practice disclosing a diagnosis or condition with others (optional assignment).	Ring Around the Rosie	Hot or Cold	None

Format of the Sessions

Parent Session Therapist Guide

- **Homework Review.** Each parent group begins with a review of the previous homework assignments. This section of each chapter provides concrete questions for group leaders to ask parents during the *Homework Review*.
- **Didactic Lesson.** The didactic material for each parent and child lesson is presented in this section of each chapter through the presentation of concrete rules and steps of social behavior, along with ***social coaching*** guidelines.
- **Homework Assignments.** To generalize the newly learned skills outside of the program setting, weekly socialization homework assignments are given. This section of each chapter provides a comprehensive description of the upcoming homework assignments along with recommendations for appropriate ***social coaching***.

Child Session Therapist Guide

- **Didactic Lesson.** This section of each chapter provides a structured outline and script for how to present the child didactic lesson. The didactic material is provided through the presentation of puppet shows highlighting role-play demonstrations of targeted skills.
- **Child Behavioral Rehearsals.** Each child lesson is followed by two child behavioral rehearsal exercises made up of familiar childhood games (i.e., Red Rover, Simon Says). These activities are intended to give children numerous opportunities to practice the newly learned skills in the context of more natural social situations.

Parent Coached Play

- *Parent Coached Play* occurs at the end of every session when parents and children are reunited in the child room and are assigned to join another parent-child dyad to have *mock playdates*. During this time, children practice newly learned friendship skills while parents provide social coaching to promote skill usage. Each dyad is assigned at least one member of the program staff to provide support and guidance on parent ***social coaching*** strategies.

Parent Handouts

- *Parent Handouts* should be distributed to parents at the beginning of each *Didactic Lesson* as a tool to help parents remember the skills being taught, provide guidelines for ***social coaching***, and provide an overview of weekly homework assignments. *Parent Handouts* should be photocopied and distributed to parents EVERY WEEK and should be given to absent group members for the corresponding missed sessions.

Parent Coached Play Cards

- *Parent Coached Play Cards* should be distributed to parents prior to *Parent Coached Play* and are intended to be used as a tool to help guide parents in their ***social coaching*** on newly learned skills. *Parent Coached Play Cards* should be photocopied and distributed to parents EVERY WEEK and should be given to absent group members for missed sessions.

Parent Homework Worksheets

- *Parent Homework Worksheets* are found at the end of every chapter and should be distributed to parents prior to discussing the homework assignments for the coming week. *Parent Homework Worksheets* provide an overview of the assignments with room for note-taking about how parents completed assignments and provided ***social coaching*** on targeted skills. *Parent Homework Worksheets* are intended to be returned to the program staff to monitor homework completion and should be photocopied and distributed to parents EVERY WEEK.

Lesson Format

PEERS® for Preschoolers is intended to be implemented as a weekly group, taught once per week for 90 minutes. Parents and children meet separately and concurrently for the first 60 minutes, followed by 30 minutes of *Parent Coached Play* and a *Final Wrap-Up*.

Format of the Parent Group

- **Homework Review (30–40 minutes).** The parent group leader reviews the homework assignments from the previous week with every family at the beginning of the group using the guidelines in the *Parent Session Therapist Guide*.
- **Didactic Lesson (20–30 minutes).** The parent group leader presents the parent and child didactic lessons following the guidelines in the *Parent Session Therapist Guide*, distributes the *Parent Handouts, Parent Coached Play Cards,* and *Parent Homework Worksheets* to parents, and reviews the upcoming *Homework Assignments*.

Format of the Child Group

- **Didactic Lesson and Role-Play Demonstrations (20 minutes).** The child group leader and behavioral coaches present the *Didactic Lesson* using the puppet show script following the guidelines in the *Child Session Therapist Guide*.
- **Group Behavioral Rehearsal 1 (10–15 minutes).** The child group leader and behavioral coaches have children practice newly learned skills in the first behavioral rehearsal exercise outlined in the section of each chapter labeled *Behavioral Rehearsal 1*.
- **Break Time (10 minutes).** It is recommended that children have a brief bathroom break between the two behavioral rehearsal activities, which is roughly halfway through the 90-minute session.
- **Group Behavioral Rehearsal 2 (10–15 minutes).** The child group leader and behavioral coaches have children practice newly learned skills in the second behavioral rehearsal exercise outlined in the section of each chapter labeled *Behavioral Rehearsal 2*. To add variety throughout the session, behavioral rehearsal exercises will typically alternate between gross motor activities and more sedentary activities.

Format of Parent Coached Play

- **Parent Coached Play (20 minutes).** Parents and children are reunited in the child room to practice newly learned skills in the context of dyadic mock ***playdates*** with other group members. Children play turn-taking games with other group members while parents provide ***social coaching*** with the support of program staff.

- **Final Wrap-Up (10 minutes).** Led by the child group leader, the *Final Wrap-Up* includes a brief review of the newly learned friendship skill and a summary of the homework assignments, followed by counting stars earned by each child for participation, which are then exchanged for prizes at the end of every session.

Group Composition

- **Group Size.** The recommended group size for *PEERS® for Preschoolers* is between eight and ten children. Running groups with fewer than six children is somewhat risky in that group members may drop out of the program and absences may occur, significantly decreasing the size of the group along with the ability to practice skills with other group members. Running groups larger than ten is possible but will likely require more personnel. More than 10 children might also increase the duration of each of the activities and not be feasible with developmental expectations for young children (attention span, etc.).
- **Age Distribution of the Group.** *PEERS® for Preschoolers* is most appropriate for children four to six years of age. Although the program may be used with slightly younger or older children, it is important to confirm that the skills taught are age-appropriate, being neither too sophisticated nor too elementary.
- **Language Distribution of the Group.** *PEERS® for Preschoolers* is most suitable for children with at least flexible use of four- to five-word spontaneous phrases. While the program may be used with children with more delayed speech, it is important to set children up for success by confirming that their receptive language is sufficient to comprehend the material and that their expressive language is sufficient to apply the skills taught.
- **Gender Distribution of the Group.** It is not necessary or advisable to separate groups based on gender identity. However, if you have only one child of a specific gender in a group, as a courtesy you may notify the family to confirm that they are comfortable participating. Anecdotally, many families will move forward with enrollment even if their child does not have a same-gendered peer in the group, but we have found they appreciate being notified in advance and given the choice to enroll.

Screening Guidelines

Screening and enrollment guidelines will be largely guided by the hosting organization. In school settings, it is unlikely that families will attend an eligibility appointment or an intake interview, as school personnel are more likely to be familiar with the family and are better able to determine the appropriateness of fit for the group. However, in medical, mental health, and therapeutic settings, eligibility appointments and intake interviews are commonplace and often occur with both the parent and child present. If a family is found to be inappropriate or ineligible for *PEERS® for Preschoolers,* it is advisable to have appropriate referrals and recommendations available.

- **Pre-Screening Appointment.** The screening process typically begins with a brief phone call or video chat with the parent and program staff. The main objective of a pre-screening appointment is to assess whether the family appears to be a good fit for *PEERS® for Preschoolers*, and/or if other services and supports are warranted. Intake clinicians are advised to pay close attention to the following screening criteria when determining the appropriateness of fit:

- Child is between four and six years of age.
- Child and parent are interested and motivated to learn the skills taught in *PEERS® for Preschoolers* related to making and keeping friends.
- Child and parent are motivated and available to attend 90-minute weekly groups over the course of 16 weeks.
- Child has adequate expressive and receptive language (i.e., the ability to speak in at least four- to five-word spontaneous phrases).
- Child has adequate behavioral and emotional regulation (i.e., the ability to participate in the group without frequent outbursts or tantrums).
- Child has adequate attentional skills (i.e., the ability to attend to a 20-minute didactic lesson presented as a puppet show, participate in two 15-minute behavioral rehearsal activities, and interact in a 20-minute parent coached play exercise)
- Child does not demonstrate physical aggression that could cause harm to self, others, or property.
- Child has an absence of significant social anxiety that would prevent participation in the group.
- Parent is willing to provide ***social coaching*** during weekly *socialization homework assignments*, including enrolling in ***playgroups*** and organizing ***playdates***.
- Child is toilet trained (if necessary, according to the setting).

Eligibility Appointments/Intake Interviews. Once the family has completed the pre-screening appointment and appears to be a good fit for the program, an eligibility appointment or intake interview should be scheduled. The objective of this appointment is to make a final determination about eligibility and/or whether other services and supports are warranted. Intake clinicians are advised to pay close attention to the screening criteria mentioned above when determining the appropriateness of fit.

Eligibility appointments or intake interviews are typically conducted in person over 60–90 minutes and may involve a brief play observation with the parent and child. Play observations may include free play, child-directed play, and/or parent-directed play to ascertain the language and play skills of the child and the current/baseline ***social coaching*** skills of the parent. The remainder of the appointment is typically conducted in the absence of the child and with the parent(s) alone. Interviews with parents typically include the developmental and background history of the child and a thorough discussion of presenting concerns relating to making and keeping friends (see Appendix A for an example of an *Intake Interview Document*). Topics typically include:

- History of present concerns.
- Child developmental history.
- Child educational history.
- Child psychiatric history.
- Family legal history (if applicable).
- Family psychiatric and medical history.
- Child medical history.
- Child current medications.

- Mental status examination.
- Diagnostic impressions.
- Assessment and plan.

While determining the appropriateness of participation in *PEERS® for Preschoolers,* it is also important to give families an overview of what to expect from the program and be prepared to answer questions. The *Sample Welcome Letter* (Appendix B) gives a summary of program expectations, including the following:

- Program objectives (including a summary of skills taught in *PEERS® for Preschoolers*).
- Format and size of the groups.
- Start and end dates.
- Time and location of the groups.
- Importance of regular attendance and coming on time.
- The need for the same parent to be present for ALL sessions.
  - To maintain consistency in ***social coaching***, discourage switching off between parents from week to week, although all parents should be welcome.
- Explanation of weekly *socialization homework assignments.*
- Policy regarding sibling childcare during the group.
- Qualifications of group leaders.
- Directions and parking information.
- Contact information.

Required Personnel

When parent groups and child groups are taught concurrently, two group leaders are needed for *PEERS® for Preschoolers.* Group leaders typically include psychologists, psychiatrists, marriage and family therapists, social workers, speech and language therapists, occupational therapists, recreational therapists, vocational counselors, and other mental health professionals and educators. Regardless of their professional background, child group leaders should have previous experience working with children with social difficulties and be familiar with behavioral management strategies, while parent group leaders should have experience working with parents and/or families. Group leaders should also be fully trained on all aspects of the *PEERS® for Preschoolers* curriculum either by reading this manual beforehand and/or attending a *PEERS® Certified Training Seminar.*

In addition to having two group leaders, it will be essential to have two to three behavioral coaches to assist with the child group. Behavioral coaches often include undergraduate students, graduate students, teacher aides, and/or trainees studying education, psychology, or some related mental health field, as well as other mental health professionals and educators. Behavioral coaches should be trained on all aspects of the *PEERS® for Preschoolers* curriculum and have a good understanding of behavior reinforcement and management strategies. Behavioral coaches are often responsible for conducting role-play demonstrations, providing performance feedback through coaching during behavioral rehearsal exercises, assisting the child group leader with reinforcement and behavior management, and providing ***social coaching*** guidance to parents during *Parent Coached Play.* The typical child-to-adult ratio in *PEERS® for Preschoolers* is two to three children per adult, but a minimum of three adults will be necessary for most of the *Child Didactic Lessons.*

Physical Facilities

The skills taught to children in *PEERS® for Preschoolers* should be presented much like a preschool or kindergarten classroom. For the child group, the room should have sufficient space for the *Listening Circle* (i.e., children sit in a semi-circle facing the child group leader to receive instructions) and gross motor activities (i.e., *Red Rover, Duck Duck Goose, Musical Chairs*). Moreover, since *Parent Coached Play* is typically conducted in the child group room, there should be adequate space for dyadic mock ***playdates*** for the entire group. For the parent group, the room should include a large conference table with chairs for the parents to sit around facing the group leader.

Materials Needed

Each *Parent Session Therapist Guide, Child Session Therapist Guide, Child Behavioral Rehearsals,* and *Parent Coached Play* section of the manual includes an overview of the materials needed. Table 0.2 includes a list of all the materials needed according to the session.

Teaching Methods

- **Didactic Lessons Using Concrete Rules and Steps.** Many neurodivergent children have a penchant for rules and are likely to follow them. Perhaps because the world is generally unpredictable, rules provide a stable means of understanding social surroundings. Considering this preference for rules, *PEERS® for Preschoolers* teaches friendship skills using concrete rules and steps of social behavior. Sophisticated social behaviors are deconstructed into smaller rules and steps to aid comprehension during *Didactic Lessons*.
- **Ecologically Valid Social Skills.** One aspect of *PEERS® for Preschoolers* that is unique from other friendship programs is the use of ***ecologically valid social skills***. This essentially involves teaching social behaviors that are naturally used by those who are socially accepted by their peers. In other words, you will not be teaching children what we *THINK* children should do in social situations, but what actually *WORKS* according to research.
- **Use of Buzzwords.** Another unique aspect of the *PEERS® for Preschoolers* curriculum is the use of ***buzzwords***. Terms that are ***bold and italicized*** in the manual are ***buzzwords*** and represent important concepts from the curriculum. The buzzwords symbolize social behaviors that can be identified in just a few simple words. Using the ***buzzwords*** as much as possible will help to develop a common language between parents, children, and the program staff.
- **Role-Play Demonstrations.** The modeling of social behavior is a critical ingredient to understanding friendship skills. Role-play demonstrations are used throughout the *PEERS® for Preschoolers* manual to illustrate specific rules and steps of social etiquette. Role-play demonstrations are provided within the context of puppet show scripts in the *Child Session Therapist Guides* and the *Behavioral Rehearsal Exercises,* and are meant to be read verbatim.
- **Behavioral Rehearsal Exercises.** To fully comprehend a particular set of social skills, it is necessary to use them through practice and repetition. The use of behavioral rehearsal exercises occurs twice in every child session through the playing of common childhood games (i.e., *Red Rover, Duck Duck Goose, Musical Chairs*). Behavioral rehearsal exercises are a critical ingredient for skill acquisition and should always be paired with ***social coaching*** with performance feedback from the program staff.

Table 0.2 Materials Needed According to the Session

Session	*Recurring Materials Needed in the Parent Group*	*Recurring Materials Needed in the Child Group*	*Unique Materials Needed in the Child Group*
1	1. Conference table and chairs. 2. Name tags. 3. *Parent Handouts*. 4. *Parent Homework Worksheets*. 5. *Parent Coached Play Cards*. 6. *Planned Absence Sheets*. 7. *Homework Compliance Sheet*. 8. Pens.	1. Carpet squares or chairs. 2. "Making Friends Helper" badge. 3. Star chart with names of children. 4. Marker for star chart. 5. Name tags. 6. Prize bins with prizes. 7. Turn-taking games.	1. Pig puppet. 2. Monkey puppet. 3. Building blocks. 4. Small container for building blocks.
2	1. Conference table and chairs. 2. Name tags. 3. *Parent Handouts*. 4. *Parent Homework Worksheets*. 5. *Parent Coached Play Cards*. 6. *Planned Absence Sheets*. 7. *Homework Compliance Sheet*. 8. Pens.	1. Carpet squares or chairs. 2. "Making Friends Helper" badge. 3. Star chart with names of children. 4. Marker for star chart. 5. Name tags. 6. Prize bins with prizes. 7. Turn-taking games	1. Lion puppet. 2. Elephant puppet. 3. Small ball. 4. Safety cones or masking tape.
3	1. Conference table and chairs. 2. Name tags. 3. *Parent Handouts*. 4. *Parent Homework Worksheets*. 5. *Parent Coached Play Cards*. 6. *Homework Compliance Sheet*. 7. Pens.	1. Carpet squares or chairs. 2. "Making Friends Helper" badge. 3. Star chart with names of children. 4. Marker for star chart. 5. Name tags. 6. Prize bins with prizes. 7. Turn-taking games.	1. Tiger puppet. 2. Frog puppet. 3. Two toy cars. 4. Small bucket. 5. Music and music player. 6. Chairs for Musical Share Chairs.
4	1. Conference table and chairs. 2. Name tags. 3. *Parent Handouts*. 4. *Parent Homework Worksheets*. 5. *Parent Coached Play Cards*. 6. *Homework Compliance Sheet*. 7. Pens.	1. Carpet squares or chairs. 2. "Making Friends Helper" badge. 3. Star chart with names of children. 4. Marker for star chart. 5. Name tags. 6. Prize bins with prizes. 7. Turn-taking games.	1. Cow puppet. 2. Lion puppet. 3. Toy plane. 4. Drawing paper. 5. Coloring tools. 6. Tables or flat surfaces to draw on.

(*Continued*)

Table 0.2 Continued

Session	*Recurring Materials Needed in the Parent Group*	*Recurring Materials Needed in the Child Group*	*Unique Materials Needed in the Child Group*
5	1. Conference table and chairs. 2. Name tags. 3. *Parent Handouts.* 4. *Parent Homework Worksheets.* 5. *Parent Coached Play Cards.* 6. *Homework Compliance Sheet.* 7. Pens.	1. Carpet squares or chairs. 2. "Making Friends Helper" badge. 3. Star chart with names of children. 4. Marker for star chart. 5. Name tags. 6. Prize bins with prizes. 7. Turn-taking games.	1. Mouse puppet. 2. Pig puppet. 3. Toy car. 4. Small animal figures. 5. Safety cones or masking tape. 6. Music and music player. 7. Chairs for Musical Share Chairs.
6	1. Conference table and chairs. 2. Name tags. 3. *Parent Handouts.* 4. *Parent Homework Worksheets.* 5. *Parent Coached Play Cards.* 6. *Homework Compliance Sheet.* 7. Pens.	1. Carpet squares or chairs. 2. "Making Friends Helper" badge. 3. Star chart with names of children. 4. Marker for star chart. 5. Name tags. 6. Prize bins with prizes. 7. Turn-taking games.	1. Frog puppet. 2. Tiger puppet. 3. Small ball. 4. Music and music player. 5. Safety cones or masking tape.
7	1. Conference table and chairs. 2. Name tags. 3. *Parent Handouts.* 4. *Parent Homework Worksheets.* 5. *Parent Coached Play Cards.* 6. *Homework Compliance Sheet.* 7. Pens.	1. Carpet squares or chairs. 2. "Making Friends Helper" badge. 3. Star chart with names of children. 4. Marker for star chart. 5. Name tags. 6. Prize bins with prizes. 7. Turn-taking games.	1. Horse puppet. 2. Duck puppet. 3. Two toy planes. 4. Two toy cars. 5. Lego Duplo sets. 6. Tables and chairs (optional).
8	1. Conference table and chairs. 2. Name tags. 3. *Parent Handouts.* 4. *Parent Homework Worksheets.* 5. *Parent Coached Play Cards.* 6. *Homework Compliance Sheet.* 7. Pens.	1. Carpet squares or chairs. 2. "Making Friends Helper" badge. 3. Star chart with names of children. 4. Marker for star chart. 5. Name tags. 6. Prize bins with prizes. 7. Turn-taking games.	1. Elephant puppet. 2. Monkey puppet. 3. Building blocks. 4. A small object for Hot or Cold. 5. Drawing paper. 6. Coloring tools. 7. Tables or flat surfaces to draw on.
9	1. Conference table and chairs. 2. Name tags. 3. *Parent Handouts.* 4. *Parent Homework Worksheets.* 5. *Parent Coached Play Cards.* 6. *Homework Compliance Sheet.* 7. Pens.	1. Carpet squares or chairs. 2. "Making Friends Helper" badge. 3. Star chart with names of children. 4. Marker for star chart. 5. Name tags. 6. Prize bins with prizes. 7. Turn-taking games.	1. Lion puppet. 2. Cow puppet. 3. Small ball. 4. Sets of toys for Swap and Play. 5. Bean bag for Hot Potato. 6. Tables and chairs for Swap and Play.

(*Continued*)

Table 0.2 Continued

Session	*Recurring Materials Needed in the Parent Group*	*Recurring Materials Needed in the Child Group*	*Unique Materials Needed in the Child Group*
10	1. Conference table and chairs. 2. Name tags. 3. *Parent Handouts.* 4. *Parent Homework Worksheets.* 5. *Parent Coached Play Cards.* 6. *Homework Compliance Sheet.* 7. Pens.	1. Carpet squares or chairs. 2. "Making Friends Helper" badge. 3. Star chart with names of children. 4. Marker for star chart. 5. Name tags. 6. Prize bins with prizes. 7. Turn-taking games.	1. Pig puppet. 2. Horse puppet. 3. Mouse puppet. 4. Hacky sack. 5. Safety cones or masking tape.
11	1. Conference table and chairs. 2. Name tags. 3. *Parent Handouts.* 4. *Parent Homework Worksheets.* 5. *Parent Coached Play Cards.* 6. *Homework Compliance Sheet.* 7. Pens.	1. Carpet squares or chairs. 2. "Making Friends Helper" badge. 3. Star chart with names of children. 4. Marker for star chart. 5. Name tags. 6. Prize bins with prizes. 7. Turn-taking games.	1. Tiger puppet. 2. Elephant puppet. 3. Small ball. 4. Two toy cars. 5. Music and music player. 6. Safety cones or masking tape. 7. Sets of toys for Swap and Play. 8. Bean bag for Hot Potato. 9. Tables and chairs for Swap and Play.
12	1. Conference table and chairs. 2. Name tags. 3. *Parent Handouts.* 4. *Parent Homework Worksheets.* 5. *Parent Coached Play Cards.* 6. *Homework Compliance Sheet.* 7. Pens.	1. Carpet squares or chairs. 2. "Making Friends Helper" badge. 3. Star chart with names of children. 4. Marker for star chart. 5. Name tags. 6. Prize bins with prizes. 7. Turn-taking games.	1. Monkey puppet. 2. Lion puppet. 3. Building blocks or Lego. 4. A toy box with lid. 5. Building blocks and Lego. 6. Sets of Tinker Toys. 7. Small object for Hot or Cold.
13	1. Conference table and chairs. 2. Name tags. 3. *Parent Handouts.* 4. *Parent Homework Worksheets.* 5. *Parent Coached Play Cards.* 6. *Homework Compliance Sheet.* 7. Pens.	1. Carpet squares or chairs. 2. "Making Friends Helper" badge. 3. Star chart with names of children. 4. Marker for star chart. 5. Name tags. 6. Prize bins with prizes. 7. Turn-taking games.	1. Mouse puppet. 2. Frog puppet. 3. Building blocks or Lego.

(*Continued*)

Table 0.2 Continued

Session	*Recurring Materials Needed in the Parent Group*	*Recurring Materials Needed in the Child Group*	*Unique Materials Needed in the Child Group*
14	1. Conference table and chairs. 2. Name tags. 3. *Parent Handouts*. 4. *Parent Homework Worksheets*. 5. *Parent Coached Play Cards*. 6. *Homework Compliance Sheet*. 7. Pens.	1. Carpet squares or chairs. 2. "Making Friends Helper" badge. 3. Star chart with names of children. 4. Marker for star chart. 5. Name tags. 6. Prize bins with prizes. 7. Turn-taking games.	1. Cow puppet. 2. Lion puppet. 3. Building blocks or Lego. 4. Small bucket.
15	1. Conference table and chairs. 2. Name tags. 3. *Parent Handouts*. 4. *Parent Homework Worksheets*. 5. *Parent Coached Play Cards*. 6. *Homework Compliance Sheet*. 7. Pens.	1. Carpet squares or chairs. 2. "Making Friends Helper" badge. 3. Star chart with names of children. 4. Marker for star chart. 5. Name tags. 6. Prize bins with prizes. 7. Turn-taking games.	1. Cow puppet. 2. Tiger puppet. 3. Two toy cars. 4. Small book. 5. Bucket with building blocks. 6. Drawing paper. 7. Tables and chairs or flat surfaces to draw on.
16	1. Conference table and chairs. 2. Name tags. 3. *Parent Handouts*. 4. *Homework Compliance Sheet*. 5. Pens. 6. Post-assessments (optional).	1. Carpet squares or chairs. 2. "Making Friends Helper" badge. 3. Star chart with names of children. 4. Marker for star chart. 5. Name tags. 6. Prize bins with prizes.	1. Cow puppet. 2. Tiger puppet. 3. Mouse puppet. 4. Three toy airplanes. 5. Bucket with building blocks. 6. Hacky sack. 7. Small object for Hot or Cold. 8. Graduation diplomas. 9. ALL the puppets for graduation.

- **Coaching with Performance Feedback.** To receive the full benefit of behavioral rehearsal opportunities, it is critical that program staff provide performance feedback through coaching. Parents are also encouraged to provide ***social coaching*** in the home and community as described in the *Parent Handouts*. ***Social coaching*** is an important component of *PEERS® for Preschoolers* because not all children will acquire these skills immediately and will instead need additional assistance in applying and generalizing the skills being taught.
- **Behavioral Reinforcement Using a Token Economy.** Child participation and attention will be reinforced and rewarded through a token economy in the form of stars given at the end of each activity. The number of stars given should be EQUAL for all attending children to avoid competition and/or behavioral disruption triggered by unequal rewards. (Note: this type of reward system is developmentally appropriate for children four to six years of age but would be different when children are school-aged.) Stars will be given after each of the following activities and are highlighted in the following sections of the *Child Session Therapist Guide*:

- Child Didactic Lesson
- Behavioral Rehearsal 1
- Break Time (optional)
- Behavioral Rehearsal 2
- Parent Coached Play

The number of stars given may vary according to the program preferences, but the total amount should increase weekly. Each week, at the end of the session during a *Final Wrap-Up* with the children and parents, the child group leader will count all the stars for one child with the help of the families. Prizes will be chosen by children based on the number of stars earned. Two prize boxes should include a wide variety of prizes to be chosen by children. For example, the *Yellow Prize Box* might include a selection of prizes when children earn 10 or more stars, while the *Blue Prize Box* might include a selection of prizes when the children earn 20 or more stars. The child group leader should ensure that children earn at least 10 stars in each group, and the number of stars earned should INCREASE EVERY WEEK. The child group leader should also ensure that the children reach at least 20 stars by the halfway point of the program, at least 30 stars by the three-quarters mark, and at least 40 stars by the end of the program. A scripted description of how to distribute stars is provided at the end of each child activity.

- **Homework Assignments.** Each lesson includes homework assignments to promote the use of skills in more natural social settings. Completion of homework assignments is critical to the generalization of skills and overall success in *PEERS® for Preschoolers*. Decades of research in *PEERS®* suggests that those who more frequently complete homework assignments have significantly better outcomes. Consequently, group leaders should strongly encourage the practicing of newly learned skills outside of the group and hold parents accountable for these assignments through the weekly *Homework Review*.
- **Homework Review.** To ensure that parents and children are using the skills outside of *PEERS® for Preschoolers*, the parent group leader will conduct *Homework Review* at the beginning of every parent session. *Homework Review* consists of an examination of completed assignments from the previous week, focused on practicing newly learned skills. A considerable amount of time is spent on *Homework Review* in each session (i.e., approximately 30–40 minutes), emphasizing the importance of behavioral rehearsal and practice in natural social settings. Friendship skills are not expected to generalize to other settings without the completion of homework assignments, so plan to spend a substantial amount of time reviewing homework. *Homework Review* is also the time in which the parent group leader will individualize the program for each family by assessing what is working and what is not working and troubleshooting any issues that may arise.
- **Flexibility with the Manual.** One of the common criticisms of manualized programs is that they represent "*one size fits all*" approaches. Obviously, very little in life is "*one size fits all,*" and manualized programs should not be treated in this manner. Instead, the *PEERS® for Preschoolers* curriculum is intended to be used flexibly. That means that rules and steps of social behavior should be modified accordingly when necessary. A good example of this relates to cultural variation in friendship skills formation and maintenance. The skills taught in *PEERS® for Preschoolers* represent the common social customs often utilized when making and keeping friends in North America and other Western cultures (although the program is used globally). However, even within Western society, there is great cultural variation.

Consequently, group leaders should modify the curriculum according to the social customs of the group members. Because not every family will affiliate with the same culture, *Homework Review* may afford an excellent opportunity to individualize the program for each family. The purpose of *Homework Review* is not only to ensure that skills are being practiced appropriately in natural settings but also to provide an opportunity to troubleshoot and adapt the program for anyone for whom it is not working. Flexibility with the manual (without too much deviation from the core curriculum) is also an essential ingredient to ensuring that all group members will benefit from *PEERS® for Preschoolers*.

Tracking Progress

Tracking progress is an essential part of determining whether your program is working. It is how a program maintains quality control. Below is a list of commonly used measures used in our published scientific studies with *PEERS® for Preschoolers*. Several standardized assessments of social functioning are included. These measures are widely available and have shown substantial change following the program. They also impose little demand upon parents and teachers to complete, and when used as a pre-, post-, and follow-up assessment of social functioning, these measures provide a good evaluation of program outcome.

Quality of Socialization Questionnaire-Preschool (QSQ-Pre; Appendix C)

The *QSQ-Pre* is a measure of social engagement completed by parents to assess the frequency of engagement in ***playdates*** and ***playgroups*** in the previous month. The *Social Initiation Scale* consists of two items – measuring the number of *hosted playdates* in the previous month and the number of different friends hosted. The *Social Reciprocity Scale* measures the number of *invited playdates* the child was invited to in the previous month and the number of different friends that invited the child. The *Social Engagement Scale* measures the frequency of attendance at ***playgroups*** in the previous month, including the number of different ***playgroups*** attended by the child. The *QSQ-Pre* was adapted from *the Quality of Play Questionnaire* (*QPQ*; Frankel & Mintz 2009), which was developed through factor analysis of 175 school-aged children. The reported frequency of *hosted* and *invited playdates* significantly discriminated community-referred from clinic samples ($p < 0.005$). The *QSQ-Pre* can be easily and affordably administered to parents before and after *PEERS® for Preschoolers* as a measure of program outcomes. The measure takes approximately five minutes to complete and can be found in *Appendix C* of this manual.

Social Responsiveness Scale Second Edition-School Age (SRS-2; Constantino & Gruber, 2012)

The *SRS-2* measures the presence and severity of autism-related social challenges (i.e., social awareness, social cognition, social communication, social motivation, and restricted interests and repetitive behaviors) as they occur in natural social settings. The *SRS-2* can be completed by parents and/or teachers before and after *PEERS® for Preschoolers* as a measure of outcome. Scores are presented as *T*-scores with a mean of 50 and a standard deviation of 10, with higher scores reflecting greater social challenges. The *SRS-2* was normed on a representative national sample and has good internal consistency ($\alpha = 0.95$), inter-rater reliability ($r = 0.61$), and convergent validity (Constantino & Gruber, 2012). The *SRS-2* takes approximately 15 minutes to complete.

Social Skills Improvement System (SSIS; Gresham & Elliot, 2008)

The *SSIS* is a standardized measure that assesses social skills and problem behaviors for children 3–18 years of age using a four-point Likert rating system. Prosocial skills are measured across seven domains: communication, cooperation, assertion, responsibility, empathy, engagement, and self-control. Problem behaviors are assessed across five domains: internalizing, externalizing, bullying, hyperactivity/inattention, and autism spectrum. *Social Skills* and *Problem Behaviors Scales* are represented using standard scores with a mean of 100 and a standard deviation of 15, with higher scores on the *Social Skills Scale* reflecting better social functioning, with the reverse for the *Problem Behaviors Scale*. The *SSIS* can be completed by parents and/or teachers prior to and following *PEERS® for Preschoolers* to assess outcome. The *SSIS* takes approximately 15 minutes to complete.

Parenting Stress Index Fourth Edition – Short Form (PSI-SF-4; Abidin, 2012)

The *PSI-SF-4* examines caregiver stress among parents of children 0–12 years of age. Total scores are summative across three domains: *Parental Distress*, *Parent–Child Dysfunctional Interaction*, and *Difficult Child*. The measure produces *T*-scores based on population data, with a normal range of T-scores falling between 39 and 57. Higher scores are indicative of greater parenting stress. The *PSI-SF-4* demonstrates robust internal reliability, with alpha coefficients ranging from 0.80 to 0.87 for each domain. The measure has been validated across multiple high-risk groups and remains a fundamental tool for measuring family functioning and caregiver stress among parents of neurodivergent children (Barroso et al., 2016; Kuhn et al., 2023; Lee et al., 2016). The *PSI-SF-4* can be administered to parents prior to and following *PEERS® for Preschoolers* to assess changes in parenting stress. The measure takes approximately 5–10 minutes to complete.

Research Evidence

Social skills programs are popular and often highly sought when building a holistic program of services for autistic and neurodivergent individuals across the lifespan. Parents often seek play and friendship-focused programs from an early age. By preschool, common social difficulties experienced by neurodivergent children may include less peer engagement, difficulty interpreting social cues, difficulty engaging in reciprocal conversations, and fewer friendships. Meta-analyses of existing group social skills programs for autistic children show mixed or inconclusive results, often reflecting gains in social knowledge rather than meaningful changes in social interactions and friendships. This manual was inspired by the growing body of systematic reviews identifying likely effective social skills strategies and approaches while highlighting a dearth of accessible evidence-based programming focused on friendship skills for young neurodivergent children and their families.

PEERS® for Preschoolers is a downward adaptation of *PEERS® for Adolescents* and *PEERS® for Young Adults*, both evidence-based programs for autistic individuals and those with other social differences. The *PEERS® for Preschoolers* program is comprised of many of the same teaching methods used in the adolescent and young adult *PEERS®* manuals, such as utilizing a caregiver-assisted approach, structured didactic lessons, role-play demonstrations, behavioral rehearsal activities, and homework assignments to promote meaningful generalization and maintenance of skills outside of the program setting. Several key modifications were made to the *PEERS® for Preschoolers* program that were informed by systematic reviews of the existing literature on social skills programs and broader child development literature. Some of these modifications include teaching skills and encouraging social interactions through play, presenting didactic lessons via puppet shows, creating behavioral rehearsal opportunities through popular childhood games, and partnering with parents via hands-on coaching and performance feedback.

Numerous studies have reported on the efficacy and feasibility of the *PEERS® for Preschoolers* program. Positive and promising gains have been reported for both children and parents. At the child level, studies have shown improvement in social behaviors, including social communication behaviors and broader autism-related behaviors (Antezana et al., 2022; Factor et al., 2021; Factor et al., 2022; Park et al., 2022; Tripathi et al., 2021; Tripathi et al., 2023). Several studies have demonstrated the durability of these child gains over time, with children continuing to show improvements in their social and friendship skills from four weeks up to five years following participation in *PEERS® for Preschoolers* (Antezana et al., 2022; Tripathi et al., 2021; Tripathi et al., 2023).

Positive changes to parent behavior have been reported as well and are likely attributed to the parent education and training received throughout the program. These gains include improvements in parenting styles and parent-child interactions, reports of greater parenting self-efficacy, and increased understanding of their children (Factor et al., 2021; Factor et al., 2022; Tripathi et al., 2024). The pivotal role of parents is highlighted in long-term follow-up studies. Research reveals that children continued to have more peer engagement as measured by playdates. Specifically, children who had gone through *PEERS® for Preschoolers* were having playdates at a comparable frequency to typically developing children one to five years after the program, likely due to parents' ongoing ***social coaching*** and involvement (Tripathi et al., 2022). Likewise, parents who reported that they continued to utilize the ***social coaching*** skills following *PEERS® for Preschoolers*, specifically ***priming*** and preparing their children for various social interactions and situations, reported greater improvements in their children's friendship skills and decreased parenting stress one to five years after participation (Tripathi et al., 2024).

With regard to implementation, studies have demonstrated feasibility and fidelity in implementation by program staff (Factor et al., 2021, 2022; Park et al., 2022). In addition, parents reported acceptability of the program as measured by their high attendance and participation in the program. These results have also been replicated in studies that administered the *PEERS® for Preschoolers* program in a shorter amount of time (i.e., twice-weekly sessions over the course of eight weeks), reflecting flexibility in the program to adapt to varying real-life clinic and community needs and resources (Antezana et al., 2022; Factor et al., 2021, 2022; Park et al., 2022).

This research overview suggests that children and parents are likely to benefit from participation in *PEERS® for Preschoolers*, with gains often maintained years after completion of the program. With careful adherence to the guidelines provided in the *PEERS® for Preschoolers* manual, it is anticipated that educators and practitioners using this program can expect similar outcomes for the families they serve.

Session 1

Introduction and Listening and Following Directions

PARENT SESSION THERAPIST GUIDE

Parent Session Agenda

- Opening Remarks (15 minutes).
- Identifying Strengths (15 minutes).
- Overview of the Program (10 minutes).
- Didactic Lesson (20 minutes).
- Parent Coached Play (20 minutes).
- Final Wrap-Up (10 minutes).

Materials Needed

- Conference room with a large table and enough chairs for the parent group leader and all parents to sit comfortably around the table.
  - Avoid sitting in a circle without a table as this creates the atmosphere of group therapy.
- Name tags for parents and treatment team.
- *Parent Handouts.*
- *Parent Homework Worksheets.*
- *Parent Coached Play Cards.*
- *Planned Absence Sheets* to be collected at the end of the session (see Appendix D).
- *Attendance and Homework Compliance Sheet* for parent group leader (see Appendix E).
- Pens for note-taking (consider having extra pens for parents who need them).

Opening Remarks (15 Minutes)

- This part of the session is primarily led by the child group leader and takes place in the child room (see *Child Session Therapist Guide*).
  - The treatment team will introduce themselves by saying their name and their role.
  - The parents will introduce themselves by saying their name and their child's name and age.
- After the *Opening Remarks* in the child room, have the parents join you in the parent room and have a seat around the conference table.
- Begin by welcoming the group.
- Introduce yourself and any other treatment team members again by sharing your name and your background (e.g., professional titles, qualifications, role in PEERS® for Preschoolers).
- Explain that in a moment we will have each parent introduce themselves to the group, but, prior to that, we will need to review rules and limits to confidentiality.

DOI: 10.4324/9781003502968-2

Review Rules and Limits of Confidentiality

- Encourage group members to keep what they hear in the group confidential.
  - Explain, *"We ask that you maintain the confidentiality of other group members. That means you should not discuss things brought up here with anyone outside of the group. Although we hope everyone will respect this rule, please remember that we can't control whether group members follow this rule."*
- Review mandated reporting guidelines and limits of confidentiality (this will vary according to region):
  - Explain, *"We also need to review our limits to confidentiality. If members of our treatment team have information that a child is being abused or neglected or that there is risk of harm to that child or others, we are required to report this information to the proper authorities. This is also true for concerns about the abuse or neglect of elders and dependents."*
  - Explain, *"Apart from these mandated reporting guidelines, we will keep what you share confidential. We also want you to maintain confidentiality. Can everyone give a verbal agreement not to share what you hear outside of this group?"*
- Have parents verbally agree to keep the information shared in the group about other families confidential.

Identifying Strengths (15 Minutes)

- Explain, *"PEERS® for Preschoolers is a skill-building group, focusing on helping children make and keep friends. Unlike other programs, it is a strengths-based approach and honors neurodiversity. The term neurodiversity essentially means that people have different ways of thinking. These differences do not make us less than or more than any other person. Arguably, there are great strengths in neurodiversity. It's often these strengths that make us better friends. When families seek services, we often spend a lot of time focusing on our children's challenges, but instead, we're going to begin this program by focusing on your child's strengths. So we're going to go around the room and have each of you reintroduce yourself and share what you like best about your child."*
- Go around the room and have parents introduce themselves by saying:
  - Their name.
  - Their child's name and age.
  - One favorite quality or characteristic they like about their child.
- If a parent focuses on something negative, redirect them to finding something positive.
- Repeat what the parent liked best about their child succinctly and reframe how that strength is important to making and keeping friendships.
- At the end of this exercise, explain, *"All of the strengths you identified in your children will be important characteristics for developing and maintaining close meaningful friendships."*

Embracing Neurodiversity

The term neurodiversity essentially means that people have different ways of thinking. These differences do not make us less than or more than any other person. Arguably, there are great strengths in neurodiversity and PEERS® is a strengths-based approach.

- **While the focus of PEERS® for Preschoolers is to help develop and enhance friendship skills for autistic and neurodivergent children, the PEERS® method is meant to be delivered using a neuroaffirming approach.**
- **In teaching social strategies for making and keeping friends, it is important to respect the role of neurodiversity.**
- **Learning and/or using the strategies taught in PEERS®:**
  - **Should NOT be about changing a person.**
  - **Should be about enhancing social interactions so others can appreciate our children for who they already are.**
  - **Will be YOUR CHOICE and the choice of your family.**

To highlight the importance of choice and respect for neurodiversity, each session begins with a Neuroaffirming Pledge. This pledge is also used in updated practice guidelines for PEERS® programs for teens and young adults as well. The PEERS® Neuroaffirming Pledge states the following principles:

- **We value neurodiversity, acceptance, and authenticity.**
- **We honor the diverse ways people experience the world.**
- **We respect each person's unique perspectives and communication styles.**
- **We recognize there is no one right way to connect with others.**
- **If using the strategies taught in PEERS® feels like camouflaging or masking and/or they don't align with your goals or the goals of your family, then you do not have to use them.**
- **Learning and using the skills taught in PEERS® is a PERSONAL CHOICE.**

Purpose and Structure of the Group

Explain the following:

- PEERS® for Preschoolers is a social skills group designed to help children make and keep friends.
- We focus on teaching the following skills:
  - How to listen and follow directions.
  - How to ask for and use peers' names.
  - How to greet friends.
  - How to share and give turns to friends.
  - How to ask for turns during play.
  - How to keep cool when feeling frustrated or angry during play.
  - How to be less bossy and more cooperative during play.
  - How to be a good sport.
  - How to maintain play interactions with peers.
  - How to ask friends to play.
  - How to join ongoing game play.
  - How to transition to new activities when playing with friends.
  - How to ask for and give help to others.
  - How to maintain appropriate body boundaries.
  - How to use an appropriate volume during play.

- Each skill builds upon the previously learned skills, so we will go in a predetermined sequence.
- Some children may already be good at some of these skills but may need instruction or refinement with others.
- We will be meeting once a week for 90 minutes for 16 weeks.
- There will be a child group and a parent group that meet in separate rooms at the same time.
- Parents will be told what the children are learning in the child group and given tips on how to ***social coach*** their child.
- Parents will also be given instruction on behavior management techniques as they relate to ***social coaching*** their child in using the newly learned skills to make and keep friends.
- Parents will practice ***social coaching*** during *Parent Coached Play* each week, which includes organized play activities with their child and other group members.
  - Parents will receive real-time feedback from the treatment team while ***social coaching*** their child during these play activities.
- Throughout the week, parents will help their child practice the newly learned skills in the home and community setting through weekly socialization homework assignments.
  - We will review completed assignments at the beginning of each week.
  - Parents will be given a *Homework Worksheet* to be completed and returned the following week.
- At the end of the 16 weeks, there will be a brief review of the skills with suggestions about where to go from here, followed by a graduation party and ceremony.
- Distribute the *Planned Absence Sheet.*
  - Remind parents that it is extremely important for all sessions to be attended.
    - If families miss three or more sessions, we do not expect them to get the full benefit of the program.
    - Explain the cancellation policy for families who need to be absent.
  - If families need to miss any sessions, parents should indicate the absence on the *Planned Absence Sheet* and return the sheet to the treatment team at the end of the current session (or before the second session at the latest).
  - The group leaders might consider rescheduling a session if there are several planned absences for a particular week.
- Explain that if families come late, children will miss the lesson, parents may miss the homework review, and both will miss out on valuable information.
  - If parents do arrive late, they should drop their children off in the child room before joining the parent session.

Overview of the Program (10 Minutes)

- Distribute the *Parent Handouts.*
  - Sections in **bold print** come directly from the *Parent Handout.*
  - Terms that are ***bold and italicized*** are buzzwords and represent important concepts from the didactic lesson.
    - The buzzwords represent social behaviors that can be identified in a few simple words.
    - Parents are strongly encouraged to use the buzzwords as much as possible to develop a common language between parents, their child, and treatment providers.

Structure of the Parent Sessions

- **Homework Review (30–40 minutes).**
  - **The session begins with a review of the previous homework assignments.**
    - **Parents will be given homework assignments each week to help their child practice the newly learned skills.**
    - Part of the homework assignments are to provide ***social coaching*** to your child on the targeted skills. This may include recording a video of your ***social coaching*** with your child which will be shown and discussed during homework review.
    - If you arrive late, you will miss part of the homework review and lose the opportunity for individualized feedback.
  - We will only focus on COMPLETED and ATTEMPTED homework assignments.
    - Time will not be spent talking about why homework assignments were not completed unless it is to troubleshoot a problem.
    - **We expect the same parent to come each week, but if other family members attend in their place, be sure to let them know the details of the homework assignments.**
    - **The success of the program depends on the completion of the homework assignments.**

- **Didactic Lesson (20–30 minutes).**
  - **The next portion of the session includes parent and child didactic lessons with corresponding homework assignments for the coming week.**
  - **Each week parents will receive:**
    - ***Parent Handout* with a brief description of the lesson and the homework assignments.**
      - Parents are encouraged to save these handouts and store them in a binder.
      - Parents are also encouraged to share the handouts with other family members, educators, and treatment providers who may help their child with their social skills.
      - If families are absent, parents will be sent an electronic version of the *Parent Handout* and expected to go over the lesson with their child prior to the next meeting.
    - ***Homework Assignment Worksheet* to be completed and returned the following week.**
    - ***Parent Coached Play Card* that provides *social coaching* tips for parents related to the corresponding lesson.**

- **Parent Coached Play (20 minutes).**
  - **Children will practice newly learned skills with other group members during organized play activities with turn-taking games brought from home.**
    - **Although the treatment team will have back-up games, families are expected to bring turn-taking games from home for their child to play during mock *playdates*.**
  - **Parents will *social coach* their child during organized mock *playdates*.**
  - **Parents will receive real-life *social coaching* from the treatment team as they facilitate these play interactions.**

- **Final Wrap-Up (10 minutes).**
  - **At the end of the session, there will be a brief wrap-up with all families during which the lesson and homework assignments for the coming week will be reviewed.**

Structure of the Child Sessions

- **Didactic Lesson (20 minutes).**
    - The didactic lesson will focus on key social skills related to making and keeping friends.
    - **Lessons will be taught using concrete rules and steps of social behavior, presented through live puppet shows conducted by the treatment team.**
    - **Children will practice newly learned skills with the puppets and other group members.**

- **Group Behavioral Rehearsal (10–15 minutes).**
    - **A behavioral rehearsal exercise will follow lessons to include additional practice of the newly learned skills within the context of familiar childhood games and sports.**
    - Children will receive reinforcement through a rewards system for practicing these skills with other group members (i.e., earning stars that can be exchanged for prizes at the end of the session).

- **Break Time (10 minutes).**
    - **Children will be given a bathroom and water break in between the two group behavioral rehearsal exercises.**

- **Group Behavioral Rehearsal (10–15 minutes).**
    - **A second behavioral rehearsal exercise will follow the bathroom break to include additional practice of the newly learned skills within the context of familiar childhood games and sports.**

- **Parent Coached Play (20 minutes).**
    - **Children will practice newly learned skills with other group members during mock *playdates* while receiving *social coaching* from their parents and the treatment team.**

- **Final Wrap-Up (10 minutes).**
    - **The lesson and homework assignments for the coming week will be reviewed.**
    - **Children will have the opportunity to exchange stars from their rewards program for prizes.**

Children's Reward System

- Children will receive stars for:
    - Participating during didactic lessons.
    - Practicing the newly learned skills during the group behavioral rehearsal activities.
    - Listening and following directions during unstructured activities (bathroom breaks, etc.).
    - Practicing the newly learned skills during *Parent Coached Play*.
- At the end of each session, children will be allowed to choose prizes from different prize bins depending on the number of stars earned.
- The group leader will ensure that children earn at least the minimum number of stars needed to earn a prize to reinforce participation and practice of the newly learned skills.
- To discourage competition among children, all children will be awarded the same number of stars.

What to Expect from the Group

- **Parents will gain knowledge in how to help their child learn to *be a good friend.***
- **Parents will learn how to be *social coaches* in supporting their child's attempts to make and keep friends.**
  - **Parents will learn how to foster more sustained, positive play interactions between their child and their child's *playmates.***
- **Parents will be given instruction and support in broadening their child's social network by joining *playgroups* and finding suitable *playmates.***
- **The four main responsibilities of parents in this group are to:**
  - **Enroll their child in social activities or *playgroups* where they can meet *potential playmates.***
  - **Arrange *playdates* for their child to practice the newly learned skills and develop friendships.**
  - **Complete weekly homework assignments with their child to support the generalization of newly learned skills in more natural settings.**
  - **Provide *social coaching* to promote the use and maintenance of skills.**

What Not to Expect from the Group

- **This is not a support group or a group to learn about broader developmental issues.**
- **Children will not improve unless families attend regularly and arrive on time.**
- **Children will not improve unless families regularly complete or attempt to complete homework assignments.**
- **This is not a "friendship matching" group.**
  - **The purpose is not to develop lasting friendships with other group members.**
- **Group members should not socialize with one another outside of the group during the program.**
  - **Families are welcome to socialize AFTER the group is over.**
  - The no-fraternizing rule helps to avoid:
    - Cliques forming between group members.
    - The exclusion of group members.
    - Conflict arising outside of the group.
    - Changing of group dynamics.
    - Failure to identify a source of friends outside of the group.
- **Other difficulties children may be having will not be addressed in the group.**
  - **The focus of treatment is on friendships only.**
  - **We will not meet our goal of helping the children make and keep friends if we get side-tracked during group.**
  - If your child is having other issues that need to be addressed, we would be happy to speak with you outside of the group and provide appropriate referrals when necessary.

Didactic Lessons (20 Minutes)

Didactic Lesson: Characteristics of Good Friendships

Explain, "*The name of this group is PEERS® for Preschoolers. PEERS® is an acronym and stands for the Program for the Education and Enrichment of Relational Skills. PEERS® is a program that includes many different types of social skills classes from childhood through adulthood, all focused on enhancing social interactions and promoting positive relationships. The program is called PEERS® because 'peers' are friends or potential playmates and the goal of this group is to help your children make and keep meaningful friendships. Another goal of this program is for you to learn how to better support your children's attempts to make and keep friends. To help your child develop meaningful friendships, it's important for us to discuss what qualities make a good friend. You will find that the characteristics of good friendships for young children are not so different from the characteristics of good friendships for all of us.*"

Ask, *"What are the characteristics that make a good friend for young children?"* (Have parents brainstorm the different characteristics of a good friendship.)

- **Sharing of Common Interests**
  - Friends share similar interests, likes, and hobbies.
  - Common interests give you things to talk about and do together.
- **Caring**
  - Good friendships are based on fondness, warmth, affection, and mutual caring.
  - Caring involves feeling and showing compassion, concern, and empathy.
- **Support**
  - Support involves providing help and assistance when needed.
  - Support includes giving encouragement and reassurance when times are hard.
- **Mutual Understanding**
  - Mutual understanding means understanding each person's perspectives, including likes and dislikes.
  - This understanding means you may even anticipate each other's thoughts and feelings.
- **Commitment and Loyalty**
  - Commitment is a promise that you will be there for each other in tough times.
  - Loyalty includes actions that show your support and allegiance.
- **Honesty and Trust**
  - Without honesty, there is little trust or security in friendship.
  - Trust is an assurance that your friend will support you and have your back.
- **Equality**
  - In equal friendships, no one person dominates the other.
  - The needs of both are equally important, and enjoyment is reciprocal and shared.
- **Ability to Self-Disclose**
  - Self-disclosure is sharing your private thoughts, feelings, and history.
  - Even casual friends may share some thoughts and feelings with one another.
- **Conflict Resolution**
  - Even close friends argue from time to time, but they can resolve the conflict.
  - Ability to resolve conflict is often determined by caring, commitment, and trust.
- **Close Proximity and Frequent Contact**
  - Close proximity includes interacting on a regular basis.
  - Frequent contact would include having regular playdates, sitting together at snack time, or playing during unstructured time.

Types of Friendships

Explain, "*There are generally four types of friendships for young children. Sometimes it can be confusing for us to know what type of friendship children have. One of the easiest ways to determine what type of friendship we have and whether this is a good choice in a friend is to consider how many characteristics of a friendship this relationship has. Just like the characteristics of good friends, the types of friendships young children have are not so different from the types of friendships we all have.*"

Present the different types of friendships for young children:

- **Acquaintances:**
  - **These are people that may know each other by name, but do not know each other well and do not usually associate outside of school or *playgroups*.**
  - Ask, *"Do acquaintances have many of the characteristics of a good friend?"*
    - Answer: No; they don't know each other well enough.
- **Casual friends:**
  - **These are people who know each other by name and interact sporadically, but do not spend a lot of time together socially.**
  - Ask, *"Do casual friends have many of the characteristics of a good friend?"*
    - Answer: Not many; they don't know each other that well.
- **Regular friends:**
  - **These are friends that play together regularly; they may go to the same social activities and spend time with each other outside of school or *playgroups*.**
  - Ask, *"Do regular friends have many of the characteristics of a good friend?"*
    - Answer: Yes; they have many, but not necessarily all.
- **Best friends:**
  - **These are friends that play together frequently and have regular *playdates*; they seek each other out even when other *playmates* are around.**
  - Ask, *"Do best friends have many of the characteristics of a good friend?"*
    - Answer: Yes; they should have most if not all.

Explain, *"The goal of PEERS® for Preschoolers is not to help your child have dozens of acquaintances or casual friends. Instead, the goal of this program is to help your children develop a few close meaningful friendships, like those we described as regular friends or best friends."*

Friendship is a Choice

Explain, *"We have a saying in PEERS® that friendship is a choice. Do we get to be friends with everyone?* (Pause to allow parents to answer "*no.*") *Does everyone get to be friends with us?* (Pause to allow parents to answer "*no.*") *The same is true for our children. One of the ways to determine if a playmate is a good choice for our children is to consider the characteristics of a good friend and the different types of friends."*

- **It is important to remember that *friendship is a choice.***
  - ***Our kids don't get to be friends with everyone.***
  - ***Everyone doesn't get to be friends with our kids.***

- **Use the Characteristics of Friendships and Types of Friendships as a guide for making good friendship choices.**

Didactic Lesson: Social Coaching

Explain, *"One of the most important roles parents have in PEERS® for Preschoolers will be to help promote your child's use of newly learned play skills. This will involve providing social coaching to your child using the 4 Ps. The 4 Ps stand for PRIMING, PROMPTING, PRAISING, and PROVIDING CORRECTIVE FEEDBACK USING A PRAISE SANDWICH. In a few moments, we will explain what these strategies involve. But before we can provide social coaching, we need to create opportunities for your child to practice newly learned skills. Here are some suggestions for creating practice opportunities to social coach your child."*

Creating Practice Opportunities

- **Practice play skills during games or activities that your child enjoys.**
  - **Practicing play skills during enjoyable preferred activities will keep your child's frustration level down and motivation level up.**
  - **Practice play skills during existing family routines.**
    - **It can be difficult to practice the skills if you feel like you need to "schedule" practice times.**
    - **Instead of trying to schedule times to practice, think about how you can creatively incorporate opportunities for practice into your existing family routine.**
      - **Mealtimes.**
      - **Weekly family activities.**
      - **School/daycare drop-off.**
    - **This will make it more likely that practice opportunities will occur and be sustained as part of your family routine.**

- ***Prime* your child about the desired behavior BEFORE naturally occurring *teachable moments.***
  - **Example: When dropping off your child at school in the morning, *prime* your child to *greet their friends* (Lesson 2) and go over the rules.**

- ***Prompt* your child about the desired behavior when it comes up DURING naturally occurring *teachable moments* throughout the week.**
  - **Example: While playing games with family members, *prompt* your child to *share and take turns* (Lesson 3) with siblings and family members.**

- ***Praise* your child by catching them being good throughout the week.**
  - **Whenever you see your child spontaneously use the skills, be sure to *praise* them using the buzzwords.**

- **Using the buzzwords is a way to relabel and reinforce the behavior while using repetition of instruction.**
- **Example: *"Great job sharing and taking turns!"* (Lesson 3)**

- **Use freebies to *social coach* new and previously learned skills.**
  - **When targeting more difficult (new) skills, incorporate more opportunities for easier (previously learned) skills to keep motivation high and frustration low.**
  - **Easier skills may include freebies.**
  - **Example: Rather than prompting to *share and give a turn* (Lesson 3) every time (i.e., say *"here"* and *use names*), allow your child to have several turns (or freebies) using the previously learned skills of *listening and following directions* (Lesson 1) while incorporating *praise.***

- **Avoid providing *social coaching* at every moment.**
  - **You do not want to over coach to the point that it takes away from the fun.**
  - **If your child becomes frustrated by your *social coaching*, you may need to modify one or both of the following:**
    - **Type of *social coaching***
      - **Example: More *praise* and less *corrective feedback.***
    - **Frequency of *social coaching***
      - **Example: More intermittent reinforcement rather than continuous reinforcement.**

Didactic Lesson: Listening and Following Directions

Explain, *"The first lesson the children are learning today is how to listen and follow directions. These are our first buzzwords. In order to learn the skills we teach in PEERS® for Preschoolers, it's important for our children to be able to listen and follow directions. Because some of your children may already be good at listening and following directions, this lesson will also be a good opportunity to put them at ease and orient them to the group."*

Snapshot of the Lesson: Listening and Following Directions

The objective of this lesson is to teach children how to *listen and follow directions.* Steps for *listening and following directions* include:

1. ***Listen with your ears* (cup your hand behind your ear).**
2. ***Be quiet with your mouth* (place your index finger in front of your mouth and say "shhh").**
3. ***Have calm hands and a calm body* (put your hands to your side).**
4. ***Do what you're told to do.***

Didactic Lesson: Parent Social Coaching using the *4 Ps*

Explain, *"As your child's social coach, you will be using several coaching techniques throughout this program. Perhaps the four most critical coaching techniques you will use to promote the use of targeted social skills include the 4 Ps. Each week, we will give you examples of how to use the 4 Ps while coaching your child on the newly learned social skills."*

- ***Priming*:**
  - ***Priming* involves preparing your child to practice newly learned skills immediately before a social opportunity.**
    - **Example: Going over the *Parent Handout* with your child to identify the rules and steps of a particular skill just before practicing.**
- ***Prompting*:**
  - ***Prompting* involves a gentle reminder for your child to use a particular skill in the moment.**
    - **Example: *"Remember to listen with your ears."***
    - **Example: *"Let's be quiet with your mouth when your friend is talking."***
    - **Example: *"What should you do with your hands and body when listening?"***
- ***Praising*:**
  - ***Praising* includes complimenting your child when they use or attempt to use a particular skill CORRECTLY.**
  - ***Praising* is one of the most powerful parenting strategies to promote behaviors that we want to see more of but is often under-utilized by parents.**
  - **The most effective way to *praise* the use of targeted skills is to incorporate buzzwords into the *praise.***
  - **Using buzzwords will help clarify exactly what they did correctly.**

Table 1.1 Examples of Praising

INAPPROPRIATE EXAMPLES	APPROPRIATE EXAMPLES
"Great job!"	***"Great job listening and following directions!"***
"Nice work!"	***"Nice work following directions and doing what you're told to do!"***
"Good job!"	***"Good job having a calm body when you were listening!"***

- ***Providing corrective feedback using a praise sandwich:***
  - ***Providing corrective feedback* is essential when your child's attempts to use a particular skill need refinement (i.e., they did not successfully use all aspects of the skill or they inappropriately used some aspect of the skill).**
  - **Giving feedback could seem punitive unless it is provided with *praise.***
  - ***Corrective feedback* should be given in the form of a *praise sandwich*:**
    1. **Start with *praise* using buzzwords.**
       - **To get their attention, consider first using your child's name if others are present.**
    2. ***Provide corrective feedback* using buzzwords.**
    3. **End with a general statement of *praise.***

Table 1.2 Examples of Corrective Feedback

INAPPROPRIATE EXAMPLES	APPROPRIATE EXAMPLES
"You didn't do it right!"	***"Good job listening. Remember to have calm hands and a calm body next time, but great job!"***
"Next time do what you're told to do!"	***"Nice try following directions. Remember to do what you're told next time, but good job!"***
"You need to follow directions!"	***"Great job listening. Don't forget to follow directions next time, but nice job!"***

Parent Coached Play

- Distribute the *Parent Coached Play Cards.*
- Explain, *"Each week we will discuss behavior management strategies to help you social coach your children. In all our discussions, the 4 Ps will be highlighted. In a moment, we will be joining the children for Parent Coached Play where we will arrange mock playdates with other group members. The Parent Coached Play Cards will provide you with some examples of how to coach your child during these play interactions. Our treatment team will be there to provide you with support, but the goal of these play interactions is for you to get some practice coaching on the newly learned skills of listening and following directions. Be sure to keep the Parent Coached Play Cards in front of you to help guide your social coaching on listening and following directions during this activity and during your homework assignments."*
- Review the examples of the ***4 Ps*** provided on the *Parent Coached Play Card.*

Homework Assignments

(Briefly review the homework assignments and troubleshoot any potential problems with parents.)

1. **Practice listening and following directions.**
   - **Practice having your child *listen and follow directions* this week during preferred and highly motivating activities while providing *social coaching* using the *4 Ps.***
     - ***Priming:* Review the rules for *listening and following directions* with your child BEFORE PRACTICING during preferred and highly motivating activities.**
     - ***Prompting:* Remind your child IN THE MOMENT to *listen and follow directions* whenever the opportunities present.**
     - ***Praising: Praise* your child for using the buzzwords whenever they *listen and follow directions* CORRECTLY.**
     - ***Providing corrective feedback: Provide corrective feedback* in the form of a *praise sandwich* whenever your child ATTEMPTS to *listen and follow directions.***
   - **Please send us a 30–60-second video of *social coaching* for *listening and following directions* with your child to be viewed during homework review.**
     - **Please include:**
       - **Skills your child did well.**
       - **Skills you would like to work on with your child.**

2. **Bring a turn-taking game.**
   - **Bring a turn-taking game that your child enjoys playing and can be played with the other children.**
     - **Common games: *Candy Land, Chutes and Ladders, Connect Four, Don't Break the Ice, Pop the Pig, Hi Ho Cherry-O, Operation, Perfection, Memory, Gone Fishin'.***
     - **Do not bring games that your child:**
       - **Will have difficulty sharing with others.**
       - **May become upset if the game pieces break or get lost.**

Parent Tips for Completing Homework Assignments

- **Suggestions for video recording on smartphones:**
  - **Test your audio and video quality.**
  - **Consider using a tripod.**
  - **Do not hold the camera while filming.**
  - **Consider using landscape mode.**
  - **Consider using the front-facing recording feature on your phone (so your child cannot see themself when filming).**
  - **Include both you and your child in the video.**
- **Suggestions for using *Parent Coached Play Cards*:**
  - **This coaching card can be used to provide support while using the *4 Ps* during your *social coaching* during homework assignments.**
  - **Consider sharing the *Parent Coached Play Cards* and *Parent Handouts* with your child's other care providers.**
- **Suggestions for using *Parent Homework Worksheets*:**
  - **This worksheet will assist you in self-monitoring your use of the *4 Ps* in your *social coaching* during weekly homework assignments.**
  - **Please remember to complete this worksheet and return it to the treatment staff at the next meeting of PEERS® for Preschoolers.**

Session 1 Continued

Introduction and Listening and Following Directions

CHILD SESSION THERAPIST GUIDE

Child Session Agenda

- Opening Remarks (10 minutes).
- Didactic Lesson: *Listening and Following Directions* (20 minutes).
- Group Behavioral Rehearsal Activity 1: *Simon Says* (10 minutes).
- Break Time (10 minutes).
- Group Behavioral Rehearsal Activity 2: *Head, Shoulders, Knees, and Toes* (10 minutes).
- Parent Coached Play: *Dyadic Playdates* (20 minutes).
- Final Wrap-Up (10 minutes).

Snapshot of the Lesson: Listening and Following Directions

The objective of this lesson is to teach children how to ***listen and follow directions***. Steps for ***listening and following directions*** include:

1. ***Listen with your ears*** (cup your hand behind your ear).
2. ***Be quiet with your mouth*** (place your index finger in front of your mouth and say "shhh").
3. ***Have calm hands and a calm body*** (put your hands to your side).
4. ***Do what you're told to do.***

Materials Needed

- Pig puppet.
- Monkey puppet.
- Building blocks.
- Small container for building blocks.
- Carpet squares or chairs.
- "Making Friends Helper" badge.
- Star chart with names of children.
- Marker for star chart.
- Name tags for families and treatment team.
- Prize bins with prizes.

Children's Reward System

- Each child should receive an equal number of stars at the end of every activity for:
  - Participating during didactic lessons.
  - Practicing the newly learned skills during group behavioral rehearsal activities.
  - Practicing the newly learned skills during *Parent Coached Play*.
  - Listening and following directions
- At the end of each session, children choose prizes from colored prize bins depending on the number of stars earned.
  - 10 stars = Yellow Prize Bin
  - 20 stars = Blue Prize Bin
- Prizes vary in value across colored prize bins based on the number of stars needed.
- Children can choose multiple prizes from one prize bin or choose one prize from one prize bin.
  - Example: 20 stars equals any of the following combinations:
    - One prize from the Blue Prize Bin
    - Two prizes from the Yellow Prize Bin
- The group leader should ensure that children earn at least 10 stars per session to reinforce participation and practice of the newly learned skills.
- To discourage competition among children, all children are awarded the same number of stars.
- The number of stars earned should increase from week to week (e.g., the final number of stars might increase from 10 stars in week one to 40 stars by week 16).

Preparing for the Lesson

- Follow the script below with the group leader using a pig puppet to play the part of "Penny Pig."
- A behavioral coach uses a monkey puppet to play the part of "Mickey Monkey."
- An additional behavioral coach assists in the behavioral rehearsal and provides encouragement and feedback to the group.
- A child is chosen at the beginning of the lesson as the "Making Friends Helper."
  - The "Making Friends Helper" wears a special badge and is the first child to practice the skill.
- The group leader and a behavioral coach sit on the floor at the front of the room.
- A special-colored carpet square (e.g., red) is placed at the front of the room next to the group leader to be used as the "Good Friend Square."
- For the children, additional carpet squares of the same color (e.g., green) are placed in a semi-circle facing the group leader and the "Good Friend Square."
- Note: If carpet squares are unavailable, the children and behavioral coaches may sit on chairs.
- The material in *italic font* should be read by the indicated person.
- The material in ***bold and italic font*** represents buzzwords.
- The material in CAPITAL LETTERS within the script should be given extra emphasis while the group is encouraged to say the words in unison.

Behavioral Coaching Techniques

Behavioral coaches should use the following coaching techniques described below throughout the lesson and the behavioral rehearsal activities. (Note: ***priming*** occurs during the introduction to the activity.)

- ***Prompting*:**
  - Use the buzzwords to ***prompt*** the children to ***listen and follow directions*** IN THE MOMENT.
    - Example: *"Remember to listen with your ears."*
    - Example: *"Let's be quiet with your mouth when your friend is talking."*
    - Example: *"What should you do with your hands and body when listening?"*
- ***Praising*:**
  - Reinforce ***listening and following directions*** by ***praising*** the children when they use the skills CORRECTLY.
    - Example: *"Great job listening and following directions!"*
    - Example: *"Great job following directions and doing what you're told to do!"*
    - Example: *"Good job having a calm body when you were listening!"*
- ***Providing corrective feedback:***
  - Reinforce ATTEMPTS to ***listen and follow directions*** by ***praising*** the children and identifying what could be done differently next time.
    - Example: *"Good job listening. Remember to have calm hands and a calm body next time, but great job!"*
    - Example: *"Nice try following directions. Remember to do what you're told next time, but good try!"*
    - Example: *"Great job listening. Don't forget to follow directions next time, but good job!"*

Opening Remarks (10 minutes)

- Allow the families to explore the room for a few moments before starting Opening Remarks.
- The child group leader begins by welcoming the families.
- Have the children sit in a semi-circle on the carpet squares facing the child group leader.
- Have the parents sit on the floor behind their children.

Group leader: *"Okay friends! Let's earn a star for sitting nicely on our carpet squares in the Listening Circle. Parents, help your child to have a seat."*

- Have the treatment team introduce themselves by saying their name and their role.
- Go around the room and have families introduce themselves by saying their name and their child's name.

Group leader: *"Parents, this is the child room where the children will be learning new skills each week. Children will earn stars* (point to the Star Chart at the front of the room) *for participating and practicing the skills. At the end of each group, children will exchange their stars for fun prizes* (show the two-colored prize bins)*."*

"Hey friends (point to the children)*, when you earn 10 stars you get to pick a prize from the yellow bin* (show a few prizes from the yellow bin) *and when you earn 20 stars you get to pick a prize from the blue bin* (show a few prizes from the blue bin)*. To start, everyone gets a star for coming in today!"* (Give each child a star on the Star Chart.)

(All behavioral coaches clap and cheer and encourage the children to clap as well. If children have sound sensitivities, consider replacing hand clapping with finger clapping or open-hand waving.)

"Okay friends, it's time to play some fun games with our puppet friends. Let's say goodbye to your parents. They'll come back soon to play some games with us. Parents, you'll head down to the parent room and we'll see you soon for Parent Coached Play!"

Allow parents to leave the room before starting the lesson. Consider distracting the children with the introduction of the puppets.

Group leader: (Sit at the front of the room and hold up puppets for the children to see.) *"Hey friends, I brought some of my fun friends to play with us today! Have you met Penny Pig and Mickey Monkey? Penny Pig and Mickey Monkey are going to be playing with us today and teaching us how to listen and follow directions. But first, we need to choose a Making Friends Helper. The Making Friends Helper will be our first friend to practice listening and following directions. Who wants to be our Making Friends Helper?"* (Choose from among the children raising their hands and place the "Making Friends Helper" badge on the child. The child stays in their seat for now.)

Didactic Lesson: Listening and Following Directions (20 Minutes)

Penny Pig: *"Hi friends! I'm Penny Pig. Oink, oink! Today we're going to practice listening and following directions. Listening and following directions is a great way to be nice to our friends!"*

"Who should we listen and follow directions with? We should listen and follow directions with our FRIENDS, TEACHERS, MOMMIES, DADDIES, BROTHERS AND SISTERS."

"Why should we listen and follow directions? We should listen and follow directions so we can learn new things."

"How should we listen and follow directions? First, we should listen with our EARS (cup your hand behind your ear), *be quiet with our MOUTHS* (place your index finger in front of your mouth and say "*shhh*") *and have calm hands and a calm BODY* (put your hands to your side). *Then, we should follow directions by doing what we're told to do."*

"Remember, listening and following directions are a nice way to be a good friend! Oink, oink!"

Role Play: Listening and Following Directions

Mickey Monkey: (Begin playing with Legos or blocks while commenting to yourself, such as *"This is such a cool tower!"* The small container is close by for clean up.)

Penny Pig:	(Turn to look at the group of children.) *"Hey friends! I see my friend Mickey Monkey playing with blocks but it's time to clean up. Let's see if Mickey Monkey can listen and follow directions."* (Turn to look at Mickey Monkey.) *"Mickey Monkey, it's time to clean up!"*
Mickey Monkey:	(Ignore Penny Pig and continue to play while commenting to yourself.)
Penny Pig:	(Turn to look at the group of children.) *"Hey friends, did Mickey Monkey listen and follow directions?"* (Shake your head no and encourage the children to say *"no."*) *"That's right! He kept playing with his toys. Let's see if Mickey Monkey can listen and follow directions this time.* (Turn to look at Mickey Monkey.) *Mickey Monkey, can you show us how to listen? Remember to listen with your EARS* (cup your hand behind your ear)*, be quiet with your MOUTH* (place your index finger in front of your mouth and say "*shhh*") *and have calm hands and a calm BODY* (put your hands to your side) *when you listen."*
Mickey Monkey:	(Stop talking and playing and put your hands on your lap.)
Penny Pig:	(Turn to look at the group of children.) *"Hey friends, is Mickey Monkey being quiet with his mouth and having calm hands and a calm body?"* (Nod your head yes and encourage the children to say *"yes."*) *"That's right! Oink, oink! Great job listening, Mickey Monkey! Now let's see if Mickey Monkey can follow directions by doing what he's told to do."* (Turn to look at Mickey Monkey.) *"Mickey Monkey, it's time to clean up!"*
Mickey Monkey:	*"Okay, Penny Pig. Ooh, ooh!"* (Place the blocks in the container.)
Penny Pig:	(Turn to look at the group of children.) *"Hey friends, did Mickey Monkey do a good job of listening and following directions?"* (Nod your head yes and encourage the children to say *"yes."*) *"That's right! Oink, oink!"*
Penny Pig and Mickey Monkey:	(Say *"good job," give a "pig high-five"* and *"monkey high-five,"* clap, cheer, and encourage the children to clap as well. Mickey Monkey takes the blocks and container and sits on the other side of the Good Friend Square (i.e., the Good Friend Square is between Penny Pig and Mickey Monkey).)
Penny Pig:	*"Now let's see _____ (behavioral coach) try! _____ (Behavioral coach), please come sit on the Good Friend Square."*
Behavioral coach:	(Sit on the Good Friend Square.)

Penny Pig: *"_____ (Behavioral coach), can you show us how to listen and follow directions with Mickey Monkey?"*

Behavioral coach: *"Okay, Penny Pig."*

Penny Pig: *"Remember to listen with your* (cup your hand behind your ear to prompt children to say "*ears*")*...EARS, be quiet with your* (place your index finger in front of your mouth to prompt children to say "*mouth*")*...MOUTH, and when you listen to Mickey Monkey have calm hands and a calm* (put your hands to your side to prompt children to say "*body*")*...BODY. Then do what you're told to do."*

Mickey Monkey: (Hand the behavioral coach several blocks. The container is close by for clean up.)

Behavioral coach: (Begin to build a tower with the blocks for a few moments while commenting to self.)

Mickey Monkey: *"_____ (Behavioral coach), it's time to clean up! Ooh, ooh!"*

Behavioral coach: *"Okay, Mickey Monkey."* (Stop talking and playing with the blocks, put the blocks in the container, and place your hands to your side.)

Penny Pig: *"Great job listening and following directions, _____ (Behavioral coach)! Oink, oink!"*

Penny Pig and Behavioral coach: (Say *"good job," give a "pig high-five"* and *"monkey high-five,"* clap, cheer, and encourage the children to clap as well.)

Behavioral coach: (Give the container of blocks back to Mickey Monkey and leave the Good Friend Square.)

Behavioral Rehearsal: Listening and Following Directions

Penny Pig: (Turn to look at the group of children.) *"Okay friends! Now let's see our Making Friends Helper _____ try! _____ (Making Friends Helper), come sit on the Good Friend Square and show us how to listen and follow directions with Mickey Monkey."* (The Making Friends Helper should sit on the Good Friend Square.)

"Remember to listen with your (cup your hand behind your ear to prompt children to say "*ears*")*...EARS, be quiet with your* (place your index finger in front of your mouth to prompt children to say "*mouth*")*...MOUTH, and when you listen to Mickey Monkey have calm hands and a calm* (put your hands to your side to prompt children to say "*body*")*...BODY. Then do what you're told to do."*

Mickey Monkey:	(Hand the Making Friends Helper several blocks. The container is close by for clean up.)
Penny Pig:	(If needed, ***social coach*** the Making Friends Helper to begin playing with the blocks.)
Mickey Monkey:	*"_____ (Making Friends Helper), it's time to clean up! Ooh, ooh!"*
Penny Pig:	(If needed, ***social coach*** the Making Friends Helper to stop playing with the blocks, put the blocks in the container, and place their hands to their side.) *"Great job listening and following directions, _____ (Making Friends Helper)! Oink, oink!"* (Say *"good job," give a "pig high-five"* and *"monkey high-five,"* clap, cheer, and encourage the children to clap as well.) (The Making Friends Helper should give the container of blocks back to Mickey Monkey.) *"Okay, _____ (Making Friends Helper), choose another friend to sit on the Good Friend Square."* (If needed, ***social coach*** the Making Friends Helper to choose another child before returning to their seat.)

Repeat the following with each child:

Penny Pig:	(Have each child take turns sitting on the Good Friend Square and practicing ***listening and following directions*** with Mickey Monkey.) *"Okay friends! Now let's see _____ (child) try! _____ (Child), come sit on the Good Friend Square and show us how to listen and follow directions with Mickey Monkey."* (The child should sit on the Good Friend Square.) *"Remember to listen with your* (cup your hand behind your ear to prompt children to say "*ears*")*...EARS, be quiet with your* (place your index finger in front of your mouth to prompt children to say "*mouth*")*...MOUTH, and when you listen to Mickey Monkey have calm hands and a calm* (put your hands to your side to prompt children to say "*body*")*...BODY. Then do what you're told to do."*
Mickey Monkey:	(Hand the child several blocks. The container is close by for clean up.)
Penny Pig:	(If needed, ***social coach*** the child to begin playing with the blocks.)
Mickey Monkey:	*"_____ (Child), it's time to clean up! Ooh, ooh!"*

Penny Pig: (If needed, ***social coach*** the child to stop playing with the blocks, put the blocks in the container, and place their hands to their side.)

"Great job listening and following directions, _____ (child)! Oink, oink!"

(Say *"good job," give a "pig high-five"* and *"monkey high-five,"* clap, cheer, and encourage the children to clap as well.)

"Okay, _____ (child), choose another friend to sit on the Good Friend Square." (If needed, ***social coach*** the child to choose another child before returning to their seat.)

Didactic Lesson Wrap-Up

Group leader: *"Well friends, you all did a great job listening and following directions by listening with your* (cup your hand behind your ear to prompt children to say *"ears")...EARS, being quiet with your* (place your index finger in front of your mouth to prompt children to say *"mouth")...MOUTH, and when you listened to Mickey Monkey, having calm hands and a calm* (put your hands to your side to prompt children to say *"body")...BODY. And great job doing what you were told to do!"*

"You each earned ____ (number) stars for listening and following directions! Let's start with _____ (child)."

Award each child the same number of stars by repeating the following with each child:

Group leader: *"Where's _____ (child)?"* (Wait until all the children are looking at the child.)

"_____ (Child), how many stars did you earn?" (Pause briefly to allow the child to respond.)

"That's right! Let's all count for _____ (child)! One, two, three... (add stars to the Star Chart as they are counted aloud)*! Everybody clap for _____ (child)!"* (All behavioral coaches clap and cheer and encourage the children to clap as well.)

Session 1 Continued

Simon Says

BEHAVIORAL REHEARSAL ACTIVITY 1

Materials Needed

- None.

Room Setup

- Remove or place all carpet squares to the side.
- The group leader stands at the front of the room facing the children.
- The children and behavioral coaches sit in the play area facing the group leader.

Rules: Simon Says

- The group leader reads the script below to explain the rules.
- Present a command to the children and behavioral coaches. The children and behavioral coaches practice ***listening and following directions*** by following the command.
- All commands begin with *"Simon says..."*
  - The purpose of the game is to practice ***listening and following directions*** rather than to eliminate group members.
  - Note: No group members will be eliminated during the game playing.
- Keep commands simple and fun. Present commands that require some movement.
  - Examples:
    - *"Simon says hop like a kangaroo!"*
    - *"Simon says stomp your feet like a giant!"*
  - The group leader and behavioral coaches may need to model the commands for the children.
- Between each command, instruct the children to freeze in place by saying, *"Simon says FREEZE!* (Pause.) *And sit."*
  - Do not present the next command until all children have stopped moving.
- Use the *Simon Say Commands* in the table below to keep the children engaged in the game.
- Optional: Once familiar with the game, allow the children to suggest new commands.

Behavioral Rehearsal: Simon Says (10 Minutes)

The group leader leads the activity. The behavioral coaches and children sit nearby as the group leader explains the rules.

Group leader: *"Hey friends! Now we're going to play Simon Says and practice listening and following directions. I'll tell each of you to do some fun and silly things like, 'Simon says hop like a frog'* (hop like a frog) *or 'Simon says waddle like a penguin'* (waddle like a penguin). *Then you will practice listening and following directions by hopping like a frog or waddling like a penguin. After a while, we'll say 'Simon says FREEZE' and you all need to listen and follow directions by freezing in place. Can everybody show me how to freeze?"* (Pause briefly to allow the children to demonstrate freezing in place.)

"Great job, friends! Okay, so let's remember to practice listening and following directions by listening with your (cup your hand behind your ear to prompt children to say "*ears*")*...EARS, being quiet with your* (place your index finger in front of your mouth to prompt children to say "*mouth*")*... MOUTH, having calm hands and a calm* (put your hands to your side to prompt children to say "*body*")*...BODY and doing what you're told to do. Okay, let's have _____ (behavioral coaches) try first!"*

Role Play: Simon Says

The group leader presents the commands. Two behavioral coaches demonstrate how to ***listen and follow directions*** by playing *Simon Says* while the other behavioral coaches and children sit nearby watching.

Group leader: *"Okay _____ (behavioral coaches), let's play Simon Says and practice listening and following directions. Remember to FREEZE when I say, 'Simon says FREEZE!' Are we ready?"*

"_____ (Behavioral coaches), Simon says walk like a penguin!"

Behavioral coaches: (Walk like penguins.)

Group leader: (Allow behavioral coaches to walk like penguins for a few seconds.) *"Great job listening and following directions _____ (behavioral coaches)!* (Wait a few more seconds.) *Simon says FREEZE!* (Pause.) *And sit."*

Behavioral coaches: (Freeze in place. Then sit on the floor.)

Group leader: *"Great job listening and following directions, _____ (behavioral coaches)! Let's keep playing. Are we ready?"*

Behavioral coaches: *"_____ (Behavioral coaches), Simon says hop like a frog!"*

(Hop like frogs.)

Group leader: (Allow behavioral coaches to hop like frogs for a few seconds.) *"Great job listening and following directions_____ (behavioral coaches)!* (Wait a few more seconds.) *Simon says FREEZE!* (Pause.) *And sit."*

Behavioral coaches: (Freeze in place. Then sit on the floor.)

Group leader: *"Great job listening and following directions, _____ (behavioral coaches)! Okay friends, now it's everybody's turn to play! Are we ready?"* (Have the children stand up to play *Simon Says.*)

Behavioral Rehearsal: Simon Says

Group leader: *"Simon says _____ (command)!"* (Model the command for the children.)

Table 1.3 Simon Says Commands

Walk like a robot	Waddle like a penguin
Peck like a chicken	Gallop like a horse
Stomp your feet like a giant	Walk backward
Shake your hips	Crawl like a baby
Hop like a kangaroo	Give a friend a high-five
Swim like a shark	Chomp like an alligator
Slither like a snake	Act like a monkey
Shake your legs	Dig like a dog
Spin like a top	Shake your whole body
Wiggle like a worm	Walk like a crab
Dance	Hop like a frog
Move slow like a turtle	Fly like a plane

Allow the children to ***listen and follow directions*** by following the command for several seconds.

Group leader: *"Simon says FREEZE!* (Pause.) *And sit."* (Allow the children to ***listen and follow directions*** by freezing in place, then sitting on the floor.)

"Great job listening and following directions! Let's keep playing. Are we ready?"

Introduce new commands following the instructions above. Eventually, consider allowing the children to suggest new commands.

Group leader: *"Who wants to pick what we should do next? Let's raise our hands and remember to listen to our friends and follow directions."*

Introduce new (appropriate) commands suggested by the children following the instructions above.

Behavioral Rehearsal Wrap-Up

Group leader: *"Well friends, great job listening and following directions! Give yourselves a big round of applause!"* (All behavioral coaches clap and cheer and encourage the children to clap as well.)

"Now everyone sit in the Listening Circle." (Have children return to the Listening Circle to sit on their carpet squares.)

"Okay friends, you did a great job listening and following directions by listening with your (cup your hand behind your ear to prompt children to say "*ears*")*...EARS, being quiet with your* (place your index finger in front of your mouth to prompt children to say "*mouth*")*...MOUTH, and when you listened, having calm hands and a calm* (put your hands to your side to prompt children to say "*body*")*...BODY. And great job doing what you were told to do!"*

"You each earned ____ (number) more stars for listening and following directions! Let's start with _____ (child)."

Award each child the same number of stars by repeating the following with each child:

Group leader: *"Where's _____ (child)?"* (Wait until all the children are looking at the child.)

"_____ (Child), how many stars did you earn?" (Pause briefly to allow the child to respond.)

"That's right! Let's all count for _____ (child)! One, two, three... (add stars to the Star Chart as they are counted aloud)*! Everybody clap for _____ (child)!"* (All behavioral coaches clap and cheer and encourage the children to clap as well.)

Break Time (10 Minutes)

- The puppets may be used to lead the children to and from the bathroom during break time.
- To assist with transitions and limit unstructured time, behavioral coaches may review the lesson with the children while waiting for the remaining children to return from the bathroom.
- You may want to award stars for good behavior after returning from the bathroom.

Session 1 Continued

Head, Shoulders, Knees, and Toes

BEHAVIORAL REHEARSAL ACTIVITY 2

Materials Needed

- None.

Room Setup

- Remove or place all carpet squares to the side.
- The group leader stands at the front of the room facing the children.
- The children and behavioral coaches stand in a semi-circle facing the group leader.

Rules: Head, Shoulders, Knees, and Toes

- The group leader reads the script below to explain the rules.
- All behavioral coaches and children (if able) sing the *Head, Shoulders, Knees, and Toes* song while acting out the lyrics:
  - *Head, shoulders, knees and toes, knees and toes…*
    Head, shoulders, knees and toes, knees and toes…
    Eyes and ears and mouth and nose…
    Head, shoulders, knees and toes, knees and toes!

- The children practice ***listening and following directions*** by acting out the lyrics.
- To begin the game and for each new modification, initially sing the song slowly until the children become familiar with the game.
- After a few repetitions, different body parts or articles of clothing may be substituted into the song.
  - Substitute only ONE body part or article of clothing at a time.
  - The new body part or article of clothing will replace the "toes."
  - Examples:
    - Head, shoulders, knees and TUMMY, knees and TUMMY!
    - Head, shoulders, knees and ANKLES, knees and ANKLES!
    - Head, shoulders, knees and BACK, knees and BACK!

Behavioral Rehearsal: Head, Shoulders, Knees, and Toes (10 Minutes)

The group leader leads the activity. The behavioral coaches and children sit nearby as the group leader explains the rules.

Group leader: *"Hey friends! Now we're going to play Head, Shoulders, Knees and Toes. The song goes like this..."* (Sing the song with the behavioral coaches while acting out the movements by touching the body part being referenced.)

"Head, shoulders, knees and toes, knees and toes...

Head, shoulders, knees and toes, knees and toes...

Eyes and ears and mouth and nose...

Head, shoulders, knees and toes, knees and toes!"

"We're going to sing the song together. As we sing, listen to the song and follow directions. After a few turns, we'll change the body parts so make sure to listen so you can follow directions."

"Remember to practice listening and following directions by listening with your (cup your hand behind your ear to prompt children to say "*ears*")... *EARS, being quiet with your* (place your index finger in front of your mouth to prompt children to say "*mouth*")*...MOUTH, and when you're listening, having calm hands and a calm* (put your hands to your side to prompt children to say "*body*")*...BODY. And don't forget to do what you're told to do. Okay, let's have _____ (behavioral coaches) try first!"*

Role Play: Head, Shoulders, Knees, and Toes

The group leader leads the role play. Two behavioral coaches demonstrate how to play *Head, Shoulders, Knees, and Toes* while the children sit nearby watching.

Group leader: *"Okay _____ (behavioral coach 1 and 2), let's play Head, Shoulders, Knees and Toes and practice listening and following directions. Are you ready?"*

Everyone sings the *Head, Shoulders, Knees, and Toes* song while the behavioral coaches act out the lyrics.

Group leader: *"Great job listening and following directions, _____ (behavioral coaches)! Let's keep playing, but THIS time we're going to change a body part. Instead of touching our 'toes' we're going to touch our 'tummy.' So make sure to listen so you can follow directions! Are you ready?"*

Everyone sings the *Head, Shoulders, Knees, and Toes* song by substituting *"toes"* for *"tummy"* while the behavioral coaches act out the lyrics.

Group leader: *"Great job listening and following directions, _____ (behavioral coaches)! Okay friends, now it's everybody's turn to play Head, Shoulders, Knees, and Toes! Are we ready?"* (Have the children stand up to play *Head, Shoulders, Knees, and Toes.*)

Behavioral Rehearsal: Head, Shoulders, Knees, and Toes

Everyone: *"Head, shoulders, knees and toes, knees and toes...*

Head, shoulders, knees and toes, knees and toes...

Eyes and ears and mouth and nose...

Head, shoulders, knees and toes, knees and toes!"

Group leader: *"Great job listening and following directions, friends! Okay, this time we're going to change a body part. Instead of touching our 'toes' we're going to touch our _______ (body part). So make sure to listen so you can follow directions! Are we ready?"*

After each song, change the lyrics to substitute "toes" for a new body part or article of clothing. Substitute only ONE body part or article of clothing at a time.

Substitutions: *Head, shoulders, knees and TUMMY, knees and TUMMY!*

Head, shoulders, knees and ANKLES, knees and ANKLES!

Head, shoulders, knees and BACK, knees and BACK!

Head, shoulders, knees and WRISTS, knees and WRISTS!

Head, shoulders, knees and HIPS, knees and HIPS!

Head, shoulders, knees and CHIN, knees and CHIN!

Head, shoulders, knees and FEET, knees and FEET!

Head, shoulders, knees and SHIRT, knees and SHIRT!

Head, shoulders, knees and SHOES, knees and SHOES!

Head, shoulders, knees and SOCKS, knees and SOCKS!

Head, shoulders, knees and PANTS, knees and PANTS!

Consider allowing children to suggest new body parts or articles of clothing.

Group leader: *"Who wants to pick the next new body part? Let's raise our hands and remember to listen and follow directions."*

Introduce new (appropriate) body parts or articles of clothing suggested by the children following the instructions above.

Behavioral Rehearsal Wrap-Up

Group leader: *"Well friends, great job listening and following directions! Give yourselves a big round of applause!"* (All behavioral coaches clap and cheer and encourage the children to clap as well.)

"Now everyone sit in the Listening Circle." (Have children return to the Listening Circle to sit on their carpet squares.)

"Okay friends, you did a great job listening and following directions by listening with your (cup your hand behind your ear to prompt children to say "*ears*")*...EARS, being quiet with your* (place your index finger in front of your mouth to prompt children to say "*mouth*")*...MOUTH, having calm hands and a calm* (put your hands to your side to prompt children to say "*body*")*...BODY when you listened. And great job doing what you were told to do!"*

"You each earned ____ (number) more stars for listening and following directions! Let's start with _____ (Child)."

Award each child the same number of stars by repeating the following with each child:

Group leader: *"Where's _____ (child)?"* (Wait until all the children are looking at the child.)

"_____ (Child), how many stars did you earn?" (Pause briefly to allow the child to respond.)

"That's right! Let's all count for _____ (child)! One, two, three... (add stars to the Star Chart as they are counted aloud)*! Everybody clap for _____ (child)!"* (All behavioral coaches clap and cheer and encourage the children to clap as well.)

"Now we're going to play some games with our parents and practice listening and following directions some more!"

Introduction and Listening and Following Directions

PARENT COACHED PLAY: DYADIC PLAYDATES

Materials Needed

- Turn-taking games provided by the treatment team.
  - Common games: *Candy Land, Chutes and Ladders, Connect Four, Don't Break the Ice, Pop the Pig, Hi Ho Cherry-O, Operation, Perfection, Memory, Gone Fishin'.*
- Tables and chairs or carpet squares.
- *Parent Coached Play Cards.*

Room Setup

- If available, organize tables in separate corners of the room with four to six chairs per table.
- If tables are unavailable, place two carpet squares in separate corners of the room to indicate where the children will sit.

Rules: Dyadic Playdates

- The group leader divides the families into groups of two families each.
  - If there are an odd number of children, pair one child with a behavioral coach who will serve as a ***playmate***. In this case, you will need an additional coach to serve as a behavioral coach for the parent.
  - To avoid social exclusion, avoid having children play in triads as much as possible.
- Assign each group to sit at a table or specific play area.
  - Children should sit next to each other.
  - Parents will act as ***social coaches*** by sitting on the other side of their child to minimize interrupting the natural flow of play between the children.
  - One behavioral coach will be assigned to each dyad to provide ***social coaching*** suggestions and feedback to parents.
- Children will select turn-taking games provided by the treatment team.
- Each child will have ten minutes to play their chosen game with their ***playmate*** and then will switch games.
- Parents will choose which child's game will be played first.
- To minimize unstructured periods, parents will help the children set up the game in a cooperative fashion (handing game pieces to each other, offering suggestions, etc.).
- Parents will ***social coach*** the children to ***listen and follow directions*** as they play using the guidelines highlighted on the *Parent Coached Play Cards.*

- Behavioral coaches will provide support to parents in their ***social coaching*** using the ***4 Ps*** (***priming, prompting, praising,*** and ***providing corrective feedback***) and will model appropriate ***social coaching*** behavior when necessary.
- After approximately nine minutes of play, instruct the parents to prepare the children for the upcoming game swap.
- After approximately one additional minute of play (ten minutes total), instruct the parents to have the children clean up and swap games.
- Repeat the cycle with the second game for the remaining ten minutes before returning to the *Listening Circle.*

Behavioral Coaching: Dyadic Playdates

Behavioral coaches will ***social coach*** parents during dyadic ***playdates*** in the following ways:

- ***Priming*:**
  - Begin the play interactions with parents going over the rules for ***listening and following directions*** BEFORE GAME PLAYING.
    - Example: "*Remember that as you play your games, we want you to practice listening and following directions by listening with your* (cup your hand behind your ear to prompt children to say "*ears*")*...EARS, being quiet with your* (place your index finger in front of your mouth to prompt children to say "*mouth*")*...MOUTH, having calm hands and a calm* (put your hands to your side to prompt children to say "*body*")*...BODY and doing what you're told to do.*"
- ***Prompting*:**
  - Remind parents to use the buzzwords to ***prompt*** their child to ***listen and follow directions*** IN THE MOMENT.
  - Help parents to identify opportunities to proactively ***prompt*** their child to ***listen and follow directions***.
    - Example: "*Your friend wants to say something. Let's listen with your ears.*"
    - Example: "*What should you do with your ears right now?*"
    - Example: "*Remember to follow directions.*"
  - Assist parents to follow through with the ***prompts*** they present to their child.
- ***Praising*:**
  - Remind parents to ***praise*** and reinforce their child whenever their child ***listens and follows directions*** CORRECTLY.
    - Example: "*Great job listening to your friend!*"
    - Example: "*Great job following directions and doing what you're told to do!*"
    - Example: "*Great job having calm hands and a calm body when you listened!*"
- ***Providing corrective feedback using a praise sandwich*:**
  - Remind parents to ***praise*** their child's ATTEMPTS to ***listen and follow directions*** and identify what could be done differently next time.
    - Example: "*Good job listening. Remember to have calm hands and a calm body next time, but great job!*"
    - Example: "*Nice try following directions. Remember to do what you're told next time, but good try!*"
    - Example: "*Great job listening. Don't forget to follow directions next time, but good job!*"

Parent Coached Play: Dyadic Playdates (20 Minutes)

- Have each child choose a turn-taking game provided by the treatment team.
- The group leader sits on the floor at the front of the room.
- The families sit on the floor in a semi-circle facing the group leader.

Group leader: *"Hey friends, we're going to have playdates and play with the cool games you picked out. As you play your games, we want you to practice listening and following directions by listening with your* (cup your hand behind your ear to prompt children to say "*ears*")*...EARS, being quiet with your* (place your index finger in front of your mouth to prompt children to say "*mouth*")*...MOUTH, having calm hands and a calm* (put your hands to your side to prompt children to say "*body*")*...BODY and doing what you're told to do. After a few minutes, we'll tell you to swap games and everybody will get to play a new game, so make sure you're listening. And parents you will be coaching your children on listening and following directions using your Parent Coached Play Cards throughout the game playing. Okay, let's play with our games!"*

- Parents will ***social coach*** their children to ***listen and follow directions*** throughout the game playing.
- After approximately nine minutes of play, instruct the parents to prepare the children for the upcoming game swap by saying, *"Parents, tell your children that we'll be swapping games in one minute."*
- After approximately one additional minute of play (ten minutes total), instruct the parents to swap games by saying, *"Parents, it's time to swap games. Social coach the children to practice listening and following directions when playing the next game."*
- After approximately nine minutes of playing the second game, instruct the parents to prepare the children for clean up by saying, *"Parents, tell your children that we'll be cleaning up in one minute."*
- After approximately one additional minute of play (ten minutes total), ***prompt*** the parents to instruct their children to clean up by saying, *"Parents, it's time to clean up. Let's social coach the children to listen and follow directions by cleaning up before sitting in the Listening Circle."*
- If needed, parents will ***social coach*** their child to ***listen and follow directions*** to clean up.

Final Wrap-Up (10 Minutes)

- The child group leader sits on the floor at the front of the room.
- The children sit on the carpet squares in a semi-circle facing the group leader, with parents sitting behind their children.

Group leader: *"Okay friends, you all did a great job playing your games and listening and following directions! When we're listening, do you think we should listen with our ears?"* (Pause briefly to allow the children to say *"yes."*)

Group leader: *"That's right, friends! And when we're listening, do you think we should have a loud mouth or a quiet mouth?"* (Pause briefly to allow the children to respond.)

"That's right, friends! And when we're listening, do you think we should have calm hands and a calm body?" (Pause briefly to allow the children to say *"yes."*)

"That's right! And when we're following directions, do you think we should do what we're told to do?" (Pause briefly to allow children to respond *"yes."*)

"That's right, friends! You all did such a great job listening and following directions that you each earned ____ (number) more stars! Let's start with _____ (child)."

Award each child the same number of stars by repeating the following with each child:

Group leader: *"Where's _____ (child)?"* (Wait until all the children are looking at the child.)

"_____ (Child), how many stars did you earn?" (Pause briefly to allow the child to respond.)

"That's right! Let's all count for _____ (child)! One, two, three... (add stars to the Star Chart as they are counted aloud)*! Everybody clap for _____ (child)!"* (All behavioral coaches clap and cheer and encourage the children to clap as well.)

"And remember you all earned those stars by listening and following directions! Everyone did a great job and parents you did an excellent job social coaching! Parents, remember your homework assignments this week are to continue practicing listening and following directions with your children using the 4 Ps and to bring a turn-taking game next week."

"Alright little friends, do you want to count ALL of our stars?" (Pause briefly to allow the children to respond.)

"Let's all count together and see how many stars we earned today! One, two, three...(count the number of stars for one child)*!"*

"You each earned ____ (total number) stars today! Round of applause for our friends!" (All behavioral coaches should clap and cheer and encourage the families to clap as well.)

"Great job, friends! Don't forget to choose your reward before you leave. See you all next week!"

Session 1 Continued

Introduction and Listening and Following Directions

PEERS® FOR PRESCHOOLERS: PARENT HANDOUT

Overview of the Program

Embracing Neurodiversity

The term neurodiversity essentially means that people have different ways of thinking. These differences do not make us less than or more than any other person. Arguably, there are great strengths in neurodiversity and PEERS® is a strengths-based approach.

- While the focus of PEERS® for Preschoolers is to help develop and enhance friendship skills for autistic and neurodivergent children, the PEERS® method is meant to be delivered using a neuroaffirming approach.
- In teaching social strategies for making and keeping friends, it is important to respect the role of neurodiversity.
- Learning and/or using the strategies taught in PEERS®:
  - Should NOT be about changing a person.
  - Should be about enhancing social interactions so others can appreciate our children for who they already are.
  - Will be YOUR CHOICE and the choice of your family.

To highlight the importance of choice and respect for neurodiversity, each session begins with a Neuroaffirming Pledge. This pledge is also used in updated practice guidelines for PEERS® programs for teens and young adults as well. The PEERS® Neuroaffirming Pledge states the following principles:

- We value neurodiversity, acceptance, and authenticity.
- We honor the diverse ways people experience the world.
- We respect each person's unique perspectives and communication styles.
- We recognize there is no one right way to connect with others.
- If using the strategies taught in PEERS® feels like camouflaging or masking and/or they don't align with your goals or the goals of your family, then you do not have to use them.
- Learning and using the skills taught in PEERS® is a PERSONAL CHOICE.

Structure of the Parent Sessions

- **Homework Review (30–40 minutes):**

- The session begins with a review of the previous homework assignments.
  - Parents will be given homework assignments each week to help their child practice the newly learned skills.
  - We expect the same parent to come each week, but if other family members attend in your place, be sure to let them know the details of the homework assignments.
  - The success of the program depends on the completion of the homework assignments.

- **Didactic Lesson (20–30 minutes):**
  - The next portion of the session includes parent and child didactic lessons with corresponding homework assignments for the coming week.
  - Each week parents will receive:
    - *Parent Handout* with a brief description of the lesson and the homework assignments.
    - *Homework Assignment Worksheet* to be completed and returned the following week.
    - *Parent Coached Play Card* that provides ***social coaching*** tips for parents related to the corresponding lesson.
- **Parent Coached Play (20 minutes):**
  - Children will practice newly learned skills with other group members during organized play activities with turn-taking games brought from home.
    - Although the treatment team will have back-up games, families are expected to bring turn-taking games from home for their child to play during mock ***playdates***.
  - Parents will ***social coach*** their child during organized mock ***playdates.***
  - Parents will receive real-life ***social coaching*** from the treatment team as they facilitate these play interactions.
- **Final Wrap-Up (10 minutes):**
  - At the end of the session, there will be a brief wrap-up with all families during which the lesson and homework assignments for the coming week will be reviewed.

Structure of the Child Sessions

- **Didactic Lesson (20 minutes):**
  - Lessons will be taught using concrete rules and steps of social behavior, presented through live puppet shows conducted by the treatment team.
  - Children will practice newly learned skills with the puppets and other group members.
- **Group Behavioral Rehearsal (10–15 minutes):**
  - A behavioral rehearsal exercise will follow lessons to include additional practice of the newly learned skills within the context of familiar childhood games and sports.
- **Break Time (10 minutes):**
  - Children will be given a bathroom and water break in between the two group behavioral rehearsal exercises.
- **Group Behavioral Rehearsal (10–15 minutes):**
  - A second behavioral rehearsal exercise will follow the bathroom break to include additional practice of the newly learned skills within the context of familiar childhood games and sports.
- **Parent Coached Play (20 minutes):**
  - Children will practice newly learned skills with other group members during mock ***playdates*** while receiving ***social coaching*** from their parents and the treatment team.
- **Final Wrap-Up (10 minutes):**

- The lesson and homework assignments for the coming week will be reviewed.
- Children will have the opportunity to exchange stars from their rewards program for prizes.

What to Expect from the Group

- Parents will gain knowledge in how to help their child learn to be a good friend.
- Parents will learn how to be ***social coaches*** in supporting their child's attempts to make and keep friends.
  - Parents will learn how to foster more sustained, positive play interactions between their child and their child's ***playmates***.
- Parents will be given instruction and support in broadening their child's social network by joining ***playgroups*** and finding suitable ***playmates.***
- The four main responsibilities of parents in this group are to:
  - Enroll their child in social activities or ***playgroups*** where they can meet potential ***playmates***.
  - Arrange ***playdates*** for their child to practice the newly learned skills and develop friendships.
  - Complete weekly homework assignments with their child to support the generalization of newly learned skills in more natural settings.
  - Provide ***social coaching*** to promote the use and maintenance of skills.

What Not to Expect from the Group

- This is not a support group or a group to learn about broader developmental issues.
- Children will not improve unless families attend regularly and arrive on time.
- Children will not improve unless families regularly complete homework assignments.
- This is not a "friendship matching" group.
  - The purpose is not to develop lasting friendships with other group members.
- Group members should not socialize with one another outside of the group during the program.
  - Families are welcome to socialize AFTER the program is over.
- Other difficulties children may be having will not be addressed in the group.
  - The focus of treatment is on friendships only.
  - We will not meet our goal of helping the children make and keep friends if we get side-tracked during the group.

Characteristics of Good Friendships

- Sharing of common interests.
- Caring.
- Support.
- Mutual understanding.
- Commitment and loyalty.
- Honesty and trust.
- Equality.
- Ability to self-disclose.
- Conflict resolution.
- Close proximity and frequent contact.

Types of Friendships

- **Acquaintances:**
  - These are people who may know each other by name, but do not know each other well and do not usually associate outside of school or ***playgroups***.
- **Casual friends:**
  - These are people who know each other by name and interact sporadically but do not spend a lot of time together socially.
- **Regular friends:**
  - These are friends who play regularly; they may go to the same social activities and spend time with each other outside of school or ***playgroups***.
- **Best friends:**
  - These are friends who play frequently and have regular ***playdates***; they seek each other out even when other ***playmates*** are around.

Friendship is a Choice

- It is important to remember that ***friendship is a choice.***
  - ***Our kids don't get to be friends with everyone.***
  - ***Everyone doesn't get to be friends with our kids.***
- Use the Characteristics of Friendships and Types of Friendships as a guide for making good choices.

Creating Practice Opportunities

- **Practice play skills during games or activities that your child enjoys.**
  - **Practicing play skills during enjoyable preferred activities will keep your child's frustration level down and motivation level up.**
  - **Practice play skills during existing family routines.**
    - It can be difficult to practice the skills if you feel like you need to "schedule" practice times.
    - Instead of trying to schedule times to practice, think about how you can creatively incorporate opportunities for practice into your existing family routine.
      - Mealtimes.
      - Weekly family activities.
      - School/daycare drop-off.
    - This will make it more likely that practice opportunities will occur and be sustained as part of your family routine.

- ***Prime*** **your child about the desired behavior BEFORE naturally occurring *teachable moments.***
  - Example: When dropping off your child at school in the morning, ***prime*** your child to ***greet their friends*** (Lesson 2) and go over the rules.

- ***Prompt*** **your child about the desired behavior when it comes up DURING naturally occurring *teachable moments* throughout the week.**
  - Example: While playing games with family members, ***prompt*** your child to ***share and take turns*** (Lesson 3) with siblings and family members.

- ***Praise* your child by catching them being good throughout the week.**
    - Whenever you see your child spontaneously use the skills, be sure to ***praise*** them using the buzzwords.
    - Using the buzzwords is a way to relabel and reinforce the behavior while using repetition of instruction.
    - Example: *"Great job sharing and taking turns!"* (Lesson 3).
- **Use freebies to *social coach* new and previously learned skills.**
    - When targeting more difficult (new) skills, incorporate more opportunities for easier (previously learned) skills to keep motivation high and frustration low.
    - Easier skills may include freebies.
    - Example: Rather than ***prompting*** to ***share and give a turn*** (Lesson 3) every time (i.e., ***say "here"*** and ***use names***), allow your child to have several turns (or *freebies*) using the previously learned skills of ***listening and following directions*** (Lesson 1) while incorporating ***praise***.
- **Avoid providing *social coaching* at every moment.**
    - You do not want to over coach to the point that it takes away from the fun.
    - If your child becomes frustrated by your ***social coaching***, you may need to modify one or both of the following:
        - Type of ***social coaching***:
            - Example: More ***praise*** and less ***corrective feedback***.
        - Frequency of ***social coaching***:
            - Example: More intermittent reinforcement rather than continuous reinforcement.

Snapshot of the Child Lesson: Listening and Following Directions

The objective of this lesson is to teach children how to ***listen and follow directions***. Steps for ***listening and following directions*** include:

1. ***Listen with your ears*** (cup your hand behind your ear).
2. ***Be quiet with your mouth*** (place your index finger in front of your mouth and say "***shhh***").
3. ***Have calm hands and a calm body*** (put your hands to your side).
4. ***Do what you're told to do***.

Parent Social Coaching Using the *4 Ps*

- ***Priming***:
    - ***Priming*** involves preparing your child to practice newly learned skills immediately before a social opportunity.
        - Example: Going over the *Parent Handout* with your child to identify the rules and steps of a particular skill just before practicing.
- ***Prompting***:
    - ***Prompting*** involves a gentle reminder for your child to use a particular skill IN THE MOMENT.
        - Example: *"Remember to listen with your ears."*

- Example: *"Let's be quiet with your mouth when your friend is talking."*
- Example: *"What should you do with your hands and body when listening?"*

- ***Praising***:
  - ***Praising*** includes complimenting your child when they use or attempt to use a particular skill CORRECTLY.

Table 1.1 Examples of Praising

INAPPROPRIATE EXAMPLES	APPROPRIATE EXAMPLES
"Great job!"	***"Great job listening and following directions!"***
"Nice work!"	***"Nice work following directions and doing what you're told to do!"***
"Good job!"	***"Good job having a calm body when you were listening!"***

  - ***Praising*** is one of the most powerful parenting strategies to promote behaviors that we want to see more of but is often under-utilized by parents.
  - The most effective way to ***praise*** the use of targeted skills is to incorporate buzzwords into the ***praise***.
  - Using buzzwords will help clarify exactly what they did correctly.
- ***Providing corrective feedback using a praise sandwich***:
  - ***Providing corrective feedback*** is essential when your child's attempts to use a particular skill needs refinement (i.e., they did not successfully use all aspects of the skill or they inappropriately used some aspect of the skill).
  - Giving feedback could seem punitive unless it is provided with ***praise***.
  - ***Corrective feedback*** should be given in the form of a ***praise sandwich***:
    1. Start with ***praise*** using buzzwords.
       - To get their attention, consider first using your child's name if others are present.
    2. ***Provide corrective feedback*** using buzzwords.
    3. End with a general statement of ***praise***.

Table 1.2 Examples of Corrective Feedback

INAPPROPRIATE EXAMPLES	APPROPRIATE EXAMPLES
"You didn't do it right!"	***"Good job listening. Remember to have calm hands and a calm body next time, but great job!"***
"Next time do what you're told to do!"	***"Nice try following directions. Remember to do what you're told next time, but good job!"***
"You need to follow directions!"	***"Great job listening. Don't forget to follow directions next time, but nice job!"***

Homework Assignments

1. **Practice listening and following directions.**
   - **Practice having your child *listen and follow directions* this week during preferred and highly motivating activities while providing *social coaching* using the *4 Ps*.**

    - ***Priming***: Review the rules for ***listening and following directions*** with your child BEFORE PRACTICING.
    - ***Prompting***: Remind your child IN THE MOMENT to ***listen and follow directions*** whenever the opportunities present.
    - ***Praising***: ***Praise*** your child for using the buzzwords whenever they ***listen and follow directions*** CORRECTLY.
    - ***Providing corrective feedback***: ***Provide corrective feedback*** in the form of a ***praise sandwich*** whenever your child ATTEMPTS to ***listen and follow directions***.
  - **Please send us a 30–60-second video of social coaching for *listening and following directions* with your child to be viewed during homework review.**
    - Please include:
      - Skills your child did well.
      - Skills you would like to work on with your child.

2. **Bring a turn-taking game.**
   - Bring a turn-taking game that your child enjoys playing and can be played with the other children.
     - Common games: *Candy Land, Chutes and Ladders, Connect Four, Don't Break the Ice, Pop the Pig, Hi Ho Cherry-O, Operation, Perfection, Memory, Gone Fishin'*.
     - Do not bring games that your child:
       - Will have difficulty sharing with others.
       - May become upset if the game pieces break or get lost.

Parent Tips for Completing Homework Assignments

- **Suggestions for video recording on smartphones:**
  - Test your audio and video quality.
  - Consider using a tripod.
  - Do not hold the camera while filming.
  - Consider using landscape mode.
  - Consider using the front-facing recording feature on your phone (so your child cannot see themself when filming).
  - Include both you and your child in the video.

- **Suggestions for using *Parent Coached Play Cards*:**
  - This coaching card can be used to provide support while using the ***4 Ps*** during your ***social coaching*** during homework assignments.
  - Consider sharing the *Parent Coached Play Cards* and *Parent Handouts* with your child's other care providers.

- **Suggestions for using *Parent Homework Worksheets*:**
  - This worksheet will assist you in self-monitoring your use of the ***4 Ps*** in your ***social coaching*** during weekly homework assignments.
  - Please remember to complete this worksheet and return it to the treatment staff at the next meeting of PEERS® for Preschoolers.

Session 1 Continued

Listening and Following Directions

PEERS® FOR PRESCHOOLERS: PARENT COACHED PLAY CARD

Snapshot of the Lesson: Listening and Following Directions

1. ***Listen with your ears*** (cup your hand behind your ear).
2. ***Be quiet with your mouth*** (place your index finger in front of your mouth and say "***shhh***").
3. ***Have calm hands and a calm body*** (put your hands to your side).
4. ***Do what you're told to do***.

Priming BEFORE Game Playing

- Example: "*Remember that as you play your game, you should practice listening and following directions by listening with your* (cup your hand behind your ear to prompt child to say "*ears*")*...EARS, being quiet with your* (place your index finger in front of your mouth to prompt child to say "*mouth*")*...MOUTH, having calm hands and a calm* (put your hands to your side to prompt child to say "*body*")*...BODY and doing what you're told to do.*"

Prompting IN THE MOMENT

- Example: *"Your friend wants to say something. Let's listen with your ears."*
- Example: *"What should you do with your ears right now?"*
- Example: *"Remember to follow directions."*

Praising for CORRECT Use of Skills

- Example: *"Great job listening to your friend!"*
- Example: *"Great job following directions and doing what you're told to do!"*
- Example: *"Great job having calm hands and a calm body when you listened!"*

Providing Corrective Feedback for ATTEMPTS Using a Praise Sandwich

- Example: *"Good job listening. Remember to have calm hands and a calm body next time, but great job!"*
- Example: *"Nice try following directions. Remember to do what you're told next time, but good try!"*
- Example: *"Great job listening. Don't forget to follow directions next time, but good job!"*

Session 1 Continued

Listening and Following Directions

PEERS® FOR PRESCHOOLERS: PARENT HOMEWORK WORKSHEET

Child's Name:	Parent's Name:		Date:	
HOMEWORK ASSIGNMENTS	PRIMING (REVIEWING RULES BEFORE PRACTICE)	PROMPTING (IN THE MOMENT)	PRAISING (USING BUZZWORDS)	PROVIDING CORRECTIVE FEEDBACK (USING A PRAISE SANDWICH)
Listen and follow directions				
Bring a turn-taking game	Did you bring a turn-taking game? YES or NO (Circle)		Which game did you bring?	

Please fill out this worksheet by describing what you did to complete the homework assignments. Worksheets will be collected during Homework Review at the next session of PEERS® for Preschoolers.

Session 2

Finding Playgroups and Meeting and Greeting Friends

PARENT SESSION THERAPIST GUIDE

Parent Session Agenda

- Homework Review (30 minutes).
- Didactic Lessons (30 minutes).
- Parent Coached Play (20 minutes).
- Final Wrap-Up (10 minutes).

Materials Needed

- Conference room with a large table and enough chairs for the parent group leader and all parents to sit comfortably around the table.
    - Avoid sitting in a circle without a table as this creates the atmosphere of group therapy.
- Name tags for parents and treatment team.
- *Parent Handouts* (for the current week and the previous week).
- *Parent Homework Worksheets* (for the current week and the previous week).
- *Parent Coached Play Cards* (for the current week and the previous week).
- *Planned Absence Sheets* (distribute to those absent in the previous week or if changes were made to the schedule due to a high number of planned absences).
- *Attendance and Homework Compliance Sheet* for parent group leader.
- Pens for note-taking (consider having extra pens for parents who need them).

Homework Review (30 Minutes)

1. **Practice listening and following directions.**
    - Review the 30–60-second video of ***social coaching*** for ***listening and following directions*** for each family. (For larger groups, you may need to review video recordings in two smaller groups with two different parent group leaders.)
        - Have parents identify:
            - Skills their child did well.
            - Skills they would like to work on with their child.
        - Provide ***social coaching*** tips as appropriate for each family.

DOI: 10.4324/9781003502968-3

- If parents did not send a video of ***social coaching***, confirm the following:
  - Parents practiced having their child ***listen and follow directions*** during preferred and highly motivating activities while providing ***social coaching*** using the ***4 Ps***.
    - ***Priming*:** Reviewed the rules for ***listening and following directions*** with their child BEFORE PRACTICING.
    - ***Prompting*:** Reminded their child IN THE MOMENT to ***listen and follow directions*** whenever the opportunity presented.
    - ***Praising*: *Praised*** their child using the buzzwords whenever they ***listened and followed directions*** CORRECTLY.
    - ***Providing corrective feedback*: *Provided corrective feedback*** in the form of a ***praise sandwich*** whenever their child ATTEMPTED to ***listen and follow directions***.

2. **Bring a turn-taking game.**
   - Confirm parents brought a turn-taking game that their child enjoys playing and can be played with the other children. (To avoid distractions, these games should be left with the parents until *Parent Coached Play*.)
     - Common games: *Candy Land, Chutes and Ladders, Connect Four, Don't Break the Ice, Pop the Pig, Hi Ho Cherry-O, Operation, Perfection, Memory, Gone Fishin'.*

Didactic Lessons (30 Minutes)

PEERS® Neuroaffirming Pledge

- We value neurodiversity, acceptance, and authenticity.
- We honor the diverse ways people experience the world.
- We respect each person's unique perspectives and communication styles.
- We recognize there is no one right way to connect with others.
- If using the strategies taught in PEERS® feels like camouflaging or masking and/or they don't align with your goals or the goals of your family, then you do not have to use them.
- Learning and using the skills taught in PEERS® is a PERSONAL CHOICE.

Didactic Lesson: Playgroups

- Distribute the *Parent Handouts*.
  - Sections in **bold print** come directly from the *Parent Handout*.
  - Terms that are ***bold and italicized*** are buzzwords and represent important concepts from the didactic lesson.
- Explain, *"Last week we talked about the characteristics that make a good friend and types of friendships for young children. Now it's important to discuss where our children will meet potential friends. Playgroups or extracurricular activities are one of the best sources of friends because they facilitate social interactions between similar-aged peers and presumably attract people with common interests. One of your main responsibilities will be to enroll your child in playgroups where they will have opportunities to practice the skills they learn in PEERS® with potential playmates."*
- Ask, *"What are some common playgroups or extracurricular activities for young children?"*
- Have parents brainstorm different ***playgroups*** (see Table 2.1 for examples of *Common Playgroups for Young Children*).

Table 2.1 Common Playgroups for Young Children

Sports camps	**Theater arts camp**	**Science camps**
Soccer league	**Drama classes**	**Space camps**
T-ball/baseball	**Art camps**	**Nature camps**
Softball	**Painting classes**	**Gardening classes**
Little League	**Finger painting groups**	**Chorus**
AYSO	**Drawing/coloring groups**	**Music classes**
Swimming classes	**Pottery classes**	**Band**
Martial arts	**Arts and crafts groups**	**Orchestra**
Karate	**Color Me Mine**	**Glee club**
Flag football	**Dance classes**	**Choir**
Basketball	**Ballet classes**	**School of Rock**
Tennis	**Tap classes**	**YMCA classes**
My Gym	**Hip hop dance classes**	**Library clubs**
Gymnastics	**Cooking classes**	**Book clubs**
Gymboree	**Baking classes**	**Story time**
Mommy and Me classes	**Lego groups**	**Cub scouts/boy scouts**
Trampoline gyms	**Pokémon groups**	**Brownies/girl scouts**
Jungle gyms	**Magic groups**	**4H**
Indoor rock climbing	**Board games groups**	**Sunday school**
Yoga classes	**Card games groups**	**Hebrew school**
Meditation classes	**Language classes**	**Religious groups**

Finding Playgroups

- Explain, *"The next step in identifying the right playgroups for your child is to think about WHERE you might find information about these groups in your community."*
- Ask, *"Where might you find information about playgroups in your area?*
- Have parents brainstorm places where they might get more information about ***playgroups*** in their community (see Table 2.2 for a list of *Common Sources of Information about Playgroups*).

Table 2.2 Common Sources of Information about Playgroups

School	**Other parents/friends**	**Local libraries**
Daycare	**Teachers/daycare**	**Recreation centers**
Preschool	**Family members**	**Community parks**
Afterschool programs	**Therapists**	**YMCA**
Head Start	**Coworkers**	**Community centers**
Sunday school	**Google search**	**Cub scouts/boy scouts**
Hebrew school	**Parent listservs**	**Brownies/girl scouts**
Jewish Community Center	**Community parent groups**	**4H**
Religious centers	**Parenting blogs**	**Natural history museums**
Local church/mosque	**Parenting magazines**	**Art museums**
Local temple/synagogue	**Meetup.com**	**Science museums**
My Gym	**Parenting message boards**	**Summer camps**
Fitness centers	**Volunteer groups**	**Art classes**
Mommy and Me groups	**Carpools**	**Music classes**
Gymboree groups	**Sports groups**	**Science classes**

Selecting Playgroups: Consider the 5 Ws

- Explain, *"The next step in selecting the right playgroup is to consider whether the activity is a good fit for your child and your family. One simple way to assess the appropriateness of a playgroup is to consider the 5 Ws."*

- **WHO:**
  - **Who are the other children and parents?**
  - **Are the children around the same age and level of support needs?**
  - **Will the other group members be accepting and inclusive?**
- **WHAT:**
  - **What is the activity?**
  - **Are the activities of the *playgroup* based on my child's interest?**
  - **Will my child be able to participate in the activities meaningfully?**
- **WHERE:**
  - **Where is the *playgroup*?**
  - **Is the location relatively close to our home or school?**
  - **Do the other families live in close proximity in order to facilitate *playdates*?**
- **WHEN:**
  - **When do the *playgroups* meet?**
  - **How soon does the next *playgroup* start?**
  - **Will we be able to consistently attend the *playgroups*?**
- **HOW:**
  - **How does my child enroll?**
  - **How will we get to the *playgroups*?**
  - **How will we pay for the *playgroups* if there is a cost?**

- Explain, *"Although it will be important to consider the 5 Ws as you investigate potential playgroups, you may have to be flexible in choosing the group that works best for your family. Next week we will talk about choosing playgroups and different criteria to consider as you make your choices."*

Didactic Lesson: Meeting and Greeting Friends

- Explain, *"This week the children are learning how to meet and greet friends by asking names and using names. Your children will need to know how to ask their friend's name when meeting a peer for the first time or if they happen to forget their friend's name. It's also important that your children consistently use their friend's name so that their friends know when they're trying to talk to them and play with them."*

Snapshot of the Lesson: Meeting and Greeting Friends

The objective of this lesson is to teach children how to *meet and greet friends* by *asking and using names* and *saying "hi" and "bye."*

Asking Names

1. ***Look at your friend with your eyes*** **(point to your eyes).**
2. ***Smile with your mouth*** **(point to your mouth and smile).**

3. ***Say, "What's your name?"***
4. ***Say your name, "I'm ____ (Name)."***

Using Names

1. ***Look at your friend with your eyes*** **(point to your eyes).**
2. ***Smile with your mouth*** **(point to your mouth and smile).**
3. ***Use names when talking to your friend.***

Saying "Hi"

1. ***Look at your friend with your eyes*** **(point to your eyes).**
2. ***Smile with your mouth*** **(point to your mouth and smile).**
3. ***Wave with your hand*** **(wave your hand).**
4. ***Say "hi" using your friend's name.***

Saying "Bye"

1. ***Look at your friend with your eyes*** **(point to your eyes).**
2. ***Smile with your mouth*** **(point to your mouth and smile).**
3. ***Wave with your hand*** **(wave your hand).**
4. ***Say "bye" using your friend's name.***

Parent Coached Play

- Distribute the *Parent Coached Play Cards*.
- Review the examples of the ***4 Ps*** provided on the *Parent Coached Play Card.*
- Remind parents that in a few moments, we will be joining the children for *Parent Coached Play* in the context of mock dyadic ***playdates***.
- Parents should keep the *Parent Coached Play Card* in front of them during the dyadic ***playdate*** for recommendations on how to ***social coach*** children on ***meeting and greeting friends***.

Homework Assignments

(Briefly review the homework assignments and troubleshoot any potential problems with parents.)

1. **Find a playgroup for your child.**
    - **Investigate and begin to enroll your child in a *playgroup* based on their interests.**
    - **Consider the *5 Ws*:**
        - **WHO will be there?**
        - **WHAT is the activity?**
        - **WHERE does the *playgroup* meet?**
        - **WHEN does the *playgroup* take place?**
        - **HOW will I enroll my child?**

2. **Practice meeting and greeting friends.**
   - **Practice having your child *meet and greet friends* this week during preferred and highly motivating activities while providing *social coaching* using the *4 Ps*.**
     - ***Priming:* Review the rules for *meeting and greeting friends* with your child BEFORE PRACTICING.**
     - ***Prompting:* Remind your child IN THE MOMENT to *meet and greet friends* whenever the opportunities present.**
     - ***Praising: Praise* your child for using the buzzwords whenever they *meet and greet friends* CORRECTLY.**
     - ***Providing corrective feedback: Provide corrective feedback* in the form of a *praise sandwich* whenever your child ATTEMPTS to *meet and greet friends*.**
   - **Please send us a 30–60-second video of *social coaching* for *meeting and greeting friends* with your child to be viewed during homework review.**
     - **Please include:**
       - **Skills your child did well.**
       - **Skills you would like to work on with your child.**

3. **Provide social coaching on previously learned skills.**
   - **Continue providing *social coaching* to your child throughout the week using the *4 Ps* for *listening and following directions*.**

4. **Bring a turn-taking game.**
   - **Bring a turn-taking game that your child enjoys playing and can be played with the other children.**
     - **Common games: *Candy Land, Chutes and Ladders, Connect Four, Don't Break the Ice, Pop the Pig, Hi Ho Cherry-O, Operation, Perfection, Memory, Gone Fishin'*.**
     - **Do not bring games that your child:**
       - **Will have difficulty sharing with others.**
       - **May become upset if the game pieces break or get lost.**

Parent Tips for Completing Homework Assignments

- **Suggestions for video recording on smartphones:**
  - **Test your audio and video quality.**
  - **Consider using a tripod.**
  - **Do not hold the camera while filming.**
  - **Consider using landscape mode.**
  - **Consider using the front-facing recording feature on your phone (so your child cannot see themself when filming).**
  - **Include both you and your child in the video.**
- **Suggestions for using *Parent Coached Play Cards:***
  - **This coaching card can be used to provide support while using the *4 Ps* during your *social coaching* during homework assignments.**

- **Consider sharing the *Parent Coached Play Cards* and *Parent Handouts* with your child's other care providers.**

- **Suggestions for using *Parent Homework Worksheets*:**
  - **This worksheet will assist you in self-monitoring your use of the *4 Ps* in your *social coaching* during weekly homework assignments.**
  - **Please remember to complete this worksheet and return it to the treatment staff at the next meeting of PEERS® for Preschoolers.**

Session 2 Continued
Meeting and Greeting Friends

CHILD SESSION THERAPIST GUIDE

Child Session Agenda

- Didactic Lesson: *Meeting and Greeting Friends* (20 minutes).
- Group Behavioral Rehearsal Activity 1: *What Time Is It, Friend?* (15 minutes).
- Break Time (10 minutes).
- Group Behavioral Rehearsal Activity 2: *Red Light, Green Light* (15 minutes).
- Parent Coached Play: *Dyadic Playdates* (20 minutes).
- Final Wrap-Up (10 minutes).

Snapshot of the Lesson: Meeting and Greeting Friends

The objective of this lesson is to teach children how to ***meet and greet friends*** by ***asking and using names*** and ***saying "hi" and "bye."*** Steps for ***meeting and greeting friends*** include:

Asking Names

1. ***Look at your friend with your eyes*** (point to your eyes).
2. ***Smile with your mouth*** (point to your mouth and smile).
3. ***Say, "What's your name?"***
4. ***Say your name, "I'm ____ (Name)."***

Using Names

1. ***Look at your friend with your eyes*** (point to your eyes).
2. ***Smile with your mouth*** (point to your mouth and smile).
3. ***Use names when talking to your friend.***

Saying "Hi"

1. ***Look at your friend with your eyes*** (point to your eyes).
2. ***Smile with your mouth*** (point to your mouth and smile).
3. ***Wave with your hand*** (wave your hand).
4. ***Say "hi" using your friend's name.***

Saying "Bye"

1. ***Look at your friend with your eyes*** (point to your eyes).
2. ***Smile with your mouth*** (point to your mouth and smile).
3. ***Wave with your hand*** (wave your hand).
4. ***Say "bye" using your friend's name.***

Materials Needed

- Lion puppet.
- Elephant puppet.
- Small ball.
- Carpet squares or chairs.
- "Making Friends Helper" badge.
- Star chart with names of children.
- Marker for star chart.
- Name tags for families and treatment team.
- Prize bins with prizes.

Preparing for the Lesson

- Follow the script below with the child group leader using a lion puppet to play the part of "Larry Lion."
- A behavioral coach uses an elephant puppet to play the part of "Ellie Elephant."
- An additional behavioral coach assists in the behavioral rehearsal and provides encouragement and feedback to the group.
- A child is chosen at the beginning of the lesson as the "Making Friends Helper."
    - The "Making Friends Helper" wears a special badge and is the first child to practice the skill.
- The child group leader and behavioral coach sit on the floor at the front of the room.
- A special-colored carpet square (e.g., red) is placed at the front of the room next to the child group leader to be used as the "Good Friend Square."
- For the children, additional carpet squares of the same color (e.g., green) are placed in a semi-circle facing the child group leader and the "Good Friend Square."
- Note: If carpet squares are unavailable, the children and behavioral coaches may sit on chairs.
- The material in *italics* should be read by the indicated person.
- The material in ***bold and italics*** represents buzzwords and should be emphasized when read.
- The material in CAPITAL LETTERS within the script should be given extra emphasis while the group is encouraged to say the words in unison.

Behavioral Coaching Techniques

Behavioral coaches should use the following ***social coaching*** techniques described below throughout the lesson and the behavioral rehearsal activities. (Note: ***priming*** occurs during the introduction to the activity.)

- ***Prompting***:
  - Use the buzzwords to ***prompt*** the children to ***ask and use names*** and ***greet friends*** IN THE MOMENT.
    - Example: *"Remember to look and smile when asking names."*
    - Example: *"Don't forget to use names when you say 'hi'."*
    - Example: *"What should you say if you don't know your friend's name?"*
- ***Praising***:
  - Reinforce ***asking and using names*** and ***greeting friends*** by ***praising*** the children when they use the skills CORRECTLY.
    - Example: *"Great job asking names!"*
    - Example: *"Great job smiling and waving when you said 'bye!'"*
    - Example: *"Good job using names when you gave a turn!"*
- ***Provide corrective feedback using a praise sandwich***:
  - Reinforce ATTEMPTS to ***ask and use names*** and ***greet friends*** by ***praising*** the children and identifying what could be done differently next time.
    - Example: *"Good job using names. Remember to look and smile next time, but nice job!"*
    - Example: *"Nice try asking names. Remember to say, 'What's your name?' next time, but good job!"*
    - Example: *"Good job saying 'bye.' Don't forget to look and wave next time, but great job!"*
- Continue to provide ***social coaching*** on previously learned skills:
  - ***Listening and following directions.***

Didactic Lesson: Meeting and Greeting Friends (20 Minutes)

Have the children sit in a semi-circle on the carpet squares facing the child group leader.

Part I: Meeting Friends

Larry Lion: (Sit at the front of the room and choose a Making Friends Helper.) *"Who wants to be our Making Friends Helper?"*

(Choose from among the children raising their hands and place the "Making Friends Helper" badge on the child. The child stays in their seat for now.)

"Hi friends! I'm Larry Lion. Grrr, Grrr! Today we're going to practice asking and using names and saying 'hi' and 'bye.' Asking and using names and saying 'hi' and 'bye' are great ways to be nice to our friends! Let's first learn about asking names."

"Who should we ask names with? We should ask names with our friends, teachers, and people we want to know better."

"Why should we ask names? We should ask names so our friends know that we're talking to them."

"How should we ask names? We should ask names by looking at our friends with our EYES (point to your eyes and then Larry Lion's eyes), *smiling with our MOUTH* (point to your mouth and smile), *and saying, 'What's your name?' Then we should say our name too."*

"Remember, asking names is a nice way to be a good friend! Grrr, grrr!"

Role Play: Meeting Friends

Ellie Elephant:	(Begin playing with the small ball.)
Larry Lion:	(Turn to look at the group of children.) *"Hey friends! I see someone playing ball. I want to play too but I don't know their name. Hmmm....* (Look confused, scratch your head, and pause.) *Hey friends, I know! Do you think I should ask their name?"* (Nod your head yes and encourage the children to say *"yes."*) *"That's a great idea! Grrr, grrr! Let's do it!* (Turn to look at Ellie Elephant and smile.) *What's your name?"*
Ellie Elephant:	(Turn to look at Larry Lion and smile.) *"Ellie Elephant."*
Larry Lion:	*"I'm Larry Lion.* (Turn to look at the group of children.) *Hey friends, did I do a good job of asking names and saying my name?"* (Nod your head yes and encourage the children to say *"yes."*) *"That's right! Grrr, grrr!"*
Larry Lion and Ellie Elephant:	(Say *"good job," give a "lion high-five" and "elephant high-five,* clap, cheer, and encourage the children to clap as well.)

Part II: Greeting Friends

Larry Lion:	(Turn to look at the group of children.) *"Hey friends, once we know our friends' names, it's also nice to greet our friends by saying 'hi' and 'bye' and using our friends' names."* *"Who should we say 'hi' and 'bye' to? We should say 'hi' and 'bye' with our FRIENDS, TEACHERS, MOMMIES, DADDIES, BROTHERS, AND SISTERS."* *"When should we say 'hi' and 'bye'? We should say 'hi'* (wave your hand) *when we see our friends, and we should say 'bye'* (wave your hand) *when we leave our friends."*

"How should we say 'hi' and 'bye'? We should say 'hi' and 'bye' by looking at our friends with our (point to your eyes to prompt the children to say "*eyes*")*...EYES, smiling with our* (point to your mouth to prompt the children to say "*mouth*")*...MOUTH, and waving with our hand* (wave your hand) *when we say 'hi' and 'bye'. And don't forget to use NAMES."*

"Remember, saying 'hi' and 'bye' are nice ways to be a good friend! Grrr, grrr!"

Role Play: Greeting Friends

Ellie Elephant:	(Begin playing with the small ball.)
Larry Lion:	(Turn to look at the group of children.) *"Hey friends, now that I know Ellie Elephant's name, do you think I should say 'hi?'"* (Nod your head yes and encourage the children to say *"yes."*) *"And do you think I should use Ellie Elephant's name so they know I'm talking to them?"* (Nod your head yes and encourage the children to say *"yes."*) *"That's a great idea! Grrr, grrr! Let's do it!* (Turn to look at Ellie Elephant and smile.) *Hi, Ellie Elephant* (wave at Ellie Elephant)*!"*
Ellie Elephant:	(Turn to look at Larry Lion and smile.) *"Hi, Larry Lion* (wave at Larry Lion)! *Do you want to play?"*
Larry Lion:	*"Okay, Ellie Elephant!"*
Ellie Elephant:	*"Okay, Larry Lion. Catch* (throw the small ball to Larry Lion)*!"*
Ellie Elephant and Larry Lion:	(Play catch for a few turns while making comments, such as *"Great throw!" or "Nice catch!")*
Larry Lion:	(Turn to look at the group of children.) *"Hey friends, did we do a good job of saying 'hi' and using names?"* (Nod your head yes and encourage the children to say *"yes."*) *"That's right! Grrr, grrr!* (Turn to look at Ellie Elephant and smile.) *Let's keep playing, Ellie Elephant!"*
Ellie Elephant:	*"Okay, Larry Lion!"*
Ellie Elephant and Larry Lion:	(Play catch for a few turns while making comments, such as *"Great throw!" or "Nice catch!")*
Behavioral coach:	*"Ellie Elephant, it's time to go home!"*
Larry Lion:	(Turn to look at the group of children.) *"Hey friends, it's time for Ellie*

Elephant to go home. Do you think I should say 'bye' (wave your hand) *to Ellie Elephant?"* (Nod your head yes and encourage the children to say *"yes."*) *"That's right, friends! Grrr, Grrr! Let's do it!* (Turn to look at Ellie Elephant and smile.) *Bye, Ellie Elephant* (wave at Ellie Elephant)!*"*

Ellie Elephant: (Ellie Elephant turns to look at Larry Lion and smiles.) *"Bye, Larry Lion (wave at Larry Lion)*!"

Larry Lion: *"Hey friends, did I do a good job of saying 'bye' and using names with Ellie Elephant?"* (Nod your head yes and encourage the children to say *"yes."*)

"That's right, friends! Grrr, grrr!"

Larry Lion and Ellie Elephant: (Say *"good job," give a "lion high-five" and "elephant high-five,"* clap, cheer, and have the children to clap as well.

Ellie Elephant takes the small ball and sits on the other side of the Good Friend Square (i.e., the Good Friend Square in between Larry Lion and Ellie Elephant). Larry Lion ***social coaches*** the children as needed while they practice ***asking and using names*** and ***greeting friends*** with Ellie Elephant.)

Larry Lion: *"Now let's see _____ (behavioral coach) try! _____ (Behavioral coach), please come sit on the Good Friend Square."*

Behavioral coach: (Sit on the Good Friend Square.)

Larry Lion: *"_____ (Behavioral coach), can you show us how to ask and use names and say 'hi' and 'bye' with Ellie Elephant?"*

Behavioral coach: *"Okay, Larry Lion."*

Larry Lion: (Turn to look at the group of children.) *"Remember to ask and use names and say 'hi' and 'bye' by looking at Ellie Elephant with your* (point to your eyes to prompt children to say "*eyes*")*...EYES, smiling with your* (point to your mouth to prompt the children to say "*mouth*")*...MOUTH, and waving with your* (wave your hand to prompt the children to say "*hand*")*...HAND."*

Ellie Elephant: (Begin to play with the small ball.)

Behavioral coach: (Turn to look at Ellie Elephant and smile.) *"What's your name?"*

Ellie Elephant: (Turn to look at the behavioral coach and smile.) *"Ellie Elephant."*

Behavioral coach: *"I'm ____ (behavioral coach)."*

Ellie Elephant: *"Hi, ____ (behavioral coach)* (wave at the behavioral coach)!*"*

Behavioral coach: *"Hi, Ellie Elephant* (wave at Ellie Elephant)!*"*

Ellie Elephant: *"____ (Behavioral coach), do you want to play* (hold up the small ball)?*"*

Behavioral coach: *"Okay, Ellie Elephant!"*

Ellie Elephant: *"Catch, ____ (behavioral coach)* (throw the small ball to the behavioral coach)*!"*

Ellie Elephant and Behavioral coach: (Play catch for a few turns while making comments, such as

"Great throw!" or "Nice catch!")

Larry Lion: *"Ellie Elephant, it's time to go home!* (Look at the behavioral coach.) *____ (Behavioral coach), it's time for Ellie Elephant to go home. What should you say?"*

Behavioral coach: (Look at Ellie Elephant and smile.) *"Bye, Ellie Elephant* (wave at Ellie Elephant)!*"*

Ellie Elephant: (Look at the behavioral coach and smile.) *"Bye, ____ (behavioral coach)* (wave at the behavioral coach)*!"*

Larry Lion: *"Great job asking and using names and saying 'hi' and 'bye' ____ (behavioral coach)! Grrr, grrr!"*

(Say *"good job," give a "lion high-five" and "elephant high-five,"* clap, cheer, and have the children to clap as well.)

Larry Lion and Behavioral coach: (Leave the Good Friend Square.)

Behavioral Rehearsal: Meeting and Greeting Friends

Larry Lion: (Turn to look at the group of children.) *"Okay friends! Now let's see our Making Friends Helper _____ try! _____ (Making Friends Helper), come sit on the Good Friend Square and show us how to ask and use names and say 'hi' and 'bye' with Ellie Elephant."* (The Making Friends Helper should sit on the Good Friend Square.)

"Remember to ask names by looking at Ellie Elephant with your (point to your eyes to prompt children to say "*eyes*")*...EYES, smiling with your* (point to your mouth to prompt children to say "*mouth*")*...MOUTH, and saying 'What's your name?'"*

"Then remember to say 'hi' and 'bye' by waving with your (wave your hand to prompt the children to say "*hand*")*...HAND. And don't forget to use* (pause briefly to prompt the children to say "*names*")*...NAMES."*

Ellie Elephant: (Begin to play with the small ball.)

Larry Lion: (If needed, ***social coach*** the Making Friends Helper to ***look, smile,*** and ***say "What's your name?"*** *to Ellie* Elephant.)

Ellie Elephant: (Look up at the Making Friends Helper and smile.) *"Ellie Elephant."*

Larry Lion: (If needed, ***social coach*** the Making Friends Helper to ***look*** and ***say "I'm ____ (Making Friends Helper)"*** to Ellie Elephant.)

Ellie Elephant: *"Hi, ____ (Making Friends Helper)* (wave at the Making Friends Helper)!*"*

Larry Lion: (If needed, ***social coach*** the Making Friends Helper to ***look, smile, wave,*** and ***say "Hi, Ellie Elephant!"*** to Ellie Elephant.)

Ellie Elephant: *"____ (Making Friends Helper), do you want to play* (hold up the small ball)?*"*

Larry Lion: (If needed, ***social coach*** the Making Friends Helper to look, smile, and say, *"Okay, Ellie Elephant"* to Ellie Elephant.)

Ellie Elephant: *"Catch, ____ (Making Friends Helper)* (throw the small ball to the Making Friends Helper)!*"*

(Play catch for a few turns while Ellie Elephant makes comments, such as *"Great throw!"* or *"Nice catch!"*)

Larry Lion: *"Ellie Elephant, it's time to go home!* (Look at the Making Friends Helper) *____ (Making Friends Helper), it's time for Ellie Elephant to go home. What should you say?"*

(If needed, ***social coach*** the Making Friends Helper to ***look, smile, wave,*** and ***say "Bye, Ellie Elephant!"*** to Ellie Elephant.)

Ellie Elephant: *"Bye, ____ (Child)* (wave at the Making Friends Helper)!*"*

Larry Lion: *"Great job asking and using names and saying 'hi' and 'bye' ____ (Making Friends Helper)! Grrr, grrr!"*

(Say *"good job," give a "lion high-five" and "elephant high-five,"* clap, cheer, and encourage the children to clap as well.)

(The Making Friends Helper should give the small ball back to Ellie Elephant.)

"Okay, Making Friends Helper, choose another friend to sit on the Good Friend Square." (If needed, ***social coach*** the Making Friends Helper to choose another child before returning to their seat.)

Repeat the following with each child:

Larry Lion: (Have each child take turns sitting on the Good Friend Square and practicing ***asking and using names*** and ***saying "hi" and "bye"*** with Ellie Elephant.)

(Turn to look at the group of children.) *"Okay friends! Now let's see _____ (Child) try! _____ (Child), come sit on the Good Friend Square and show us how to ask and use names and how to say 'hi' and 'bye' with Ellie Elephant."*

(The child should sit on the Good Friend Square.)

"Remember to ask names by looking at Ellie Elephant with your (point to your eyes to prompt children to say "*eyes*")...*EYES, smiling with your* (point to your mouth to prompt children to say "*mouth*")...*MOUTH, and saying 'What's your name?'"*

"And remember to say 'hi' and 'bye' by waving with your (wave your hand to prompt the children to say "*hand*")...*HAND. And don't forget to use* (pause briefly to prompt the children to say "*names*")...*NAMES."*

Ellie Elephant: (Begin to play with the small ball.)

Larry Lion: (If needed, ***social coach*** the child to ***look, smile,*** and ***say "What's your name?"*** to Ellie Elephant.)

Ellie Elephant: (Look up at the child and smile.) *"Ellie Elephant."*

Larry Lion: (If needed, ***social coach*** the child to ***look*** and ***say "I'm ____ (Child)"*** to Ellie Elephant.)

Ellie Elephant: *"Hi, ____ (Child)* (wave at the child)*!"*

Larry Lion: (If needed, ***social coach*** the child to ***look, smile, wave,*** and ***say "Hi, Ellie Elephant!"*** to Ellie Elephant.)

Ellie Elephant: *"____ (Child), do you want to play* (hold up the small ball)*?"*

Larry Lion: (If needed, ***social coach*** the child to look, smile, and say, *"Okay, Ellie Elephant"* to Ellie Elephant.)

Ellie Elephant: *"Catch, ____ (child)* (throw the small ball to the Making Friends Helper)*!"*

Ellie Elephant: (Play catch for a few turns while Ellie Elephant makes comments, such as *"Great throw!"* or *"Nice catch!"*)

Larry Lion: *"Ellie Elephant, it's time to go home!* (Look at the child.) *____ (Child), it's time for Ellie Elephant to go home. What should you say?"*

(If needed, ***social coach*** the child to ***look, smile, wave,*** and ***say "Bye, Ellie Elephant!"*** to Ellie Elephant.)

Ellie Elephant: *"Bye, ____ (child)* (wave at the child)*!"*

Larry Lion: *"Great job asking and using names and saying 'hi' and 'bye' ____ (child)! Grrr, grrr!"*

(Say *"good job," give a "lion high-five" and "elephant high-five,"* clap, cheer, and encourage the children to clap as well.)

(The child should give the small ball back to Ellie Elephant.)

"Okay, ____ (child), choose another friend to sit on the Good Friend Square." (If needed, ***social coach*** the child to choose another child before returning to their seat.)

Didactic Lesson Wrap-Up

Group leader: *"Well friends, you all did a great job asking names by looking at your friend with your* (point to your eyes to prompt children to say "*eyes*")*...EYES, smiling with your* (point to your mouth to prompt children to say "*mouth*")*... MOUTH, and asking 'What's your name?' And great job using names* and *saying 'hi' and 'bye' too!"*

"You each earned ____ (number) stars for listening and following directions! Let's start with _____ (child)."

Award each child the same number of stars by repeating the following with each child:

Group leader: *"Where's _____ (child)?"* (Wait until all the children are looking at the child.)

"_____ (Child), how many stars did you earn?" (Pause briefly to allow the child to respond.)

"That's right! Let's all count for _____ (child)! One, two, three... (add stars to the Star Chart as they are counted aloud)*! Everybody clap for _____ (child)!"* (All behavioral coaches clap and cheer and encourage the children to clap as well.)

Session 2 Continued

What Time Is It, Friend?

BEHAVIORAL REHEARSAL ACTIVITY 1

Materials Needed

- Safety cones or masking tape.

Room Setup

- Remove or place all carpet squares to the side.
- Use the safety cones or masking tape to delineate a *"friend zone"* at one end of the room and a *"safe zone"* at the opposite end of the room.

Rules: What Time Is It, Friend?

- The child group leader reads the script below to explain the rules, which are based on the popular game, *What Time Is It, Mr. Fox?*
- Pick a child to be the first *"friend."*
    - The *friend* should stand next to the child group leader.
- The children and behavioral coaches are standing next to one other while holding hands in the *safe zone*.
- Instruct the children to ***ask*** the *friend* their ***name***.
- The *friend* should respond by ***saying their name***.
- Then instruct the children and the *friend* to practice ***greeting friends*** by ***saying "hi"*** and ***using names***.
- When playing the game, the children should call out in unison "*What time is it _____?*" and practice ***using names***.
- The *friend* should respond by calling out a time (e.g., "It's 2 o'clock" or "It's 4 o'clock").
- The children and behavioral coach should take the specified number of steps forward (e.g., two steps or four steps) while counting aloud.
- After a few repetitions, the *friend* should say, "It's tag time!" and chase the children back to the *safe zone*.
- If the *friend* tags a child, then that child will be the new *friend.*
    - The *friend* cannot tag a child once a child is behind the *safe zone*.
- If the *friend* is unable to tag a child, then ask the *friend* to choose the next *friend*.
- As the new *friend* leaves the *safe zone*, the children should practice ***saying "bye"*** and ***using names***.

- As the old *friend* approaches the *safe zone*, the children should practice ***saying "hi"*** and ***using names***.
- Repeat this cycle until all children have had at least one turn being the *friend*.

Behavioral Rehearsal: What Time Is It, Friend? (15 minutes)

The group leader leads the activity. The behavioral coaches and children sit in the *safe zone* as the group leader explains the rules.

Group leader: *"Hey friends, now we're going to play What Time Is It, Friend? It's like the game called What Time Is It, Mr. Fox? I'll pick the first friend to stand next to me in the friend zone* (point to the *friend zone). Everyone else will stand in the safe zone* (point to the *safe zone) and hold hands. First, you need to ask the friend their name by looking at your friend with your* (point to your eyes to prompt children to say *"eyes")...EYES, smiling with your* (point to your mouth to prompt children to say *"mouth")...MOUTH, and saying 'What's your name?' The friend will then say their name. Then do you think you should greet your friend by saying 'hi' while using their name and waving your hand?"* (Nod your head yes and encourage the children to say *"yes.")*

"That's right, friends! Then all of you in the safe zone (point to the *safe zone*) *will ask the friend, 'What time is it?' using the friend's name. If the friend says, '2 o'clock' then you all take TWO steps forward* (demonstrate taking two steps forward while counting aloud). *If the friend says, '4 o'clock' then you all take FOUR steps forward* (demonstrate taking four steps forward while counting aloud). *If the friend says, 'It's tag time!' then run back to the safe zone* (point to the *safe zone*) *before you're tagged. If you get tagged, then you're the new friend. Each time we choose a new friend, do you think it's a good idea to say 'bye'* (wave your hand) *to our friend?"* (Nod your head yes and encourage the children to say *"yes."*)

"That's right, friends! And remember to say 'hi' and 'bye' by waving with your (wave your hand to prompt the children to say "*hand*")...*HAND. And don't forget to use* (pause briefly to prompt the children to say "*names*")... *NAMES. Okay, let's have _____ (behavioral coaches) try first!"*

Role Play: What Time Is It, Friend?

The child group leader is the first *friend*, with two behavioral coaches helping to demonstrate how to play *What Time Is It, Friend?* The other behavioral coaches and children sit in the *safe zone* watching.

Group leader: *"Okay _____ (behavioral coaches), let's play What Time Is It, Friend? and practice asking and using names and greeting friends. I'll be the first friend. Remember to first ask my name."*

Behavioral coaches: *"What's your name?"*

Group leader: *"I'm _____ (group leader)."*

Behavioral coaches: *"Hi, ____ (group leader)* (wave your hands)*!"*

Group leader: *"Hi, friends* (wave your hand)*! Great job asking and using names and saying 'hi'! Okay _____ (behavioral coaches), now you can ask me 'What time is it, _____ (group leader)?' Remember to use names and follow directions by holding hands when you step forward."*

Behavioral coaches: (Behavioral coaches are holding hands.) *"What time is it, _____ (group leader)?"*

Group leader: *"It's 2 o'clock, friends."*

Behavioral coaches: (Take two steps forward while counting aloud and holding hands.)

"What time is it, _____ (group leader)?"

Group leader: *"It's 4 o'clock, friends."*

Behavioral coaches: (Take four steps forward while counting aloud and holding hands.)

"What time is it, _____ (group leader)?"

Group leader: *"It's tag time!"* (Chase the behavioral coaches back toward the *safe zone*.)

Behavioral coaches: (Run toward the *safe zone* to avoid being tagged.)

Group leader: (Return to the *friend zone* and face the children.) *"Great job using names and following directions! Okay friends, now it's everyone's turn to play. Who wants to be our first friend in the friend zone?"* (Choose a child among those with their hands raised and have them stand in the *friend zone* with the group leader. The behavioral coaches and children stand in the *safe zone* holding hands.)

Behavioral Rehearsal: What Time Is It, Friend?

Group leader: *"Okay everyone, let's practice asking names with our new friend."* (If needed, ***social coach*** the children to ***ask names*** and ***say their name***.)

"Hey friends, can everyone say '*hi*' *to our new friend ____ (child)?"*

Group leader: (If needed, ***social coach*** the children to ***say "hi"*** to one another.)

"Great job asking and using names and saying 'hi'! Are we ready? All together now." (If needed, ***social coach*** the children in the *safe zone* to call out in unison, *"What time is it, ____ (child)?"* and ***social coach*** the *friend* to respond.)

(The behavioral coaches and children should take the specified number of steps forward until the *friend* says, *"It's tag time"* and the behavioral coaches and children run back to the *safe zone*.)

*"Great job using names and listening and following directions! ____ (Child), choose someone else to be the next friend. Remember to look and smile and use names when you pick a new friend!" (If needed, the group leader **social coaches** the child to **look, smile,** and **use names** when choosing the next friend.)*

"____ (Old child) is going to join you in the safe zone and ____ (new child) is going to be our new friend in the friend zone."

*"Everyone say 'hi' to ____ (old child)." (If needed, **social coach** the children to **say "hi" using names** to the friend returning to the safe zone.)*

"Everyone say 'bye' to ____ (new child), our new friend!" (If needed, ***social coach*** the children and the *new friend* to ***say "bye"*** to one another while ***using names*** as the *new friend* joins the *friend zone*.)

"Great job greeting friends! Let's keep on playing. Are we ready? All together now."

(Have each child take turns being the *friend* in the *friend zone* while practicing ***asking and using names and greeting friends*** in the manner described above.)

Behavioral Rehearsal Wrap-Up

Group leader: *"Well friends, great job asking and using names and saying 'hi' and 'bye'! Give yourselves a big round of applause!"* (All behavioral coaches clap and cheer and encourage the children to clap as well.)

"Now everyone sit in the Listening Circle." (Have children return to the Listening Circle to sit on their carpet squares.)

"Okay friends, you all did a great job asking names by looking at your friend with your (point to your eyes to prompt children to say *"eyes"*)*...EYES, smiling with your* (point to your mouth to prompt children to say *"mouth"*)*... MOUTH, and asking 'What's your name?' And great job using names and saying 'hi' and 'bye' too!"*

"You each earned ____ (number) stars for listening and following directions! Let's start with _____ (child)."

Award each child the same number of stars by repeating the following with each child:

Group leader: *"Where's _____ (child)?"* (Wait until all the children are looking at the child.)

"_____ (Child), how many stars did you earn?" (Pause briefly to allow the child to respond.)

"That's right! Let's all count for _____ (child)! One, two, three... (add stars to the Star Chart as they are counted aloud)*! Everybody clap for _____ (child)!"* (All behavioral coaches clap and cheer and encourage the children to clap as well.)

Break Time (10 Minutes)

- The puppets may be used to lead the children to and from the bathroom during break time.
- To assist with transitions and limit unstructured time, behavioral coaches may review the lesson with the children while waiting for the remaining children to return from the bathroom.
- You may want to award stars for good behavior after returning from the bathroom.

Session 2 Continued

Red Light, Green Light

BEHAVIORAL REHEARSAL ACTIVITY 2

Materials Needed

- Safety cones or masking tape.

Room Setup

- Remove or place all carpet squares to the side.
- Place safety cones or masking tape at the front of the room to delineate the *"starting zone."*
- Place safety cones or masking tape at the opposite end of the room to delineate the *"finishing zone."*

Rules: Red Light, Green Light

- The child group leader reads the script below to explain the rules.
- Pick a child to be the first *"stoplight friend."*
  - The *stoplight friend* stands in the *finishing zone* with the child group leader.
- The remaining children and behavioral coaches will be the *"car friends."* They should stand in the *starting zone* while holding hands and facing the *finishing zone*.
- Announce the *stoplight friend* to the group and ***social coach*** the children to ***say "bye" using names***.
- To begin the game, the *stoplight friend* may need ***prompting*** to say, "*Green light.*"
- The *car friends* should take small steps toward the *stoplight friend* while holding hands.
- Every few seconds, the *stoplight friend* should say a different command.
  - *"Green light"* means taking small steps at a normal walking speed.
  - *"Yellow light"* means taking small steps in slow motion.
  - *"Red light"* means stopping and freezing in place.
- Once the *car friends* reach the *finishing zone*, ***social coach*** the *stoplight friend* to practice ***using names*** while choosing the next *stoplight friend.*
- As the current *stoplight friend* approaches the *finishing zone*, the children should practice ***saying "hi"*** and ***using names***.
- As the new *stoplight friend* leaves the *finishing zone*, the children should practice ***saying "bye"*** and ***using names***.
- Repeat this cycle until all children have had at least one turn being the *stoplight friend.*
- Plan to play *Red Light, Green Light* for approximately 15 minutes or until *Parent Coached Play* begins.

Behavioral Rehearsal: "Red Light, Green Light" (15 Minutes)

The group leader leads the activity. The behavioral coaches and children stand in the *starting zone* as the group leader explains the rules.

Group leader: *"Hey friends, now we're going to play a game called Red Light, Green Light. One friend will be the stoplight friend, and everyone else will be the car friends. The car friends will stand in the 'starting zone'* (point to the *starting zone*) *while holding hands, and the stoplight friend will stand in the 'finishing zone'* (point to the *finishing zone*). *The stoplight friend will tell us what to do so we need to listen and follow directions. If the stoplight friend says, 'Green light' then we take small steps forward walking normally like this* (demonstrate taking three small steps forward at a normal speed). *Can everybody show me walking normally?* (Pause briefly to allow the children to demonstrate.)*"*

"Great job listening and following directions! And if our stoplight friend says, 'Yellow light' then we take small steps forward in SLOW motion (demonstrate taking three small steps forward in slow motion). *Can everybody show me walking in SLOW motion?* (Pause briefly to allow the children to demonstrate.)*"*

"That's right, friends! And if our stoplight friend says, 'Red light' then we need to FREEZE (demonstrate freezing in place)*! Can everybody show me freezing?* (Pause briefly to allow the children to demonstrate.)*"*

"Great job listening and following directions! Now everyone go back to the starting zone." (Pause briefly to allow children to return to the *starting zone.*)*"*

"Everybody will get to be the stoplight friend. When we have a new stoplight friend, we'll practice saying 'hi' and 'bye' and using names. Remember to say 'hi' and 'bye' by looking at your friends with your (point to your eyes to prompt children to say "*eyes*")*...EYES, smiling with your* (point to your mouth and smile to prompt children to say "*mouth*")*...MOUTH, and waving with your HAND* (wave your hand). *And don't forget to use* (pause briefly to prompt the children to say "*names*")*...NAMES. Okay, let's have _____ (behavioral coach) try first!"*

Role Play: Red Light, Green Light

The group leader leads the role play. One behavioral coach is the first *stoplight friend*, while another behavioral coach is the *car friend.* The two behavioral coaches will demonstrate how to play *Red Light, Green Light*. The remaining behavioral coaches and children should be sitting in the *starting zone*.

Group leader:	*"Okay friends, _____ (behavioral coach 1) is our first stoplight friend and _____ (behavioral coach 2) is our first car friend. _____ (behavioral coach 1), come stand next to me in the finishing zone. As you leave the starting zone, let's practice saying 'bye' while using names."*
Behavioral coach 1:	*"Bye, ____ (behavioral coach 2)!"* (Wave to the behavioral coach 2 while leaving the *starting zone*. Walk to the *finishing zone* and stand next to the group leader.)
Behavioral coach 2:	*"Bye, ____ (behavioral coach 1)!"* (Wave to behavioral coach 1.)
Group leader:	*"Great job saying 'bye' and using names! Let's begin."*
Behavioral coach 1:	*"Green light!"*
Behavioral coach 2:	(Take a few steps forward at normal walking speed.)
Behavioral coach 1:	*"Red light!"*
Behavioral coach 2:	(Freeze in place.)
Group leader:	*"Great job listening and following directions, ____ (behavioral coach 2)! Let's keep playing."*
Behavioral coach 1:	*"Yellow light!"*
Behavioral coach 2:	(Take a few steps forward at a SLOW pace.)
Behavioral coach 1:	*"Red light!"*
Behavioral coach 2:	(Freeze in place.)
Group leader:	*"Great job listening and following directions, ____ (behavioral coach 2)!" Let's keep playing.*
Behavioral coach 1:	*"Green light!"*
Behavioral coach 2:	(Take steps forward at normal walking speed until you reach the *finishing zone*.)
Group leader:	*"You made it to the finishing zone! Great job, ____ (behavioral coaches 1 and 2)! Okay friends, now it's everybody's turn to play Red Light, Green Light! Are we ready?"* (Pause briefly to allow the children to say "*yes*.")

Behavioral Rehearsal: "Red Light, Green Light"

Have the behavioral coaches and children stand in the *starting zone* while holding hands. The group leader and behavioral coach 1 (former *stoplight friend*) will stand in the *finishing zone* and select the next *stoplight friend.*

Group leader: *"Who wants to be our next stoplight friend?"* (Choose a child among those with their hands raised and have them stand in the *finishing zone* with the group leader.)

"____ (Child), come stand next to me in the finishing zone. Let's all practice saying 'bye' using names to the new stoplight friend ____ (child) and saying 'hi' using names to the old stoplight friend ____ (behavioral coach 1)." (If needed, ***social coach*** the children to ***say "bye" using names*** as the new *stoplight friend* leaves the *starting zone* and to ***say "hi" using names*** as the old *stoplight friend* approaches the *starting zone.*)

"Car friends, let's remember to ***listen and follow directions*** *when we're playing Red Light, Green Light. Are we ready?"* (If needed, ***social coach*** the *stoplight friend* to give stoplight commands and children to ***listen and follow directions.*** Play until the *car friends* reach the *finishing zone.*)

"Okay ____ (child), choose the next stoplight friend. Remember to look and smile and use names when you pick a new stoplight friend!" (If needed, ***social coach*** the child to ***use names*** when choosing the next *stoplight friend.*)

(Repeat the sequence above until each child has at least one turn at being the *stoplight friend.*)

Behavioral Rehearsal Wrap-Up

Group leader: *"Well friends, great job greeting your friends by using names and saying 'hi' and 'bye!' Give yourselves a big round of applause!"* (All behavioral coaches clap and cheer and encourage the children to clap as well.)

"Now everyone sit in the Listening Circle." (Have children return to the Listening Circle to sit on their carpet squares.)

"Okay friends, you all did a great job greeting your friends by looking at your friend with your (point to your eyes to prompt children to say "*eyes*")... *EYES, smiling with your* (point to your mouth to prompt children to say "*mouth*")*...MOUTH, and saying 'hi' and 'bye' while using names!"*

"You each earned ____ (number) stars for greeting your friends and listening and following directions! Let's start with _____ (child)."

Award each child the same number of stars by repeating the following with each child:

Group leader: *"Where's _____ (child)?"* (Wait until all the children are looking at the child.)

"_____ (Child), how many stars did you earn?" (Pause briefly to allow the child to respond.)

"That's right! Let's all count for _____ (child)! One, two, three… (add stars to the Star Chart as they are counted aloud)! *Everybody clap for _____ (child)!"* (All behavioral coaches clap and cheer and encourage the children to clap as well.)

"Now we're going to play some games with our parents and practice listening and following directions, asking and using names, and greeting friends!"

Session 2 Continued
Meeting and Greeting Friends

PARENT COACHED PLAY: DYADIC PLAYDATES

Materials Needed

- Games brought by children and parents from home.
- Turn-taking games provided by the treatment team:
  - Common games: *Candy Land, Chutes and Ladders, Connect Four, Don't Break the Ice, Pop the Pig, Hi Ho Cherry-O, Operation, Perfection, Memory, Gone Fishin'.*
- Tables and chairs or carpet squares.
- *Parent Coached Play Cards.*

Room Setup

- If available, organize tables in separate corners of the room with four to six chairs per table.
- If tables are unavailable, place two carpet squares in separate corners of the room to indicate where the children will sit.
- The group leader sits on the floor at the front of the room.
- The families sit on the floor in a semi-circle facing the group leader.

Rules for Dyadic Playdates

- The child group leader divides the families into groups of two families each.
  - If there are an odd number of children, pair one child with a behavioral coach who will serve as a ***playmate***. In this case, you will need an additional coach to serve as a behavioral coach for the parent.
  - To avoid social exclusion, avoid having children play in triads as much as possible.
- Assign each group to sit at a table or specific play area.
  - Children should sit next to each other.
  - Parents will act as ***social coaches*** by sitting on the other side of their child to minimize interrupting the natural flow of play between the children.
  - One behavioral coach will be assigned to each dyad to provide ***social coaching*** suggestions and feedback to parents.
- Children will take turns playing the games brought from home or games provided by the treatment team.
- Each child will have ten minutes to play their chosen game with their ***playmate*** and will then switch games.

- Parents will choose which child's game will be played first.
- To minimize unstructured periods, parents will help the children set up the game in a cooperative fashion (handing game pieces to each other, offering suggestions, etc.).
- As they play, parents will ***social coach*** the children on previously learned and newly learned skills using the guidelines highlighted on the *Parent Coached Play Cards.*
- Behavioral coaches will provide support to parents in their ***social coaching*** using the ***4 Ps*** (***priming, prompting, praising,*** and ***providing corrective feedback***) and will model appropriate ***social coaching*** behavior when necessary.
- After approximately nine minutes of play, instruct the parents to prepare the children for the upcoming game swap.
- After approximately one additional minute of play (ten minutes total), instruct the parents to have the children clean up and swap games.
- Repeat the cycle with the second game for the remaining ten minutes before returning to the *Listening Circle.*

Behavioral Coaching: Dyadic Playdates

Behavioral coaches will ***social coach*** parents during dyadic ***playdates*** in the following ways:

- ***Priming*:**
  - Begin the play interactions with parents going over the rules for ***meeting and greeting friends*** BEFORE GAME PLAYING.
    - Example: "*Remember that before you play your games, we want you to practice asking your friend their name by looking at your friend with your* (point to your eyes to prompt children to say "*eyes*")...*EYES, smiling with your* (point to your mouth to prompt children to say "*mouth*")...*MOUTH, and saying 'What's your name?' When your friend tells you their name, you should say your name. Then do you think you should greet friends by saying 'hi' while using their name and waving* (wave your hand) *to each other?"*
- ***Prompting*:**
  - Remind parents to use the buzzwords to ***prompt*** their child to ***ask and use names*** and ***greet their friends*** IN THE MOMENT.
  - Help parents to identify opportunities to proactively ***prompt*** their child to ***ask and use names*** and ***greet their friends***.
    - Example: *"Let's use names when playing with our friends."*
    - Example: *"Remember to say 'hi' before we start playing."*
    - Example: *"Should you use names when you ask your friend to play?"*
  - Assist parents to follow through with the ***prompts*** they present to their child.
- ***Praising*:**
  - Remind parents to ***praise*** and reinforce their child whenever their child ***asks and uses names*** and ***greets friends*** CORRECTLY.
    - Example: *"Great job saying 'bye' and waving to your friend!"*
    - Example: *"Great job using names when you gave a turn!"*
    - Example: *"Great job asking names!"*
- ***Provide corrective feedback using a praise sandwich*:**
  - Remind parents to ***praise*** their child's ATTEMPTS to ***ask and use names*** and ***greet friends*** and identify what could be done differently next time.

    - Example: *"Good job using names. Remember to look at your friend next time, but nice job!"*
    - Example: *"Nice job saying 'hi.' Don't forget to use names next time, but good job!"*
    - Example: *"Nice try asking names. Remember to say 'What's your name?' next time, but good try!"*
- Remind parents to continue to ***social coach*** on previously learned skills:
    - ***Listening and following directions.***

Parent Coached Play: Dyadic Playdates (20 Minutes)

- Have each child choose a turn-taking game brought from home or provided by the treatment team.
- The child group leader sits on the floor at the front of the room.
- The families sit on the floor in a semi-circle facing the child group leader.

Group leader: *"Hey friends, we're going to have playdates and play with the fun games you brought today. We want you to practice using names while you play with your friend. If you forget your friend's name, you can ask names by looking at your friend with your (point to your eyes to prompt children to say "eyes")...EYES, smiling with your (point to your mouth to prompt children to say "mouth")...MOUTH, and asking 'What's your name?' Then you can say your name too. And friends, remember to say 'hi' (wave your hand) before you start playing and say 'bye' (wave your hand) when you finish playing. And don't forget to use (pause briefly to prompt the children to say "names")...NAMES. Parents, remember to social coach your children by using your Parent Coached Play Cards. Okay, let's play with our games!"*

- Before playing, parents will ***social coach*** their child to say, ***"What's your name?"*** and then ***say their name*** if their ***playmate's*** name is unknown. Parents will also ***social coach*** their child to ***say "hi"*** to one another ***using names***.
- Parents will ***social coach*** their children to ***use names*** throughout the game playing.
- After approximately nine minutes of play, instruct the parents to prepare the children for the upcoming game swap by saying, *"Parents, tell your children that we'll be swapping games in one minute."*
- After approximately one additional minute of play (ten minutes total), instruct the parents to swap games by saying, *"Parents, it's time to swap games. Social coach the children to practice listening and following directions when playing the next game."*
- After approximately nine minutes of playing the second game, instruct the parents to prepare the children for clean up by saying, *"Parents, tell your children that we'll be cleaning up in one minute."*
- After approximately one additional minute of play (ten minutes total), ***prompt*** the parents to instruct their children to clean up by saying, *"Parents, it's time to clean up. Let's social coach the children to listen and follow directions by cleaning up and then say 'bye' to their friend using names before sitting in the Listening Circle."*

- If needed, parents will ***social coach*** their child to ***listen and follow directions*** to clean up.
- Then parents will ***social coach*** their child to ***say "bye"*** to their friend ***using nam***es.

Final Wrap-Up (10 Minutes)

- The child group leader sits on the floor at the front of the room.
- The children sit on the carpet squares in a semi-circle facing the child group leader, with parents sitting behind their children.

Group leader: *"Okay friends, you all did a great job playing your games and asking and using names and saying 'hi' and 'bye.' When we're asking and using names, do you think we should LOOK with our EYES and SMILE with our MOUTH?"* (Pause briefly to allow the children to say *"yes.")*

"That's right, friends! And when we're asking names, do you think we should say 'What's your name?' and then say our names too?" (Pause briefly to allow the children to say "*yes*.")

"That's right, friends! And when we're saying 'hi' and 'bye,' do you think we should wave our hand to our friend (wave your hand)*?"* (Pause briefly to allow the children to say "*yes*.")

"That's right, friends! You all did such a great job asking and using names and greeting friends today that you each earned ____ (number) more stars! Let's start with ____ (child)."

Award each child the same number of stars by repeating the following with each child:

Group leader: *"Where's _____ (child)?" (Wait until all the children are looking at the child.)*

"_____ (Child), how many stars did you earn?" (Pause briefly to allow the child to respond.)

"That's right! Let's all count for _____ (child)! One, two, three... (add stars to the Star Chart as they are counted aloud)*! Everybody clap for _____ (child)!"* (All behavioral coaches clap and cheer and encourage the children to clap as well.) *"And remember you all earned those stars by asking and using names and greeting friends! Everyone did a great job and parents you did an excellent job social coaching! Parents, remember your homework assignments this week are to continue practicing asking and using names, greeting friends, and listening and following directions with your children using the 4 Ps. And don't forget to investigate and begin to enroll your children in playgroups and to bring a turn-taking game next week."*

"Alright little friends, do you want to count our stars?" (Pause briefly to allow the children to respond "*yes*.")

Group leader: *"Let's all count together and see how many stars we earned today! One, two, three... (count the number of stars for one child)!"*

"You each earned ____ (total number) stars today! Round of applause for our friends!" (All behavioral coaches should clap and cheer and encourage the families to clap as well.)

"Great job, friends! Don't forget to choose your reward before you leave.

See you all next week!"

Session 2 Continued

Finding Playgroups and Meeting and Greeting Friends

PEERS® FOR PRESCHOOLERS: PARENT HANDOUT

Table 2.1 Common Playgroups for Young Children

Sports camps	Theater arts camp	Science camps
Soccer league	Drama classes	Space camps
T-ball/baseball	Art camps	Nature camps
Softball	Painting classes	Gardening classes
Little League	Finger painting groups	Chorus
AYSO	Drawing/coloring groups	Music classes
Swimming classes	Pottery classes	Band
Martial arts	Arts and crafts groups	Orchestra
Karate	Color Me Mine	Glee club
Flag football	Dance classes	Choir
Basketball	Ballet classes	School of Rock
Tennis	Tap classes	YMCA classes
My Gym	Hip hop dance classes	Library clubs
Gymnastics	Cooking classes	Book clubs
Gymboree	Baking classes	Story time
Mommy and Me classes	Lego groups	Cub scouts/boy scouts
Trampoline gyms	Pokémon groups	Brownies/girl scouts
Jungle gyms	Magic groups	4H
Indoor rock climbing	Board games groups	Sunday school
Yoga classes	Card games groups	Hebrew school
Meditation classes	Language classes	Religious groups

Table 2.2 Common Sources of Information about Playgroups

School	Other parents/friends	Local libraries
Daycare	Teachers/daycare	Recreation centers
Preschool	Family members	Community parks
Afterschool programs	Therapists	YMCA
Head Start	Coworkers	Community centers
Sunday school	Google search	Cub scouts/boy scouts
Hebrew school	Parent listservs	Brownies/girl scouts
Jewish Community Center	Community parent groups	4H
Religious centers	Parenting blogs	Natural history museums
Local church/mosque	Parenting magazines	Art museums
Local temple/synagogue	Meetup.com	Science museums
My Gym	Parenting message boards	Summer camps
Fitness centers	Volunteer groups	Art classes
Mommy and Me groups	Carpools	Music classes
Gymboree groups	Sports groups	Science classes

Selecting Playgroups: Consider the 5 Ws

- **WHO:**
  - Who are the other children and parents?
  - Are the children around the same age and level of support needs?
  - Will the other group members be accepting and inclusive?
- **WHAT:**
  - What is the activity?
  - Are the activities of the ***playgroup*** based on my child's interest?
  - Will my child be able to participate in the activities meaningfully?
- **WHERE:**
  - Where is the ***playgroup***?
  - Is the location relatively close to our home or school?
  - Do the other families live in close proximity in order to facilitate ***playdates***?
- **WHEN:**
  - When do the ***playgroups*** meet?
  - How soon does the next ***playgroup*** start?
  - Will we be able to consistently attend the ***playgroups***?
- **HOW:**
  - How does my child enroll?
  - How will we get to the ***playgroups***?
  - How will we pay for the ***playgroups*** if there is a cost?

Snapshot of the Lesson: Meeting and Greeting Friends

The objective of this lesson is to teach children how to ***meet and greet friends*** by ***asking and using names*** and ***saying "hi" and "bye."***

Asking Names

1. ***Look at your friend with your eyes*** (point to your eyes).
2. ***Smile with your mouth*** (point to your mouth and smile).
3. ***Say, "What's your name?"***
4. ***Say your name, "I'm ____ (Name)."***

Using Names

1. ***Look at your friend with your eyes*** (point to your eyes).
2. ***Smile with your mouth*** (point to your mouth and smile).
3. ***Use names when talking to your friend.***

Saying "Hi"

1. ***Look at your friend with your eyes*** (point to your eyes).
2. ***Smile with your mouth*** (point to your mouth and smile).

3. ***Wave with your hand*** (wave your hand).
4. ***Say "hi" using your friend's name.***

Saying "Bye"

1. ***Look at your friend with your eyes*** (point to your eyes).
2. ***Smile with your mouth*** (point to your mouth and smile).
3. ***Wave with your hand*** (wave your hand).
4. ***Say "bye" using your friend's name.***

Homework Assignments

1. **Find a playgroup for your child.**
   - Investigate and begin to enroll your child in a ***playgroup*** based on their interests.
   - Consider the ***5 Ws*:**
     - **WHO** will be there?
     - **WHAT** is the activity?
     - **WHERE** does the ***playgroup*** meet?
     - **WHEN** does the ***playgroup*** take place?
     - **HOW** will I enroll my child?

2. **Practice meeting and greeting friends.**
   - **Practice having your child *meet and greet friends* this week during preferred and highly motivating activities while providing *social coaching* using the *4 Ps*.**
     - ***Priming:*** Review the rules for ***meeting and greeting friends*** with your child BEFORE PRACTICING.
     - ***Prompting:*** Remind your child IN THE MOMENT to ***ask and use names*** and ***say "hi" and "bye"*** whenever the opportunities present.
     - ***Praising: Praise*** your child for using the buzzwords whenever they ***meet and greet friends*** CORRECTLY.
     - ***Providing corrective feedback: Provide corrective feedback*** in the form of a ***praise sandwich*** whenever your child ATTEMPTS to ***meet and greet friends***.
   - **Please send us a 30–60-second video of *social coaching* for *meeting and greeting friends* with your child to be viewed during homework review.**
     - Please include:
       - Skills your child did well.
       - Skills you would like to work on with your child.

3. **Provide social coaching on previously learned skills.**
   - Continue providing ***social coaching*** to your child throughout the week using the ***4 Ps*** for ***listening and following directions***.

4. **Bring a turn-taking game**.
   - Bring a turn-taking game that your child enjoys playing and can be played with the other children.
     - Common games: *Candy Land, Chutes and Ladders, Connect Four, Don't Break the Ice, Pop the Pig, Hi Ho Cherry-O, Operation, Perfection, Memory, Gone Fishin'.*
     - Do not bring games that your child:
       - Will have difficulty sharing with others.
       - May become upset if the game pieces break or get lost.

Parent Tips for Completing Homework Assignments

- **Suggestions for video recordings on smartphones:**
  - Test your audio and video quality.
  - Consider using a tripod.
  - Do not hold the camera while filming.
  - Consider using landscape mode.
  - Consider using the front-facing recording feature on your phone (so your child cannot see themself when filming).
  - Include both you and your child in the video.
- **Suggestions for using *Parent Coached Play Cards:***
  - This coaching card can be used to provide support while using the *4 Ps* during your ***social coaching*** during homework assignments.
  - Consider sharing the *Parent Coached Play Cards* and *Parent Handouts* with your child's other care providers.
- **Suggestions for using *Parent Homework Worksheets:***
  - This worksheet will assist you in self-monitoring your use of the *4 Ps* in your ***social coaching*** during weekly homework assignments.
  - Please remember to complete this worksheet and return it to the treatment staff at the next meeting of PEERS® for Preschoolers.

Session 2 Continued

Finding Playgroups and Meeting and Greeting Friends

PEERS® FOR PRESCHOOLERS: PARENT COACHED PLAY CARD

Snapshot of the Lesson: Meeting and Greeting Friends

Asking Names

1. ***Look at your friend with your eyes*** (point to your eyes).
2. ***Smile with your mouth*** (point to your mouth and smile).
3. ***Say, "What's your name?"***
4. ***Say your name, "I'm ____ (Name)."***

Using Names

1. ***Look at your friend with your eyes*** (point to your eyes).
2. ***Smile with your mouth*** (point to your mouth and smile).
3. ***Use names when talking to your friend.***

Saying "Hi"

1. ***Look at your friend with your eyes*** (point to your eyes).
2. ***Smile with your mouth*** (point to your mouth and smile).
3. ***Wave with your hand*** (wave your hand).
4. ***Say "hi" using your friend's name.***

Saying "Bye"

1. ***Look at your friend with your eyes*** (point to your eyes).
2. ***Smile with your mouth*** (point to your mouth and smile).
3. ***Wave with your hand*** (wave your hand).
4. ***Say "bye" using your friend's name.***

Priming BEFORE Game Playing

- Example: *"Remember that before you play your games, we want you to practice asking names by looking at your friend with your* (point to your eyes to prompt child to say "*eyes*")*...EYES, smiling with your* (point to your mouth to prompt child to say "*mouth*")*...MOUTH, and saying 'What's your name?' then tell them your name by saying, 'I'm ______ (name).'"*

Prompting IN THE MOMENT

- Example: *"Remember to look and smile when asking names."*
- Example: *"Don't forget to use names when you say 'hi.'"*
- Example: *"What should you say if you don't know your friend's name?"*

Praising for CORRECT Use of Skills

- Example: *"Great job asking names!"*
- Example: *"Great job smiling and waving when you said 'bye!'"*
- Example: *"Good job using names when you gave a turn!"*

Providing Corrective Feedback for ATTEMPTS Using a Praise Sandwich

- Example: *"Good job using names. Remember to look and smile next time, but nice job!"*
- Example: *"Nice try asking names. Remember to say, 'What's your name?' next time, but good try!"*
- Example: *"Good job saying 'bye.' Don't forget to look and wave next time, but great job!"*

- Continue to provide ***social coaching*** on previously learned skills:
  - ***Listening and following directions.***

Finding Playgroups and Meeting and Greeting Friends

PEERS® FOR PRESCHOOLERS: PARENT HOMEWORK WORKSHEET

Child's Name:	*Parent's Name:*		*Date:*	
HOMEWORK ASSIGNMENTS	PRIMING (REVIEWING RULES BEFORE PRACTICE)	PROMPTING (IN THE MOMENT)	PRAISING (USING BUZZWORDS)	PROVIDING CORRECTIVE FEEDBACK (USING A PRAISE SANDWICH)
Meeting and greeting friends				
Listen and follow directions				
Playgroups	Which playgroups did you investigate and enroll in?			
Bring a turn-taking game	Did you bring a turn-taking game? YES or NO (Circle)		Which game did you bring?	

Please fill out this worksheet by describing what you did to complete the homework assignments. Worksheets will be collected during Homework Review at the next session of PEERS® for Preschoolers.

Session 3

Choosing Playgroups and Sharing and Giving a Turn

PARENT SESSION THERAPIST GUIDE

Parent Session Agenda

- Homework Review (40 minutes).
- Didactic Lessons (20 minutes).
- Parent Coached Play (20 minutes).
- Final Wrap-Up (10 minutes).

Materials Needed

- Conference room with a large table and enough chairs for the parent group leader and all parents to sit comfortably around the table.
  - Avoid sitting in a circle without a table as this creates the atmosphere of group therapy.
- Name tags for parents and treatment team.
- *Parent Handouts* (for the current week and the previous weeks).
- *Parent Homework Worksheets* (for the current week and the previous weeks).
- *Parent Coached Play Cards* (for the current week and the previous weeks).
- *Attendance and Homework Compliance Sheets* for parent group leader.
- Pens for note taking (consider having extra pens for parents who need them).

Homework Review (40 Minutes)

1. **Find a playgroup for your child.**
   - Confirm parents investigated and began to enroll their child in a ***playgroup.***
     - If the child is currently enrolled in appropriate ***playgroups*** with potential ***playmates***, they do not need to enroll in new ***playgroups***.
     - Confirm parents considered the ***5 Ws***
       - **WHO** will be there?
       - **WHAT** is the activity?
       - **WHERE** does the ***playgroup*** meet?
       - **WHEN** does the ***playgroup*** take place?
       - **HOW** will I enroll my child?

DOI: 10.4324/9781003502968-4

2. **Practice meeting and greeting friends.**
   - Review the 30–60-second video of ***social coaching*** for ***meeting and greeting friends*** for each family. (For larger groups, you may need to review video recordings in two smaller groups with two different parent group leaders.)
     - Have parents identify:
       - Skills their child did well.
       - Skills they would like to work on with their child.
     - Provide ***social coaching*** tips as appropriate for each family.
   - If parents did not send a video of ***social coaching***, confirm the following:
     - Parents practiced having their child ***meet and greet friends*** during preferred and highly motivating activities while providing ***social coaching*** using the ***4 Ps***.
       - ***Priming*:** Reviewed the rules for ***meeting and greeting friends*** with their child BEFORE PRACTICING.
       - ***Prompting*:** Reminded their child IN THE MOMENT to ***meet and greet friends*** whenever the opportunity presented.
       - ***Praising*: *Praised*** their child for using the buzzwords whenever they ***met and greeted friends*** CORRECTLY.
       - ***Providing corrective feedback*: *Provided corrective feedback*** in the form of a ***praise sandwich*** whenever their child ATTEMPTED to ***meet and greet friends***.

3. **Provide social coaching on previously learned skills.**
   - Confirm parents continued to provide ***social coaching*** to their child throughout the week using the ***4 Ps*** for ***listening and following directions.***

4. **Bring a turn-taking game.**
   - Confirm parents brought a turn-taking game that their child enjoys playing and can be played with the other children. (To avoid distractions, these games should be left with the parents until *Parent Coached Play*.)
     - Common games: *Candy Land, Chutes and Ladders, Connect Four, Don't Break the Ice, Pop the Pig, Hi Ho Cherry-O, Operation, Perfection, Memory, Gone Fishin'.*

Didactic Lessons (20 Minutes)

PEERS® Neuroaffirming Pledge:

- We value neurodiversity, acceptance, and authenticity.
- We honor the diverse ways people experience the world.
- We respect each person's unique perspectives and communication styles.
- We recognize there is no one right way to connect with others.
- If using the strategies taught in PEERS® feels like camouflaging or masking and/or they don't align with your goals or the goals of your family, then you do not have to use them.
- Learning and using the skills taught in PEERS® is a PERSONAL CHOICE.

Didactic Lesson: Choosing Playgroups

- Distribute *Parent Handouts*.
  - Sections in **bold print** come directly from the *Parent Handout*.
  - Terms that are ***bold and italicized*** are buzzwords and represent important concepts from the didactic lesson.
- Explain, *"Last week we discussed how to find playgroups and considered how to select playgroups based on the 5 Ws. Finding the right playgroup is important as it will serve as a source of potential playmates with whom to potentially have playdates. Just as adolescents and adults often find their friends through involvement in extracurricular activities and social activities, so do younger children. Because friendships are based on common interests, it will be critical that playgroups be based on your child's interests. Today we're going to talk about the criteria for a good playgroup and how to assess whether a playgroup is appropriate for your child."*

Criteria for Good Playgroups

- Explain, *"When considering the 5 Ws and deciding which playgroups to enroll your child in, there are several additional factors to keep in mind. While it is unlikely that you will find the perfect playgroup that fulfills all your child's interests and needs, it is still helpful to consider the criteria for good playgroups and then be willing to be flexible if needed. Here are some of the criteria for a good playgroup."*

- **Meets regularly (preferably weekly).**
- **Located close to your home.**
  - **It will be difficult to arrange regularly occurring *playdates* with other families if the *playgroup* is far from your home.**
- **Includes other children in the same age range and level of support needs as your child.**
- **Includes informal time so that your child will have opportunities to interact and play with other children naturally.**
- **Activities are based on your child's interests, likes, or hobbies.**
  - **Avoid activities your child dislikes, may be difficult for them, or may trigger their sensitivities.**
- **Begins within the next few weeks.**
- **Permits some parent involvement in order to facilitate peer interactions and organize *playdates* with other families.**
  - **At a minimum, this may include drop-off and pickup times.**

Assessing Appropriateness of Playgroups

- Explain, *"While some of these considerations may be fairly simple to determine, others may require more investigation. For example, assessing the age and level of support needs of the other children may require some direct observation. Even if the children appear to be at the same developmental stage as your child, this is not a guarantee that these peers or their parents will be a good fit for your child or for you. Additionally, even though the focus of the playgroup activity may seem like an interest to your child, there are no guarantees that your child will find the playgroup fun and engaging. Consider the following recommendations when assessing the appropriateness of a playgroup for your child."*

- **Observe the group composition.**
  - **Ask yourself if this is a good *playgroup* for your child based on these factors:**
    - **Common interests of group members.**
    - **Language or communication abilities.**
    - **Age range and support needs.**
    - **Gender distribution of the group (if relevant).**
    - **Developmental level of the group.**
    - **Social functioning and expectations of the group.**
    - **Physical activity level.**

- **Notice your child's reaction to the group.**
  - **Notice which *playgroup* activities your child enjoys.**
  - **Notice if there are aspects of the *playgroup* your child dislikes.**
  - **Observe whether your child becomes more or less comfortable over time and exposure.**
  - **Consider asking your child what they thought of the group.**

- **Identify potential *playmates*.**
  - **Observe which children your child plays with or appears to be interested in getting to know.**
  - **Notice which children may be a good fit and potential *playmate* for your child.**
  - **Observe which children appear to show a positive interest in your child.**
  - **Notice which activities, games, or toys your child and their potential *playmate(s)* enjoy playing.**
    - **These activities, games, or toys may be incorporated into future *playdates*.**

- **Identify preferred social activities.**
  - **Take note of which activities, games, or toys your child enjoys.**
    - **These preferred social activities might be used as an enticement to return to the group.**
    - **These activities, games, or toys may be incorporated into future *playdates* with related or unrelated *playmates*.**
  - **Notice which activities your child dislikes and consider whether some accommodation can or should be made to make the activities less aversive.**

- **Observe the *playgroup* facilitators.**
  - **Notice how attuned the *playgroup* facilitators are to your child.**
  - **Consider whether your child will receive adequate support during the *playgroup* activities.**
  - **Observe the appropriateness of parent participation or involvement in the activities.**

- **Engage with other parents.**
  - **Engage in light social chit-chat with other parents.**
    - **Make a point to chat with the parents of the *potential playmates* you have identified for your child.**
    - **Use the *playgroup* as a reason for talking to other parents (e.g., "*So how long have you and your child been coming here?*")**

    - **Assess your interest in and compatibility with the other parents.**
    - **The goal is to build a foundation for potential *playdates* so you will need to earn the other parents' trust.**
    - **Talking with other parents is also a great way to gather information about other *playgroups* and social activities.**
    - **You may want to hold off on suggesting a *playdate* until you have had a few interactions with the other parent(s) and the potential *playmate(s)*.**
        - We will teach you how to ask for a ***playdate*** in a future lesson.

- Explain, *"So these are some of the strategies that you might consider using to assess the appropriateness of a playgroup for your child. Many of these considerations will require direct observation of the playgroup, which may not be possible in some cases. Remember that although the criteria mentioned make up the gold standard for playgroups, you may have to be flexible in choosing the group that works best for your family."*

Didactic Lesson: Sharing and Giving a Turn

Explain, *"This week the children are learning how to share and give a turn when playing with their friends. This is an important skill to help your children sustain positive play interactions with their friends and to increase reciprocity in their play. Next week's child lesson will focus on how to ask for a turn."*

Snapshot of the Lesson: Sharing and Giving a Turn

The objective of this lesson is to teach children how to *share and give a turn* when playing with friends and potential *playmates*.

1. ***Look at your friends with your eyes*** **(point to your eyes).**
2. ***Smile with your mouth*** **(point to your mouth and smile).**
3. ***Say "here" using names*** **when you *share and give a turn*.**

Parent Coached Play

- Distribute the *Parent Coached Play Cards*.
- Review the examples of the ***4 Ps*** provided on the *Parent Coached Play Card*.
- Remind parents that in a few moments, we will be joining the children for *Parent Coached Play* in the context of mock dyadic ***playdates***.
- Parents should keep the *Parent Coached Play Card* in front of them during the dyadic ***playdate*** for recommendations on how to ***social coach*** children on ***sharing and giving a turn***.

Homework Assignments

(Briefly review the homework assignments and troubleshoot any potential problems with parents.)

1. **Find a playgroup for your child.**
   - **Investigate and begin to enroll your child in a *playgroup* using the criteria for a good *playgroup*:**
     - **Meets regularly (preferably weekly).**
     - **Located close to your home.**
     - **Includes other children in the same age range and level of support needs as your child.**
     - **Includes informal time so that your child will have opportunities to interact and play with other children naturally.**
     - **Activities are based on your child's interests, likes, or hobbies.**
     - **Begins within the next few weeks.**
     - **Permits some parent involvement in order to facilitate peer interactions and organize *playdates* with other families.**

2. **Practice sharing and giving a turn.**
   - **Practice having your child *share and give turns* this week during preferred and highly motivating activities while providing *social coaching* using the *4 Ps*.**
     - ***Priming*: Review the rules for *sharing and giving turns* with your child BEFORE PRACTICING.**
     - ***Prompting*: Remind your child IN THE MOMENT to *share and give turns* whenever the opportunities present.**
     - ***Praising*: *Praise* your child for using the buzzwords whenever they *share and give turns* CORRECTLY.**
     - ***Providing corrective feedback*: *Provide corrective feedback* in the form of a *praise sandwich* whenever your child ATTEMPTS to *share and give turns*.**
   - **Please send us a 30–60-second video of *social coaching* for *sharing and giving turns* with your child to be viewed during homework review.**
     - **Please include:**
       - **Skills your child did well.**
       - **Skills you would like to work on with your child.**

3. **Provide social coaching on previously learned skills.**
   - **Continue providing *social coaching* to your child throughout the week using the *4 Ps*.**
   - **Previous skills include:**
     - ***Listening and following directions*.**
     - ***Meeting and greeting friends*.**

4. **Bring a turn-taking game.**
   - **Bring a turn-taking game that your child enjoys playing and can be played with the other children.**
     - **Common games: *Candy Land, Chutes and Ladders, Connect Four, Don't Break the Ice, Pop the Pig, Hi Ho Cherry-O, Operation, Perfection, Memory, Gone Fishin'.***
     - **Do not bring games that your child:**
       - **Will have difficulty sharing with others.**
       - **May become upset if the game pieces break or get lost.**

Parent Tips for Completing Homework Assignments

- **Suggestions for video recording on smartphones:**
  - **Test your audio and video quality.**
  - **Consider using a tripod.**
  - **Do not hold the camera while filming.**
  - **Consider using landscape mode.**
  - **Consider using the front-facing recording feature on your phone (so your child cannot see themself when filming).**
  - **Include both you and your child in the video.**
- **Suggestions for using *Parent Coached Play Cards*:**
  - **This coaching card can be used to provide support while using the *4 Ps* during your *social coaching* during homework assignments.**
  - **Consider sharing the *Parent Coached Play Cards* and *Parent Handouts* with your child's other care providers.**
- **Suggestions for using *Parent Homework Worksheets:***
  - **This worksheet will assist you in self-monitoring your use of the *4 Ps* in your *social coaching* during weekly homework assignments.**
  - **Please remember to complete this worksheet and return it to the treatment staff at the next meeting of PEERS® for Preschoolers.**

Session 3 Continued

Choosing Playgroups and Sharing and Giving a Turn

CHILD SESSION THERAPIST GUIDE

Child Session Agenda

- Didactic Lesson: *Sharing and Giving a Turn* (20 minutes).
- Group Behavioral Rehearsal Activity 1: *Sweet Potato Soup* (15 minutes).
- Break Time (10 minutes).
- Group Behavioral Rehearsal Activity 2: *Musical Share Chairs* (15 minutes).
- Parent Coached Play: *Dyadic Playdates* (20 minutes).
- Final Wrap-Up (10 minutes).

Snapshot of the Lesson: Sharing and Giving a Turn

The objective of this lesson is to teach children how to *share and give a turn*. Steps for *sharing and giving a turn* include:

1. ***Look at your friend with your eyes* (point to your eyes).**
2. ***Smile with your mouth* (point to your mouth and smile).**
3. ***Say "here" using names* (demonstrate handing over a toy) when you *share and give a turn*.**

Materials Needed

- Tiger puppet.
- Frog puppet.
- Two toy cars.
- Carpet squares or chairs.
- "Making Friends Helper" badge.
- Star chart with names of children.
- Marker for star chart.
- Name tags for families and treatment team.
- Prize bins with prizes.

Preparing for the Lesson

- Follow the script below with the group leader using a tiger puppet to play the part of "Timmy Tiger."
- A behavioral coach uses a frog puppet to play the part of "Franny Frog."

- An additional behavioral coach assists in the behavioral rehearsal and provides encouragement and feedback to the group.
- A child is chosen at the beginning of the lesson as the "Making Friends Helper."
  - The "Making Friends Helper" wears a special badge and is the first child to practice the skill.
- The group leader and the behavioral coach sit on the floor at the front of the room.
- A special-colored carpet square (e.g., red) is placed at the front of the room next to the group leader to be used as the "Good Friend Square."
- For the children, additional carpet squares of the same color (e.g., green) are placed in a semi-circle facing the group leader and the "Good Friend Square."
- Note: If carpet squares are unavailable, the children and behavioral coaches may sit on chairs.
- The material in *italics* should be read by the indicated person.
- The material in ***bold and italics*** represents buzzwords and should be emphasized when read.
- The material in CAPITAL LETTERS within the script should be given extra emphasis while the group is encouraged to say the words in unison.

Behavioral Coaching Techniques

Behavioral coaches should use the following ***social coaching*** techniques described below throughout the lesson and the behavioral rehearsal activities. (Note: ***priming*** occurs during the introduction to the activity.)

- ***Prompting***:
  - Use the buzzwords to ***prompt*** the children to ***share and give a turn*** IN THE MOMENT.
    - Example: *"Remember to give a turn."*
    - Example: *"Don't forget to say 'here' and use names when sharing."*
    - Example: *"Your friend wants a turn. What should you do?"*
- ***Praising***:
  - Reinforce ***sharing and giving a turn*** by ***praising*** the children when they use the skills CORRECTLY.
    - Example: *"Great job using names when you shared with your friend!"*
    - Example: *"Great job sharing nicely!"*
    - Example: *"Good job sharing when your friend asked for a turn!"*
- ***Providing corrective feedback using a praise sandwich***:
  - Reinforce ATTEMPTS to ***share and give a turn*** by ***praising*** the children and identifying what could be done differently next time.
    - Example: *"Good job sharing. Remember to say 'here' next time, but nice job!"*
    - Example: *"Nice try sharing. Remember to share nicely next time, but good try!"*
    - Example: *"Great job giving a turn. Don't forget to look next time, but good job!"*
- Continue to provide ***social coaching*** on previously learned skills:
  - ***Listening and following directions.***
  - ***Meeting and greeting friends.***

Didactic Lesson: Sharing and Giving a Turn (20 Minutes)

Have the children sit in a semi-circle on the carpet squares facing the group leader.

Timmy Tiger: (Sit at the front of the room and choose a Making Friends Helper.) *"Who wants to be our Making Friends Helper?"*

(Choose from among the children raising their hands and place the "Making Friends Helper" badge on the child. The child stays in their seat for now.)

"Hi friends! I'm Timmy Tiger. Grrr, grrr! Today we're going to practice sharing and giving a turn. Sharing and giving turns are great ways to be nice to our friends!"

"Who should we share and give a turn with? We should share and give a turn with our FRIENDS, TEACHERS, PARENTS, BROTHERS, AND SISTERS."

"When should we share and give a turn? We should share and give a turn when our friends ask to play with our toys."

"How should we share and give a turn? We should share and give a turn by looking at our friends with our (point to your eyes and then Timmy Tiger's eyes)*...EYES, smiling with our* (point to your mouth and smile)*...MOUTH, saying 'here'* (demonstrate handing over a toy), *when we share our toys, don't forget to use NAMES."*

"Remember, sharing and giving a turn are nice ways to be a good friend! Grrr, grrr!"

Role Play: Sharing and Giving a Turn

Timmy Tiger: (Play with the two toy cars while making car noises and commenting to yourself.)

Franny Frog: (Turn to look at the group of children.) *"Hey friends! I see my friend Timmy Tiger playing with some cool cars! I want to play, too. I'm going to ask for a turn. Ribbit, ribbit!* (Turn to look at Timmy Tiger and smile.) *Timmy Tiger, can I play with your cars? Ribbit, ribbit!"*

Timmy Tiger: (Turn to look at the group of children.) *"Hey friends! My friend Franny Frog wants to play with my cars. Do you think I should share and give a turn?"* (Nod your head yes and encourage the children to say *"yes."*) *"That's a great idea! Grrr, grrr! Let's do it!* (Turn to look at Franny Frog and smile.) *Okay. Here, Franny Frog!"* (Hand one of the cars to Franny Frog.)

Franny Frog: (Look at Timmy Tiger and smile.) *"Thanks, Timmy Tiger! Ribbit, ribbit!"*

Timmy Tiger and Franny Frog: (Play together with the cars for a few moments while commenting, such as *"Cool car, Timmy Tiger!"* or *"Watch me, Franny Frog!"*)

Timmy Tiger:	(Turn to look at the group of children.) *"Hey friends, did I do a good job sharing and giving a turn?"* (Nod your head yes and encourage the children to say *"yes."*) *"That's right! Grrr, grrr!"*
Timmy Tiger and Franny Frog:	(Say *"good job," give a "tiger high-five"* and *"frog high-five,"* clap, cheer, and encourage the children to clap as well. Franny Frog sits on the other side of the Good Friend Square (i.e., the Good Friend Square is between Timmy Tiger and Franny Frog). Timmy Tiger ***social coaches*** the children as needed while they practice ***sharing and giving a turn*** with Franny Frog.)
Timmy Tiger:	(Hold onto both cars.) *"Now let's see _____ (behavioral coach) try! _____ (Behavioral coach), please come sit on the Good Friend Square."*
Behavioral coach:	(Sit on the Good Friend Square.)
Timmy Tiger:	*"_____ (Behavioral coach), can you show us how to share and give a turn with Franny Frog?"*
Behavioral coach:	*"Okay, Timmy Tiger."*
Timmy Tiger:	(Turn to look at the group of children.) *"Remember to look at Franny Frog with your* (point to your eyes to prompt children to say "*eyes*")*...EYES, smile with your* (point to your mouth to prompt children to say "*mouth*")*... MOUTH, and say 'here'* (demonstrate handing over a toy) *when you share and give a turn. And don't forget to use* (pause briefly to prompt the children to say "*names*")*...NAMES."* (Give both cars to the behavioral coach.)
Behavioral coach:	(Play with the toy cars while making car noises and commenting to yourself.)
Franny Frog:	(Look at the behavioral coach member and smile.) *"____ (Behavioral coach), can I play with your cars?"*
Behavioral coach:	(Look at Franny Frog and smile.) *"Okay. Here, Franny Frog."* (Hand one of the cars to Franny Frog.)
Franny Frog:	*"Thanks, ____ (Behavioral coach)! Ribbit, ribbit!"*
Franny Frog and behavioral coach:	(Play together with the cars for a few moments while commenting, such as *"Cool car, Franny Frog!"* or *"Watch me, ____ (behavioral coach)!"*)
Timmy Tiger:	*"Great job sharing and giving a turn, ____ (behavioral coach)! Grrr, grrr!"*

Franny Frog and behavioral coach: (Say *"good job," give a "tiger high-five"* and *"frog high-five,"* clap, cheer, and encourage the children to clap as well. Then return both cars to Timmy Tiger.)

Behavior coach: (Leave the Good Friend Square.)

Behavioral Rehearsal: Sharing and Giving a Turn

Timmy Tiger: (Turn to look at the group of children.) *"Okay friends! Now let's see our Making Friends Helper _____ try! _____ (Making Friends Helper), come sit on the Good Friend Square and show us how to share and give a turn with Franny Frog."*

(The Making Friends Helper should sit on the Good Friend Square.)

"Remember to look at Franny Frog with your (point to your eyes to prompt children to say "*eyes*")*…EYES, smile with your* (point to your mouth to prompt children to say "*mouth*")*…MOUTH, and say 'here'* (demonstrate handing over a toy) *when you share and give a turn. And don't forget to use* (pause briefly to prompt the children to say "*names*")*…NAMES."*

(Give both cars to the Making Friends Helper. If needed, ***social coach*** the Making Friends Helper to play with the toy cars.)

Franny Frog: (Turn to look at the Making Friends Helper and smile.) *"____ (Making Friends Helper), can I play with your cars?"*

Timmy Tiger: (If needed, ***social coach*** the Making Friends Helper to ***look, smile,*** and ***say "Here, Franny Frog,"*** while ***sharing*** one of the cars with Franny Frog.)

Franny Frog: *"Thanks, ____ (Making Friends Helper)! Ribbit, ribbit!"*

(Franny Frog and the Making Friends Helper play together with the cars for a few moments while Franny Frog makes comments while playing, such as *"Cool car, ____ (Making Friends Helper)!"* or *"Look at this, ____ (Making Friends Helper)!"*)

Timmy Tiger: *"Great job sharing and giving a turn, ____ (Making Friends Helper)! Grrr, grrr!"*

Franny Frog: (Say *"good job," give a "tiger high-five"* and *"frog high-five,"* clap, cheer, and encourage the children to clap as well. Franny Frog and the Making Friends Helper should return the cars back to Timmy Tiger.)

Timmy Tiger: *"Okay, Making Friends Helper, choose another friend to sit on the Good Friend Square."* (If needed, ***social coach*** the Making Friends Helper to choose another child before returning to their seat.)

Repeat the following with each child:

Timmy Tiger: (Have each child take turns sitting on the Good Friend Square and practice ***sharing and giving a turn*** with Franny Frog.)

(Turn to look at the group of children.) *"Okay friends! Now let's see _____ (Child) try! _____ (Child), come sit on the Good Friend Square and show us how to share and give a turn with Franny Frog."*

(The child should sit on the Good Friend Square.) *"Remember to look at Franny Frog with your* (point to your eyes to prompt children to say "*eyes*")*...EYES, smile with your* (point to your mouth to prompt children to say "*mouth*")*...MOUTH, and say 'here'* (demonstrate handing over a toy) *when you share and give a turn. And don't forget to use* (pause briefly to prompt the children to say "*names*")*...NAMES."*

(Give both cars to the child. If needed, ***social coach*** the child to play with the toy cars.)

Franny Frog: (Turn to look at the child and smile.) *"____ (Child), can I play with your cars?"*

Timmy Tiger: (If needed, ***social coach*** the child to ***look, smile,*** and ***say "Here, Franny Frog,"*** while ***sharing*** one of the cars with Franny Frog.)

Franny Frog: *"Thanks, ____ (Child)! Ribbit, ribbit!"*

(Franny Frog and the child play together with the cars for a few moments while Franny Frog makes comments while playing, such as *"Cool car, ____ (Child)!"* or *"Look at this, ____ (Child)!"*)

Timmy Tiger: *"Great job sharing and giving a turn, ____ (Child)! Grrreat!"*

Franny Frog: (Say *"good job," give a "tiger high-five"* and *"frog high-five,"* clap, cheer, and encourage the children to clap as well. Franny Frog and the child should return the cars back to Timmy Tiger.)

Timmy Tiger: *"Okay, ____ (Child), choose another friend to sit on the Good Friend Square."* (If needed, ***social coach*** the child to choose another child before returning to their seat.)

Didactic Lesson Wrap-Up

Group leader: *"Well friends, you all did a great job sharing and giving a turn by looking at your friend with your* (point to your eyes to prompt children to say *"eyes"*)*...EYES, smiling with your* (point to your mouth to prompt children to say *"mouth"*)*...MOUTH, and saying 'here'* (demonstrate handing over a toy) *when you shared and gave a turn. And great job using* (pause briefly to prompt the children to say *"names"*)*...NAMES!"*

"You each earned ____ (number) stars for sharing and giving a turn! Let's start with ____ (child)."

Award each child the same number of stars by repeating the following with each child:

Group leader: *"Where's ____ (Child)?"* (Wait until all the children are looking at the child.)

"____ (Child), how many stars did you earn?" (Pause briefly to allow the child to respond.)

"That's right! Let's all count for ____ (Child)! One, two, three... (add stars to the Star Chart as they are counted aloud)*! Everybody clap for ____ (Child)!"* (All behavioral coaches clap and cheer and encourage the children to clap as well.)

Session 3 Continued

Sweet Potato Soup

BEHAVIORAL REHEARSAL ACTIVITY 1

Materials Needed

- Small bucket.

Room Setup

- Remove or place all carpet squares to the side.
- The group leader sits on the floor at the front of the room holding the small bucket.
- The behavioral coaches and children sit on the floor in a circle with the group leader.

Rules: Sweet Potato Soup

- The group leader reads the script below to explain the rules.
- All behavioral coaches and children lightly tap their laps while singing the *Sweet Potato Soup* song:
    - *"Sweet potato, sweet potato, oop, oop, oop! What did ____ (person holding the bucket) put in that soup?"*
- The child or behavioral coach holding the bucket then pretends to place an item into the bucket while naming it.
    - If needed, the behavioral coaches will help the children to think of items.
- The child should then practice ***sharing and giving a turn*** by passing the bucket to the person sitting next to them while ***looking, saying "here"*** and ***using names***.
- After one round, have the children place other categories of objects into the soup.
    - Examples: Insects, toys, favorite snacks, etc.
    - Have all children practice using the same category before introducing new categories.
- Optional: Children may also be allowed to suggest additional (appropriate) categories of objects.

Behavioral Rehearsal: Sweet Potato Soup (15 Minutes)

The group leader leads the activity. The behavioral coaches and children sit in a circle on the floor with the group leader while the rules are explained.

Group leader: *"Hey friends! Now we're going to play a game called Sweet Potato Soup! We're going to sing a fun song that goes like this, 'Sweet potato, sweet potato, oop, oop, oop! What did ____ (behavioral coach)* (point to behavioral coach*) put in that soup? We're going to use this bucket* (hold up the bucket) *to make our yummy soup. When your friends call your name, say what food you want to put in the bucket and then put it in the bucket* (demonstrate placing pretend food in the bucket and stirring). *You can put in carrots* (demonstrate placing pretend carrots in the bucket) *or potatoes* (demonstrate placing pretend potatoes in the bucket) *or whatever yummy food you like! Then do you think it's a good idea for us to share and give a turn to our friends?"* (Nod your head yes and encourage the children to say "*yes*.")

"That's right, friends! And remember to share and give a turn by giving the bucket to the friend next to you and looking at your friend with your (point to your eyes to prompt children to say "*eyes*")*...EYES, smiling with your* (point to your mouth to prompt children to say "*mouth*")*...MOUTH, and saying 'here'* (hand the bucket to the person sitting next to you). *And don't forget to use* (pause briefly to prompt the children to say "*names*")*...NAMES!"*

"And remember to listen and follow directions because sometimes we're going to put some silly things like bugs or candy into the soup. Okay, _____ (behavioral coaches) and I will go first!"

Role Play: Sweet Potato Soup

The group leader leads the role play. Two behavioral coaches demonstrate how to play *Sweet Potato Soup*. The two behavioral coaches sit next to each other to one side of the group leader.

Group leader: *"Let's play Sweet Potato Soup and practice sharing and giving a turn. _____ (Behavioral coach 1), you'll go first. Are we ready?"* (Hand the small bucket to behavioral coach 1.)

Everyone: *"Sweet potato, sweet potato, oop, oop, oop! What did _____ (behavioral coach 1) put in that soup?"*

Behavioral coach 1: *"I'm going to put _____ (food) into the soup* (demonstrate placing food in the bucket and stirring)*."*

Group leader: *"Great job, _____ (behavioral coach 1)! Now remember to share and give a turn by giving the bucket to _____ (behavioral coach 2)."*

Behavioral coach 1: *"Okay, _____ (group leader)."* (Turn to look at the behavioral coach 2 and smile.) *"Here, _____ (behavioral coach 2), it's your turn!"* (Hand the small bucket to behavioral coach 2.)

Behavioral coach 2: (Take the small bucket from the behavioral coach.) *"Thanks, _____ (behavioral coach 1)!"*

Group leader: *"Great job sharing and giving a turn, _____ (behavioral coach 1)! Let's keep playing. Are we ready?"* (Pause to allow children to say "*yes*.")

Everyone: *"Sweet potato, sweet potato, oop, oop, oop! What did _____ (behavioral coach 2) put in that soup?"*

Behavioral coach 2: *"I'm going to put _____ (food) in the soup* (demonstrate placing food in the bucket and stirring)*."*

Group leader: *"Great job, _____ (behavioral coach 2)! Now remember to share and give a turn by giving the bucket to _____ (child sitting next to behavioral coach 2)."*

Behavioral coach 2: *"Okay, _____ (group leader).* (Turn to look at the child sitting next to you and smile.) *Here, _____ (child), it's your turn!"* (Hand the small bucket to the child. If needed, ***prompt*** the child to take the small bucket.)

Group leader: *"Great job sharing and giving a turn, _____ (behavioral coach 2)! Okay friends, now it's everybody's turn to play Sweet Potato Soup. Are we ready?"*

Behavioral Rehearsal: Sweet Potato Soup

Everyone: *"Sweet potato, sweet potato, oop, oop, oop! What did _____ (child holding the bucket) put in that soup?"*

Group leader: (If needed, ***social coach*** the child to pick an item and pretend to place the item in the bucket.) *"Good job listening and following directions, ____ (child)!"*

"Now let's share and give a turn with ____ (person sitting next to the child)." (If needed, ***social coach*** the child to ***share and give a turn*** by ***saying "Here, _____ (child or behavioral coach)"*** and handing them the bucket.)

"Great job sharing and giving a turn, ____ (child)! Let's keep playing. Are we ready?"

Continue in the manner described above until everyone has had a turn to choose an item for the soup. Finish one round before introducing new categories of objects. Children may also be allowed to suggest additional categories of objects when appropriate.

Group leader: *"Okay friends, let's listen and follow directions because this time we're going to put ____ (new category) into the soup! Are we ready?"*

Table 3.1 Examples of New Categories

Insects	Articles of clothing	Toys
Favorite snacks	Candy	Body parts
Animals	Things at the zoo	Things at the park
Things that are furry	Things that smell good	Anything you want

Behavioral Rehearsal Wrap-Up

Group leader: *"Well friends, great job sharing and giving a turn! Give yourselves a big round of applause!"* (All behavioral coaches clap and cheer and encourage the children to clap as well.)

"Now everyone should come sit in the Listening Circle." (Have children return to the Listening Circle to sit on their carpet squares.)

"Okay friends, you did a great job sharing and giving a turn by looking

at your friends with your (point to your eyes to prompt children to say "*eyes*")*...EYES, smiling with your* (point to your mouth to prompt children to say "*mouth*")*...MOUTH, and saying 'here'* (demonstrate handing over the bucket) *when you shared and gave a turn. And great job using* (pause briefly to prompt the children to say "*names*")*...NAMES!"*

"You each earned ____ (number) more stars for sharing and giving a turn! So let's start with ____ (child)."

Award each child the same number of stars by repeating the following with each child:

Group leader: *"Where's _____ (child)?"* (Wait until all the children are looking at the child.)

"_____ (Child), how many stars did you earn?" (Pause briefly to allow the child to respond.)

"That's right! Let's all count for _____ (child)! One, two, three... (add stars to the Star Chart as they are counted aloud)*! Everybody clap for _____ (child)!"* (All behavioral coaches clap and cheer and encourage the children to clap as well.)

Break Time (10 Minutes)

- The puppets may be used to lead the children to and from the bathroom during break time.
- To assist with transitions and limit unstructured time, behavioral coaches may review the lesson with the children while waiting for the remaining children to return from the bathroom.
- You may want to award stars for good behavior after returning from the bathroom.

Session 3 Continued

Musical Share Chairs

BEHAVIORAL REHEARSAL ACTIVITY 2

Materials Needed

- Music and music player.
- Chairs (two chairs less than the total number of children and behavioral coaches).

Room Setup

- Arrange the chairs in one large circle facing outward with some space in between the chairs.
- The group leader stands at the front of the room.
- The children and behavioral coaches stand around the circle of chairs facing the group leader.

Rules: Musical Share Chairs

- The group leader reads the script below to explain the rules.
- Once the music begins to play, the children and behavioral coaches begin to slowly walk around the chairs in the same direction.
- Stop the music after 10–15 seconds and instruct the children to quickly find a chair.
  - The children and behavioral coaches should quickly sit in one of the chairs.
  - Only children (no behavioral coaches) should be left standing when the music is stopped.
- Then announce which children do not have a chair and ***social coach*** the seated children to offer to ***share*** their chair.
  - The focus of the game is to practice ***sharing and giving a turn*** and not to ***ask for a turn***.
- All children should be seated before the music is resumed.
  - Do not remove any chairs. The point of the game is to practice ***sharing and giving a turn*** rather than to eliminate group members.
- Repeat this cycle until all children have had several turns ***sharing and giving a turn***.
- Throughout the game, behavioral coaches will need to ensure that all children have had an equal number of opportunities to practice ***sharing and giving a turn***.
- Optional: After the children are familiar with the game, instruct the children to move around the circle in different ways.
  - Examples: hop on one foot, hop like a bunny, stomp like a giant, tiptoe like a cat, etc.

Behavioral Rehearsal: Musical Share Chairs (15 Minutes)

The group leader leads the activity. The children are sitting in the chairs and the behavioral coaches are standing as the group leader explains the rules.

Group leader: *"Hey friends, now we're going to play a game called Musical Share Chairs. When* you hear the music, everyone walks around the chairs. Can every*body show me how to walk around the chairs?"* (Pause briefly to allow the children to demonstrate walking around the circle of chairs.)

"That's right, friends! And when the music stops, quickly find a chair and sit down (sit down in one of the chairs to demonstrate). *But you have to be fast because we don't have enough chairs for everybody! Do you think it's a good idea to share your share if a friend doesn't have a chair?"* (Encourage the children to say *"yes."*)

"That's right friends! So remember to look at your friends with your (point to your eyes to prompt children to say "*eyes*")*...EYES, smile with your* (point to your mouth and smile to prompt children to say "*mouth*")*...MOUTH, and say 'here' when you share your chair. And don't forget to use* (pause briefly to prompt the children to say "*names*")*...NAMES!"*

"And remember to listen because we'll move around the chairs in different silly ways like stomping like a giant (demonstrate stomping) *or tip-toeing like a cat* (demonstrate walking on your tiptoes). *Okay, let's play Musical Share Chairs!"*

Role Play: Musical Share Chairs

The group leader leads the role play and controls the music. Two behavioral coaches demonstrate how to play *Musical Share Chairs*. The children walk around the circle with the behavioral coaches. For the role play, have ONE less chair than there are players.

Group leader: (Play the music.) *"Okay friends, everybody start walking around the circle."*

(Allow the children and behavioral coaches to walk slowly around the chairs, then pause the music after 10–15 seconds.) *"The music stopped! Everybody find a chair and sit!"*

Behavioral coach 1: (Walk slowly when finding a chair in order to be left standing.)

Group leader: *"Hey friends, _____ (behavioral coach 1) doesn't have a chair. _____ (Behavioral coach 2), can you show us how to share and give a turn by sharing your chair? Remember to say 'here' and don't forget to use names!"*

Behavioral coach 2: *"Here, _____ (behavioral coach 1), you can share my chair."*

Behavioral coach 1: *"Thanks, _____ (behavioral coach 2)!"*

Group leader: *"Great job sharing and giving a turn, _____ (behavioral coach 1 and 2)! Now everybody stand up so we can keep playing! Ready?"*

Behavioral Rehearsal: Musical Share Chairs

Remove ONE ADDITIONAL chair, so there are TWO chairs less than there are players.

Group leader: (Play the music.) *"Okay friends, everybody start walking around the circle."*

(Allow the children and behavioral coaches to walk slowly around the chairs, then pause the music after 10–15 seconds.) *"The music stopped! Everybody find a chair and sit!"* (Behavioral coaches should be quick to find a chair so children must practice ***sharing*** their chairs with their friends.)

"Hey friends, _____ (children) don't have chairs. Which little friends will share their chairs?" (If needed, ***social coach*** the children to ***share and give a turn***.)

"Great job sharing and giving a turn! Everybody stand up so we can keep playing. Are we ready?"

After several rounds of the sequence above, you may introduce new ways of moving around the circle of chairs.

Group leader: *"Okay friends, let's listen and follow directions because this time we're going to _____ (new movement) around the chairs!"* (Each new movement should be modeled by the group leader and the behavioral coaches before playing.)

Table 3.2 Examples of New Movements

Hope like a bunny	Stomp like a giant	Hop on one foot
Tip-toe like a cat	Fly like a bird	Swim like a fish
Walk sideways like a crab	Walk backward slowly	Take small baby steps
Slither like a snake	Walk in slow motion	Take giant steps

Behavioral Rehearsal Wrap-Up

Group leader: *"Well friends, great job sharing and giving a turn! Give yourselves a big round of applause!"* (All behavioral coaches clap and cheer and encourage the children to clap as well.)

"Now everyone should sit in the Listening Circle." (Have children return to the Listening Circle to sit on their carpet squares.)

"Okay friends, you did a great job sharing and giving a turn by looking at your friends with your (point to your eyes to prompt children to say "*eyes*")*...EYES, smiling with your* (point to your mouth to prompt children to say "*mouth*")*...MOUTH, and saying 'here'* (demonstrate handing over the bucket) *when you shared and gave a turn. And great job using* (pause briefly to prompt the children to say "*names*")*...NAMES!"*

You each earned ____ (number) more stars for sharing and giving a turn! So let's start with ____ (child)."

Award each child the same number of stars by repeating the following with each child:

Group leader: *"Where's _____ (child)?"* (Wait until all the children are looking at the child.)

"_____ (Child), how many stars did you earn?" (Pause briefly to allow the child to respond.)

"That's right! Let's all count for _____ (child)! One, two, three... (add stars to the Star Chart as they are counted aloud)*! Everybody clap for _____ (child)!"* (All behavioral coaches clap and cheer and encourage the children to clap as well.)

"Now we're going to play some games with our parents and practice sharing and giving a turn some more!"

Session 3 Continued

Sharing and Giving a Turn

PARENT COACHED PLAY: DYADIC PLAYDATES

Materials Needed

- Games brought by children and parents from home.
- Turn-taking games provided by the treatment team.
  - Common games: *Candy Land, Chutes and Ladders, Connect Four, Don't Break the Ice, Pop the Pig, Hi Ho Cherry-O, Operation, Perfection, Memory, Gone Fishin'.*
- Tables and chairs or carpet squares.
- *Parent Coached Play Cards.*

Room Setup

- If available, organize tables in separate corners of the room with 4–6 chairs per table.
- If tables are unavailable, place two carpet squares in separate corners of the room to indicate where the children will sit.
- The group leader sits on the floor at the front of the room.
- The families sit on the floor in a semi-circle facing the group leader.

Rules: Dyadic Playdates

- The group leader divides the families into groups of two families each.
  - If there are an odd number of children, pair one child with a behavioral coach who will serve as a ***playmate***. In this case, you will need an additional coach to serve as a behavioral coach for the parent.
  - To avoid social exclusion, avoid having children play in triads as much as possible.
- Assign each group to sit at a table or specific play area.
  - Children should sit next to each other.
  - Parents will act as ***social coaches*** by sitting on the other side of their child to minimize interrupting the natural flow of play between the children.
  - One behavioral coach will be assigned to each dyad to provide ***social coaching*** suggestions and feedback to parents.
- Children will take turns playing the games brought from home or games provided by the treatment team.

- Each child will have ten minutes to play their chosen game with their ***playmate*** and will then switch games.
- Parents will choose which child's game will be played first.
- To minimize unstructured periods, parents will help the children set up the game in a cooperative fashion (handing game pieces to each other, offering suggestions, etc.).
- As they play, parents will ***social coach*** the children on previously learned and newly learned skills using the guidelines highlighted on the *Parent Coached Play Cards.*
- Behavioral coaches will provide support to parents in their ***social coaching*** using the ***4 Ps*** (***priming, prompting, praising,*** and ***providing corrective feedback***) and will model appropriate ***social coaching*** behavior when necessary.
- After approximately nine minutes of play, instruct the parents to prepare the children for the upcoming game swap.
- After approximately one additional minute of play (ten minutes total), instruct the parents to have the children clean up and swap games.
- Repeat the cycle with the second game for the remaining ten minutes before returning to the *Listening Circle.*

Behavioral Coaching: Dyadic Playdates

Behavioral coaches will ***social coach*** parents during dyadic ***playdates*** in the following ways:

- ***Priming*:**
  - Begin the play interactions with parents going over the rules for ***sharing and giving a turn*** BEFORE GAME PLAYING.
    - Example: *"Remember that while you're playing games with your friend we want you to share and give a turn. You can do that by looking at your friend with your* (point to your eyes to prompt children to say *"eyes")...EYES, smiling with your* (point to your mouth to prompt children to say *"mouth")...MOUTH, and saying 'here'* (demonstrate handing over a toy) *when you share and give a turn. And don't forget to use* (pause briefly to prompt the children to say *"names")...NAMES."*
- ***Prompting*:**
  - Remind parents to use the buzzwords to ***prompt*** their child to ***share and give a turn*** IN THE MOMENT.
  - Help parents to identify opportunities to proactively ***prompt*** their child to ***share and give turns***.
    - Example: *"Don't forget to share and give turns when our friends ask for a turn."*
    - Example: *"Remember to say 'here' when sharing."*
    - Example: *"Let's share and give a turn nicely."*
  - Assisting parents to follow through with the ***prompts*** they present to their child.
- ***Praising*:**
  - Remind parents to ***praise*** and reinforce their child whenever their child ***shares and gives a turn*** CORRECTLY.
    - Example: *"Great job sharing your toy!"*
    - Example: *"Great job giving a turn nicely to your friend!"*

    - Example: *"Good job looking when you shared your toy!"*
- ***Providing corrective feedback using a praise sandwich*:**
    - Remind parents to ***praise*** their child's ATTEMPTS to ***share and give a turn*** and identify what could be done differently next time.
        - Example: *"Good job sharing. Remember to say 'here' next time, but nice job!"*
        - Example: *"Nice try giving a turn. Let's try to share nicely next time, but good try!"*
        - Example: *"Good job sharing. Don't forget to look next time, but great job!"*
- Remind parents to continue to ***social coach*** on previously learned skills:
    - ***Listening and following directions.***
    - ***Meeting and greeting friends.***

Parent Coached Play: Dyadic Playdates (20 Minutes)

- Have each child choose a turn-taking game brought from home or provided by the treatment team.
- The group leader sits on the floor at the front of the room.
- The families sit on the floor in a semi-circle facing the group leader.

Group leader: *"Hey friends, we're going to have more playdates and play with the cool games you brought from home. This time we want you to practice sharing and giving a turn when playing with your friend. Remember to share and give a turn by looking at your friend with your* (point to your eyes to prompt children to say *"eyes"*)*...EYES, smiling with your* (point to your mouth to prompt children to say *"mouth"*)*...MOUTH, and saying 'here'* (demonstrate handing over a toy) *when you share and give a turn. And don't forget to use* (pause briefly to prompt the children to say *"names"*)*...NAMES."*

"And friends, don't forget to say 'hi' (wave your hand) *before you start playing and say 'bye'* (wave your hand) *when you finish playing. And if you don't remember your friend's name, you can ask, 'What's your name?' and then say your name too. Parents, remember to social coach your children by using your Parent Coached Play Cards. Okay, let's play with our games!"*

- Before playing, parents will ***social coach*** their child to say, "***What's your name?***" and then ***say their name*** if their ***playmate***'s name is unknown. Parents will also ***social coach*** their child to ***say*** "***hi***" to one another ***using names***.
- Parents will ***social coach*** their children to ***share and take turns*** throughout the game playing.
- After approximately nine minutes of play, instruct the parents to prepare the children for the upcoming game swap by saying, *"Parents, tell your children that we'll be swapping games in one minute."*
- After approximately one additional minute of play (ten minutes total), instruct the parents to swap games by saying, *"Parents, it's time to swap games. Social coach the children to share and give a turn when playing the next game."*

- After approximately nine minutes of playing the second game, instruct the parents to prepare the children for clean up by saying, *"Parents, tell your children that we'll be cleaning up in one minute."*
- After approximately one additional minute of play (ten minutes total), ***prompt*** the parents to instruct their children to clean up by saying, *"Parents, it's time to clean up. Let's social coach the children to listen and follow directions by cleaning up and then say 'bye' to their friend using names before sitting in the Listening Circle."*
- If needed, parents will ***social coach*** their child to ***listen and follow directions*** to clean up.
- Then parents will ***social coach*** their child to ***say*** "***bye***" to their friend ***using names***.

Final Wrap-Up (10 Minutes)

- The group leader sits on the floor at the front of the room.
- The children sit on the carpet squares in a semi-circle facing the group leader, with parents sitting behind their children.

Group leader: *"Okay friends, you all did a great job playing your games and sharing and giving a turn. When we're sharing and giving a turn, do you think we should LOOK with our EYES and SMILE with our MOUTHS?"* (Pause briefly to allow the children to say *"yes."*)

"That's right, friends! And when we're sharing and giving a turn, do you think we should say 'here' (demonstrate handing over a toy) *and use names?"* (Pause briefly to allow the children to say *"yes."*).

"That's right, friends! You all did such a great job sharing and giving a turn today that you each earned ____ (number) more stars! Let's start with ____ (child)."

Award each child the same number of stars by repeating the following with each child:

Group leader: *"Where's _____ (child)?"* (Wait until all the children are looking at the child.)

"_____ (Child), how many stars did you earn?" (Pause briefly to allow the child to respond.)

"That's right! Let's all count for _____ (child)! One, two, three... (add stars to the Star Chart as they are counted aloud)*! Everybody clap for _____ (child)!"* (All behavioral coaches clap and cheer and encourage the children to clap as well.)

"And remember you all earned those stars by sharing and giving a turn! Everyone did a great job and parents, you did an excellent job social coaching! Parents, remember your homework assignments this week are for you

and your children to practice sharing and giving a turn and to continue practicing all the other things we've learned to be a good friend using the 4 Ps. And don't forget to investigate and begin to enroll your children in playgroups."

"Alright little friends, do you want to count our stars?" (Pause briefly to allow the children to respond *"yes."*)

"Let's all count together and see how many stars we earned today! One, two, three... (count the number of stars for one child)*!"*

"You each earned ____ (total number) stars today! Round of applause for our friends!" (All behavioral coaches should clap and cheer and encourage the families to clap as well.)

"Great job, friends! Don't forget to choose your reward before you leave. See you all next week!"

Session 3 Continued

Choosing Playgroups and Sharing and Giving a Turn

PEERS® FOR PRESCHOOLERS: PARENT HANDOUT

Didactic Lesson: Choosing Playgroups

Criteria for Good Playgroups

- Meets regularly (preferably weekly).
- Located close to your home.
  - It will be difficult to arrange regularly occurring ***playdates*** with other families if the ***playgroup*** is far from your home.
- Includes other children in the same age range and level of support needs as your child.
- Includes informal time so that your child will have opportunities to interact and play with other children naturally.
- Activities are based on your child's interests, likes, or hobbies.
  - Avoid activities your child dislikes, may be difficult for them, or may trigger their sensitivities.
- Begins within the next few weeks.
- Permits some parent involvement in order to facilitate peer interactions and organize ***playdates*** with other families.
  - At a minimum, this may include drop-off and pickup times.

Assessing Appropriateness of Playgroups

- **Observe the group composition.**
  - Ask yourself if this is a good ***playgroup*** for your child based on these factors:
    - Common interests of group members.
    - Language or communication abilities.
    - Age range and support needs.
    - Gender distribution of the group (if relevant).
    - Developmental level of the group.
    - Social functioning and expectations of the group.
    - Physical activity level.

- **Notice your child's reaction to the group.**
  - Notice which ***playgroup*** activities your child enjoys.
  - Notice if there are aspects of the ***playgroup*** your child dislikes.

- Observe whether your child becomes more or less comfortable over time and exposure.
- Consider asking your child what they thought of the group.

- **Identify potential *playmates*.**
  - Observe which children your child plays with or appears to be interested in getting to know.
  - Notice which children may be a good fit and potential ***playmate*** for your child.
  - Observe which children appear to show a positive interest in your child.
  - Notice which activities, games, or toys your child and their potential ***playmate(s)*** enjoy playing.
    - These activities, games, or toys may be incorporated into future ***playdates***.

- **Identify preferred social activities.**
  - Take note of which activities, games, or toys your child enjoys.
    - These preferred social activities might be used as an enticement to return to the group.
    - These activities, games, or toys may be incorporated into future ***playdates*** with related or unrelated ***playmates***.
  - Notice which activities your child dislikes and consider whether some accommodation can or should be made to make the activities less aversive.

- **Observe the *playgroup* facilitators.**
  - Notice how attuned the ***playgroup*** facilitators are to your child.
  - Consider whether your child will receive adequate support during the ***playgroup*** activities.
  - Observe the appropriateness of parent participation or involvement in the activities.

- **Engage with other parents.**
  - Engage in light social chit-chat with other parents.
    - Make a point to chat with the parents of the potential ***playmates*** you have identified for your child.
    - Use the ***playgroup*** as a reason for talking to other parents (e.g., *"So how long have you and your child been coming here?"*)
  - Assess your interest in and compatibility with the other parents.
  - The goal is to build a foundation for potential ***playdates*** so you will need to earn the other parents' trust.
  - Talking with other parents is also a great way to gather information about other ***playgroups*** and social activities.
  - You may want to hold off on suggesting a ***playdate*** until you have had a few interactions with the other parent(s) and the potential ***playmate(s)***.

Snapshot of the Lesson: Sharing and Giving a Turn

The objective of this lesson is to teach children how to ***share and give a turn*** when playing with friends and potential ***playmates***.

1. ***Look at your friends with your eyes*** (point to your eyes).
2. ***Smile with your mouth*** (point to your mouth and smile).
3. ***Say "here" using names*** when you ***share and give a turn.***

Homework Assignments

1. **Find a playgroup for your child.**
   - Investigate and begin to enroll your child in a ***playgroup*** using the criteria for a good ***playgroup***:
     - Meets regularly (preferably weekly).
     - Located close to your home.
     - Includes other children in the same age range and level of support needs as your child.
     - Includes informal time so that your child will have opportunities to interact and play with other children naturally.
     - Activities are based on your child's interests, likes, or hobbies.
     - Begins within the next few weeks.
     - Permits some parent involvement in order to facilitate peer interactions and organize ***playdates*** with other families.
2. **Practice sharing and giving a turn.**
   - **Practice having your child *share and give turns* this week during preferred and highly motivating activities while providing *social coaching* using the *4 Ps.***
     - ***Priming:*** Review the rules for ***sharing and giving turns*** with your child BEFORE PRACTICING.
     - ***Prompting:*** Remind your child IN THE MOMENT to ***share and give turns*** whenever the opportunities present.
     - ***Praising: Praise*** your child for using the buzzwords whenever they ***share and give turns*** CORRECTLY.
     - ***Providing corrective feedback: Provide corrective feedback*** in the form of a ***praise sandwich*** whenever your child ATTEMPTS to ***share and give turns***.
   - **Please send us a 30–60-second video of *social coaching* for *sharing and giving turns* with your child to be viewed during homework review.**
     - Please include:
       - Skills your child did well
       - Skills you would like to work on with your child
3. **Provide social coaching on previously learned skills.**
   1. Continue providing ***social coaching*** to your child throughout the week using the ***4 Ps***.
   2. Previous skills include:
      - ***Listening and following directions***.
      - ***Meeting and greeting friends***.

4. **Bring a turn-taking game.**
    - Bring a turn-taking game that your child enjoys playing and can be played with the other children.
        - Common games: *Candy Land, Chutes and Ladders, Connect Four, Don't Break the Ice, Pop the Pig, Hi Ho Cherry-O, Operation, Perfection, Memory, Gone Fishin'.*
        - Do not bring games that your child:
            - Will have difficulty sharing with others.
            - May become upset if the game pieces break or get lost.

Parent Tips for Completing Homework Assignments

- **Suggestions for video recording on smartphones:**
    - Test your audio and video quality.
    - Consider using a tripod.
    - Do not hold the camera while filming.
    - Consider using landscape mode.
    - Consider using the front-facing recording feature on your phone (so your child cannot see themself when filming).
    - Include both you and your child in the video.

- **Suggestions for using *Parent Coached Play Cards*:**
    - This coaching card can be used to provide support while using the ***4 Ps*** during your ***social coaching*** during homework assignments.
    - Consider sharing the *Parent Coached Play Cards* and *Parent Handouts* with your child's other care providers.

- **Suggestions for using *Parent Homework Worksheets*:**
    - This worksheet will assist you in self-monitoring your use of the ***4 Ps*** in your ***social coaching*** during weekly homework assignments.
    - Please remember to complete this worksheet and return it to the treatment staff at the next meeting of PEERS® for Preschoolers.

Session 3 Continued
Sharing and Giving a Turn

PEERS® FOR PRESCHOOLERS: PARENT COACHED PLAY CARD

Snapshot of the Lesson: Sharing and Giving a Turn

1. ***Look at your friends with your eyes*** (point to your eyes).
2. ***Smile with your mouth*** (point to your mouth and smile).
3. ***Say "here" using names*** when you ***share and give a turn.***

Priming BEFORE Game Playing

- Example: *"Remember that while you're playing games with your friend we want you to share and give a turn. You can do that by looking at your friend with your* (point to your eyes to prompt your child to say "*eyes*")*...EYES, smiling with your* (point to your mouth to prompt your child to say "*mouth*")*...MOUTH, and saying 'here'* (demonstrate handing over a toy) *when you share and give a turn. And don't forget to use* (pause briefly to prompt your child to say "*names*")*...NAMES."*

Prompting IN THE MOMENT

- Example: *"Remember to give a turn."*
- Example: *"Don't forget to say 'here' and use names when sharing."*
- Example: *"Your friend wants a turn. What should you do?"*

Praising for CORRECT Use of Skills

- Example: *"Great job using names when you shared with your friend!"*
- Example: *"Great job sharing nicely!"*
- Example: *"Good job sharing when your friend asked for a turn!"*

Providing Corrective Feedback for ATTEMPTS Using a Praise Sandwich

- Example: *"Good job sharing. Remember to say 'here' next time, but nice job!"*
- Example: *"Nice try sharing. Remember to share nicely next time, but good try!"*
- Example: *"Great job giving a turn. Don't forget to look next time, but good job!"*

- Continue to provide ***social coaching*** on previously learned skills:
  - ***Listening and following directions.***
  - ***Meeting and greeting friends.***

Session 3 Continued

Choosing Playgroups and Sharing and Giving a Turn

PEERS® FOR PRESCHOOLERS: PARENT HOMEWORK WORKSHEET

<table>
<tr><td>Child's Name:</td><td colspan="2">Parent's Name:</td><td colspan="2">Date:</td></tr>
<tr><td>HOMEWORK ASSIGNMENTS</td><td>PRIMING (REVIEWING RULES BEFORE PRACTICE)</td><td>PROMPTING (IN THE MOMENT)</td><td>PRAISING (USING BUZZWORDS)</td><td>PROVIDING CORRECTIVE FEEDBACK (USING A PRAISE SANDWICH)</td></tr>
<tr><td>Sharing and giving turns</td><td></td><td></td><td></td><td></td></tr>
<tr><td>Practice previous skills:
• Meeting and greeting friends
• Listening and following directions</td><td></td><td></td><td></td><td></td></tr>
<tr><td>Playgroups
Investigate and enroll in playgroup(s).</td><td colspan="4">Which playgroups did you investigate and enroll in?</td></tr>
<tr><td>Bring a turn-taking game</td><td colspan="2">Did you bring a turn-taking game?
YES or NO
(Circle)</td><td colspan="2">Which game did you bring?</td></tr>
</table>

Please fill out this worksheet by describing what you did to complete the homework assignments. Worksheets will be collected during Homework Review at the next session of PEERS® for Preschoolers.

Session 4

Preparing for Playgroups and Asking for a Turn

PARENT SESSION THERAPIST GUIDE

Parent Session Agenda

- Homework Review (40 minutes).
- Didactic Lessons (20 minutes).
- Parent Coached Play (20 minutes).
- Final Wrap-Up (10 minutes).

Materials Needed

- Conference room with a large table and enough chairs for the parent group leader and all parents to sit comfortably around the table.
    - Avoid sitting in a circle without a table as this creates the atmosphere of group therapy.
- Name tags for parents and treatment team.
- *Parent Handouts* (for the current week and the previous weeks).
- *Parent Homework Worksheets* (for the current week and the previous weeks).
- *Parent Coached Play Cards* (for the current week and the previous weeks).
- *Attendance and Homework Compliance Sheets* for parent group leader.
- Pens for note taking (consider having extra pens for parents who need them).

Homework Review (40 Minutes)

1. **Find a playgroup for your child.**
    - Confirm parents investigated and began to enroll their child in a ***playgroup***.
        - If the child is currently enrolled in appropriate ***playgroups*** with potential ***playmates***, they do not need to enroll in new ***playgroups***.
        - Confirm parents considered the criteria for a good ***playgroup***:
            - Meets regularly (preferably weekly).
            - Located close to their home.
            - Includes other children in the same age range and level of support needs as their child.
            - Includes informal time so that their child will have opportunities to interact and play with other children naturally.
            - Activities are based on their child's interests, likes, or hobbies.
            - Begins within the next few weeks.
            - Permits some parent involvement in order to facilitate peer interactions and organize ***playdates*** with other families.

DOI: 10.4324/9781003502968-5

2. **Practice sharing and giving a turn.**
   - Review the 30–60-second video of social coaching for ***sharing and giving a turn*** for each family. (For larger groups, you may need to review video recordings in two smaller groups with two different parent group leaders).
     - Have parents identify:
       - Skills their child did well.
       - Skills they would like to work on with their child.
     - Provide ***social coaching*** tips as appropriate for each family.
   - If parents did not send a video of ***social coaching***, confirm the following:
     - Parents practiced having their child ***share and give turns*** during preferred and highly motivating activities while providing ***social coaching*** using the ***4 Ps.***
       - ***Priming:*** Reviewed the rules for ***sharing and giving turns*** with their child BEFORE PRACTICING.
       - ***Prompting:*** Reminded their child IN THE MOMENT to ***share and give turns*** whenever the opportunity presented.
       - ***Praising: Praised*** their child using the buzzwords whenever they ***shared and gave turns*** CORRECTLY.
       - ***Providing corrective feedback:*** ***Provided corrective feedback*** in the form of a ***praise sandwich*** whenever their child ATTEMPTED to ***share and give turns***.

3. **Provide social coaching on previously learned skills.**
   - Confirm parents continued to provide ***social coaching*** to their child throughout the week using the ***4 Ps*** for previously learned skills:
     - ***Listening and following directions***.
     - ***Meeting and greeting friends***.

4. **Bring a turn-taking game.**
   - Confirm the following:
     - Brought a turn-taking game that their child enjoys playing and can be played with the other children. (To avoid distractions, these games should be left with the parents until *Parent Coached Play*.)

Didactic Lessons (20 Minutes)

PEERS® Neuroaffirming Pledge:

- We value neurodiversity, acceptance, and authenticity.
- We honor the diverse ways people experience the world.
- We respect each person's unique perspectives and communication styles.
- We recognize there is no one right way to connect with others.
- If using the strategies taught in PEERS® feels like camouflaging or masking and/or they don't align with your goals or the goals of your family, then you do not have to use them.
- Learning and using the skills taught in PEERS® is a PERSONAL CHOICE.

Didactic Lesson: Preparing for Playgroups

- Distribute *Parent Handouts*.
  - Sections in **bold print** come directly from the *Parent Handout*.
  - Terms that are ***bold and italicized*** are buzzwords and represent important concepts from the didactic lesson.
- Explain, "*Last week we discussed assessing whether a playgroup is appropriate for your child and may be a good source for potential playmates. Once an appropriate playgroup has been identified, it will be important to do several things to prepare your child in order to decrease anxiety, promote a positive experience, and enrich social interactions. Consider previewing the 5 Ws with your child to guide the conversation and preparations.*"

Preview the 5 Ws with Your Child

- **WHO will be there?**
  - **Point out other children that your child knows and likes that will be present or have been to the *playgroup*.**
    - **Karate Example: Your child's older sibling went to the same karate class.**
    - **Swimming Example: Your child's preschool classmate will also be at the swimming class.**
  - **Point out positive relationships that the *playgroup* instructor may have with your child or persons that your child is familiar with and/or likes.**
  - **Karate Example: The karate instructor is a family member of a friend of your child.**
  - **Swimming Example: The swimming instructor is the physical education teacher of your child's sibling.**
  - **Once your child has attended the *playgroup* and other children are known:**
    - **Have your child identify which peers they would like to play with during the *playgroup*.**
    - **Remind your child at drop-off which *playmates* they enjoy playing with.**
    - **Listen for recurring names of *playmates* your child mentions and name-drop them when talking about the *playgroup*.**

- **WHAT are the activities?**
  - **The activities of the *playgroup* should be preferred activities for your child to make the experience rewarding and pleasurable.**
    - **Remind your child how much they enjoy the activity when referencing the *playgroup*.**
  - **Preview games and activities with your child once the *playgroup* is chosen.**
  - **Practice games, activities, and playing with toys that may be new to your child.**
    - **Familiarize your child with the new games, activities, toys, or materials prior to the playgroup.**
      - **Karate Example: Show them their karate uniform, drive them by the dojo.**
      - **Swimming Example: Show them their swimsuit and goggles, drive them by the pool.**
    - **Present the rules of the game or activity if unknown to your child.**
      - **Karate Example: Listening, following directions, imitating, taking turns.**
      - **Swimming Example: Listening, following directions, no running by the pool, no splashing others, no jumping into the pool.**
    - **Highlight which elements of the game or activity that your child is already familiar with and/or does well.**
      - **Karate Example: Good balance, excellent imitation skills.**

        - **Swimming Example: Enjoyment of water, good ability to listen and follow directions.**
    - **Pointing out these elements to your child may reduce your child's anxiety and increase excitement about the *playgroup*.**

- **WHERE will the playgroup take place?**
    - **Mention the location of the *playgroup* if it is a familiar or preferred setting.**
        - **Karate Example: Karate classes take place at their favorite community recreation center.**
        - **Swimming Example: Swimming classes take place at the local YMCA where they have enjoyed other classes.**

- **WHEN will the *playgroup* take place?**
    - **Attempt to choose *playgroups* that do not interfere with other preferred activities.**
        - **Your child should not have to give up a favorite activity or pastime to attend the *playgroup* (e.g., your child must miss a recurring *playdate* to attend karate classes).**
    - **Try to limit the number of competing obligations for your child prior to attending the *playgroup.***
        - **Your child should not be overscheduled on the day they are to attend a *playgroup* (e.g., taking swimming classes after a long day of preschool and therapy).**

- **HOW will you get your child to attend?**
    - **Consider linking the *playgroup* to some other preferred activity or reward.**
    - **The reward should be contingent on meaningful participation in the *playgroup*.**
        - **Karate Example: Visiting the park after karate.**
        - **Swimming Example: Getting ice cream after swimming classes.**

Explain, "*So these are some of the ways you can prepare for and promote your child's attendance at playgroups. Previewing the 5 Ws will enable you to prepare your child for this new activity, which may reduce feelings of anxiety and uncertainty while focusing on the familiar and pleasurable aspects of the activities.*"

Didactic Lesson: Asking for a Turn

Explain, "*Last week we focused on sharing and giving a turn during play. This week the children are learning how to ask for a turn when playing with their friends. This is an important skill for initiating play with friends and for promoting reciprocity in play.*"

Snapshot of the Lesson: Asking for a Turn

The objective of this lesson is to teach children how to *ask for a turn*. Steps for *asking for a turn* include:

1. ***Look at your friend with your eyes* (point to your eyes).**
2. ***Smile with your mouth* (point to your mouth and smile).**
3. ***Say "Can I have a turn please?" using names.***

Parent Coached Play

- Distribute the *Parent Coached Play Cards*.
- Review the examples of the ***4 Ps*** provided on the *Parent Coached Play Card.*
- Remind parents that in a few moments, we will be joining the children for *Parent Coached Play* in the context of mock dyadic ***playdates***.
- Parents should keep the *Parent Coached Play Card* in front of them during the dyadic ***playdate*** for recommendations on how to ***social coach*** children on ***asking for a turn***.

Homework Assignments

(Briefly review the homework assignments and troubleshoot any potential problems with parents.)

1. **Find a playgroup for your child.**
   - **Investigate and begin to enroll your child in a *playgroup* using the criteria for a good *playgroup*:**
     - **Meets regularly (preferably weekly).**
     - **Located close to your home.**
     - **Includes other children in the same age range and level of support needs as your child.**
     - **Includes informal time so that your child will have opportunities to interact and play with other children naturally.**
     - **Activities are based on your child's interests, likes, or hobbies.**
     - **Begins within the next few weeks.**
     - **Permits some parent involvement in order to facilitate peer interactions and organize *playdates* with other families.**

2. **Practice asking for a turn.**
   - **Practice having your child *ask for a turn* this week during preferred and highly motivating activities while providing *social coaching* using the *4 Ps*.**
     - ***Priming:* Review the rules for *asking for a turn* with your child BEFORE PRACTICING.**
     - ***Prompting:* Remind your child IN THE MOMENT to *ask for a turn* whenever the opportunities present.**
     - ***Praising: Praise* your child for using the buzzwords whenever they *ask for a turn* CORRECTLY.**
     - ***Providing corrective feedback: Provide corrective feedback* in the form of a *praise sandwich* whenever your child ATTEMPTS to *ask for a turn*.**
   - **Please send us a 30–60-second video of *social coaching* for *asking for a turn* with your child to be viewed during homework review.**
     - **Please include:**
       - **Skills your child did well.**
       - **Skills you would like to work on with your child.**

3. **Provide social coaching on previously learned skills.**
   - **Continue providing *social coaching* to your child throughout the week using the *4 Ps.***
   - **Previous skills include:**
     - ***Listening and following directions.***
     - ***Meeting and greeting friends.***
     - ***Sharing and giving a turn.***

4. **Bring a turn-taking game.**
   - **Bring a turn-taking game that your child enjoys playing and can be played with the other children.**

Session 4 Continued

Asking for a Turn

CHILD SESSION THERAPIST GUIDE

Child Session Agenda

- Didactic Lesson: *Asking for a Turn* (20 minutes).
- Group Behavioral Rehearsal Activity 1: *Duck, Duck, Goose* (15 minutes).
- Break Time (10 minutes).
- Group Behavioral Rehearsal Activity 2: *Swap Draw* (15 minutes).
- Parent Coached Play: *Dyadic Playdates* (20 minutes).
- Final Wrap-Up (10 minutes).

Snapshot of the Lesson: Asking for a Turn

The objective of this lesson is to teach children how to ***ask for a turn***. Steps for ***asking for a turn*** include:

1. ***Look at your friend with your eyes*** (point to your eyes).
2. ***Smile with your mouth*** (point to your mouth and smile).
3. ***Say "Can I have a turn please?" using names.***

Materials Needed

- Cow puppet.
- Lion puppet.
- Toy plane.
- Carpet squares or chairs.
- "Making Friends Helper" badge.
- Star chart with names of children.
- Marker for star chart.
- Name tags for families and treatment team.
- Prize bins with prizes.

Preparing for the Lesson

- Follow the script below with the group leader using a cow puppet to play the part of "Kelly Cow."
- A behavioral coach member uses a lion puppet to play the part of "Larry Lion."

- An additional behavioral coach assists in the behavioral rehearsal and provides encouragement and feedback to the group.
- A child is chosen at the beginning of the lesson as the "Making Friends Helper."
  - The "Making Friends Helper" wears a special badge and is the first child to practice the skill.
- The group leader and the behavioral coach sit on the floor at the front of the room.
- A special-colored carpet square (e.g., red) is placed at the front of the room next to the group leader to be used as the "Good Friend Square."
- For the children, additional carpet squares of the same color (e.g., green) are placed in a semi-circle facing the group leader and the "Good Friend Square."
- Note: If carpet squares are unavailable, the children and behavioral coaches may sit on chairs.
- The material in *italics* should be read by the indicated person.
- The material in ***bold and italics*** represents buzzwords and should be emphasized when read.
- The material in CAPITAL LETTERS with the script should be given extra emphasis while the group is encouraged to say the words in unison.

Behavioral Coaching Techniques

Behavioral coaches should use the following coaching techniques described below throughout the lesson and the behavioral rehearsal activities. (Note: ***priming*** occurs during the introduction to the activity.)

- ***Prompting***
  - Use the buzzwords to ***prompt*** the children to ***ask for a turn*** IN THE MOMENT.
    - Example: *"Remember to ask for a turn."*
    - Example: *"Where should you look when you ask for a turn?"*
    - Example: *"What should you say if you want a turn?"*
- ***Praising***
  - Reinforce ***asking for a turn*** by ***praising*** the children when they use the skills CORRECTLY.
    - Example: *"Great job asking for a turn!"*
    - Example: *"Great job saying, 'Can I have a turn please?'"*
    - Example: *"Good job using names when you asked for a turn!"*
- ***Providing corrective feedback using a praise sandwich***
  - Reinforce ATTEMPTS to ***ask for a turn*** by ***praising*** the children and identifying what could be done differently next time.
    - Example: *"Good job asking for a turn. Remember to look next time, but nice job!"*
    - Example: *"Nice try asking for a turn. Remember to say, 'Can I have a turn please?' next time, but good try!"*
    - Example: *"Great job asking for a turn. Don't forget to use names next time, but good job!"*
- Continue to provide ***social coaching*** on previously learned skills:
  - ***Listening and following directions.***
  - ***Meeting and greeting friends.***
  - ***Sharing and giving a turn.***

Didactic Lesson: Asking for a Turn (20 Minutes)

Have the children sit in a semi-circle on the carpet squares facing the group leader.

Kelly Cow: (Sit at the front of the room and choose a Making Friends Helper.) "*Who wants to be our Making Friends Helper?*"

(Choose from among the children raising their hands and place the "Making Friends Helper" badge on the child. The child stays in their seat for now.)

"*Hi friends! I'm Kelly Cow. Moo, moo! Today we're going to practice asking for a turn. Asking for a turn is a great way to be nice to our friends!*"

"*Who should we ask for a turn with? We should ask for a turn with our FRIENDS, TEACHERS, MOMMIES, DADDIES, BROTHERS, AND SISTERS.*"

"*When should we ask for a turn? We should ask for a turn when we want to play with our friends' toys or games.*"

"*How should we ask for a turn? We should ask for a turn by looking at our friends with our* (point to your eyes and then Kelly Cow's eyes)*...EYES, smiling with our* (point to your mouth and smile)*...MOUTH, and then saying, 'Can I have a turn please?' And don't forget to use* (pause briefly to prompt the children to say *"names"*)*...NAMES.*"

"*Remember, asking for a turn is a nice way to be a good friend! Moo, moo!*"

Role Play: Asking for a Turn

Larry Lion and Kelly Cow: (Larry Lion plays with the toy plane. Kelly Cow does not have a toy and is watching Larry Lion play.)

Larry Lion: (Comment to self while flying the toy plane.) *"Whoa! This plane is so cool! Grrr, Grrr!"*

Kelly Cow: (Turn to look at the group of children.) *"Hey friends! My friend Larry Lion is playing with a cool plane. I wish I could play with it, too. Do you think I should ask Larry Lion for a turn?"* (Nod your head yes and encourage the children to say *"yes."*)

Kelly Cow: *"That's a great idea! Moo, moo! Let's do it!* (Turn to look at Larry Lion and smile.) *Larry Lion* (point to the toy plane), *can I have a turn please?"*

Larry Lion:	(Turn to look at Kelly Cow and smile.) *"Okay, here Kelly Cow."* (Hand the plane to Kelly Cow.)
Kelly Cow:	*"Thanks, Larry Lion!* (Turn to look at the group of children.) *Hey friends, did I do a good job asking for a turn?"* (Nod your head yes and encourage the children to say *"yes.")* *"That's right! Moo, moo!"*
Kelly Cow and Larry Lion:	(Say *"good job," give a "cow high-five" and "lion high-five,"* clap, cheer, and encourage the children to clap as well. Larry Lion sits on the other side of the Good Friend Square (i.e., the Good Friend Square is between Kelly Cow and Larry Lion). (Kelly Cow ***social coaches*** the children as needed while they practice ***asking for a turn*** with Larry Lion.)
Kelly Cow:	*"Now let's see _____ (behavioral coach) try! _____ (behavioral coach), please come sit on the Good Friend Square."*
Behavioral coach:	(Sit on the Good Friend Square.)
Kelly Cow:	"*_____ (Behavioral coach), can you show us how to ask for a turn with Larry Lion?*"
Behavioral coach:	*"Okay, Kelly Cow."*
Kelly Cow:	(Turn to look at the group of children.) "*Remember to look at Larry Lion with your* (point to your eyes to prompt children to say "*eyes*")*…EYES, smile with your* (point to your mouth to prompt children to say "*mouth*")*…MOUTH, and then say, 'Larry Lion, can I have a turn please?' And don't forget to use* (pause briefly to prompt the children to say *"names"*)*...NAMES.*"
Larry Lion:	(Comment to self while flying the toy plane.) *"Whoa! This plane is so* *cool! Grrr, Grrr!"*
Behavioral coach:	(Turn to look at Larry Lion and smile.) *"Larry Lion* (point to the toy plane), *can I have a turn please?"*
Larry Lion:	(Turn to look at the behavioral coach member and smile.) *"Okay, here _____ (behavioral coach). Grrr, Grrr!"* (Hand the plane to the behavioral coach member.)
Behavioral coach:	*"Thanks, Larry Lion!"*
Kelly Cow:	*"Great job asking for a turn, _____ (behavioral coach)! Moo, moo!"*

Larry Lion and Behavioral coach: (Say *"good job," give a "cow high-five"* and *"lion high-five,"* clap, cheer, and encourage the children to clap as well.)

Behavioral coach: (Return the toy plane to Larry Lion and leave the Good Friend Square.)

Behavioral Rehearsal: Asking for a Turn

Kelly Cow: (Turn to look at the group of children.) *"Okay friends! Now let's see our Making Friends Helper _____ try! _____ (Making Friends Helper), come sit on the Good Friend Square and show us how to ask for a turn with Larry Lion."*

(The Making Friends Helper should sit on the Good Friend Square.)

"Remember to look at Larry Lion with your (point to your eyes to prompt children to say *"eyes"*)*...EYES, smile with your* (point to your mouth to prompt children to say *"mouth"*)*...MOUTH, and then say, 'Larry Lion, can I have a turn please?' And don't forget to use* (pause briefly to prompt the children to say *"names"*)*...NAMES."*

Larry Lion: (Comment to self while flying the toy plane.) *"Whoa! This plane is so cool! Grrr, Grrr!"*

Kelly Cow: (If needed, ***social coach*** the Making Friends Helper to ***look*** at Larry Lion, ***smile***, and ***say, "Larry Lion, can I have a turn please?"***)

Larry Lion: (Turn to look at the Making Friends Helper and smile.) *"Okay, here ____ (Making Friends Helper). Grrr, Grrr!"* (Hand the toy plane to the Making Friends Helper.)

Kelly Cow: *"Great job asking for a turn, ____ (Making Friends Helper)! Moo, moo!"*

(Say *"good job," give a "cow high-five"* and *"lion high-five,"* clap, cheer, and encourage the children to clap as well. The Making Friends Helper should return the toy plane to Kelly Cow.)

"Okay, Making Friends Helper, choose another friend to sit on the Good Friend Square." (If needed, ***social coach*** the Making Friends Helper to choose another child before returning to their seat.)

Repeat the following with each child:

Kelly Cow: (Have each child take turns sitting on the Good Friend Square and practicing ***asking for a turn*** with Larry Lion.)

(Turn to look at the group of children.) *"Okay friends! Now let's see ____ (Child) try! ____ (Child), come sit on the Good Friend Square and show us how to ask for a turn with Larry Lion."*

(The child should sit on the Good Friend Square.) "*Remember to look at Larry Lion with your* (point to your eyes to prompt children to say *"eyes"*)*...EYES, smile with your* (point to your mouth to prompt children to say *"mouth"*)*...MOUTH, and then say, 'Larry Lion, can I have a turn please?' And don't forget to use* (pause briefly to prompt the children to say *"names"*)*...NAMES.*"

Larry Lion: (Comment to self while flying the toy plane.) *"Whoa! This plane is so cool! Grrr, Grrr!"*

Kelly Cow: (If needed, ***social coach*** the child to ***look, smile,*** and ***say, "Larry Lion, can I have a turn please?"*** to Larry Lion.)

Larry Lion: (Turn to look at the child and smile.) *"Okay, here ____ (Child). Grrr, Grrr!"* (Hand the toy plane to the child.)

Kelly Cow: *"Great job asking for a turn, ____ (Child)! Moo, moo!"*

(Say *"good job,"* give a *"cow high-five"* and *"lion high-five,"* clap, cheer, and encourage the children to clap as well. The child should return the toy plane to Larry Lion.)

"Okay, ____ (child), choose another friend to sit on the Good Friend Square." (If needed, ***social coach*** the child to choose another child before returning to their seat.)

Didactic Lesson Wrap-Up

Group leader: "*Well friends, you all did a great job asking for a turn by looking at your friend with your* (point to your eyes to prompt children to say *"eyes"*)*... EYES, smiling with your* (point to your mouth to prompt children to say *"mouth"*)*...MOUTH, and saying, 'Can I have a turn please?' And great job using* (pause briefly to prompt the children to say *"names"*)*...NAMES!*"

Group leader: *"You each earned ____ (number) stars for asking for a turn! Let's start with ____ (Child)."*

Award each child the same number of stars by repeating the following with each child:

Group leader: "*Where's ____ (Child)?"* (Wait until all the children are looking at the child.)

"____ *(Child), how many stars did you earn?*" (Pause briefly to allow the child to respond.)

"*That's* right*! Let's all count for ____ (Child)! One, two, three…* (add stars to the Star Chart as they are counted aloud)*! Everybody clap for ____ (Child)!*" (All behavioral coaches clap and cheer and encourage the children to clap as well.)

Session 4 Continued

Duck, Duck, Goose

BEHAVIORAL REHEARSAL ACTIVITY 1

Materials Needed

- None.

Room Setup

- Remove or place all carpet squares to the side.
- The group leader stands at the front of the room facing the children.
- The children and behavioral coaches sit in a circle on the floor.

Rules: Duck, Duck, Goose

- The group leader reads the script below to explain the rules.
- The group leader chooses a child to be a "*farmer.*"
- The *farmer* walks around the circle, softly tapping each child on the head while saying, "*duck.*"
  - The group leader walks next to the *farmer* to **social coach** as needed.
- The *farmer* randomly selects a child by tapping the child's head and saying, "*goose!*"
- The "*goose*" stands up and chases the *farmer* around the circle.
- The *farmer* runs around the circle and tries to sit in the *goose's* seat without being tagged.
- To continue the game, the *goose* is the next *farmer* and ***asks for a turn*** from the current *farmer.*
  - The purpose of the game is to practice ***asking for a turn*** and ***sharing and giving a turn*** rather than to eliminate group members.
- The next *farmer* ***asks for a turn*** by saying, "_______ ***(Child), can I have a turn please?"***
- The current *farmer* ***shares and gives a turn*** by saying, **"*Okay,* _______ *(child).*"**
- To ensure all children have an opportunity to ***ask for a turn***, help the current *farmer* choose which child will be the *goose* based on various attributes.
  - Example: "*Let's choose a friend who wears glasses. Who is wearing glasses?*"
  - Example: "*Let's choose a friend wearing red shoes. Which friend is wearing red shoes?*"

Behavioral Rehearsal: Duck, Duck, Goose (15 Minutes)

The group leader leads the activity. The behavioral coaches and children sit in a circle on the floor while the group leader explains the rules.

Group leader: *"Hey friends, now we're going to play a game called Duck, Duck, Goose. One friend will be the farmer. The farmer walks around the circle, taps our heads, and says, 'duck, duck…'* (Demonstrate by tapping two children on the head while saying *"duck."*) *If the farmer taps your head and says, 'goose,' get up and chase the farmer around the circle.* (Demonstrate running around the circle.) *The farmer will run around the circle and will try to sit in your seat before being tagged. If your head was tapped, you'll be the next farmer. Then do you think it would be a good idea to ask for a turn?"* (Nod your head yes and encourage the children to say *"yes."*)

"That's right, friends! And remember to ask for a turn by looking at your friends with your (point to your eyes to prompt children to say *"eyes"*)*… EYES, smiling with your* (point to your mouth to prompt children to say *"mouth"*)*…MOUTH, and saying, 'Can I have a turn please?' And don't forget to use* (pause briefly to prompt the children to say *"names"*)*…NAMES."*

"And when you share and give a turn, remember to say 'okay' while using names. Okay, _____ (behavioral coaches 1 and 2) will go first!"

Role Play: Duck, Duck, Goose

The group leader leads the role play. The two behavioral coaches demonstrate how to play *Duck, Duck, Goose*.

Group leader:	*"____ (Behavioral coach 1), you're our first farmer. Are you ready?"*
Behavioral coach 1:	*"Yes, ____ (group leader)."* (Walk around the circle and softly tap the heads of the children while saying *"duck."* Then tap behavioral coach 2 on the head and say, *"Goose!")*
Behavioral coach 1 and 2:	(Run around the circle. Behavioral coach 1 (the *farmer*) sits down in the seat of behavioral coach 2 before being tagged.)
Group leader:	*"Great job playing ____ (behavioral coaches 1 and 2)! ____ (Behavioral coach 2), you're the next farmer. Remember to ask for a turn by looking at your friends with your eyes, smiling with your mouth, and saying, ____ (behavioral coach 1), can I have a turn please?' And ____ (behavioral coach 1), remember to share and give a turn by saying, 'Okay, ____ (behavioral coach 2)'. And don't forget to use names."*
Behavioral coach 2:	(Look and smile at behavioral coach 1.) *"____ (Behavioral coach 1), can I have a turn please?"*
Behavioral coach 1:	*"Okay, ____ (behavioral coach 2)."*
Group leader:	*"Great job asking for a turn and sharing and giving a turn! Okay friends, now it's everybody's turn to play Duck, Duck, Goose."*

Behavioral Rehearsal: Duck, Duck, Goose

Group leader: *"Our next farmer is ____ (child). Remember to ask for a turn by looking at your friends with your eyes, smiling with your mouth, and saying, ____ (behavioral coach 2), can I have a turn please?' And ____ (behavioral coach 2), remember to share and give a turn by saying, 'Okay, ____ (child)'. And don't forget to use names."*

(If needed, ***social coach*** the child acting as the *farmer* to ***look*** and ***smile*** at behavioral coach 2 and ***say, "____ (Behavioral coach 2), can I have a turn please?"***)

Behavioral coach 2: *"Okay, ____ (child)."*

Group leader: *"Great job asking for a turn and sharing and giving a turn! Let's keep playing. Are we ready?"* (If needed, ***social coach*** the child acting as the *farmer* to follow the rules for *Duck, Duck, Goose.)*

"Great job playing (children)! ____ (second child), you're the next farmer. Remember to ask for a turn by looking at your friends with your eyes, smiling with your mouth, and saying, '_______ (first child), can I have a turn please?' And ____ (first child), remember to share and give a turn by saying, 'Okay, ____ (second child).' And don't forget to use names."

Continue in the manner described above making sure all the children have equal opportunities to be the *farmer*.

Behavioral Rehearsal Wrap-Up

Group leader: *"Well friends, great job asking for a turn and sharing and giving a turn! Give yourselves a big round of applause!"* (All behavioral coaches clap and cheer and encourage the children to clap as well.)

"Now everyone should come sit in the Listening Circle." (Have children return to the Listening Circle to sit on their carpet squares.)

"Okay friends, you did a great job asking for a turn by looking at your friends with your (point to your eyes to prompt children to say *"eyes"*)...*EYES, smiling with your* (point to your mouth to prompt children to say *"mouth"*)... *MOUTH, and saying, 'Can I have a turn please?' And nice job using* (pause briefly to prompt the children to say *"names"*)...*NAMES!"*

"You each earned ____ (number) more stars for asking for a turn! Let's start with ____ (Child)."

Award each child the same number of stars by repeating the following with each child:

Group leader: *"Where's _____ (child)?"* (Wait until all the children are looking at the child.)

"_____ (Child), how many stars did you earn?" (Pause briefly to allow the child to respond.)

"That's right! Let's all count for _____ (child)! One, two, three... (add stars to the Star Chart as they are counted aloud)*! Everybody clap for _____ (child)!"* (All behavioral coaches clap and cheer and encourage the children to clap as well.)

Break Time (10 Minutes)

- The puppets may be used to lead the children to and from the bathroom during break time.
- To assist with transitions and limit unstructured time, behavioral coaches may review the lesson with the children while waiting for the remaining children to return from the bathroom.
- You may want to award stars for good behavior after returning from the bathroom.

Session 4 Continued

Swap Draw

BEHAVIORAL REHEARSAL ACTIVITY 2

Materials Needed

- Drawing paper (approximately four to five sheets per group).
- Coloring tools (approximately three to four per group).
  - Examples: washable markers, crayons, and colored pencils.
- Tables or hard, flat surfaces to draw on.

Room Setup

- Organize tables or drawing surfaces around the room with three to five chairs around each table.
- Place sets of paper and coloring tools on the tables or drawing surfaces, providing enough space for children and at least one behavioral coach to sit around the materials.
- The group leader sits on the floor at the front of the room to begin.
- The children and behavioral coaches sit on the floor in a semi-circle facing the group leader to receive instructions.

Rules: Swap Draw

- The group leader reads the script below to explain the rules.
- The group leader divides the children into dyads.
  - If there is an odd number of children, pair one child with a behavioral coach.
  - Assign at least one behavioral coach per dyad to ***social coach***.
- Direct each group to sit at a table around the set of drawing materials.
- Behavioral coaches should ***social coach*** the children to ***share and give a turn*** by picking one child to choose the first theme to be drawn.
  - Behavioral coaches may need to help the children identify a theme.
- Behavioral coaches place one piece of paper and the coloring tools in front of the chosen child and instruct the child to begin drawing.
- If needed, behavioral coaches should ***social coach*** the second child to watch as the first child draws.
- Behavioral coaches help facilitate positive play interactions by asking questions and making comments (e.g., *"What do you think _______ (first child) is drawing?"* or *"That's so cool!"*).
- After approximately 30 seconds, behavioral coaches should prepare the children for the upcoming swap during which the children practice ***asking for a turn*** and ***sharing and giving a turn*** (e.g., *"Okay friends, we're going to swap in 5 seconds"*).

- After approximately 5 additional seconds, behavioral coaches instruct the children to swap materials.
- The child that was watching then ***asks for a turn***, and the child that was drawing ***shares and gives a turn*** by handing the paper and coloring tools to the other child.
- The children continue to draw on the shared piece of paper following the same drawing theme.

Table 4.1 Examples of Drawing Themes

Outer space	Beach	Schoolyard
Home	Friends	Family
Farm	Zoo	Jungle
Playground	Park	Swimming pool
Dinosaurs	Animals	Under the sea

- Repeat the cycle every 30 seconds.
- After approximately five minutes, behavioral coaches should ***social coach*** the children to ***share and give a turn*** by allowing the other child to choose the theme for the next drawing.
- Behavioral coaches provide new paper to the children each time a new theme is chosen.

Behavioral Rehearsal: Swap Draw (15 Minutes)

The group leader leads the activity. The children and behavioral coaches are sitting in a semi-circle facing the group leader as the rules are explained.

Group leader: *"Hey friends, now we're going to play Swap Draw. You'll get to draw some fun pictures with your friend, like the beach or the jungle or the park. But only one friend* (hold up one finger) *will draw at a time, so let's be a good friend by watching* (point to your eyes) *our friends draw. And remember to wait nicely. When you hear the word 'swap,' you'll practice asking for a turn or sharing and giving a turn. If you were waiting, you'll ask your friend for a turn by looking at your friend with your* (point to your eyes to prompt children to say *"eyes"*)...*EYES, smiling with your* (point to your mouth to prompt children to say *"mouth"*)...*MOUTH, and saying, 'Can I have a turn please?' And when our friends ask for a turn, do you think it's a good idea to share and give a turn?* (Nod your head yes and encourage the children to say *"yes."*)

"That's right friends! So remember if your friend asks for a turn, you should share and give a turn by saying 'okay.' And don't forget to use (pause briefly to prompt the children to say '*names*')...*NAMES. Okay, let's play Swap Draw!"*

Place children into dyads with at least one behavioral coach.

Behavioral coach: *"Okay friends, let's practice sharing and giving a turn by letting ____ (first child) choose the first picture we'll draw."* (If needed, ***social coach*** the children to ***share and give a turn***.)

After approximately 30 seconds, prepare the children to swap:

Behavioral coach: *"Okay friends, in about five seconds we're going to swap the paper and markers and practice asking for a turn and sharing and giving a turn."*

After approximately five additional seconds, have the children swap the drawing materials while continuing to add to the current drawing theme on the same sheet of paper:

Behavioral coach: *"And...swap!"* (If needed, ***social coach*** the children to ***ask for a turn*** and ***share and give a turn***. Then have the children swap the drawing materials.)

Repeat this cycle every 30 seconds for approximately five minutes before having the other child choose a new drawing theme with a new sheet of paper.

Behavioral coach: *"Friends, let's practice sharing and giving a turn by letting ____ (second child) choose the next picture we'll draw."* (If needed, ***social coach*** the children to ***share and give a turn***.)

Behavioral Rehearsal Wrap-Up

Group leader: *"Well friends, great job asking for a turn and sharing and giving a turn!*

Give yourselves a big round of applause!" (All behavioral coaches clap and cheer and encourage the children to clap as well.)

"Now everyone should come sit in the Listening Circle." (Have children return to the Listening Circle to sit on their carpet squares.)

"Okay friends, you did a great job asking for a turn by looking at your friends with your (point to your eyes to prompt children to say *"eyes"*)*...EYES, smiling with your* (point to your mouth to prompt children to say *"mouth"*)*... MOUTH, and saying, 'Can I have a turn please?' And nice job using* (pause briefly to prompt the children to say *"names"*)*...NAMES!"*

"You each earned ____ (number) more stars for asking for a turn! Let's start with ____ (Child)."

Award each child the same number of stars by repeating the following with each child:

Group leader: *"Where's _____ (child)?"* (Wait until all the children are looking at the child.)

"_____ (Child), how many stars did you earn?" (Pause briefly to allow the child to respond.)

"That's right! Let's all count for _____ (child)! One, two, three... (add stars to the Star Chart as they are counted aloud)*! Everybody clap for _____ (child)!"* (All behavioral coaches clap and cheer and encourage the children to clap as well.)

"Now we're going to play some games with our parents and practice sharing and giving a turn some more!"

Session 4 Continued

Asking for a Turn

PARENT COACHED PLAY: DYADIC PLAYDATES

Materials Needed

- Games brought by children and parents from home.
- Turn-taking games provided by the treatment team.
- Tables and chairs or carpet squares.
- *Parent Coached Play Cards.*

Room Setup

- If available, organize tables in separate corners of the room with four to six chairs per table.
- If tables are unavailable, place two carpet squares in separate corners of the room to indicate where the children will sit.

Rules: Dyadic Playdates

- The group leader divides the families into groups of two families each.
  - If there are an odd number of children, pair one child with a behavioral coach who will serve as a ***playmate***. In this case, you will need an additional coach to serve as a behavioral coach for the parent.
  - To avoid social exclusion, avoid having children play in triads as much as possible.
- Assign each group to sit at a table or specific play area.
  - Children should sit next to each other.
  - Parents will act as ***social coaches*** by sitting on the other side of their child to minimize interrupting the natural flow of play between the children.
  - One behavioral coach will be assigned to each dyad to provide ***social coaching*** suggestions and feedback to parents.
- Children will take turns playing the games brought from home or games provided by the treatment team.
- Each child will have ten minutes to play their chosen game with their ***playmate*** and then will switch games.
- Parents will choose which child's game will be played first.
- To minimize unstructured periods, parents will help the children set up the game in a cooperative fashion (handing game pieces to each other, offering suggestions, etc.).
- As they play, parents will ***social coach*** the children on previously learned and newly learned skills using the guidelines highlighted on the *Parent Coached Play Cards.*
- Behavioral coaches will provide support to parents in their ***social coaching*** using the ***4 Ps*** (***priming, prompting, praising,*** and ***providing corrective feedback***) and will model appropriate coaching behavior when necessary.

- After approximately nine minutes of play, instruct the parents to prepare the children for the upcoming game swap.
- After approximately one additional minute of play (ten minutes total), instruct the parents to have the children clean up and swap games.
- Repeat the cycle with the second game for the remaining ten minutes before returning to the *Listening Circle*.

Behavioral Coaching: Dyadic Playdates

Behavioral coaches will ***social coach*** parents during dyadic ***playdates*** in the following ways:

- ***Priming***:
  - Begin the play interactions with parents going over the rules for ***asking for a turn*** BEFORE GAME PLAYING.
    - Example: "*Remember that before playing games with your friend we want you to ask for a turn by looking at your friend with your* (point to your eyes to prompt children to say *"eyes"*)...*EYES, smiling with your* (point to your mouth to prompt children to say *"mouth"*)...*MOUTH, and then saying, 'Can I have a turn please?' And don't forget to use* (pause briefly to prompt the children to say *"names"*)...*NAMES.*"
- ***Prompting***:
  - Remind parents to use the buzzwords to ***prompt*** their child to ***ask for a turn*** IN THE MOMENT.
  - Help parents to identify opportunities to proactively ***prompt*** their child to ***ask for a turn***.
    - Example: "*Remember to ask for a turn.*"
    - Example: "*Where should you look when you ask for a turn?*"
    - Example: "*What should you say if you want a turn?*"
  - Assisting parents to follow through with the ***prompts*** they present to their child.
- ***Praising***:
  - Remind parents to praise and reinforce their child whenever their child ***asks for a turn*** CORRECTLY.
    - Example: "*Great job asking for a turn!*"
    - Example: "*Great job saying, 'Can I have a turn please?'*"
    - Example: "*Good job using names when you asked for a turn!*"
- ***Providing corrective feedback using a praise sandwich***:
  - Remind parents to ***praise*** their child's ATTEMPTS to ***ask for a turn*** and identify what could be done differently next time.
    - Example: "*Good job asking for a turn. Remember to look next time, but nice job!*"
    - Example: "*Nice try asking for a turn. Remember to say, 'Can I have a turn please?' next time, but good try!*"
    - Example: "*Great job asking for a turn. Don't forget to use names next time, but good job!*"
- Remind parents to continue to ***social coach*** on previously learned skills:
  - ***Listening and following directions.***
  - ***Meeting and greeting friends.***
  - ***Sharing and giving a turn.***

Parent Coached Play: Dyadic Playdates (20 Minutes)

- Have each child choose a turn-taking game brought from home or provided by the treatment team.
- The group leader sits on the floor at the front of the room.
- The families sit on the floor in a semi-circle facing the group leader.

Group leader: "*Hey friends, we're going to have more playdates and play with the fun games you brought from home. While you play, we want you to practice asking for a turn by looking at your friend with your* (point to your eyes to prompt children to say *"eyes"*)*...EYES, smiling with your* (point to your mouth to prompt children to say *"mouth"*)*...MOUTH, and saying, 'Can I have a turn please? And if your friend asks for a turn, do you think we should share and give a turn?*" (Pause briefly to allow the children to respond "*yes*.")

"*That's right, friends! Remember to share and give a turn by saying, 'Okay, it's your turn' or 'Okay, here.' And don't forget to use names when you ask for a turn and share and give a turn. Parents, remember to social coach your children by using your Parent Coached Play Cards. Okay, let's play with our games!*"

- Before playing, parents will ***social coach*** their child to say, "***What's your name?***" and then ***say their name*** if their ***playmate's*** name is unknown. Parents will also ***social coach*** their child to ***say*** "***hi***" to one another ***using names***.
- Parents will ***social coach*** their children to ***ask for a turn*** and ***share and take turns*** throughout the game playing.
- After approximately nine minutes of play, instruct the parents to prepare the children for the upcoming game swap by saying, "*Parents, tell your children that we'll be swapping games in one minute.*"
- After approximately one additional minute of play (ten minutes total), instruct the parents to swap games by saying, "*Parents, it's time to swap games. Social coach the children to ask for a turn and share and give a turn before playing the next game.*"
- After approximately nine minutes of playing the second game, instruct the parents to prepare the children for clean up by saying, "*Parents, tell your children that we'll be cleaning up in one minute.*"
- After approximately one additional minute of play (ten minutes total), ***prompt*** the parents to instruct their children to clean up by saying, "*Parents, it's time to clean up. Let's social coach the children to listen and follow directions by cleaning up and then say 'bye' to their friend using names before sitting in the Listening Circle.*"
- If needed, parents will ***social coach*** their child to ***listen and follow directions*** to clean up.
- Then parents will ***social coach*** their child to ***say*** "***bye***" to their friend ***using names***.

Final Wrap-Up (10 Minutes)

- The group leader sits on the floor at the front of the room.
- The children sit on the carpet squares in a semi-circle facing the group leader, with parents sitting behind their children.

Group leader: *"Okay friends, you all did a great job playing your games and asking for a turn. When we're asking for a turn, do you think we should LOOK with our EYES and SMILE with our MOUTH?"* (Pause briefly to allow the children to say *"yes."*)

"That's right, friends! And when we're asking for a turn, do you think we should take our friend's toy without asking?" (Demonstrate swiftly taking away a toy and pause for the children to say *"no."*)

"That's right friends! Instead, do you think we should say, 'Can I have a turn please?' and use names?" (Pause briefly to allow the children to say *"yes."*)

"That's right, friends! You all did such a great job asking for a turn today that you each earned ____ (number) more stars! Let's start with ____ (child)."

Award each child the same number of stars by repeating the following with each child:

Group leader: *"Where's _____ (child)?"* (Wait until all the children are looking at the child.)

"_____ (child), how many stars did you earn?" (Pause briefly to allow the child to respond.)

"That's right! Let's all count for _____ (child)! One, two, three... (add stars to the Star Chart as they are counted aloud)*! Everybody clap for _____ (child)!"* (All behavioral coaches clap and cheer and encourage the children to clap as well.)

"And remember you all earned those stars by asking for a turn and sharing and giving a turn! Everyone did a great job, and parents, you did an excellent job social coaching! Parents, remember your homework assignments this week are for you and your children to practice asking for a turn and to continue practicing all the other things we've learned to be a good friend using the 4 Ps. And don't forget to investigate and begin to enroll your children in playgroups."

"Alright little friends, do you want to count our stars?" (Pause briefly to allow the children to respond *"yes."*)

"Let's all count together and see how many stars we earned today! One, two, three...(count the number of stars for one child)*!"*

"You each earned ____ (total number) stars today! Round of applause for our friends!" (All behavioral coaches should clap and cheer and encourage the families to clap as well.)

"Great job, friends! Don't forget to choose your reward before you leave. See you all next week!"

Session 4 Continued

Preparing for Playgroups and Asking for a Turn

PEERS® FOR PRESCHOOLERS: PARENT HANDOUT

Didactic Lesson: Preparing for Playgroups

Preview the 5 Ws with Your Child

- **WHO will be there?**
  - Point out other children that your child knows and likes that will be present or have been to the ***playgroup***.
    - Karate Example: Your child's older sibling went to the same karate class.
    - Swimming Example: Your child's preschool classmate will also be at the swimming class.
  - Point out positive relationships that the ***playgroup*** instructor may have with your child or persons that your child is familiar with and/or likes.
    - Karate Example: The karate instructor is a family member of a friend of your child.
    - Swimming Example: The swimming instructor is the physical education teacher of your child's sibling.
  - Once your child has attended the ***playgroup*** and other children are known:
    - Have your child identify which peers they would like to play with during the ***playgroup***.
    - Remind your child at drop-off which ***playmates*** they enjoy playing with.
    - Listen for recurring names of ***playmates*** your child mentions and name-drop them when talking about the ***playgroup.***

- **WHAT are the activities?**
  - The activities of the ***playgroup*** should be preferred activities for your child to make the experience rewarding and pleasurable.
    - Remind your child how much they enjoy the activity when referencing the ***playgroup.***
  - Preview games and activities with your child once the ***playgroup*** is chosen.
  - Practice games, activities, and playing with toys that may be new to your child.
    - Familiarize your child with the new games, activities, toys, or materials prior to the ***playgroup***.
      - Karate Example: Show them their karate uniform, drive them by the dojo.
      - Swimming Example: Show them their swimsuit and goggles, drive them by the pool.
    - Present the rules of the game or activity if unknown to your child.

- Karate Example: Listening, following directions, imitating, taking turns.
- Swimming Example: Listening, following directions, no running by the pool, no splashing others, no jumping into the pool.

▪ Highlight which elements of the game or activity that your child is already familiar with and/or does well.

- Karate Example: Good balance, excellent imitation skills.
- Swimming Example: Enjoyment of water, good ability to listen and follow directions.

▪ Pointing out these elements to your child may reduce your child's anxiety and increase excitement about the ***playgroup***.

- **WHERE will the playgroup take place?**
  - Mention the location of the ***playgroup*** if it is a familiar or preferred setting.
    - Karate Example: Karate classes take place at their favorite community recreation center.
    - Swimming Example: Swimming classes take place at the local YMCA where they have enjoyed other classes.

- **WHEN will the *playgroup* take place?**
  - Attempt to choose ***playgroups*** that do not interfere with other preferred activities.
    - Your child should not have to give up a favorite activity or pastime to attend the ***playgroup*** (e.g., your child must miss a recurring ***playdate*** to attend karate classes).
  - Try to limit the number of competing obligations for your child prior to attending the ***playgroup***.
    - Your child should not be overscheduled on the day they are to attend a ***playgroup*** (e.g., taking swimming classes after a long day of preschool and therapy).

- **HOW will you get your child to attend?**
  - Consider linking the ***playgroup*** to some other preferred activity or reward.
  - The reward should be contingent on meaningful participation in the ***playgroup***.
    - Karate Example: Visiting the park after karate.
    - Swimming Example: Getting ice cream after swimming classes.

Snapshot of the Lesson: Asking for a Turn

The objective for this lesson is to teach children how to ***ask for a turn***. Steps for ***asking for a turn*** include:

1. ***Look at your friend with your eyes*** (point to your eyes).
2. ***Smile with your mouth*** (point to your mouth and smile).
3. ***Say "Can I have a turn please?" using names***.

Homework Assignments

1. **Find a playgroup for your child.**
    - Investigate and begin to enroll your child in a ***playgroup*** using the criteria for a good ***playgroup***:
        - Meets regularly (preferably weekly).
        - Located close to your home.
        - Includes other children in the same age range and level of support needs as your child.
        - Includes informal time so that your child will have opportunities to interact and play with other children naturally.
        - Activities are based on your child's interests, likes, or hobbies.
        - Begins within the next few weeks.
        - Permits some parent involvement in order to facilitate peer interactions and organize ***playdates*** with other families.

2. **Practice asking for a turn.**
    - **Practice having your child *ask for a turn* this week during preferred and highly motivating activities while providing *social coaching* using the *4 Ps*.**
        - ***Priming***: Review the rules for ***asking for a turn*** with your child BEFORE PRACTICING.
        - ***Prompting***: Remind your child IN THE MOMENT to ***ask for a turn*** whenever the opportunities present.
        - ***Praising***: ***Praise*** your child for using the buzzwords whenever they ***ask for a turn*** CORRECTLY.
        - ***Providing corrective feedback***: ***Provide corrective feedback*** in the form of a ***praise sandwich*** whenever your child ATTEMPTS to ***ask for a turn.***
    - **Please send us a 30–60-second video of *social coaching* for *asking for a turn* with your child to be viewed during homework review.**
        - Please include:
            - Skills your child did well.
            - Skills you would like to work on with your child.

3. **Provide social coaching on previously learned skills.**
    - Continue providing ***social coaching*** to your child throughout the week using the ***4 Ps.***
    - Previous skills include:
        - ***Listening and following directions***.
        - ***Meeting and greeting friends***.
        - ***Sharing and giving a turn***.

4. **Bring a turn-taking game.**
    - Bring a turn-taking game that your child enjoys playing and can be played with the other children.

Session 4 Continued

Asking for a Turn

PEERS® FOR PRESCHOOLERS: PARENT COACHED PLAY CARD

Snapshot of the Lesson: Asking for a Turn

1. ***Look at your friend with your eyes*** (point to your eyes).
2. ***Smile with your mouth*** (point to your mouth and smile).
3. ***Say "Can I have a turn please?" using names***.

Priming BEFORE Game Playing

- Example: "*Remember to practice asking for a turn by looking at your friend with your* (point to your eyes to prompt children to say *"eyes"*)*...EYES, smiling with your* (point to your mouth to prompt children to say *"mouth"*)*...MOUTH, and saying, 'Can I have a turn please?' And don't forget to use names.*"

Prompting IN THE MOMENT

- Example: "*Remember to ask for a turn.*"
- Example: "*Where should you look when you ask for a turn?*"
- Example: "*What should you say if you want a turn?*"

Praising for CORRECT Use of Skills

- Example: "*Great job asking for a turn!*"
- Example: "*Great job saying, 'Can I have a turn please?'*"
- Example: "*Good job using names when you asked for a turn!*"

Providing Corrective Feedback for ATTEMPTS Using a Praise Sandwich

- Example: "*Good job asking for a turn. Remember to look next time, but nice job!*"
- Example: "*Nice try asking for a turn. Remember to say, 'Can I have a turn please?' next time, but good try!*"
- Example: "*Great job asking for a turn. Don't forget to use names next time, but good job!*"

- Continue to provide ***social coaching*** on previously learned skills:
  - ***Listening and following directions***.
  - ***Meeting and greeting friends***.
  - ***Sharing and giving a turn***.

Session 4 Continued

Preparing for Playgroups and Asking for a Turn

PEERS® FOR PRESCHOOLERS: PARENT HOMEWORK WORKSHEET

Child's Name:	*Parent's Name:*		*Date:*	
HOMEWORK ASSIGNMENTS	PRIMING (REVIEWING RULES BEFORE PRACTICE)	PROMPTING (IN THE MOMENT)	PRAISING (USING BUZZWORDS)	PROVIDING CORRECTIVE FEEDBACK (USING A PRAISE SANDWICH)
Asking for a turn				
Practice previous skills: • **Sharing and giving turns** • **Meeting and greeting friends** • **Listening and following directions**				
Playgroups Investigate and enroll in playgroup(s).	Which playgroups did you investigate and enroll in?			
Bring a turn-taking game	Did you bring a turn-taking game? YES or NO (Circle)		Which game did you bring?	

Please fill out this worksheet by describing what you did to complete the homework assignments. Worksheets will be collected during Homework Review at the next session of PEERS® for Preschoolers.

Session 5

Planning Playdates and Keeping Cool

PARENT SESSION THERAPIST GUIDE

Parent Session Agenda

- Homework Review (40 minutes).
- Didactic Lesson (20 minutes).
- Parent Coached Play (20 minutes).
- Final Wrap-Up (10 minutes).

Materials Needed

- Conference room with a large table and enough chairs for the parent group leader and all parents to sit comfortably around the table.
  - Avoid sitting in a circle without a table as this creates the atmosphere of group therapy.
- Name tags for parents and treatment team.
- *Parent Handouts* (for the current week and the previous weeks).
- *Parent Homework Worksheets* (for the current week and the previous weeks).
- *Parent Coached Play Cards* (for the current week and the previous weeks).
- *Attendance and Homework Compliance Sheets* for parent group leader.
- Pens for note-taking (consider having extra pens for parents who need them).

Homework Review (40 Minutes)

1. **Find a playgroup for your child.**
   - Confirm parents investigated and began to enroll their child in a ***playgroup.***
     - If the child is currently enrolled in appropriate ***playgroups*** with potential ***playmates***, they do not need to enroll in new ***playgroups***.
     - Confirm parents considered the criteria for a good ***playgroup***:
       - Meets regularly (preferably weekly).
       - Located close to their home.
       - Includes other children in the same age range and level of support needs as their child.
       - Includes informal time so that their child will have opportunities to interact and play with other children naturally.
       - Activities are based on their child's interests, likes, or hobbies.
       - Begins within the next few weeks.
       - Permits some parent involvement in order to facilitate peer interactions and organize ***playdates*** with other families.

DOI: 10.4324/9781003502968-6

2. **Practice asking for a turn.**
    - Review the 30–60-second video of ***social coaching*** for ***asking for a turn*** for each family. (For larger groups, you may need to review video recordings in two smaller groups with two different parent group leaders).
        - Have parents identify:
            - Skills their child did well.
            - Skills they would like to work on with their child.
        - Provide ***social coaching*** tips as appropriate for each family.
    - If parents did not send a video of ***social coaching***, confirm the following:
        - Parents practiced having their child ***ask for a turn*** during preferred and highly motivating activities while providing ***social coaching*** using the ***4 Ps.***
            - ***Priming:*** Reviewed the rules for ***asking for a turn*** with their child BEFORE PRACTICING.
            - ***Prompting:*** Reminded their child IN THE MOMENT to ***ask for a turn*** whenever the opportunity presented.
            - ***Praising: Praised*** their child using the buzzwords whenever they ***asked for a turn*** CORRECTLY.
            - ***Providing corrective feedback: Provided corrective feedback*** in the form of a ***praise sandwich*** whenever their child ATTEMPTED to ***ask for a turn***.

3. **Provide social coaching on previously learned skills.**
    - Confirm parents continued to provide ***social coaching*** to their child throughout the week using the ***4 Ps*** for previously learned skills:
        - ***Listening and following directions.***
        - ***Meeting and greeting friends.***
        - ***Sharing and giving turns.***

4. **Bring a turn-taking game.**
    - Confirm the following:
        - Brought a turn-taking game that their child enjoys playing and can be played with the other children. (To avoid distractions, these games should be left with the parents until *Parent Coached Play*.)

Didactic Lessons (20 Minutes)

PEERS® Neuroaffirming Pledge

- We value neurodiversity, acceptance, and authenticity.
- We honor the diverse ways people experience the world.
- We respect each person's unique perspectives and communication styles.
- We recognize there is no one right way to connect with others.
- If using the strategies taught in PEERS® feels like camouflaging or masking and/or they don't align with your goals or the goals of your family, then you do not have to use them.
- Learning and using the skills taught in PEERS® is a PERSONAL CHOICE.

Didactic Lesson: Planning Playdates

- Distribute *Parent Handouts*.
  - Sections in **bold print** come directly from the *Parent Handout*.
  - Terms that are ***bold and italicized*** are buzzwords and represent important concepts from the didactic lesson.
- Explain, *"Last week we discussed what you could do to prepare your child for their playgroups to enhance their interest in the experience and enrich their interactions with potential playmates. The hope is that eventually these playmates will become friends. One common way parents can assist their children in developing close friendships with playmates is by arranging playdates. Today, we're going to talk about how to plan for playdates with potential playmates."*

Consider the 5 Ws

- **WHO will attend the *playdate*.**
  - **Identify *potential playmates* for *playdates*.**
    - **Identify peers who get along well with your child.**
      - **Recall whom your child has been playing with consistently and nicely at school or their *playgroup(s)*.**
      - **You may want to talk to your child's teacher or daycare provider to identify *potential playmates*.**
    - **Consider how the *potential playmate* is likely to respond to your *social coaching* during the *playdate*.**
      - Children who are more oppositional and require behavior management may not be appropriate.
    - **Consider whether the parent(s) of the *potential playmate*:**
      - **Is someone you are comfortable and/or willing to interact with and disclose personal information to about your child (if relevant).**
      - **Will be open to your *social coaching*.**
        - You may be able to predict their openness by having observed how they reacted to your ***social coaching*** at school or daycare or during the ***playgroup***.
  - **Consider whether the parent(s) of the *potential playmate* will be present at the *playdate*.**
    - Some parents will want to be at the ***playdate*** (especially during the first few ***playdates***) and others will be fine dropping off their child at your home.
    - It may be easier to ***social coach*** your child during the ***playdate*** if the other parent is not present.
    - **If present, inform the parent that you will be more actively involved during the *playdate*, especially until the children become more comfortable with one another.**
      - Many parents expect to chat with adults and may be less involved during ***playdates***.
    - **Tips on ways to speak to other parents regarding your *social coaching* during *playdates*:**
      - **Acknowledge that the *playdate* may be different from what they are used to because of your *social coaching*.**
      - **Consider whether you want to disclose your child's diagnoses and/or social challenges, which is a personal choice.**

  - ***Playdates* should ideally be one-on-one.**
    - **Try to avoid or limit group activities or *playdates* with multiple children at first.**
    - **One-on-one *playdates* will allow parents to *social coach* more effectively.**
    - Group activities or ***playdates*** with multiple children may be overwhelming for your child, especially as they are attempting to use the newly learned skills and if they do not have regularly occurring ***playdates***.
  - **Avoid having siblings join the *playdate* if possible.**
    - **Try not to allow your child's siblings to join the *playdate* when possible.**
      - **Prearrange other *playdates* or activities for your child's siblings.**
      - **It may be more challenging to effectively *social coach* your child if other siblings are present.**
      - If sibling conflict is common, it may decrease opportunities for your child and their peers to sustain positive play interactions.
      - If the sibling is more socially adept, they may also take over the ***playdate***.
    - **Try to avoid having the *playmate's* siblings attend the *playdate.***
      - **Recall if siblings typically accompanied parents of *playmates* to school, daycare, or the *playgroup.***
        - **If so, siblings are also likely to be present during the *playdate.***
    - **If other parents and siblings will be present during the *playdate*, think about how you may need to adapt your *social coaching* and plan on having enough snacks, activities, and supplies available for everyone to participate.**

- **WHAT will the children do during the *playdate.***
  - ***Playdates* should be activity-based.**
    - **"Free play" or "down time" is not an activity.**
      - Unstructured activities can be particularly difficult for children with social challenges.
    - **Activities should be based on the *common interests* of your child and their *playmate.***
      - ***Common interests* are those games and activities that are fun for BOTH your child and their *playmate.***
        - **Choose games or activities your child and their *playmate* commonly play at school or daycare or during the *playgroup* if appropriate.**

- **WHEN will the *playdate* happen.**
  - **Identify the exact day and time of the *playdate* with the *playmate's* parent(s).**
  - **Try to keep initial *playdates* to no more than 1–1.5 hours.**
    - ***Playdates* can be longer as your child improves in their skills and has had more *playdates* with the *playmate.***
  - **Schedule *playdates* around routines (nap times, meals, etc.).**

- **WHERE will the *playdate* take place.**
  - **Identify the location of the *playdate* with the *playmate's* parent(s).**
  - **Schedule initial *playdates* to take place in your home if possible.**
    - **It will be easier to *social coach* if the *playdate* takes place in your home.**
    - **It may be less overwhelming for your child to be in a familiar environment at first.**
    - **If the *playdate* cannot be in your home, try to choose a location where you will have the opportunity to *social coach* your child.**

        - **Try to avoid having *playdates* in other children's homes initially as you will have less control over the activities.**
    - **Be present if the *playdate* will take place outside of the home.**
        - **You need to be present to provide *social coaching* in the moment.**
        - **Your presence will likely increase your child's comfort if in a new setting.**

- **HOW will the children get to and from the *playdate.***
    - **Arrange transportation to and from the *playdate* for your child and their *playmate* (if relevant).**
    - Offering to pick up the ***playmate*** will help ensure that the ***playdate*** happens.
    - Offering to drop off the ***playmate*** will help ensure that the ***playdate*** does not exceed the 1–1.5 hour limit.

Didactic Lesson: Keeping Cool

Explain, *"Last week the children learned how to ask for a turn. This week we're going to teach them how to keep cool. It's important that they practice keeping cool because sometimes their friends won't want to share or give turns or maybe even allow your children to join the game. If your child can keep cool in the moment rather than get angry or upset, they may be more likely to be accepted into future play interactions."*

Snapshot of the Lesson: Keeping Cool

The objective of this lesson is to teach children how to *keep cool.* Steps for *keeping cool* include:

1. ***Look at your friends with your eyes* (point to your eyes).**
2. ***Nicely say "okay" using names.***
3. ***Find something else to do.***
4. ***If you're still feeling upset, take deep breaths* to *keep cool* (take two slow *deep breaths*).**
    a. ***Smell the flowers* (example of breathing in).**
    b. ***Blow out the candles* (example of breathing out).**

Parent Coached Play

- Distribute the *Parent Coached Play Cards.*
- Review the examples of the ***4 Ps*** provided on the *Parent Coached Play Card.*
- Remind parents that in a few moments, we will be joining the children for *Parent Coached Play* in the context of mock dyadic ***playdates***.
- Parents should keep the *Parent Coached Play Card* in front of them during the dyadic ***playdate*** for recommendations on how to ***social coach*** children on ***keeping cool***.

Homework Assignments

(Briefly review the homework assignments and troubleshoot any potential problems with parents.)

1. **Identify playmates for playdates.**
   - **Parents should identify one or two *potential playmates* for a *playdate.***
     - **Pay attention to whether the children seem to like each other, play nicely together, and have *common interests.***
     - **Consider whether you would be comfortable and willing to interact with the parent(s) of the *potential playmate.***
     - **Consider whether the *potential playmate* and the parent(s) would be open to your *social coaching.***
   - **Parents should identify possible games and activities for the *playdate* based on the children's *common interests.***
   - **Note: Unless your child is already having successful *playdates* with these *playmates*, hold off on scheduling a *playdate* until we get through all the playdate lessons.**

2. **Playgroups.**
   - **If not yet accomplished, enroll your child in a *playgroup* using the criteria for a good *playgroup.***
   - **During the *playgroup*, parents should identify:**
     - ***Potential playmates* for *playdates.***
     - **Your compatibility with the parents of *potential playmates.***
     - **Which peers regularly attend the *playgroup.***
     - **Popular activities, games, or toys.**
     - **Whether this is a good *playgroup* for your child.**

3. **Practice keeping cool.**
   - **Practice having your child *keep cool* this week during preferred and highly motivating activities while providing *social coaching* using the *4 Ps.***
     - ***Priming:* Review the rules for *keeping cool* with your child BEFORE PRACTICING.**
     - ***Prompting:* Remind your child IN THE MOMENT to *keep cool* whenever the opportunities present.**
     - ***Praising: Praise* your child using the buzzwords whenever they *keep cool* CORRECTLY.**
     - ***Providing corrective feedback: Provide corrective feedback* in the form of a *praise sandwich* whenever your child ATTEMPTS to *keep cool.***
   - **Please send us a 30–60-second video of *social coaching* for *keeping cool* with your child to be viewed during homework review.**
     - **Please include:**
       - **Skills your child did well.**
       - **Skills you would like to work on with your child.**

4. **Provide social coaching on previously learned skills.**
    - **Continue providing *social coaching* to your child throughout the week using the *4 Ps*.**
    - **Previous skills include:**
        - ***Listening and following directions.***
        - ***Meeting and greeting friends.***
        - ***Sharing and giving a turn.***
        - ***Asking for a turn.***

5. **Bring a turn-taking game.**
    - **Bring a turn-taking game that your child enjoys playing and can be played with the other children.**

Session 5 Continued
Keeping Cool

CHILD SESSION THERAPIST GUIDE

Child Session Agenda

- Didactic Lesson: *Keeping Cool* (20 minutes).
- Group Behavioral Rehearsal Activity 1: *Mother, May I?* (15 minutes).
- Break Time (10 minutes).
- Group Behavioral Rehearsal Activity 2: *Musical Share Chairs* (15 minutes).
- Parent Coached Play: *Dyadic Playdates* (20 minutes).
- Final Wrap-Up (10 minutes).

Snapshot of the Lesson: Keeping Cool

The objective of this lesson is to teach children how to ***keep cool***. Steps for ***keeping cool*** include:

1. ***Look at your friends with your eyes*** (point to your eyes).
2. ***Nicely say "okay" using names***.
3. ***Find something else to do***.
4. ***If you're still feeling upset, take deep breaths to keep cool*** (take two slow ***deep breaths***).
   a. ***Smell the flowers*** (example of breathing in).
   b. ***Blow out the candles*** (example of breathing out).

Materials Needed

- Mouse puppet.
- Pig puppet.
- Toy car.
- Small animal figures.
- Carpet squares or chairs.
- "Making Friends Helper" badge.
- Star chart with names of children.
- Marker for star chart.
- Name tags for families and treatment team.
- Prize bins with prizes.

Preparing for the Lesson

- Follow the script below with the group leader using a mouse puppet to play the part of "Marty Mouse."
- A behavioral coach uses a pig puppet to play the part of "Penny Pig."

- An additional behavioral coach assists in the behavioral rehearsal and provides encouragement and feedback to the group.
- A child is chosen at the beginning of the lesson as the "Making Friends Helper."
  - The "Making Friends Helper" wears a special badge and is the first child to practice the skill.
- The group leader and the behavioral coach sit on the floor at the front of the room.
- A special-colored carpet square (e.g., red) is placed at the front of the room next to the group leader to be used as the "Good Friend Square."
- For the children, additional carpet squares of the same color (e.g., green) are placed in a semi-circle facing the group leader and the "Good Friend Square."
- Note: If carpet squares are unavailable, the children and behavioral coaches may sit on chairs.
- The material in *italics* should be read by the indicated person.
- The material in ***bold and italics*** represents buzzwords and should be emphasized when read.
- The material in CAPITAL LETTERS with the script should be given extra emphasis while the group is encouraged to say the words in unison.

Behavioral Coaching Techniques

Behavioral coaches should use the following coaching techniques described below throughout the lesson and the behavioral rehearsal activities. (Note: ***priming*** occurs during the introduction to the activity.)

- ***Prompting***:
  - Use the buzzwords to ***prompt*** the children to ***keep cool*** IN THE MOMENT.
    - Example: *"Remember to keep cool."*
    - Example: *"Remember to find something else to do if your friend isn't ready to share."*
    - Example: *"What should you do if you're still upset?"*
- ***Praising***:
  - Reinforce ***keeping cool*** by ***praising*** the children when they use the skills CORRECTLY.
    - Example: *"Great job keeping cool!"*
    - Example: *"Great job nicely saying 'okay'!"*
    - Example: *"Good job taking deep breaths to keep cool!"*
- ***Providing corrective feedback using a praise sandwich***:
  - Reinforce ATTEMPTS to ***keep cool*** by ***praising*** the children and identifying what could be done differently next time.
    - Example: *"Good job keeping cool. Remember to nicely say 'okay' next time, but nice job!"*
    - Example: *"Nice try keeping cool. Remember to take deep breaths if you're still upset next time, but good try!"*
    - Example: *"Nice job keeping cool. Don't forget to find something else to do next time, but good job!"*
- Continue to provide ***social coaching*** on previously learned skills:
  - ***Listening and following directions***.
  - ***Meeting and greeting friends***.
  - ***Sharing and giving a turn***.
  - ***Asking for a turn.***

Didactic Lesson: Keeping Cool (20 Minutes)

Have the children sit in a semi-circle on the carpet squares facing the group leader.

Marty Mouse: (Sit at the front of the room and choose a Making Friends Helper.) *"Who wants to be our Making Friends Helper?"*

(Choose from among the children raising their hands and place the "Making Friends Helper" badge on the child. The child stays in their seat for now.)

"Hi friends! I'm Marty Mouse. Squeak, squeak! Today we're going to practice keeping cool. Keeping cool is a great way to be nice to our friends!"

"Who should we keep cool with? We should keep cool with our FRIENDS, TEACHERS, MOMMIES, DADDIES, BROTHERS, AND SISTERS."

"When should we keep cool? We should keep cool when we're feeling sad or angry or upset, like when our friends don't share or when we don't get what we want."

"How should we keep cool? Instead of crying or yelling or hitting, we should look at our friend with our (point to your eyes and then Marty Mouse's eyes)*...EYES, nicely say 'okay' using our friend's name, and then find something else to do. If we're still feeling sad or angry or upset, we can take deep breaths* (demonstrate taking two ***deep breaths***) *to keep cool."*

"When we're breathing in it's like we're smelling the flowers. Can everyone show me smelling the flowers? (Pause briefly to allow the children and behavioral coaches to breathe in.) *Nice job smelling the flowers, friends!"*

"When we're breathing out it's like we're blowing out the candles on a birthday cake. Can everyone show me blowing out the candles? (Pause briefly to allow the children and behavioral coaches to breathe out.) *Nice job blowing out the candles, friends!"*

"Now can everybody show me taking two deep breaths in and out?" (Pause briefly to allow the children and behavioral coaches to take two ***deep breaths***.)

"Great job, friends! Remember, even though it can be hard, it's important to keep cool to be a good friend! Squeak, squeak!"

Role Play: Keeping Cool

Marty Mouse and Penny Pig:	(Marty Mouse looks at Penny Pig, who is nearby playing with a toy car. Penny Pig comments to herself while playing. The small animal figures are off to the side within an arm's reach of Marty Mouse.)
Marty Mouse:	(Turn to the group of children.) *"Hey friends! Squeak, squeak! I see my friend Penny Pig playing with a really cool car! I'm going to ask for a turn."* (Look at Penny Pig and smile.) *"Penny Pig, can I have a turn please?"*
Penny Pig:	(Ignore Marty Mouse and continue to play while commenting to yourself.)
Marty Mouse:	(Turn to look at the group of children.) *"Hey friends, it looks like Penny Pig isn't ready to share. Do you think I should cry or yell or hit?"* (Shake your head no and encourage the children to say *"no."*) *"That's right! Squeak, squeak! I should keep cool! Do you think I should nicely say 'Okay, Penny Pig,' and then find something else to do?"* (Nod your head yes and encourage the children to say *"yes."*) *"That's a great idea! Squeak, squeak! Let's do it!* (Look at Penny Pig and smile.) *Penny Pig, can I have a turn please?"*
Penny Pig:	(Look at Marty Mouse.) *"Maybe later. Oink, oink."*
Marty Mouse:	*"Okay, Penny Pig."*
Penny Pig:	(Continue to play with the toy car while commenting to yourself.)
Marty Mouse:	*"I'm going to find something else to do. I know! I'll play with these cool animals."* (Play with the animal figures for a few moments.) (Turn to look at the group of children and use a sad voice.) *"Hey friends, I'm still sad my friend Penny Pig wouldn't share. Do you think I should take some deep breaths to keep cool?"* (Nod your head yes and encourage the children to say *"yes."*) *"That's a great idea! Squeak, squeak! Let's do it together!"* (***Prompt*** the children to take two ***deep breaths*** in unison with you.) *"That was great, friends! I feel so much better! Squeak, squeak!"*
Marty Mouse and Penny Pig:	(Say *"good job," give a "mouse high-five"* and *"pig high-five,"* clap, cheer, and encourage the children to clap as well. Marty Mouse returns the animal figures to their original position. Penny Pig sits on the other side of the Good Friend Square (i.e., the Good Friend Square is between Marty Mouse and

Penny Pig). Marty Mouse ***social coaches*** the children as needed while they practice ***keeping cool*** with Penny Pig.)

Marty Mouse:	*"Now let's see _____ (behavioral coach) try! _____ (Behavioral coach), please come sit on the Good Friend Square."*
Behavioral coach:	(Sit on the Good Friend Square.)
Marty Mouse:	*"_____ (Behavioral coach), can you show us how to keep cool with Penny Pig?"*
Behavioral coach:	*"Okay, Marty Mouse."*
Marty Mouse:	(Turn to look at the group of children.) *"Remember, if Penny Pig doesn't want to share, you can keep cool by looking at Penny Pig with your* (point to your eyes to prompt children to say *"eyes"*)*…EYES, nicely saying 'Okay, Penny Pig,' and finding something else to do. And don't forget to take deep breaths to keep cool* (demonstrate taking two ***deep breaths***)*."*
Penny Pig:	(Play with the toy car while commenting to yourself.)
Behavioral coach:	(Look at Penny Pig and smile.) *"Penny Pig, can I have a turn please?"*
Penny Pig:	(Look at the behavioral coach member.) *"Maybe later. Oink, oink."* (Resume playing with the toy car while commenting to yourself.)
Behavioral coach:	(Look at Penny Pig.) *"Okay, Penny Pig."* (Turn to look at the group of children.) *"I'm going to find something else to do. I know! I'll play with these cool animals."* (Play with the animal figures while commenting to yourself for a few moments.) (Turn to look at the group of children.) *"Hey friends, I'm still sad my friend Penny Pig wouldn't share. I'll take some deep breaths to keep cool."* (Demonstrate taking two ***deep breaths*** and continue to play while commenting to yourself for a few moments.)
Marty Mouse:	(Look at the behavioral coach member and smile.) *"Great job keeping cool, _____ (behavioral coach)! Squeak, squeak!"*
Marty Mouse and Behavioral coach:	(Say *"good job," give a "mouse high-five"* and *"pig high-five,"* clap, cheer, and encourage the children to clap as well.)

Behavioral coach:	(Give the animal figures to Marty Mouse and leave the Good Friend Square.)
Marty Mouse:	(Place the animal figures within arm's reach of the Good Friend Square.)

Behavioral Rehearsal: Keeping Cool

Marty Mouse:	(Turn to look at the group of children.) *"Okay friends! Now let's see our Making Friends Helper _____ try! _____ (Making Friends Helper), come sit on the Good Friend Square and show us how to keep cool with Penny Pig."* (The Making Friends Helper should sit on the Good Friend Square.) *"Remember when you ask Penny Pig for a turn, if Penny Pig doesn't want to share, you can keep cool by looking at Penny Pig with your* (point to your eyes to prompt children to say *"eyes"*)*...EYES, nicely saying 'Okay, Penny Pig,' and finding something else to do. And don't forget to take deep breaths to keep cool."* (Demonstrate taking two ***deep breaths.***)
Penny Pig:	(Play with the toy car while commenting to yourself.)
Marty Mouse:	(If needed, ***social coach*** the Making Friends Helper to ***look, smile,*** and ***say "Penny Pig, can I have a turn please?"***)
Penny Pig:	(Look at the Making Friends Helper.) *"Maybe later. Oink, oink."* (Resume playing with the toy car while commenting to yourself.)
Marty Mouse:	(If needed, ***social coach*** the Making Friends Helper to look at Penny Pig, nicely ***say "Okay, Penny Pig," take two deep breaths***, and ***find something else to do*** by playing with the animal figures nearby.) *"Great job keeping cool, _____ (Making Friends Helper)! Squeak, squeak!"* (Say *"good job," give a "mouse high-five"* and *"pig high-five,"* clap, cheer, and encourage the children to clap as well. The Making Friends Helper should give the animal figures to Marty Mouse, who returns them to their original place.) *"Okay, Making Friends Helper, choose another friend to sit on the Good Friend Square."* (If needed, ***social coach*** the Making Friends Helper to choose another child before returning to their seat.)

Repeat the following with each child:

Marty Mouse:	(Have each child take turns sitting on the Good Friend Square and practicing ***keeping cool*** with Penny Pig.)

(Turn to look at the group of children.) *"Okay friends! Now let's see ____ (child) try! ____ (Child), come sit on the Good Friend Square and show us how to keep cool with Penny Pig."*

(The child should sit on the Good Friend Square.) *"Remember when you ask Penny Pig for a turn, if Penny Pig doesn't want to share, you can keep cool by looking at Penny Pig with your* (point to your eyes to prompt children to say *"eyes"*)*...EYES, nicely saying 'Okay, Penny Pig,' and finding something else to do. And don't forget to take deep breaths to keep cool."* (Demonstrate taking two ***deep breaths***.)

Penny Pig: (Play with the toy car while commenting to yourself.)

Marty Mouse: (If needed, ***social coach*** the child to ***look, smile,*** and ***say "Penny Pig, can I have a turn please?"***)

Penny Pig: (Look at the child.) *"Maybe later. Oink, oink."* (Resume playing with the toy car while commenting to yourself.)

Marty Mouse: (If needed, ***social coach*** the child to look, nicely ***say "Okay, Penny Pig," take two deep breaths***, and ***find something else to do*** by playing with the animal figures nearby.)

"Great job keeping cool, _____ (child)! Squeak, squeak!"

(Say *"good job," give a "mouse high-five"* and *"pig high-five,"* clap, cheer, and encourage the children to clap as well. The child should give the animal figures to Marty Mouse, who returns them to their original place.)

"Okay, ____ (child), choose another friend to sit on the Good Friend Square." (If needed, ***social coach*** the child to choose another child before returning to their seat.)

Didactic Lesson Wrap-Up

Group leader: *"Well friends, you all did a great job keeping cool by looking at Penny Pig with your* (point to your eyes to prompt children to say *"eyes")...EYES, nicely saying 'Okay, Penny Pig,' and finding something else to do. And nice job taking deep breaths to keep cool!"*

"You each earned ____ (number) stars for keeping cool! Let's start with ____ (child)."

Award each child the same number of stars by repeating the following with each child:

Group leader: *"Where's ____ (child)?"* (Wait until all the children are looking at the child.)

"____ (child), how many stars did you earn?" (Pause briefly to allow the child to respond.)

"That's right! Let's all count for ____ (child)! One, two, three... (add stars to the Star Chart as they are counted aloud)*! Everybody clap for ____ (child)!"* (All behavioral coaches clap and cheer and encourage the children to clap as well.)

Session 5 Continued

Mother, May I?

BEHAVIORAL REHEARSAL ACTIVITY 1

Materials Needed

- Safety cones or masking tape.

Room Setup

- Remove or place all carpet squares to the side.
- Use the safety cones or masking tape to delineate a *starting zone* at one end of the room and a *finishing zone* at the opposite end of the room.
- The group leader stands in the *finishing zone* facing the children.
- The children and behavioral coaches stand next to each other in the *starting zone* facing the group leader.

Rules: Mother, May I?

- The group leader reads the script below to explain the rules.
- The group leader always assumes the role of "Mother" (i.e., deciding whether a child may step forward) and stands in the *finishing zone.*
- The group leader chooses a child from the *starting zone* to begin the game.
- The chosen player asks the group leader if they may take a certain number of steps forward by saying, "*Mother, may I take ____ steps forward?*"
- Permit or do not permit the child to take steps forward.
  - If the children ask to take more than three steps, never permit the child to step forward to allow for sufficient practice opportunities.
- If permitted, the child takes the specified number of steps forward.
- If not permitted, the child remains in their place and practices ***keeping cool***.
- Call on each child individually to take a turn.
- Repeat this cycle with each child until a child reaches the *finishing zone.*
- Once a child reaches the *finishing zone*, restart the game.
- Consider modifying the game by describing the characteristics of the next chosen player and having the children guess who it is.
  - Examples: "The next player is someone…
    - …with brown hair."
    - …wearing green pants."
    - …with a dinosaur on their shirt."

- Consider modifying the game by introducing new ways to move forward.
    - Examples: Walk sideways like a crab, tip-toe like a cat, crawl like a baby, etc.

Behavioral Rehearsal: Mother, May I? (15 Minutes)

The group leader leads the activity from the *finishing zone*. The behavioral coaches and children sit on the floor at the *starting zone* while the group leader explains the rules.

Group leader: *"Hey friends, now we're going to play a game called 'Mother, May I'? You'll stand behind the starting zone* (point to the designated area) *and face me. I'm standing in the finishing zone* (point to the designated area). *When I call your name, you should ask me, 'Mother, may I take steps forward?' You can ask to take ONE step* (hold up one finger and take one step forward) *or TWO steps* (hold up two fingers and take two steps forward) *or THREE steps* (hold up three fingers and take three steps forward). *But you CAN'T ask to take more than three steps."*

"Sometimes I'll say 'yes' when you ask to step forward, and sometimes I'll say 'no' when you ask to step forward. If I say, 'Yes, you may,' (nod your head yes) *then you can say, 'Thanks, ____ (group leader)!' and take two steps forward like this* (take two steps forward).*"*

"But if I say, 'No, you may not,' (shake your head no)*, then you should stay in place and keep cool by looking at me with your* (point to your eyes to prompt children to say *"eyes"*)*...EYES, nicely saying 'Okay, ____ (group leader)' and taking deep breaths* (demonstrate taking two ***deep breaths***).*"*

"We'll play until one of our little friends reaches me at the finishing zone. Okay, _____ (behavioral coaches 1 and 2) go first!"

Role Play: Mother, May I?

The group leader leads the role play. The two behavioral coaches demonstrate how to play *Mother, May I* while the children sit and watch from the *starting zone*.

Group leader: *"____ (Behavioral coach 1), it's your turn. Are you ready?"*

Behavioral coach 1: *"Okay, ____ (group leader). Mother, may I take two steps forward?"*

Group leader: *"Yes, you may!"*

Behavioral coach 1: *"Thanks,* ____ (group leader)! (Take two small steps forward while counting aloud.) *One. Two."*

Group leader:	*"Great job using names and listening and following directions, ____ (behavioral coach 1)! ____ (Behavioral coach 2), it's your turn."*
Behavioral coach 2:	*"Okay, ____ (group leader). Mother, may I take one step forward?"*
Group leader:	*"No, you may not."*
Behavioral coach 2:	*"Okay, ____ (group leader)."* (Take two ***deep breaths***.)
Group leader:	*"Great job keeping cool, ____ (behavioral coach 2)!"*

(The group leader should alternate between saying *"yes"* and *"no"* until one of the behavioral coaches quickly reaches the *finishing zone.*)

"Great job listening and following directions and keeping cool, ____ (behavioral coaches 1 and 2)! Okay friends, now it's time for everyone to stand up and play Mother, May I. Are we ready?"

Behavioral Rehearsal: Mother, May I?

Group leader: *"____ (Child), it's your turn. Are you ready?"*

(If needed, ***social coach*** the child to look at the group leader and say, *"Mother, may I take ____ steps forward?"*)

(The group leader should alternate between saying *"yes"* and *"no"* until one of the children reaches the *finishing zone.* Always say *"no"* to any requests over three steps.)

(If needed, ***social coach*** the child to ***say "Okay, ____ (group leader)"*** and either take the appropriate steps forward or practice ***keeping cool*** by taking ***deep breaths***.)

(When the answer is *yes*, follow up by saying, *"Great job using names and listening and following directions, ____ (child)!"*)

(When the answer is *no*, follow up by saying, *"Great job keeping cool, ____ (child)!"*)

Be sure every child is told *"no"* at least once per round to practice ***keeping cool***. Continue in this manner until one of the children reaches the *finishing zone.*

Consider modifying the game by describing the characteristics of the next chosen player and having the children guess who it is by saying, *"The next player is someone with ____ (describe characteristic of the child). Who has ____ (describe characteristic)?"*

Group leader: Introduce new actions after the first round by saying, *"Okay friends, this time we're going to move forward by ____ (new movement).* (Demonstrate moving in the way described in the new action.) *Can everybody show me ____ (new movement)?"*

Table 5.1 Examples of New Movements

Walk like a crab	Hop on one foot	Hop like a bunny
Crawl like a baby	Tip-toe like a cat	Stomp like a giant
Walk backward	Hop like a frog	Jump like a kangaroo

Behavioral Rehearsal Wrap-Up

Group leader: *"Well friends, great job keeping cool and listening and following directions! Give yourselves a big round of applause!"* (All behavioral coaches clap and cheer and encourage the children to clap as well.)

"Now everyone should come sit in the Listening Circle." (Have children return to the Listening Circle to sit on their carpet squares.)

"Okay friends, you did a great job keeping cool by looking at me with your (point to your eyes to prompt children to say *"eyes")...EYES, nicely saying 'Okay, ____ (group leader),' and taking deep breaths!"* (Take two ***deep breaths***.)

"You each earned ____ (number) more stars for keeping cool! Let's start with ____ (child)."

Award each child the same number of stars by repeating the following with each child:

Group leader: *"Where's _____ (child)?"* (Wait until all the children are looking at the child.)

"_____ (Child), how many stars did you earn?" (Pause briefly to allow the child to respond.)

"That's right! Let's all count for _____ (child)! One, two, three... (add stars to the Star Chart as they are counted aloud)*! Everybody clap for _____ (child)!"* (All behavioral coaches clap and cheer and encourage the children to clap as well.)

Break Time (10 Minutes)

- The puppets may be used to lead the children to and from the bathroom during break time.
- To assist with transitions and limit unstructured time, behavioral coaches may review the lesson with the children while waiting for the remaining children to return from the bathroom.
- You may want to award stars for good behavior after returning from the bathroom.

Session 5 Continued

Musical Share Chairs

BEHAVIORAL REHEARSAL ACTIVITY 2

Materials Needed

- Music and music player.
- Chairs (two chairs less than the total number of children and behavioral coaches).

Room Setup

- Arrange the chairs in one large circle facing outward with some space in between the chairs.
- The group leader stands at the front of the room.
- The children and behavioral coaches stand around the circle of chairs facing the group leader.

Rules: Musical Share Chairs

- The group leader reads the script below to explain the rules.
- Once the music begins to play, the children and behavioral coaches begin to slowly walk around the chairs in the same direction.
- Stop the music after 10–15 seconds and instruct the children to quickly find a chair.
  - The children and behavioral coaches should quickly sit in one of the chairs.
  - Only children (no behavioral coaches) should be left standing when the music is stopped.
- Then announce which children do not have a chair and ***social coach*** the children to ask a behavioral coach to ***share*** their chair.
- Behavioral coaches should alternate between accepting and declining the children's requests.
  - Behavioral coaches can accept the request by saying, "*Okay,* ______ *(child)*" and making room on their chair for the child.
  - Behavioral coaches can decline the request by saying, "*Not this time.*"
  - If behavioral coaches decline the request, the children are to practice ***keeping cool***.
- All children are to be seated before the music is resumed.
  - Do not remove any chairs. The point of the game is to practice ***keeping cool*** rather than to eliminate group members.
- Throughout the game, behavioral coaches should ensure that all children have had an equal number of opportunities to practice ***keeping cool***.
- Optional: After the children are familiar with the game, instruct the children to move around the circle in different ways.
  - Examples: hop on one foot, hop like a bunny, stomp like a giant, tip-toe like a cat, etc.

Behavioral Rehearsal: Musical Share Chairs (15 Minutes)

The group leader leads the activity. The children are sitting in the chairs and the behavioral coaches are standing as the group leader explains the rules.

Group leader:	*"Hey friends, now we're going to play Musical Share Chairs! When you hear the music, everyone walks around the chairs.* (Demonstrate walking around the circle of chairs.*) When the music stops, quickly find a chair and sit down.* (Demonstrate sitting down on one of the chairs.*) You have to be fast because there aren't enough chairs for everybody! If you don't have a chair, you'll ask one of our big friends (behavioral coaches) to share their chair by saying, "____ (Behavioral coach), can you share your chair with me? If they say yes, then you can sit with them. But, if they say no, then you should keep cool by looking at them with your* (point to your eyes to prompt children to say *"eyes"*)*...EYES, nicely saying 'Okay, ____ (behavioral coach).' And don't forget you can take deep breaths to keep cool."* (Demonstrate taking two ***deep breaths***.) *We'll keep playing so that everyone can practice keeping cool. Remember you can only ask our big friends if you can sit with them. Okay, let's play Musical Share Chairs!"*

Role Play: Musical Share Chairs

The group leader leads the role play and controls the music. Two behavioral coaches demonstrate how to play *Musical Share Chairs*. The children walk around the circle with the behavioral coaches. For the role play, have ONE less chair than there are players.

Group leader:	(Play the music.) *"Okay friends, everybody start walking around the circle."*
	(Allow the children and behavioral coaches to walk slowly around the chairs, then pause the music after 10–15 seconds.) *"The music stopped! Everybody find a chair and sit!"*
Behavioral coach:	(Walk slowly to find a chair in order to be left standing.)
Group leader:	*"Hey friends, ____ (Behavioral coach 1) doesn't have a chair. ____ (Behavioral coach 1), ask ____ (behavioral coach 2) if they will share their chair. If ____ (behavioral coach 2) says no, then remember to keep cool by looking at them with your eyes, nicely saying 'Okay, ____ (behavioral coach 2)' and taking deep breaths."*
Behavioral coach 1:	*"Can I share your chair, ____ (behavioral coach 2)?"*
Behavioral coach 2:	*"Okay, ____ (behavioral coach 1)."* (***Share*** your chair with behavioral coach 1.)

Group leader: *"Great job sharing and giving a turn! Everybody stand up so we can keep playing. Are we ready?"*

(Play the music.) *"Okay friends, everybody start walking around the circle."*

(Allow the children and behavioral coaches to walk slowly around the chairs, then pause the music after 10–15 seconds.) *"The music stopped! Everybody find a chair and sit!"*

Behavioral coach 1: (Walk slowly when finding a chair in order to be left standing.)

Group leader: *"Hey friends, ____ (behavioral coach 1) doesn't have a chair again. ____ (Behavioral coach 1), ask ____ (behavioral coach 2) if they will share their chair. If ____ (behavioral coach 2) says no, then remember to keep cool by looking at them with your eyes, nicely saying 'Okay, ____ (behavioral coach 2)' and taking deep breaths."*

Behavioral coach 1: *"Can I share your chair, ____ (behavioral coach 2)?"*

Behavioral coach 2: *"Not this time."*

Behavioral coach 1: *"Okay, ____ (behavioral coach 2)."* (Take two ***deep breaths***.)

Group leader: *"Great job keeping cool, ____ (behavioral coach 1)! Everybody should stand up so we can keep playing. Are we ready?"*

Behavioral Rehearsal: Musical Share Chairs

Remove ONE ADDITIONAL chair, so there are TWO chairs less than there are players.

Group leader: (Play the music.) *"Okay friends, everybody start walking around the circle."*

(Allow the children and behavioral coaches to walk slowly around the chairs, then pause the music after 10–15 seconds.) *"The music stopped! Everybody find a chair and sit!"* (Behavioral coaches should be quick to find a chair so children must practice asking to ***share*** chairs and ***keeping cool***.)

"Hey friends, _____ (children) don't have chairs. Ask ____ (behavioral coaches) to share their chair. If they say no, then remember to keep cool by looking at them with your eyes, nicely saying 'okay' while using names and taking deep breaths."

Behavioral coaches: (Alternate between saying, *"Okay, ____ (child)."* or *"Not this time."* If needed, behavioral coaches should ***social coach*** the children to ***keep cool***.)

Group leader: *"Great job sharing chairs and keeping cool! Everybody should stand up so we can keep playing. Are we ready?"*

(After several rounds of the sequence above, you may introduce new ways of moving around the circle of chairs by saying, *"Okay friends, let's listen and follow directions because this time we're going to _____ (movement) around the chairs!"* Each movement should be modeled by the group leader and the behavioral coaches before playing.)

Table 5.2 Examples of Movements

Hop like a bunny	Stomp like a giant	Hop on one foot
Tip-toe like a cat	Fly like a bird	Swim like a fish
Walk sideways like a crab	Walk backward slowly	Take small baby steps
Slither like a snake	Walk in slow motion	Take giant steps

Behavioral Rehearsal Wrap-Up

Group leader: *"Well friends, great job keeping cool and listening and following directions! Give yourselves a big round of applause!"* (All behavioral coaches clap and cheer and encourage the children to clap as well.)

"Now everyone should come sit in the Listening Circle." (Have children return to the Listening Circle to sit on their carpet squares.)

"Okay friends, you did a great job keeping cool by looking at your friends with your (point to your eyes to prompt children to say *"eyes")...EYES and nicely saying 'okay' while using names. And nice job taking deep breaths to keep cool!"* (Demonstrate taking two ***deep breaths***.)

"You each earned ____ (number) more stars for keeping cool! Let's start with ____ (child)."

Award each child the same number of stars by repeating the following with each child:

Group leader: *"Where's _____ (child)?"* (Wait until all the children are looking at the child.)

"_____ (Child), how many stars did you earn?" (Pause briefly to allow the child to respond.)

"That's right! Let's all count for _____ (child)! One, two, three... (add stars to the Star Chart as they are counted aloud)*! Everybody clap for _____ (child)!"* (All behavioral coaches clap and cheer and encourage the children to clap as well.)

"Now we're going to play some games with our parents and practice keeping cool some more!"

Session 5 Continued

Keeping Cool

PARENT COACHED PLAY: DYADIC PLAYDATES

Materials Needed

- Games brought by children and parents from home.
- Turn-taking games provided by the treatment team.
- Tables and chairs or carpet squares.
- *Parent Coached Play Cards*.

Room Setup

- If available, organize tables in separate corners of the room with 4–6 chairs per table.
- If tables are unavailable, place two carpet squares in separate corners of the room to indicate where the children will sit.

Rules: Dyadic Playdates

- The group leader divides the families into groups of two families each.
    - If there are an odd number of children, pair one child with a behavioral coach who will serve as a ***playmate***. In this case, you will need an additional coach to serve as a behavioral coach for the parent.
    - To avoid social exclusion, avoid having children play in triads as much as possible.
- Assign each group to sit at a table or specific play area.
    - Children should sit next to each other.
    - Parents will act as ***social coaches*** by sitting on the other side of their child to minimize interrupting the natural flow of play between the children.
    - One behavioral coach will be assigned to each dyad to provide ***social coaching*** suggestions and feedback to parents.
- Children will take turns playing the games brought from home or games provided by the treatment team.
- Each child will have ten minutes to play their chosen game with their playmate and will then switch games.
- Parents will choose which child's game will be played first.
- To minimize unstructured periods, parents will help the children set up the game in a cooperative fashion (handing game pieces to each other, offering suggestions, etc.).

- As they play, parents will ***social coach*** the children on previously learned and newly learned skills using the guidelines highlighted on the *Parent Coached Play Cards.*
- Behavioral coaches will provide support to parents in their ***social coaching*** using the ***4 Ps (priming, prompting, praising,*** and ***providing corrective feedback***) and will model appropriate coaching behavior when necessary.
- After approximately nine minutes of play, instruct the parents to prepare the children for the upcoming game swap.
- After approximately one additional minute of play (ten minutes total), instruct the parents to have the children clean up and swap games.
- Repeat the cycle with the second game for the remaining ten minutes before returning to the *Listening Circle.*

Behavioral Coaching: Dyadic Playdates

Behavioral coaches will ***social coach*** parents during dyadic ***playdates*** in the following ways:

- ***Priming*:**
  - Begin the play interactions with parents going over the rules for ***keeping cool*** BEFORE GAME PLAYING.
    - Example: *"Remember that when playing your games if you ever get sad or angry or upset because you don't get your way, we want you to keep cool by looking at your friend with your* (point to your eyes to prompt child to say *"eyes"*)*...EYES, nicely saying 'okay.' And don't forget to take deep breaths to keep cool* (demonstrate taking two ***deep breaths***)*."*
- ***Prompting*:**
  - Remind parents to use the buzzwords to ***prompt*** their child to ***keep cool*** IN THE MOMENT.
  - Help parents to identify opportunities to proactively ***prompt*** their child to ***keep cool.***
    - Example: *"Remember to keep cool if your friend says no."*
    - Example: *"Remember to nicely say 'okay' if your friend isn't ready to share."*
    - Example: *"What should you do if you're still feeling upset?"*
- ***Praising*:**
  - Remind parents to ***praise*** and reinforce their child whenever their child ***keeps cool*** CORRECTLY.
    - Example: *"Great job keeping cool!"*
    - Example: *"Great job keeping cool and saying 'okay'!"*
    - Example: *"Good job taking deep breaths to keep cool!"*
- ***Providing corrective feedback using a praise sandwich*:**
  - Remind parents to ***praise*** their child's ATTEMPTS to ***keep cool*** and identify what could be done differently next time.
    - Example: *"Nice try keeping cool. Remember to take deep breaths if you're still upset next time, but good job!"*
    - Example: *"Good job keeping cool. Don't forget to nicely say 'okay' next time, but nice try!"*
    - Example: *"Nice try keeping cool. Remember to listen if your friend says no, but good job!"*

- Remind parents to continue to ***social coach*** on previously learned skills:
  - ***Listening and following directions.***
  - ***Meeting and greeting friends.***
  - ***Sharing and giving a turn.***
  - ***Asking for a turn.***

Parent Coached Play: Dyadic Playdates (20 Minutes)

- Have each child choose a turn-taking game brought from home or provided by the treatment team.
- The group leader sits on the floor at the front of the room.
- The families sit on the floor in a semi-circle facing the group leader.

Group leader: *"Hey friends, we're going to have more playdates and play with the fun games you brought from home. While you play, we want you to practice keeping cool if your friend says 'no' or 'maybe later' or when it's time to swap games. Remember to keep cool by looking at your friend with your* (point to your eyes to prompt children to say "*eyes*")*...EYES, nicely saying 'okay' while using names and taking deep breaths* (take two ***deep breaths***)*. And if your friend asks for a turn, do you think we should share and give a turn?"* (Pause briefly to allow the children to respond *"yes.")*

"That's right, friends! Parents, remember to social coach your children by using your Parent Coached Play Cards. Okay, let's play with our games!"

- Before playing, parents will ***social coach*** their child to ***say "hi"*** to one another ***using names***.
- Parents will ***social coach*** their children to ***ask for a turn***, ***share and take turns,*** and ***keep cool*** throughout the game playing.
- After approximately nine minutes of play, instruct the parents to prepare the children for the upcoming game swap by saying, *"Parents, tell your children that we'll be swapping games in one minute."*
- After approximately one additional minute of play (ten minutes total), instruct the parents to swap games by saying, *"Parents, it's time to swap games. Social coach the children to ask for a turn and share and give a turn before playing the next game."*
- After approximately nine minutes of playing the second game, instruct the parents to prepare the children for clean up by saying, *"Parents, tell your children that we'll be cleaning up in one minute."*
- After approximately one additional minute of play (ten minutes total), ***prompt*** the parents to instruct their children to clean up by saying, *"Parents, it's time to clean up. Let's social coach the children to listen and follow directions by cleaning up and then say 'bye' to their friend using names before sitting in the Listening Circle."*
- If needed, parents will ***social coach*** their child to ***listen and follow directions*** to clean up.
- Then parents will ***social coach*** their child to ***say "bye"*** to their friend ***using names***.

Final Wrap-Up (10 Minutes)

- The group leader sits on the floor at the front of the room.
- The children sit on the carpet squares in a semi-circle facing the group leader, with parents sitting behind their children.

Group leader: *"Okay friends, you all did a great job playing your games and keeping cool. When we're keeping cool, do you think we should get mad or cry or yell or hit if our friends aren't ready to share with us or play with us?"* (Pause briefly to allow children to respond "no.")

"That's right, friends! Instead, we need to keep our cool! And when we're keeping cool, do you think we should nicely say 'okay' while using names and then find something else to do?" (Pause briefly to allow the children to say *"yes."*)

"That's right, friends! Do you think we should we take deep breaths to help us keep cool?" (Pause briefly to allow children to respond *"yes."*)

"That's right, friends! Let's take two deep breaths together!" (***Prompt*** the children and parents to take two ***deep breaths*** in unison with the group leader.)

"You all did such a great job keeping cool today that you each earned ____ (number) more stars! Let's start with ____ (child)."

Award each child the same number of stars by repeating the following with each child:

Group leader: *"Where's _____ (child)?"* (Wait until all the children are looking at the child.)

"_____ (Child), how many stars did you earn?" (Pause briefly to allow the child to respond.)

"That's right! Let's all count for _____ (child)! One, two, three... (add stars to the Star Chart as they are counted aloud)*! Everybody clap for _____ (child)!"* (All behavioral coaches clap and cheer and encourage the children to clap as well.)

"And remember you all earned those stars by keeping cool! Everyone did a great job, and parents, you did an excellent job social coaching! Parents, remember your homework assignments this week are for you and your children to practice keeping cool and to continue practicing all the other things we've learned to be a good friend using the 4 Ps. And don't forget to enroll your children in playgroups if you haven't already."

"Alright little friends, do you want to count our stars?" (Pause briefly to allow the children to respond *"yes."*)

"Let's all count together and see how many stars we earned today! One, two, three...(count the number of stars for one child)*!"*

"You each earned ____ (total number) stars today! Round of applause for our friends!" (All behavioral coaches should clap and cheer and encourage the families to clap as well.)

"Great job, friends! Don't forget to choose your reward before you leave. See you all next week!"

Session 5 Continued

Planning Playdates and Keeping Cool

PEERS® FOR PRESCHOOLERS: PARENT HANDOUT

Didactic Lesson: Planning Playdates

Consider the 5 Ws

- **WHO will attend the *playdate.***
    - **Identify *potential playmates* for *playdates.***
        - Identify peers who get along well with your child.
            - Recall whom your child has been playing with consistently and nicely at school or their ***playgroup(s)***.
            - You may want to talk to your child's teacher or daycare provider to identify ***potential playmates***.
        - Consider how the ***potential playmate*** is likely to respond to your ***social coaching*** during the ***playdate***.
        - Consider whether the parent(s) of the ***potential playmate***:
            - Is someone you are comfortable and/or willing to interact with and disclose personal information to about your child (if relevant).
            - Will be open to your ***social coaching***.
    - **Consider whether the parent(s) of the *potential playmate* will be present at the *playdate*.**
        - If present, inform the parent that you will be more actively involved during the ***playdate***, especially until the children become more comfortable with one another.
        - Tips on ways to speak to other parents regarding your ***social coaching*** during ***playdates***:
            - Acknowledge that the ***playdate*** may be different from what they are used to because of your ***social coaching***.
            - Consider whether you want to disclose your child's diagnoses and/or social challenges, which is a personal choice.
    - ***Playdates* should ideally be one-on-one.**
        - Try to avoid or limit group activities or ***playdates*** with multiple children at first.
        - One-on-one ***playdates*** will allow parents to ***social coach*** more effectively.

    - **Avoid having siblings join the *playdate* if possible.**
        - Try not to allow your child's siblings to join the ***playdate*** when possible.
            - Prearrange other ***playdates*** or activities for your child's siblings.
            - It may be more challenging to effectively ***social coach*** your child if other siblings are present.
        - Try to avoid having the ***playmate's*** siblings attend the ***playdate***.
            - Recall if siblings typically accompanied parents of ***playmates*** to school, daycare, or the ***playgroup***.
                - If so, siblings are also likely to be present during the ***playdate***.
        - If other parents and siblings will be present during the ***playdate***, think about how you may need to adapt your ***social coaching*** and plan on having enough snacks, activities, and supplies available for everyone to participate.

- **WHAT will the children do during the *playdate.***
    - ***Playdates* should be activity-based.**
        - "Free play" or "down time" is not an activity.
        - Activities should be based on the ***common interests*** of your child and their ***playmate***.
            - ***Common interests*** are those games and activities that are fun for BOTH your child and their ***playmate***.
                - Choose games or activities your child and their ***playmate*** commonly play at school or daycare or during the ***playgroup*** if appropriate.

- **WHEN will the *playdate* happen.**
    - **Identify the exact day and time of the *playdate* with the *playmate's* parent(s).**
    - **Try to keep initial *playdates* to no more than 1–1.5 hours**.
        - ***Playdates*** can be longer as your child improves in their skills and has had more ***playdates*** with the ***playmate***.
    - **Schedule *playdates* around routines (nap times, meals, etc.).**

- **WHERE will the *playdate* take place.**
    - **Identify the location of the *playdate* with the *playmate's* parent(s).**
    - **Schedule initial *playdates* to take place in your home if possible.**
        - It will be easier to ***social coach*** if the ***playdate*** takes place in your home.
        - It may be less overwhelming for your child to be in a familiar environment at first.
        - If the ***playdate*** cannot be in your home, try to choose a location where you will have the opportunity to ***social coach*** your child.
        - Try to avoid having ***playdates*** in other parents' homes initially as you will have less control over the activities.
    - **Be present if the *playdate* will take place outside of the home.**
        - You need to be present to provide ***social coaching*** in the moment.
        - Your presence will likely increase your child's comfort if in a new setting.

- **HOW will the children get to and from the *playdate.***
    - Arrange transportation to and from the ***playdate*** for your child and their ***playmate*** (if relevant).

Snapshot of the Lesson: Keeping Cool

The objective of this lesson is to teach children how to ***keep cool***. Steps for ***keeping cool*** include:

1. ***Look at your friends with your eyes*** (point to your eyes).
2. ***Nicely say "okay" using names.***
3. ***Find something else to do.***
4. ***If you're still feeling upset, take deep breaths*** to ***keep cool*** (take two slow ***deep breaths***):
   a. ***Smell the flowers*** (example of breathing in).
   b. ***Blow out the candles*** (example of brcathing out).

Homework Assignments

1. **Identify playmates for playdates.**
   - Parents should identify one or two ***potential playmates*** for a ***playdate***.
     - Pay attention to whether the children seem to like each other, play nicely together, and have ***common interests***.
     - Consider whether you would be comfortable and willing to interact with the parent(s) of the ***potential playmate***.
     - Consider whether the ***potential playmate*** and the parent(s) would be open to your ***social coaching***.
   - Parents should identify possible games and activities for the ***playdate*** based on the children's ***common interests***.
   - Note: Unless your child is already having successful ***playdates*** with these ***playmates***, hold off on scheduling a ***playdate*** until we get through all the **playdate** lessons.
2. **Playgroups.**
   - If not yet accomplished, enroll your child in a ***playgroup*** using the criteria for a good ***playgroup***.
   - During the ***playgroup***, parents should identify:
     - ***Potential playmates*** for ***playdates***.
     - Your compatibility with the parents of ***potential playmates***.
     - Which peers regularly attend the ***playgroup.***
     - Popular activities, games, or toys.
     - Whether this is a good ***playgroup*** for your child.
3. **Practice keeping cool**
   - **Practice having your child *keep cool* this week during preferred and highly motivating activities while providing *social coaching* using the *4 Ps*.**
     - ***Priming***: Review the rules for ***keeping cool*** with your child BEFORE PRACTICING.
     - ***Prompting***: Remind your child IN THE MOMENT to ***keep cool*** whenever the opportunities present.
     - ***Praising***: ***Praise*** your child using the buzzwords whenever they ***keep cool*** CORRECTLY.
     - ***Providing corrective feedback***: ***Provide corrective feedback*** in the form of a ***praise sandwich*** whenever your child ATTEMPTS to ***keep cool***.

- **Please send us a 30–60-second video of *social coaching* for *keeping cool* with your child to be viewed during homework review.**
    - Please include:
        - Skills your child did well.
        - Skills you would like to work on with your child.

4. **Provide social coaching on previously learned skills.**
    - Continue providing ***social coaching*** to your child throughout the week using the ***4 Ps.***
    - Previous skills include:
        - ***Listening and following directions.***
        - ***Meeting and greeting friends.***
        - ***Sharing and giving a turn.***
        - ***Asking for a turn.***
5. **Bring a turn-taking game.**
    - Bring a turn-taking game that your child enjoys playing and can be played with the other children.

Session 5 Continued

Keeping Cool

PEERS® FOR PRESCHOOLERS: PARENT COACHED PLAY CARD

Snapshot of the Lesson: Keeping Cool

1. ***Look at your friends with your eyes*** (point to your eyes).
2. ***Nicely say "okay" using names.***
3. ***Find something else to do.***
4. ***If you're still feeling upset, take deep breaths*** to ***keep cool*** (take two slow ***deep breaths***):
   a. ***Smell the flowers*** (example of breathing in).
   b. ***Blow out the candles*** (example of breathing out).

Priming BEFORE Game Playing

- Example: *"Remember to practice keeping cool by looking at your friend with your* (point to your eyes to prompt child to say *"eyes"*)*...EYES, nicely saying 'okay' while using names and finding something else to do. And don't forget to take deep breaths to keep cool* (demonstrate taking two ***deep breaths***)*."*

Prompting IN THE MOMENT

- Example: *"Remember to keep cool."*
- Example: *"Remember to find something else to do if your friend isn't ready to share."*
- Example: *"What should you do if you're still upset?"*

Praising for CORRECT Use of Skills

- Example: *"Great job keeping cool!"*
- Example: *"Great job nicely saying 'okay'!"*
- Example: *"Good job taking deep breaths to keep cool!"*

Providing Corrective Feedback for ATTEMPTS Using a Praise Sandwich

- Example: *"Good job keeping cool. Remember to nicely say 'okay' next time, but great job!"*
- Example: *"Nice try keeping cool. Remember to take deep breaths if you're still upset next time, but good try!"*

- Example: *"Nice job keeping cool. Don't forget to find something else to do next time, but good job!*

- Continue to provide ***social coaching*** on previously learned skills:
    - ***Listening and following directions.***
    - ***Meeting and greeting friends.***
    - ***Sharing and giving a turn.***
    - ***Asking for a turn.***

Session 5 Continued

Planning Playdates and Keeping Cool

PEERS® FOR PRESCHOOLERS: PARENT HOMEWORK WORKSHEET

<table>
<tr><td>Child's Name:</td><td colspan="2">Parent's Name:</td><td colspan="2">Date:</td></tr>
<tr><td>HOMEWORK ASSIGNMENTS</td><td>PRIMING (REVIEWING RULES BEFORE PRACTICE)</td><td>PROMPTING (IN THE MOMENT)</td><td>PRAISING (USING BUZZWORDS)</td><td>PROVIDING CORRECTIVE FEEDBACK (USING A PRAISE SANDWICH)</td></tr>
<tr><td>Keeping cool</td><td></td><td></td><td></td><td></td></tr>
<tr><td>Practice previous skills:
• Asking for a turn
• Sharing and giving turns
• Meeting and greeting friends
• Listening and following directions</td><td></td><td></td><td></td><td></td></tr>
<tr><td>Potential playmates</td><td colspan="4">Which potential playmates did you identify for playdates?
What games or activities did you identify for potential playdates?</td></tr>
<tr><td>Playgroups
Investigate and enroll in playgroup(s).</td><td colspan="4">Which playgroups did you investigate and enroll in?</td></tr>
<tr><td>Bring a turn-taking game</td><td colspan="2">Did you bring a turn-taking game?
YES or NO
(Circle)</td><td colspan="2">Which game did you bring?</td></tr>
</table>

Please fill out this worksheet by describing what you did to complete the homework assignments. Worksheets will be collected during Homework Review at the next session of PEERS® for Preschoolers.

Session 6

Suggesting Playdates and Being a Good Sport

PARENT SESSION THERAPIST GUIDE

Parent Session Agenda

- Homework Review (40 minutes).
- Didactic Lessons (20 minutes).
- Parent Coached Play (20 minutes).
- Final Wrap-Up (10 minutes).

Materials Needed

- Conference room with a large table and enough chairs for the parent group leader and all parents to sit comfortably around the table.
  - Avoid sitting in a circle without a table as this creates the atmosphere of group therapy.
- Name tags for parents and treatment team.
- *Parent Handouts* (for the current week and the previous weeks).
- *Parent Homework Worksheets* (for the current week and the previous weeks).
- *Parent Coached Play Cards* (for the current week and the previous weeks).
- *Attendance and Homework Compliance Sheets* for parent group leader.
- Pens for note-taking (consider having extra pens for parents who need them).

Homework Review (40 Minutes)

1. **Identify potential playmates.**
   - Have parents identify one or two ***potential playmates*** for ***playdates***.
   - Assess whether parents:
     - Paid attention to whether the children seemed to like each other, played nicely together, and had ***common interests***.
     - Considered whether they would be comfortable and willing to interact with the parent(s) of the ***potential playmate(s)***.
     - Considered whether the ***potential playmate(s)*** and the parent(s) would be open to their ***social coaching***.
   - Have parents identify possible games and activities for the ***playdate*** based on the children's ***common interests***.

DOI: 10.4324/9781003502968-7

2. **Find a playgroup for your child.**
   - Confirm parents have enrolled their child in a ***playgroup*** and have identified:
     - ***Potential playmates*** for ***playdates***.
     - Their compatibility with the parents of ***potential playmates***.
     - Which peers regularly attend the ***playgroup***.
     - Popular activities, games, or toys.
     - Whether this is a good ***playgroup*** for their child.

3. **Practice keeping cool.**
   - Review the 30–60-second video of ***social coaching*** for ***keeping cool*** for each family. (For larger groups, you may need to review video recordings in two smaller groups with two different parent group leaders).
     - Have parents identify:
       - Skills their child did well.
       - Skills they would like to work on with their child.
     - Provide ***social coaching*** tips as appropriate for each family.
   - If parents did not send a video of ***social coaching***, confirm the following:
     - Parents practiced having their child ***keep cool*** during preferred and highly motivating activities while providing ***social coaching*** using the ***4 Ps***.
       - ***Priming*****:** Reviewed the rules for ***keeping cool*** with their child BEFORE PRACTICING.
       - ***Prompting*****:** Reminded their child IN THE MOMENT to ***keep cool*** whenever the opportunity presented.
       - ***Praising*****:** ***Praised*** their child using the buzzwords whenever they ***kept cool*** CORRECTLY.
       - ***Providing corrective feedback*****:** ***Provided corrective feedback*** in the form of a ***praise sandwich*** whenever their child ATTEMPTED to ***keep cool***.

4. **Provide social coaching on previously learned skills.**
   - Confirm parents continued to provide ***social coaching*** to their child throughout the week using the ***4 Ps*** for previously learned skills:
     - ***Listening and following directions.***
     - ***Meeting and greeting friends.***
     - ***Sharing and giving turns.***
     - ***Asking for a turn.***

5. **Bring a turn-taking game.**
   - Confirm the following:
     - Brought a turn-taking game that their child enjoys playing and can be played with the other children. (To avoid distractions, these games should be left with the parents until *Parent Coached Play*.)

Didactic Lessons (20 Minutes)

PEERS® Neuroaffirming Pledge:

- We value neurodiversity, acceptance, and authenticity.
- We honor the diverse ways people experience the world.
- We respect each person's unique perspectives and communication styles.

- We recognize there is no one right way to connect with others.
- If using the strategies taught in PEERS® feels like camouflaging or masking and/or they don't align with your goals or the goals of your family, then you do not have to use them.
- Learning and using the skills taught in PEERS® is a PERSONAL CHOICE.

Didactic Lesson: Suggesting Playdates

- Distribute *Parent Handouts.*
  - Sections in **bold print** come directly from the *Parent Handout.*
  - Terms that are ***bold and italicized*** are buzzwords and represent important concepts from the didactic lesson.
- Explain, *"Last week we discussed how to plan playdates with potential playmates. Today we'll talk about how to suggest playdates with the parent(s) of these potential playmates and assess if they might be interested in having a playdate."*

Steps for Suggesting Playdates

1. **Wait for an appropriate time to ask.**
   - **Appropriate times:**
     - **When you're having a light social conversation with them.**
     - **When they're observing the *playgroup.***
     - **When they're not busy or preoccupied.**
     - **When other parents are not present.**
   - **Inappropriate times:**
     - **Drop-off or pick-up times at the *playgroup* when the other parent(s) are busy or distracted.**
     - **Group conversations with other parents.**
       - **This may make the other parents feel excluded.**
2. **Engage in casual conversation with the other parent(s).**
   - **Keep the conversation friendly and casual.**
     - **This reduces the pressure on the other parent(s).**
3. **Mention your children's *common interest(s).***
   - **Comments about GENERAL *common interest.***
     - **Example: "It seems like our kids really enjoy playing together."**
     - **Example: "I noticed our kids play together really nicely."**
     - **Example: "I noticed our kids really seem to get along."**
   - **Comments about SPECIFIC *common interest.***
     - **Example: "It seems like our kids really enjoy playing chase together."**
     - **Example: "I noticed both of our kids enjoy playing board games together."**
     - **Example: "I noticed our kids seem to have fun doing arts and crafts together."**
4. **Use the *common interest* as a reason for the potential *playdate.***
   - **Example: "*_____ (Potential playmate) and _______ (your child) seem to have a lot of fun playing together. It might be fun to get together for a playdate sometime."***
   - **Example: "*_____ (Potential playmate) and _______ (your child) seem to have a lot of fun playing chase. It might be fun to get together for a playdate sometime."***

- **Example: *"I noticed _____ (potential playmate) and _______ (your child) seem to have a lot of fun doing arts and crafts together. Maybe we should schedule a playdate sometime."***

5. **If the parent(s) seems interested, exchange contact information to set up a *playdate.***
   - **In the moment, you may tentatively choose a day and time for the *playdate* if the parent(s) are particularly enthusiastic.**
     - **Be sure to follow up with a text or email (or a phone call when appropriate) to confirm the *5 Ws* (i.e., who, what, where, when, how).**
   - **If the parent(s) do not seem interested, casually change the topic of conversation to avoid an uncomfortable situation.**
     - **Remember that *friendship is a choice.***
       - ***Our children don't get to be friends with everyone.***
       - ***Everyone doesn't get to be friends with our children.***

Assessing Interest When Suggesting Playdates

Explain, *"It can be difficult to assess the interest of other parents when suggesting a playdate, particularly if they don't outright agree or disagree. Here are some signs of interest or disinterest that you might consider when suggesting a playdate. Again, if other families don't seem interested in having playdates, it's important to remember that friendship is a choice."*

Table 6.1 Assessing Parent Interest for Playdates

SIGNS OF INTEREST	SIGNS OF DISINTEREST
Making eye contact	Not making eye contact/looking away
Smiling	Not smiling/looking uncomfortable
Turned toward you	Turned away from you
Talking to you/asking questions	Not talking to you/saying very little
Seem eager to make plans	Are reluctant/hesitant to make plans
Agree about children's mutual interest	Seem confused/distracted
Agree (even without finalizing)	Are busy or unavailable
Exchange contact information	Don't exchange contact information
Agree and they follow up later	Agree but never follow up

Didactic Lesson: Being a Good Sport

Explain, *"Last week the children learned how to keep cool if their friend isn't ready to share and give a turn, or if things aren't going their way while playing. This week we will focus on how to be a good sport when playing with friends. Being a good sport is one important way to sustain or maintain play. Like the skills for sharing and giving a turn, asking for a turn, and keeping cool, following the rules for being a good sport will help increase reciprocity in your children's play interactions."*

Snapshot of the Lesson: Being a Good Sport

The objective of this lesson is to teach children how to *be a good sport.* Steps for *being a good sport* include:

1. ***Look at your friends with your eyes* (point to your eyes).**
2. ***Smile with your mouth* (point to your mouth and smile).**
3. ***Say "good job" while using names.***
4. ***Give a high-five.***

Parent Coached Play

- Distribute the *Parent Coached Play Cards.*
- Review the examples of the ***4 Ps*** provided on the *Parent Coached Play Card.*
- Remind parents that in a few moments, we will be joining the children for *Parent Coached Play* in the context of mock dyadic ***playdates***.
- Parents should keep the *Parent Coached Play Card* in front of them during the dyadic ***playdate*** for recommendations on how to ***social coach*** children on ***being a good sport.***

Homework Assignments

(Briefly review the homework assignments and troubleshoot any potential problems with parents.)

1. **Identify potential playmates.**
   - **Have parents identify one or two *potential playmates* for *playdates.***
   - **Assess whether parents:**
     - **Paid attention to whether the children seemed to like each other, played nicely together, and had *common interests.***
     - **Considered whether they would be comfortable and willing to interact with the parent(s) of the *potential playmate(s).***
     - **Considered whether the *potential playmate(s)* and the parent(s) would be open to their *social coaching.***
   - **Have parents identify possible games and activities for the *playdate* based on the children's *common interests.***
   - **Note: Unless your child is already having successful *playdates* with these *playmates*, hold off on scheduling a *playdate* until we get through all the *playdate* lessons (next week).**

2. **Playgroups.**
   - **If not yet accomplished, enroll your child in a *playgroup* using the criteria for a good *playgroup.***
   - **During the *playgroup*, parents should identify:**
     - ***Potential playmates* for *playdates.***
     - **Your compatibility with the parents of *potential playmates.***

- **Which peers regularly attend the *playgroup.***
- **Popular activities, games, or toys.**
- **Whether this is a good *playgroup* for your child.**

3. **Practice being a good sport.**
    - **Practice having your child *be a good sport* this week during preferred and highly motivating activities while providing *social coaching* using the *4 Ps.***
        - ***Priming:* Review the rules for *being a good sport* with your child BEFORE PRACTICING.**
        - ***Prompting:* Remind your child IN THE MOMENT to *be a good sport* whenever the opportunities present.**
        - ***Praising: Praise* your child using the buzzwords whenever they are *being a good sport* CORRECTLY.**
        - ***Providing corrective feedback: Provide corrective feedback* in the form of a *praise sandwich* whenever your child ATTEMPTS to *be a good sport.***
    - **Please send us a 30–60-second video of *social coaching* for *being a good sport* with your child to be viewed during homework review.**
        - **Please include:**
            - **Skills your child did well.**
            - **Skills you would like to work on with your child.**

4. **Provide social coaching on previously learned skills.**
    - **Continue providing *social coaching* to your child throughout the week using the *4 Ps.***
    - **Previous skills include:**
        - ***Listening and following directions.***
        - ***Meeting and greeting friends.***
        - ***Sharing and giving a turn.***
        - ***Asking for a turn.***
        - ***Keeping cool.***

5. **Bring a turn-taking game.**
    - **Bring a turn-taking game that your child enjoys playing and can be played with the other children.**

Session 6 Continued

Being a Good Sport

CHILD SESSION THERAPIST GUIDE

Child Session Agenda

- Didactic Lesson: *Being a Good Sport* (20 minutes).
- Group Behavioral Rehearsal Activity 1: *Elbow to Elbow* (15 minutes).
- Break Time (10 minutes).
- Group Behavioral Rehearsal Activity 2: *Head, Shoulders, Knees, and Toes* (15 minutes).
- Parent Coached Play: *Dyadic Playdates* (20 minutes).
- Final Wrap-Up (10 minutes).

Snapshot of the Lesson: Being a Good Sport

The objective of this lesson is to teach children how to ***be a good sport***. Steps for ***being a good sport*** include:

1. ***Look at your friend with your eyes*** (point to your eyes).
2. ***Smile with your mouth*** (point to your mouth and smile).
3. ***Say "good job" using names.***
4. ***Give a high-five.***

Materials Needed

- Frog puppet.
- Tiger puppet.
- Small ball.
- Carpet squares or chairs.
- "Making Friends Helper" badge.
- Star chart with names of children.
- Marker for star chart.
- Name tags for families and treatment team.
- Prize bins with prizes.

Preparing for the Lesson

- Use the script below with the group leader using a frog puppet to play the part of "Franny Frog."
- A behavioral coach uses a tiger puppet to play the part of "Timmy Tiger."

- An additional behavioral coach assists in the behavioral rehearsal and provides encouragement and feedback to the group.
- A child is chosen at the beginning of the lesson as the "Making Friends Helper."
  - The "Making Friends Helper" wears a special badge and is the first child to practice the skill.
- The group leader and the behavioral coach sit on the floor at the front of the room.
- A special-colored carpet square (e.g., red) is placed at the front of the room next to the group leader to be used as the "Good Friend Square."
- For the children, additional carpet squares of the same color (e.g., green) are placed in a semi-circle facing the group leader and the "Good Friend Square."
- Note: If carpet squares are unavailable, the children and behavioral coaches may sit on chairs.
- The material in *italics* should be read by the indicated person.
- The material in ***bold and italics*** represents buzzwords and should be emphasized when read.
- The material in CAPITAL LETTERS within the script should be given extra emphasis while the group is encouraged to say the words in unison.

Behavioral Coaching Techniques

Behavioral coaches should use the following coaching techniques described below throughout the lesson and the behavioral rehearsal activities. (Note: ***priming*** occurs during the introduction to the activity.)

- **Prompting:**
  - Use the buzzwords to ***prompt*** the children to ***be a good sport*** IN THE MOMENT.
    - Example: *"Remember to be a good sport."*
    - Example: *"Remember to say 'good job' and use names."*
    - Example: *"What can you do with your hand when being a good sport?"*
- **Praising:**
  - Reinforce ***being a good sport*** by ***praising*** the children when they use the skills CORRECTLY.
    - Example: *"Great job being a good sport!"*
    - Example: *"Great job saying 'good job'!"*
    - Example: *"Good job looking and smiling at your friend!"*
- **Providing corrective feedback using a praise sandwich:**
  - Reinforce ATTEMPTS to ***be a good sport*** by ***praising*** the children and identifying what could be done differently next time.
    - Example: *"Good job being a good sport. Remember to say 'good job' next time, but nice job!"*
    - Example: *"Nice try being a good sport. Remember to give a high-five next time, but good try!"*
    - Example: *"Great job being a good sport. Don't forget to look and use names next time, but good job!"*
- Continue to provide ***social coaching*** on previously learned skills:
  - ***Listening and following directions.***
  - ***Meeting and greeting friends.***
  - ***Sharing and giving a turn.***
  - ***Asking for a turn.***
  - ***Keeping cool.***

Didactic Lesson: Being a Good Sport (20 Minutes)

Have the children sit in a semi-circle on the carpet squares facing the group leader.

Franny Frog:	(Sit at the front of the room and choose a Making Friends Helper.) *"Who wants to be our Making Friends Helper?"* (Choose from among the children raising their hands and place the "Making Friends Helper" badge on the child. The child stays in their seat for now.) *"Hi friends! I'm Franny Frog. Ribbit, ribbit! Today we're going to practice being a good sport. Being a good sport is a great way to be nice to our friends!"* *"Who should we be a good sport with? We should be a good sport with our FRIENDS, TEACHERS, MOMMIES, DADDIES, BROTHERS, AND SISTERS."* *"When should we be a good sport? We should be a good sport when someone does a good job, like when our friends catch a ball or finish a puzzle."* *"How should we be a good sport? We should be a good sport by looking at our friend with our* (point to your eyes and then to Franny Frog's eyes)*...EYES, smiling with our* (point to your mouth and smile)*...MOUTH, saying 'good job' and giving a high-five* (***give a high-five*** to Timmy Tiger). *And don't forget to use* (pause briefly to prompt the children to say *"names"*)*...NAMES."* *"Remember, being a good sport is a nice way to be a good friend! Ribbit, ribbit!"*

Role Play: Being a Good Sport

Franny Frog and Timmy Tiger:	(Franny Frog holds the small ball. Timmy Tiger is nearby and does not have a toy.)
Franny Frog:	(Turn to look at the group of children.) *"Hey friends! I want to play with my friend Timmy Tiger. I think I'll ask him to play catch.* (Turn to Timmy Tiger and smile.) *Timmy Tiger, let's play catch! Ribbit, ribbit!"*
Timmy Tiger:	(Turn to look at Franny Frog and smile.) *"Okay, Franny Frog! Grr, grr!"*
Franny Frog:	*"Catch, Timmy Tiger! Ribbit, ribbit!"* (Throw the small ball to Timmy Tiger.)
Timmy Tiger:	(Catch the small ball and smile.) *"Nice throw, Franny Frog! Grrr, grrr!"*

Franny Frog:	(Turn to look at the group of children.) *"Hey friends, Timmy Tiger did a great job catching the ball! Do you think I should be a good sport by saying, 'Good job, Timmy Tiger!' and giving him a high-five?"* (Nod your head yes and encourage the children to say *"yes."*) *"That's a great idea! Ribbit, ribbit! Let's do it!* (Turn to look at Timmy Tiger and smile.) *Good job, Timmy Tiger* (***give a high-five*** to Timmy Tiger)*! Ribbit, ribbit!"*
Timmy Tiger:	(Turn to look at Franny Frog and smile.) *"Thanks, Franny Frog! Grr, grr!"*
Franny Frog and Timmy Tiger:	(Say *"good job," give a "frog high-five"* and *"tiger high-five,"* clap, cheer, and encourage the children to clap as well. Timmy Tiger sits on the other side of the Good Friend Square (i.e., the Good Friend Square is between Franny Frog and Timmy Tiger) and holds the small ball. Franny Frog ***social coaches*** the children as needed while they practice ***being a good sport*** with Timmy Tiger.)
Franny Frog:	*"Now let's see _____ (behavioral coach) try! _____ (Behavioral coach), please come sit on the Good Friend Square."*
Behavioral coach:	(Sit on the Good Friend Square.)
Franny Frog:	*"_____ (Behavioral coach), can you show us how to be a good sport with Timmy Tiger?"*
Behavioral coach:	*"Okay, Franny Frog."*
Franny Frog:	(Turn to look at the group of children.) *"Remember to look at Timmy Tiger with your* (point to your eyes to prompt the children to say *"eyes"*)*... EYES, smile with your* (point to your mouth to prompt the children to say *"mouth"*)*...MOUTH, say 'Good job, Timmy Tiger!' and give him a high-five* (***give a high-five*** to Timmy Tiger). *And don't forget to use* (pause briefly to prompt the children to say *"names"*)*...NAMES."*
Timmy Tiger:	(Turn to look at the behavioral coach and smile.) *"Catch, _____ (behavioral coach)! Grr, grr!"* (Throw the small ball to the behavioral coach.)
Behavioral coach:	(Catch the small ball and smile.) *"Nice throw! Catch, Timmy Tiger!"* (Throw the small ball to Timmy Tiger.)
Timmy Tiger and Behavioral coach:	(Throw the small ball to one another for a few turns. Timmy Tiger holds onto the ball at the end.)
Behavioral coach:	*"Good job, Timmy Tiger* (***give a high-five*** to Timmy Tiger)*!"*

Timmy Tiger:	*"Thanks! Good job, _____ (behavioral coach)!"*
Franny Frog:	*"Great job being a good sport, _____ (behavioral coach)! Ribbit, ribbit!"*
Franny Frog and Behavioral coach:	(Say *"good job," give a "frog high-five"* and *"tiger high-five,"* clap, cheer, and encourage the children to clap as well.)
Behavioral coach:	(Leave the Good Friend Square.)

Behavioral Rehearsal: Being a Good Sport

Franny Frog:	(Turn to look at the group of children.) *"Okay friends! Now let's see our Making Friends Helper _____ try! _____ (Making Friends Helper), come sit on the Good Friend Square and show us how to be a good sport with Timmy Tiger."* (The Making Friends Helper should sit on the Good Friend Square.) *"Remember to look at Timmy Tiger with your* (point to your eyes to prompt the children to say *"eyes"*)*...EYES, smile with your* (point to your mouth to prompt the children to say *"mouth"*)*...MOUTH, say 'Good job, Timmy Tiger!' and give him a high-five* (***give a high-five*** to Timmy Tiger). *And don't forget to use* (pause briefly to prompt the children to say *"names"*)*...NAMES."*
Timmy Tiger:	(Turn to look at the Making Friends Helper and smile.) *"Catch, _____ (Making Friends Helper)! Grr, grr!"* (Throw the small ball to the Making Friends Helper.)
Franny Frog:	(If needed, ***social coach*** the Making Friends Helper to catch the small ball and throw it back to Timmy Tiger.)
Timmy Tiger:	(Timmy Tiger catches the small ball, looks at the Making Friends Helper, and smiles.) *"Cool throw, _____ (Making Friends Helper)!"*
Franny Frog:	(If needed, ***social coach*** the Making Friends Helper to ***look, smile,*** and ***say "Good job, Timmy Tiger!"*** while ***giving a high-five***.)
Timmy Tiger:	*"Thanks! Good job, _____ (Making Friends Helper)!"*
Franny Frog:	*"Great job being a good sport, _____ (Making Friends Helper)! Ribbit, ribbit!"*
Timmy Tiger:	(Say *"good job," give a "frog high-five"* and *"tiger high-five,"* clap, cheer, and encourage the children to clap as well. The Making Friends Helper should return the small ball to Timmy Tiger.)

Franny Frog: *"Okay, Making Friends Helper, choose another friend to sit on the Good Friend Square."* (If needed, ***social coach*** the Making Friends Helper to choose another child before returning to his or her seat.)

Repeat the following with each child:

Franny Frog: (Have each child take turns sitting on the Good Friend Square and practicing ***being a good sport*** with Timmy Tiger.)

(Turn to look at the group of children.) *"Okay friends! Now let's see ____ (child) try! ____ (Child), come sit on the Good Friend Square and show us how to be a good sport with Timmy Tiger."*

(The child should sit on the Good Friend Square.) *"Remember to look at Timmy Tiger with your* (point to your eyes to prompt the children to say *"eyes"*)*...EYES, smile with your* (point to your mouth to prompt the children to say *"mouth"*)*...MOUTH, say 'Good job, Timmy Tiger!' and give him a high-five* (***give a high-five*** to Timmy Tiger). *And don't forget to use* (pause briefly to prompt the children to say *"names"*)*...NAMES."*

Timmy Tiger: (Turn to look at the child and smile.) *"Catch, _____ (child)! Grr, grr!"* (Throw the small ball to the child.)

Franny Frog: (If needed, ***social coach*** the child to catch the small ball and throw it back to Timmy Tiger.)

Timmy Tiger: (Timmy Tiger catches the small ball, looks at the child, and smiles.) *"Cool throw, _____ (child)!"*

Franny Frog: (If needed, ***social coach*** the child to ***look, smile,*** and say **"Good job, Timmy Tiger!"** while ***giving a high-five***.)

Timmy Tiger: *"Thanks! Good job, _____ (child)!"*

Franny Frog: *"Great job being a good sport, _____ (child)! Ribbit, ribbit!"*

Timmy Tiger: (Say *"good job," give a "frog high-five"* and *"tiger high-five,"* clap, cheer, and encourage the children to clap as well. The child should return the small ball to Timmy Tiger.)

Franny Frog: *"Okay, ____ (Child), choose another friend to sit on the Good Friend Square."* (If needed, ***social coach*** the child to choose another child before returning to their seat.)

Didactic Lesson Wrap-Up

Group leader: *"Well friends, you all did a great job being a good sport by looking at your friend with your* (point to your eyes to prompt the children to say *"eyes"*)*... EYES, smiling with your* (point to your mouth to prompt the children to say *"mouth"*)*...MOUTH, saying 'good job,' while using names, and giving high-fives."*

"You each earned ____ (number) stars for being a good sport! Let's start with ____ (child)."

Award each child the same number of stars by repeating the following with each child:

Group leader: *"Where's ____ (child)?"* (Wait until all the children are looking at the child.)

"____ (Child), how many stars did you earn?" (Pause briefly to allow the child to respond.)

"That's right! Let's all count for ____ (child)! One, two, three... (add stars to the Star Chart as they are counted aloud)*! Everybody clap for ____ (child)!"* (All behavioral coaches clap and cheer and encourage the children to clap as well.)

Session 6 Continued

Elbow to Elbow

BEHAVIORAL REHEARSAL ACTIVITY 1

Materials Needed

- Music and music player.
- Safety cones or masking tape.

Room Setup

- Remove or place all carpet squares to the side.
- Use the safety cones or masking tape to designate a large play area called the *dancing zone.*
- The group leader stands at the front of the room.
- The children and behavioral coaches stand in the *dancing zone* facing the group leader.

Rules: Elbow to Elbow

- The group leader reads the script below to explain the rules.
- The group leader will play the music and the children will begin to dance.
- Pause the music every ten seconds.
- Instruct the children to *"Freeze!"* and stop dancing when the music stops.
- Immediately present a command, and the children will practice ***listening and following directions***.
    - Present one command per pause.
    - Avoid commands involving the face.
    - Examples: Elbow to elbow, foot to foot, thumb to thumb, etc.
- The children quickly look for a friend and ***follow directions*** by acting out the command.
    - Examples:
        - For *"elbow to elbow,"* the children touch elbows.
        - For *"toe to toe,"* the children touch toes.
    - If there is an odd number of children, the children form a triad.
- After each command, ***social coach*** the children to ***be a good sport*** with one another.
- Once all the children are demonstrating the command, restart the music and the children resume dancing.
- Optional: Modify the game by varying the commands.
    - Examples: Hand to wrist, toe to ankle, knee to foot, etc.

Behavioral Rehearsal: Elbow to Elbow (15 Minutes)

The group leader leads the activity. The behavioral coaches and children sit on the floor in the *dancing zone* while the group leader explains the rules.

Group leader: *"Hey friends, we're going to play a game called Elbow to Elbow. We'll play some music, and you'll dance with your friends in the dancing zone* (point to the *dancing zone*). *When the music stops, you have to FREEZE* (demonstrate freezing in place) *and listen to what I say. Can you all show me how to freeze?"* (Pause briefly to allow the children and behavioral coaches to freeze in place.)

"Nice job friends! I'm going to tell you to do silly things. If I say, 'Stand elbow to elbow,' then find a little friend and touch your elbows together like this (stand elbow to elbow with a nearby behavioral coach). *Or if I say, 'Stand toe to toe,' then find a little friend and touch your toes together like this* (stand toe to toe with a nearby behavioral coach)*."*

"Then you'll practice being a good sport by looking at your friends with your (point to your eyes to prompt the children to say *"eyes")...EYES, smiling with your* (point to your mouth to prompt the children to say *"mouth")...MOUTH, saying 'good job' while using names, and giving high-fives*." (Demonstrate ***giving a high-five*** with a nearby behavioral coach.)

"And remember to listen and follow directions because we're going to change the rules after a few turns! Okay, _____ (behavioral coaches 1 and 2) will go first!"

Role Play: Elbow to Elbow

The group leader leads the role play. The two behavioral coaches demonstrate how to play *Elbow to Elbow* while the children sit and watch in the *dancing zone.*

Group leader: (Start playing the music.) *"The music is playing. _____ (Behavioral coaches 1 and 2) begin dancing!"*

Behavioral coaches 1 and 2: (Dance in the *dancing zone.*)

Group leader: (Pause the music after ten seconds). *"The music stopped. Everybody FREEZE!"*

Behavioral coaches 1 and 2: (Freeze in place.)

Group leader: *"Great job listening and following directions, _____ (behavioral coaches 1 and 2)! Now find a friend and stand elbow to elbow!"*

Behavioral coaches 1 and 2: (Stand elbow to elbow.)

Group leader: *"Great job listening and following directions, _____ (behavioral coaches 1 and 2)! Now let's practice being a good sport! Remember to look, smile, and say 'good job' while using names and giving a high-five."*

Behavioral coach 1: (Look and smile.) *"Good job, _____ (behavioral coach 2)!"*

Behavioral coach 2: (Look and smile.) *"Good job, _____ (behavioral coach 1)* (***give a high-five*** to each other)*!"*

Group leader: *"Great job being good sports, _____ (behavioral coaches 1 and 2)! Okay friends, now it's everybody's turn to play Elbow to Elbow. Are we ready?"*

Behavioral Rehearsal: Elbow to Elbow

Group leader: (Once the children and behavioral coaches are all standing in the *dancing zone*, begin to play the music.) *"The music is playing. Everybody begin dancing!"*

(Pause the music after ten seconds.) *"The music stopped. Everybody FREEZE!"* (If needed, behavioral coaches should ***social coach*** the children to ***listen and follow directions***.)

"Great job listening and following directions! Now everyone find a little friend and stand _____ (command)!" (If needed, behavioral coaches should ***social coach*** the children to ***listen and follow directions***.)

"Great job listening and following directions! Now let's practice being a good sport! Remember to look, smile, and say 'good job' while using names and giving a high-five." (Pause briefly to allow children and behavioral coaches to ***give high-fives*** and ***be good sports*** with each other.)

"Great job being good sports! Okay friends, let's keep playing! Are we ready?"

Play *Elbow to Elbow* in this manner for several minutes using the *Sample Commands* below.

Table 6.2 Sample Commands

Elbow to elbow	Knee to knee	Toe to toe
Heel to heel	Finger to finger	Shoulder to shoulder
Back to back	Thumb to thumb	Hand to Hand
Arm to arm	Foot to foot	Ankle to ankle

Group leader: Consider adding new complex commands to play *Elbow to Elbow* by saying, *"Now I want you all to listen carefully because we're going to use TWO DIFFERENT body parts. I might say, 'hand to foot'* (stand hand to foot with a nearby behavioral coach) *or I might say, 'elbow to finger'* (stand elbow to finder with a nearby behavioral coach). *Are we ready?"*

"The music is playing. Everybody begin dancing! (Pause the music after ten seconds.) *"The music stopped. Everybody FREEZE!"* (If needed, behavioral coaches should ***social coach*** the children to ***listen and follow directions***.)

"Great job listening and following directions! Now everyone find a little friend and stand _____ (complex command)!" (If needed, behavioral coaches should ***social coach*** the children to ***listen and follow directions***.)

"Great job listening and following directions! Now let's practice being a good sport! Remember to look, smile, and say 'good job' while using names and giving a high-five." (Pause briefly to allow children and behavioral coaches to ***give high-fives*** and ***be good sports*** with each other.)

"Great job being good sports! Okay friends, let's keep playing! Are we ready?"

Play *Elbow to Elbow* in this manner for several minutes using the *Sample Complex Commands* below.

Table 6.3 Complex Sample Commands

Hand to wrist	Shoulder to elbow	Ankle to foot
Hand to shoulder	Hand to thumb	Thumb to shoulder
Elbow to knee	Elbow to pinky finger	Knee to foot
Shoulder to wrist	Ankle to knee	Back to thumb
Toe to ankle	Wrist to knee	Knee to pinky finger

Behavioral Rehearsal Wrap-Up

Group leader: *"Well friends, great job being good sports and listening and following directions! Give yourselves a big round of applause!"* (All behavioral coaches clap and cheer and encourage the children to clap as well.)

"Now everyone should come sit in the Listening Circle." (Have children return to the Listening Circle to sit on their carpet squares.)

"Okay friends, you did a great job being good sports by looking at your friends with your (point to your eyes to prompt the children to say *"eyes")... EYES, smiling with your* (point to your mouth to prompt the children to say *"mouth")...MOUTH, saying 'good job,' while using names, and giving high-fives."*

"You each earned ____ (number) more stars for being a good sport! Let's start with ____ (child)."

Award each child the same number of stars by repeating the following with each child:

Group leader: *"Where's _____ (child)?"* (Wait until all the children are looking at the child.)

"_____ (Child), how many stars did you earn?" (Pause briefly to allow the child to respond.)

"That's right! Let's all count for _____ (child)! One, two, three... (add stars to the Star Chart as they are counted aloud)*! Everybody clap for _____ (child)!"* (All behavioral coaches clap and cheer and encourage the children to clap as well.)

Break Time (10 Minutes)

- The puppets may be used to lead the children to and from the bathroom during break time.
- To assist with transitions and limit unstructured time, behavioral coaches may review the lesson with the children while waiting for the remaining children to return from the bathroom.
- You may want to award stars for good behavior after returning from the bathroom.

Session 6 Continued

Head, Shoulders, Knees, and Toes

BEHAVIORAL REHEARSAL ACTIVITY 2

Materials Needed

- None.

Room Setup

- Remove or place all carpet squares to the side.
- The group leader stands at the front of the room facing the children.
- The children and behavioral coaches stand in a semi-circle facing the group leader.

Rules: Head, Shoulders, Knees, and Toes

- The group leader reads the script below to explain the rules.
- All behavioral coaches and children (if able) sing the *Head, Shoulders, Knees, and Toes* song while acting out the lyrics:
  - *Head, shoulders, knees and toes, knees and toes...*
    Head, shoulders, knees and toes, knees and toes...
    Eyes and ears and mouth and nose...
    Head, shoulders, knees and toes, knees and toes!
- The children practice ***listening and following directions*** by acting out the lyrics.
- To begin the game and for each new modification, initially sing the song slowly until the children become familiar with the game.
- After each repetition, the children practice ***being a good sport*** with one another.
- After a few repetitions, different body parts or articles of clothing may be substituted into the song.
  - Substitute only ONE body part or article of clothing at a time.
  - The new body part or article of clothing will replace the *"toes."*
  - Examples:
    - *Head, shoulders, knees and TUMMY, knees and TUMMY!*
    - *Head, shoulders, knees and ANKLES, knees and ANKLES!*
    - *Head, shoulders, knees and BACK, knees and BACK!*

Behavioral Rehearsal: Head, Shoulders, Knees, and Toes (15 Minutes)

The group leader leads the activity. The behavioral coaches and children sit on the floor in the *play zone* while the group leader explains the rules.

Group leader: *"Hey friends! Now we're going to play Head, Shoulders, Knees, and Toes. The song goes like this..."* (Sing the song with the behavioral coaches while acting out the movements by touching the body part being referenced.)

"Head, shoulders, knees and toes, knees and toes...

Head, shoulders, knees and toes, knees and toes...

Eyes and ears and mouth and nose...

Head, shoulders, knees and toes, knees and toes!"

"We're going to sing the song together. As we sing, listen to the song and follow directions. After a few turns, we'll change the body parts so make sure to listen so you can follow directions."

"Each time we finish singing, you'll practice being a good sport by looking at your friends with your (point to your eyes to prompt the children to say *"eyes"*)*...EYES, smiling with your* (point to your mouth to prompt the children to say *"mouth"*)*...MOUTH, saying 'good job' while using names, and giving high-fives."* (Demonstrate ***giving a high-five*** with a nearby behavioral coach.)

"After a few turns, we'll change the rules so make sure to listen so you can follow directions. Okay, let's have _____ (behavioral coaches) try first!"

Role Play: Head, Shoulders, Knees, and Toes

The group leader leads the role play. The two behavioral coaches demonstrate how to play *Head, Shoulders, Knees, and Toes* while the children sit and watch in the *play zone.*

Group leader: *"Okay _____ (behavioral coaches 1 and 2), let's play Head, Shoulders, Knees, and Toes and practice being a good sport. Are we ready?"*

Everyone sings the *Head, Shoulders, Knees, and Toes* song while the behavioral coaches act out the lyrics.

Group leader: *"Great job listening and following directions _____ (behavioral coaches 1 and 2)! Now let's practice being good sports! Remember to look, smile, say 'good job' using names, and give high-fives."*

Behavioral coach 1: (Look and smile.) *"Good job, _____ (behavioral coach 2)!"*

Behavioral coach 2: (Look and smile.) *"Good job, _____ (behavioral coach 1)* (***give a high-five*** to each other)*!"*

Group leader: *"Great job being good sports! Let's keep playing, but THIS time we're going to change a body part. Instead of touching our 'toes' we're going to touch our 'tummy.' So make sure to listen so you can follow directions! Are you ready?"*

Everyone sings the *Head, Shoulders, Knees, and Toes* song by substituting *"toes"* for *"tummy"* while the behavioral coaches act out the lyrics.

Group leader: *"Great job listening and following directions! Now let's practice being good sports! Remember to look, smile, say 'good job' using names, and give high-fives."*

Behavioral coach 1: (Look and smile.) *"Good job, _____ (behavioral coach 2)!"*

Behavioral coach 2: (Look and smile.) *"Good job, _____ (behavioral coach 1)* (***give a high-five*** to each other)*!"*

Group leader: *"Great job being good sports! Okay friends, now it's everybody's turn to play Head, Shoulders, Knees, and Toes. Are we ready?"*

Behavioral Rehearsal: Head, Shoulders, Knees, and Toes

Everyone: *"Head, shoulders, knees and toes, knees and toes...*

Head, shoulders, knees and toes, knees and toes...

Eyes and ears and mouth and nose...

Head, shoulders, knees and toes, knees and toes!"

Group leader: *"Great job listening and following directions! Now let's all practice being a good sport with the little friends standing next to us!"* (If needed, behavioral coaches should ***social coach*** the children to ***be a good sport***.)

"Great job being good sports, friends! Okay, let's keep playing! This time I'm going to change a body part so make sure to listen so you can follow directions! This time instead of touching our toes we're going to touch our _______ (new body part). Are we ready?" (If needed, behavioral coaches should ***social coach*** the children to ***listen and follow directions***.)

After each song, change the lyrics to substitute *"toes"* for a new body part or article of clothing. Substitute only ONE body part or article of clothing at a time.

Substitutions: *Head, shoulders, knees and TUMMY, knees and TUMMY!*

Head, shoulders, knees and ANKLES, knees and ANKLES!

Head, shoulders, knees and BACK, knees and BACK!

Head, shoulders, knees and WRISTS, knees and WRISTS!

Head, shoulders, knees and HIPS, knees and HIPS!

Head, shoulders, knees and CHIN, knees and CHIN!

Head, shoulders, knees and FEET, knees and FEET!

Head, shoulders, knees and SHIRT, knees and SHIRT!

Head, shoulders, knees and SHOES, knees and SHOES!

Head, shoulders, knees and SOCKS, knees and SOCKS!

Head, shoulders, knees and PANTS, knees and PANTS!

Consider allowing children to suggest new body parts or articles of clothing.

Group leader: *"Who wants to pick the next new body part? Let's raise our hands and remember to listen and follow directions."*

Introduce new (appropriate) body parts or articles of clothing suggested by the children following the instructions above.

Behavioral Rehearsal Wrap-Up

Group leader: *"Well friends, great job being good sports and listening and following directions! Give yourselves a big round of applause!"* (All behavioral coaches clap and cheer and encourage the children to clap as well.)

"Now everyone should come sit in the Listening Circle." (Have children return to the Listening Circle to sit on their carpet squares.)

"Okay friends, you did a great job being a good sport by looking at your friends with your (point to your eyes to prompt the children to say *"eyes")... EYES, smiling with your* (point to your mouth to prompt the children to say *"mouth")...MOUTH, saying 'good job,' while using names and giving high-fives."*

"You each earned ____ (number) more stars for being a good sport! Let's start with ____ (child)."

Award each child the same number of stars by repeating the following with each child:

Group leader: *"Where's _____ (child)?"* (Wait until all the children are looking at the child.)

"_____ (Child), how many stars did you earn?" (Pause briefly to allow the child to respond.)

"That's right! Let's all count for _____ (child)! One, two, three... (add stars to the Star Chart as they are counted aloud)*! Everybody clap for _____ (child)!"* (All behavioral coaches clap and cheer and encourage the children to clap as well.)

"Now we're going to play some games with our parents and practice being a good sport some more!"

Session 6 Continued

Being a Good Sport

PARENT COACHED PLAY: DYADIC PLAYDATES

Materials Needed

- Games brought by children and parents from home.
- Turn-taking games provided by the treatment team.
- Tables and chairs or carpet squares.
- *Parent Coached Play Cards*.

Room Setup

- If available, organize tables in separate corners of the room with four to six chairs per table.
- If tables are unavailable, place two carpet squares in separate corners of the room to indicate where the children will sit.

Rules: Dyadic Playdates

- The group leader divides the families into groups of two families each.
    - If there are an odd number of children, pair one child with a behavioral coach who will serve as a ***playmate***. In this case, you will need an additional coach to serve as a behavioral coach for the parent.
    - To avoid social exclusion, avoid having children play in triads as much as possible.
- Assign each group to sit at a table or specific play area.
    - Children should sit next to each other.
    - Parents will act as ***social coaches*** by sitting on the other side of their child to minimize interrupting the natural flow of play between the children.
    - One behavioral coach will be assigned to each dyad to provide ***social coaching*** suggestions and feedback to parents.
- Children will take turns playing the games brought from home or games provided by the treatment team.
- Each child will have ten minutes to play their chosen game with their ***playmate*** and will then switch games.
- Parents will choose which child's game will be played first.
- To minimize unstructured periods, parents will help the children set up the game in a cooperative fashion (handing game pieces to each other, offering suggestions, etc.).

- As they play, parents will ***social coach*** the children on previously learned and newly learned skills using the guidelines highlighted on the *Parent Coached Play Cards.*
- Behavioral coaches will provide support to parents in their ***social coaching*** using the ***4 Ps (priming, prompting, praising,*** and ***providing corrective feedback***) and will model appropriate coaching behavior when necessary.
- After approximately nine minutes of play, instruct the parents to prepare the children for the upcoming game swap.
- After approximately one additional minute of play (ten minutes total), instruct the parents to have the children clean up and swap games.
- Repeat the cycle with the second game for the remaining ten minutes before returning to the *Listening Circle.*

Behavioral Coaching: Dyadic Playdates

Behavioral coaches will ***social coach*** parents during dyadic ***playdates*** in the following ways:

- ***Priming***:
  - Begin the play interactions with parents going over the rules for ***being a good sport*** BEFORE GAME PLAYING.
    - Example: *"Remember to practice being a good sport by looking at your friend with your* (point to your eyes to prompt the children to say *"eyes"*)*...EYES, smiling with your* (point to your mouth to prompt the children to say *"mouth"*)*...MOUTH, saying 'good job' while using names, and giving high-fives."*
- ***Prompting***:
  - Remind parents to use the buzzwords to ***prompt*** their child to ***be a good sport*** IN THE MOMENT.
  - Help parents to identify opportunities to proactively ***prompt*** their child to ***be a good sport***.
    - Example: *"Remember to be a good sport."*
    - Example: *"Remember to say 'good job' and use names."*
    - Example: *"What can you do with your hand when being a good sport?"*
- ***Praising***:
  - Remind parents to ***praise*** and reinforce their child whenever their child ***is a good sport*** CORRECTLY.
    - Example: *"Great job being a good sport!"*
    - Example: *"Great job saying 'good job'!"*
    - Example: *"Good job looking and smiling at your friend!"*
- ***Providing corrective feedback using a praise sandwich***:
  - Remind parents to ***praise*** their child's ATTEMPTS to ***be a good sport*** and identify what could be done differently next time.
    - Example: *"Nice job being a good sport. Remember to say 'good job' next time, but nice job!"*
    - Example: *"Nice try being a good sport. Remember to give a high-five next time, but good job!"*
    - Example: *"Great job being a good sport. Don't forget to look and use names next time, but good job!"*

- Remind parents to continue to ***social coach*** on previously learned skills:
  - ***Listening and following directions.***
  - ***Meeting and greeting friends.***
  - ***Sharing and giving a turn.***
  - ***Asking for a turn.***
  - ***Keeping cool.***

Parent Coached Play: Dyadic Playdates (20 Minutes)

- Have each child choose a turn-taking game brought from home or provided by the treatment team.
- The group leader sits on the floor at the front of the room.
- The families sit on the floor in a semi-circle facing the group leader.

Group leader: *"Hey friends, we're going to have more playdates and play with the cool games you brought from home. As you play with your friends, you'll practice being a good sport by looking at your friend with your* (point to your eyes to prompt the children to say *"eyes"*)*...EYES, smiling with your* (point to your mouth to prompt the children to say *"mouth"*)*...MOUTH, saying 'good job' while using names, and giving high-fives."*

"And don't forget to keep cool and ask for a turn and share and give a turn so that everyone has fun playing together. Parents, remember to social coach your children by using your Parent Coached Play Cards. Okay, let's play with our games!"

- Before playing, parents will ***social coach*** their child to ***say "hi"*** to one another ***using names***.
- Parents will ***social coach*** their children to ***ask for a turn***, ***share and take turns, keep cool,*** and ***be a good sport*** throughout the game playing.
- After approximately nine minutes of play, instruct the parents to prepare the children for the upcoming game swap by saying, *"Parents, tell your children that we'll be swapping games in one minute."*
- After approximately one additional minute of play (ten minutes total), instruct the parents to swap games by saying, *"Parents, it's time to swap games. Social coach the children to ask for a turn and share and give a turn before playing the next game."*
- After approximately nine minutes of playing the second game, instruct the parents to prepare the children for clean up by saying, *"Parents, tell your children that we'll be cleaning up in one minute."*
- After approximately one additional minute of play (ten minutes total), ***prompt*** the parents to instruct their children to clean up by saying, *"Parents, it's time to clean up. Let's social coach the children to listen and follow directions by cleaning up and then say 'bye' to their friend using names before sitting in the Listening Circle."*
- If needed, parents will ***social coach*** their child to ***listen and follow directions*** to clean up.
- Then parents will ***social coach*** their child to ***say "bye"*** to their friend ***using names***.

Final Wrap-Up (10 Minutes)

- The group leader sits on the floor at the front of the room.
- The children sit on the carpet squares in a semi-circle facing the group leader, with parents sitting behind their children.

Group leader: *"Okay friends, you all did a great job playing your games and being good sports. When we're being a good sport, do you think we should LOOK at our friend with our EYES and SMILE with our MOUTH?"* (Pause briefly to allow children to respond *"yes."*)

"That's right, friends! And when we're being a good sport, do you think we should say 'good job' and use our friend's name?" (Pause briefly to allow children to respond *"yes."*)

"That's right, friends! And when we're being a good sport, do you think we should give a high-five to our friend?" (Demonstrate ***giving a high-five***. Pause briefly to allow children to respond *"yes."*)

"You're right, friends! Let's give high-fives to all the little friends sitting next to us!" (Prompt the children to ***give a high-five*** to the children sitting next to them.)

"You all did such a great job being a good sport today that you each earned ____ (number) more stars! Let's start with ____ (child)."

Award each child the same number of stars by repeating the following with each child:

Group leader: *"Where's _____ (child)?"* (Wait until all the children are looking at the child.)

"_____ (Child), how many stars did you earn?" (Pause briefly to allow the child to respond.)

"That's right! Let's all count for _____ (child)! One, two, three... (add stars to the Star Chart as they are counted aloud)*! Everybody clap for _____ (child)!"* (All behavioral coaches clap and cheer and encourage the children to clap as well.)

"And remember you all earned those stars by being good sports!

Everyone did a great job, and parents you did an excellent job social coaching! Parents, remember your homework assignments this week are for you and your children to practice being a good sport and to continue practicing all the other things we've learned to be a good friend using the 4 Ps. And don't forget to enroll your children in playgroups if you haven't already."

"Alright little friends, do you want to count our stars?" (Pause briefly to allow the children to respond.)

"Let's all count together and see how many stars we earned today! One, two, three...(count the number of stars for one child)*!"*

"You each earned ____ (total number) stars today! Round of applause for our friends!" (All behavioral coaches should clap and cheer and encourage the families to clap as well.)

"Great job, friends! Don't forget to choose your reward before you leave. See you all next week!"

Session 6 Continued

Suggesting Playdates and Being a Good Sport

PEERS® FOR PRESCHOOLERS: PARENT HANDOUT

Steps for Suggesting Playdates

1. **Wait for an appropriate time to ask.**
   - **Appropriate times:**
     - When you're having a light social conversation with them.
     - When they're observing the ***playgroup.***
     - When they're not busy or preoccupied.
     - When other parents are not present.
   - **Inappropriate times:**
     - Drop-off or pick-up times at the ***playgroup*** when the other parent(s) are busy or distracted.
     - Group conversations with other parents.
       - This may make the other parents feel excluded.

2. **Engage in casual conversation with the other parent(s).**
   - Keep the conversation friendly and casual.
     - This reduces the pressure on the other parent(s).

3. **Mention your children's *common interest(s).***
   - **Comments about GENERAL *common interest.***
     - Example: "It seems like our kids really enjoy playing together."
     - Example: "I noticed our kids play together really nicely."
     - Example: "I noticed our kids really seem to get along."
   - **Comments about SPECIFIC *common interest.***
     - Example: "It seems like our kids really enjoy playing chase together."
     - Example: "I noticed both of our kids enjoy playing board games together."
     - Example: "I noticed our kids seem to have fun doing arts and crafts together."

4. **Use the *common interest* as a reason for the potential *playdate*.**
    - Example: *"_____ (Potential playmate) and _______ (your child) seem to have a lot of fun playing together. It might be fun to get together for a playdate sometime."*
    - Example: *"_____ (Potential playmate) and _______ (your child) seem to have a lot of fun playing chase. It might be fun to get together for a playdate sometime."*
    - Example: *"I noticed _____ (potential playmate) and _______ (your child) seem to have a lot of fun doing arts and crafts together. Maybe we should schedule a playdate sometime."*
5. **If the parent(s) seems interested, exchange contact information to setup a *playdate*.**
    - In the moment, you may tentatively choose a day and time for the ***playdate*** if the parent(s) are particularly enthusiastic.
        - Be sure to follow up with a text or email (or a phone call when appropriate) to confirm the ***5 Ws*** (i.e., who, what, where, when, how).
    - If the parent(s) do not seem interested, casually change the topic of conversation to avoid an uncomfortable situation.
        - Remember that ***friendship is a choice.***
            - ***Our children don't get to be friends with everyone.***
            - ***Everyone doesn't get to be friends with our children.***

Table 6.1 Assessing Parent Interest for Playdates

SIGNS OF INTEREST	SIGNS OF DISINTEREST
Making eye contact	Not making eye contact/looking away
Smiling	Not smiling/looking uncomfortable
Turned toward you	Turned away from you
Talking to you/asking questions	Not talking to you/saying very little
Seem eager to make plans	Are reluctant/hesitant to make plans
Agree about children's mutual interest	Seem confused/distracted
Agree (even without finalizing)	Are busy or unavailable
Exchange contact information	Don't exchange contact information
Agree and they follow up later	Agree but never follow up

Snapshot of the Lesson: Being a Good Sport

The objective of this lesson is to teach children how to ***be a good sport.*** Steps for ***being a good sport*** include:

1. ***Look at your friends with your eyes*** (point to your eyes).
2. ***Smile with your mouth*** (point to your mouth and smile).
3. ***Say "good job" while using names***.
4. ***Give a high-five***.

Homework Assignments

1. **Identify potential playmates.**
   - Have parents identify one or two ***potential playmates*** for ***playdates***.
   - Assess whether parents:
     - Paid attention to whether the children seemed to like each other, played nicely together, and had ***common interests***.
     - Considered whether they would be comfortable and willing to interact with the parent(s) of the ***potential playmate(s)***.
     - Considered whether the ***potential playmate(s)*** and the parent(s) would be open to their ***social coaching***.
   - Have parents identify possible games and activities for the ***playdate*** based on the children's ***common interests***.

2. **Playgroups.**
   - If not yet accomplished, enroll your child in a ***playgroup*** using the criteria for a good ***playgroup***.
   - During the ***playgroup***, parents should identify:
     - ***Potential playmates*** for ***playdates***.
     - Your compatibility with the parents of ***potential playmates***.
     - Which peers regularly attend the ***playgroup***.
     - Popular activities, games, or toys.
     - Whether this is a good ***playgroup*** for your child.

3. **Practice being a good sport.**
   - Practice having your child ***be a good sport*** this week during preferred and highly motivating activities while providing ***social coaching*** using the ***4 Ps***.
     - ***Priming:*** Review the rules for ***being a good sport*** with your child BEFORE PRACTICING.
     - ***Prompting:*** Remind your child IN THE MOMENT to ***be a good sport*** whenever the opportunities present.
     - ***Praising: Praise*** your child using the buzzwords whenever they are ***being a good sport*** CORRECTLY.
     - ***Providing corrective feedback: Provide corrective feedback*** in the form of a ***praise sandwich*** whenever your child ATTEMPTS to ***be a good sport***.
   - Please send us a 30–60-second video of ***social coaching*** for ***being a good sport*** with your child to be viewed during homework review.
     - Please include:
       - Skills your child did well.
       - Skills you would like to work on with your child.

4. **Provide social coaching on previously learned skills.**
    - Continue providing ***social coaching*** to your child throughout the week using the ***4 Ps.***
    - Previous skills include:
        - ***Listening and following directions.***
        - ***Meeting and greeting friends.***
        - ***Sharing and giving a turn.***
        - ***Asking for a turn.***
        - ***Keeping cool.***

5. **Bring a turn-taking game.**
    - Bring a turn-taking game that your child enjoys playing and can be played with the other children.

Session 6 Continued

Being a Good Sport

PEERS® FOR PRESCHOOLERS: PARENT COACHED PLAY CARD

Snapshot of the Lesson: Being a Good Sport

1. ***Look at your friends with your eyes*** (point to your eyes).
2. ***Smile with your mouth*** (point to your mouth and smile).
3. ***Say "good job" while using names.***
4. ***Give a high-five.***

Priming BEFORE Game Playing

- Example: *"Remember to practice being a good sport by looking at your friend with your* (point to your eyes to prompt the children to say *"eyes"*)*...EYES, smiling with your* (point to your mouth to prompt the children to say *"mouth"*)*...MOUTH, saying 'good job' while using names, and giving high-fives."*

Prompting IN THE MOMENT

- Example: *"Remember to be a good sport."*
- Example: *"Remember to say 'good job' and use names."*
- Example: *"What can you do with your hand when being a good sport?"*

Praising for CORRECT Use of Skills

- Example: *"Great job being a good sport!"*
- Example: *"Great job saying, 'good job'!"*
- Example: *"Good job looking and smiling at your friend!"*

Providing Corrective Feedback for ATTEMPTS Using a Praise Sandwich

- Example: *"Nice job being a good sport. Remember to say, 'good job' next time, but nice job!"*
- Example: *"Nice try being a good sport. Remember to give a high-five next time, but good job!"*
- Example: *"Great job being a good sport. Don't forget to look and use names next time, but good job!"*

- Continue to provide ***social coaching*** on previously learned skills:
    - ***Listening and following directions.***
    - ***Meeting and greeting friends.***
    - ***Sharing and giving a turn.***
    - ***Asking for a turn.***
    - ***Keeping cool.***

Session 6 Continued

Suggesting Playdates and Being a Good Sport

PEERS® FOR PRESCHOOLERS: PARENT HOMEWORK WORKSHEET

Child's Name:	Parent's Name:		Date:	
HOMEWORK ASSIGNMENTS	PRIMING (REVIEWING RULES BEFORE PRACTICE)	PROMPTING (IN THE MOMENT)	PRAISING (USING BUZZWORDS)	PROVIDING CORRECTIVE FEEDBACK (USING A PRAISE SANDWICH)
Being a good sport				
Practice previous skills: • **Keeping cool** • **Asking for a turn** • **Sharing and giving turns** • **Meeting and greeting friends** • **Listening and following directions**				
Potential playmates	Which potential playmates did you identify for playdates? What games or activities did you identify for potential playdates?			
Playgroups Investigate and enroll in playgroup(s).	Which playgroups did you investigate and enroll in?			
Bring a turn-taking game	Did you bring a turn-taking game? YES or NO (Circle)		Which game did you bring?	

Please fill out this worksheet by describing what you did to complete the homework assignments. Worksheets will be collected during Homework Review at the next session of PEERS® for Preschoolers.

Session 7

Preparing for Playdates and Show and Tell During Play

PARENT SESSION THERAPIST GUIDE

Parent Session Agenda

- Homework Review (40 minutes).
- Didactic Lessons (20 minutes).
- Parent Coached Play (20 minutes).
- Final Wrap-Up (10 minutes).

Materials Needed

- Conference room with a large table and enough chairs for the parent group leader and all parents to sit comfortably around the table.
  - Avoid sitting in a circle without a table as this creates the atmosphere of group therapy.
- Name tags for parents and treatment team.
- *Parent Handouts* (for the current week and the previous weeks).
- *Parent Homework Worksheets* (for the current week and the previous weeks).
- *Parent Coached Play Cards* (for the current week and the previous weeks).
- *Attendance and Homework Compliance Sheets* for the parent group leader.
- Pens for note taking (consider having extra pens for parents who need them).

Homework Review (40 Minutes)

1. **Identify potential playmates.**
   - Have parents identify one or two ***potential playmates*** for ***playdates***.
   - Assess whether parents:
     - Paid attention to whether the children seemed to like each other, played nicely together, and had ***common interests***.
     - Considered whether they would be comfortable and willing to interact with the parent(s) of the ***potential playmate(s)***.
     - Considered whether the ***potential playmate(s)*** and the parent(s) would be open to their ***social coaching***.
   - Have parents identify possible games and activities for the ***playdate*** based on the children's ***common interests***.

DOI: 10.4324/9781003502968-8

2. **Find a playgroup for your child.**
    - Confirm parents have enrolled their child in a ***playgroup*** and have identified:
        - ***Potential playmates*** for ***playdates.***
        - Their compatibility with the parents of ***potential playmates***.
        - Which peers regularly attend the ***playgroup.***
        - Popular activities, games, or toys.
        - Whether this is a good ***playgroup*** for their child.

3. **Practice being a good sport.**
    - Review the 30–60-second video of ***social coaching*** for ***being a good sport*** for each family. (For larger groups, you may need to review video recordings in two smaller groups with two different parent group leaders).
        - Have parents identify:
            - Skills their child did well.
            - Skills they would like to work on with their child.
        - Provide ***social coaching*** tips as appropriate for each family.
    - If parents did not send a video of ***social coaching***, confirm the following:
        - Parents practiced having their child ***be a good sport*** during preferred and highly motivating activities while providing ***social coaching*** using the ***4 Ps.***
            - ***Priming*****:** Reviewed the rules for ***being a good sport*** with their child BEFORE PRACTICING.
            - ***Prompting*****:** Reminded their child IN THE MOMENT to ***be a good sport*** whenever the opportunity presented.
            - ***Praising*****:** ***Praised*** their child using the buzzwords whenever they were ***being a good sport*** CORRECTLY.
            - ***Providing corrective feedback*****:** ***Provided corrective feedback*** in the form of a ***praise sandwich*** whenever their child ATTEMPTED to ***be a good sport***.

4. **Provide social coaching on previously learned skills.**
    - Confirm parents continued to provide ***social coaching*** to their child throughout the week using the ***4 Ps*** for previously learned skills:
        - ***Listening and following directions.***
        - ***Meeting and greeting friends.***
        - ***Sharing and giving turns.***
        - ***Asking for a turn.***
        - ***Keeping cool.***

5. **Bring a turn-taking game.**
    - Confirm the following:
        - Brought a turn-taking game that their child enjoys playing and can be played with the other children. (To avoid distractions, these games should be left with the parents until *Parent Coached Play*.)

Didactic Lessons (20 Minutes)

PEERS® Neuroaffirming Pledge:

- We value neurodiversity, acceptance, and authenticity.
- We honor the diverse ways people experience the world.
- We respect each person's unique perspectives and communication styles.
- We recognize there is no one right way to connect with others.
- If using the strategies taught in PEERS® feels like camouflaging or masking and/or they don't align with your goals or the goals of your family, then you do not have to use them.
- Learning and using the skills taught in PEERS® is a PERSONAL CHOICE.

Didactic Lesson: Preparing for Playdates

- Distribute *Parent Handouts*.
  - Sections in **bold print** come directly from the *Parent Handout*.
  - Terms that are ***bold and italicized*** are buzzwords and represent important concepts from the didactic lesson.
- Explain, *"Last week we started to discuss how to casually suggest having a playdate and how to assess if parents of your children's potential playmates might be interested in having a playdate. Today we're going to discuss how to best prepare for playdates."*

Planning Playdate Activities

- **Activities should be based on the *common interests* of your child and their *playmate*.**
  - ***Common interests* are those games and activities that are fun for BOTH your child and their *playmate*.**
    - **Choose games or activities your child and their *playmate* commonly play at school or daycare or during the *playgroup*, if possible.**
      - **If it is not possible to play these games or activities, you may ask the parent(s) of the *potential playmate* what games or activities their child likes and choose from among those that are *common interests* for both children.**
    - **Avoid trying to increase your child's flexibility in play interests by introducing new games or activities during the *playdate*.**
      - **This may decrease your child's motivation, increase their frustration, and decrease your child's social engagement with their peer during the *playdate*.**
      - This, in turn, may decrease the likelihood that future ***playdates*** will occur.
      - Remember, the goal of these initial ***playdates*** is to increase the quality and frequency of positive peer interactions, not to expand their play interests.
      - **Increasing your child's flexibility in play interests may occur during parent-child play during the week (if this is a goal).**

- **Choose a range of indoor and/or outdoor games and activities that:**
  - **Require social interaction between your child and their *potential playmate*.**

- **Provide adult supervision, but do not heavily rely on adult facilitation.**
  - **Adult supervision (monitoring play) should be constant during the *playdate.***
  - **Adult facilitation (organizing and intervening in play) will vary according to the needs of your child and should lessen as your child builds their play skills.**
    - **Constant adult facilitation may interfere with the natural flow of the children's play.**
    - **At first, you may need to be more active in *social coaching.***

- **Avoid games and activities that:**
  - **Require extensive setup during the *playdate.***
    - This may lead to lengthy unstructured, transitional periods.
  - **Your child may have difficulty *sharing or giving a turn.***
    - For example, you may need to avoid preferred toys at first if your child is unable to share the toy with peers.
  - **Your child or their *playmate* may have difficulty transitioning away from.**
    - This may lead to a tantrum.
  - **May trigger your child's or their *playmate's* sensitivities.**
    - For example, if your child or their ***playmate*** is sensitive to sound, avoid games and activities that may be loud.

Preparing for Playdates

- **Make sure you have practiced playing the games and activities that will be available during the *playdate* with your child before the *playdate.***
  - **Practice as close to the *playdate* as possible (e.g., the evening before or the morning of the *playdate*).**
    - **Practice allows you to assess what potential problems may arise (challenging behaviors, issues around unstructured time, excessive language demands, etc.).**
    - Practice presents opportunities to strengthen expected social behaviors.
    - Practice decreases the level of parent involvement which may disrupt the natural flow of positive play interactions between the children during the ***playdate***.

- **Games and activity materials should be visible but NOT accessible to the children.**
  - **Gather all the games and activity materials you'll need for the *playdate* in one area that is VISIBLE to the children so they can see what their play options are.**
    - **This will reduce unstructured or "down time" in between activities.**
    - **Have "back up" or additional games and activities ready in case the children are not interested in the primary activity, lose interest in the activity, or the activity ends sooner than expected.**
  - **Be sure games and activity materials are NOT accessible to the children, but easily accessible to YOU during the *playdate.***
    - It may be difficult for your child or their ***playmate*** to engage in a cooperative activity if they are able to access alternative activities independently.
    - If your child and their ***playmate*** can access games and activity materials without adult facilitation, they may end up engaging in parallel play instead of cooperative play.

- **Put away toys and items you or your child are unwilling to share, such as:**
  - **Highly preferred items that would be difficult for your child to transition away from or *share* cooperatively with the *playmate.***
  - **Items you or your child would be upset if lost, broken, or damaged.**

- **Be prepared to have snacks for the children and parent(s).**
  - **Find out about the *playmate's* dietary restrictions and preferences.**
  - **Snack time can be useful in providing a "break" during the *playdate.***
  - **Create opportunities for cooperative interactions during snack time.**
    - **For example, children can:**
      - **Ask each other what they would like to eat or drink.**
      - **Help each other make snacks.**
      - **Help each other distribute snacks.**
      - **Help each other clean up.**

- **Remember to keep it short and sweet at first.**
  - **Initial *playdates* should be no more than 1–1.5 hours.**
  - **Longer *playdates* run the risk of children getting tired or bored.**
  - **Leave the *playmate* and your child wanting more.**
  - **The best time to end a *playdate* is when everyone is having fun.**
  - **You may choose to pick-up and drop-off the other child if you are concerned the other parent will be late (if not present).**
  - **Be prepared with a reason for ending the *playdate.***
    - **Example: *"Well it's getting late, and we need to make dinner soon."***
    - **Example: *"It's almost nap time, so I guess we need to wrap things up."***
    - **Example: *"We have some afternoon plans, so we're going to have to wrap things up soon."***

Didactic Lesson: Show and Tell During Play

Explain, *"Last week we introduced how to be a good sport during play. Today's child lesson will focus on how to show and tell during play. Like being a good sport, show and tell is a way of sustaining or maintaining play interactions. Showing often involves showing toys or games to friends, and may include comments like, 'Look at this cool toy car!' Telling often involves telling friends what we are doing, and may include requesting statements like, 'Look at me!' or "Watch this!' Showing and telling helps children to avoid parallel play, which is the act of children sitting side by side while playing but never interacting. Teaching children how to comment during play and directing their playmate's attention through show and tell may lead to greater shared experiences, which in turn is likely to further enhance their play reciprocity and strengthen their friendships."*

Snapshot of the Lesson: Show and Tell During Play

The objective of this lesson is to teach children how to *show and tell during play.* There are two ways that children can *show and tell during play*. Steps for *showing and telling* include:

A. ***Showing your toy*:**
   1. ***Look at your friend with your eyes* (point to your eyes).**
   2. ***Smile with your mouth* (point to your mouth and smile).**
   3. ***Show your toy to your friend* (wave your toy in front of your friend).**
   4. ***Tell your friend to look* at your toy by saying, *"Look at my (cool toy)!"* while *using names.***

B. ***"Watch me!"* or *"Look at me!"*:**
   1. ***Look at your friend with your eyes* (point to your eyes).**
   2. ***Smile with your mouth* (point to your mouth and smile).**
   3. ***Tell your friend to look* at you by saying, *"Watch me!"* or *"Look at me!"* while *using names.***
   4. ***Do something fun with your toy* (e.g., fly a toy plane through the air).**

Parent Coached Play

- Distribute the *Parent Coached Play Cards*.
- Review the examples of the ***4 Ps*** provided on the *Parent Coached Play Card.*
- Remind parents that in a few moments we will be joining the children for *Parent Coached Play* in the context of mock dyadic ***playdates***.
- Parents should keep the *Parent Coached Play Card* in front of them during the dyadic ***playdate*** for recommendations on how to ***social coach*** children on ***showing and telling during play.***

Homework Assignments

(Briefly review the homework assignments and troubleshoot any potential problems with parents.)

1. **Playdates.**
   - **Schedule and have a *playdate* with a *playmate.***
   - **Prepare for the *playdate* using the *5 Ws.***
     - ***WHO: Playdates* should be one-on-one.**
     - ***WHAT: Playdates* should be activity-based.**
     - ***WHERE:* Schedule initial *playdates* to take place in your home or somewhere you can provide *social coaching.***
     - ***WHEN:* Try to keep initial *playdates* to no more than 1–1.5 hours.**
     - ***HOW:* Coordinate how the children will get to and from the *playdate.***

- **Do a final practice with your child of the games and activities that will be available during the *playdate.***
- **Gather all the games and activity materials for the *playdate* in one area that is VISIBLE and easily accessible to YOU but not the children.**
- **Provide *social coaching* during the *playdate* and assess if this is a good *playmate* for your child.**

2. **Practice show and tell during play.**
   - **Practice having your child *show and tell* this week during preferred and highly motivating activities while providing *social coaching* using the *4 Ps.***
     - ***Priming:* Review the rules for *showing and telling* with your child BEFORE PRACTICING.**
     - ***Prompting:* Remind your child IN THE MOMENT to *show and tell* whenever the opportunities present.**
     - ***Praising: Praise* your child using the buzzwords whenever they are *showing and telling* CORRECTLY.**
     - ***Providing corrective feedback: Provide corrective feedback* in the form of a *praise sandwich* whenever your child ATTEMPTS to *show and tell.***
   - **Please send us a 30–60-second video of *social coaching* for *showing and telling* with your child to be viewed during homework review.**
     - **Please include:**
       - **Skills your child did well**
       - **Skills you would like to work on with your child**

3. **Provide social coaching on previously learned skills.**
   - **Continue providing *social coaching* to your child throughout the week using the *4 Ps***
   - **Previous skills include:**
     - ***Listening and following directions.***
     - ***Meeting and greeting friends.***
     - ***Sharing and giving a turn.***
     - ***Asking for a turn.***
     - ***Keeping cool.***
     - ***Being a good sport.***

4. **Bring a turn-taking game.**
   - **Bring a turn-taking game that your child enjoys playing and can be played with the other children.**

Session 7 Continued

Show and Tell During Play

CHILD SESSION THERAPIST GUIDE

Child Session Agenda

- Didactic Lesson: *Show and Tell During Play* (20 minutes).
- Group Behavioral Rehearsal Activity 1: *Simon Says* (15 minutes).
- Break Time (10 minutes).
- Group Behavioral Rehearsal Activity 2: *Show Go Lego* (15 minutes).
- Parent Coached Play: *Dyadic Playdates* (20 minutes).
- Final Wrap-Up (10 minutes).

Snapshot of the Lesson: Show and Tell During Play

The objective of this lesson is to teach children how to ***show and tell during play.*** There are two ways that children can ***show and tell during play***. Steps for ***showing and telling*** include:

A. ***Showing your toy***:
   1. ***Look at your friend with your eyes*** (point to your eyes).
   2. ***Smile with your mouth*** (point to your mouth and smile).
   3. ***Show your toy to your friend*** (wave your toy in front of your friend).
   4. ***Tell your friend to look*** at your toy by saying, ***"Look at my (cool toy)!"*** while ***using names.***

B. ***"Watch me!"*** **or** ***"Look at me!"***:
   1. ***Look at your friend with your eyes*** (point to your eyes).
   2. ***Smile with your mouth*** (point to your mouth and smile).
   3. ***Tell your friend to look*** at you by saying, ***"Watch me!"*** or ***"Look at me!"*** while ***using names.***
   4. ***Do something fun with your toy*** (e.g., fly a toy plane through the air).

Materials Needed

- Horse puppet.
- Duck puppet.
- Two toy planes.
- Two toy cars.
- Carpet squares or chairs.
- "Making Friends Helper" badge.

- Star chart with names of children.
- Marker for star chart.
- Name tags for families and treatment team.
- Prize bins with prizes.

Preparing for the Lesson

- Use the script below with the group leader using a horse puppet to play the part of "Harry Horse."
- A behavioral coach uses a duck puppet to play the part of "Dottie Duck."
- An additional behavioral coach assists in the behavioral rehearsal and provides encouragement and feedback to the group.
- A child is chosen at the beginning of the lesson as the "Making Friends Helper."
  - The "Making Friends Helper" wears a special badge and is the first child to practice the skill.
- The group leader and the behavioral coach sit on the floor at the front of the room.
- A special-colored carpet square (e.g., red) is placed at the front of the room next to the group leader to be used as the "Good Friend Square."
- For the children, additional carpet squares of the same color (e.g., green) are placed in a semi-circle facing the group leader and the "Good Friend Square."
- Note: If carpet squares are unavailable, the children and behavioral coaches may sit on chairs.
- The material in *italics* should be read by the indicated person.
- The material in ***bold and italics*** represents buzzwords and should be emphasized when read.
- The material in CAPITAL LETTERS within the script should be given extra emphasis while the group is encouraged to say the words in unison.

Behavioral Coaching Techniques

Behavioral coaches should use the following coaching techniques described below throughout the lesson and the behavioral rehearsal activities. (Note: ***priming*** occurs during the introduction to the activity.)

- ***Prompting***:
  - Use the buzzwords to ***prompt*** the children to ***show and tell*** IN THE MOMENT.
    - Example: *"Remember to show and tell."*
    - Example: *"Don't forget to look at your friend when you show your toy."*
    - Example: *"What can you do to show your toy?"*
- ***Praising***:
  - Reinforce ***showing and telling*** by ***praising*** the children when they use the skills CORRECTLY.
    - Example: *"Great job showing and telling!"*
    - Example: *"Great job saying, 'watch me'!"*
    - Example: *"Good job telling your friend to look at your toy!"*
- ***Providing corrective feedback using a praise sandwich***:
  - Reinforce ATTEMPTS to ***show and tell*** by ***praising*** the children and identifying what could be done differently next time.
    - Example: *"Good job telling your friend to look at your toy. Remember to show your toy next time, but nice job!"*

- Example: *"Nice try showing and telling. Don't forget to tell your friend to 'watch me' next time, but good job!"*
- Example: *"Good job showing and telling. Don't forget to look and smile next time, but good try!"*

• Continue to provide ***social coaching*** on previously learned skills:
  - ***Listening and following directions.***
  - ***Meeting and greeting friends.***
  - ***Sharing and giving a turn.***
  - ***Asking for a turn.***
  - ***Keeping cool.***
  - ***Being a good sport.***

Didactic Lesson: Show and Tell During Play (20 Minutes)

Have the children sit in a semi-circle on the carpet squares facing the group leader.

Harry Horse: (Sit at the front of the room and choose a Making Friends Helper.) *"Who wants to be our Making Friends Helper?"*

(Choose from among the children raising their hands and place the "Making Friends Helper" badge on the child. The child stays in their seat for now.)

"Hi friends! I'm Harry Horse. Neigh, neigh! Today we're going to practice how to show and tell when we're playing. Show and tell is a great way to be nice to our friends!"

"*Who should we show and tell with? We should show and tell with our FRIENDS, TEACHERS, MOMMIES, DADDIES, BROTHERS, AND SISTERS."*

"When should we show and tell? We should show and tell when we play with our friends, and when we want to show them cool things."

"How should we show and tell? We can show and tell by looking at our friend with our (point to your eyes and then to Harry Horse's eyes)*...EYES, smiling with our* (point to your mouth and smile)*...MOUTH, and showing our friend our toys* (wave the toy plane in front of the children) *or telling our friend to look at our toys. We can say, 'look at this cool plane' or 'look at me' or 'watch me'* (wave the toy plane in front of the children and make the sound of an airplane flying)*!' And when we're showing and telling, don't forget to use* (pause briefly to prompt the children to say *"names"*)*...NAMES."*

"Remember, show and tell is a nice way to be a good friend! Neigh, neigh!"

Role Play: Show and Tell During Play (Showing Your Toy)

Harry Horse and Dottie Duck:	(Harry Horse and Dottie Duck engage in parallel play with the toy planes.)
Harry Horse:	(Turn to look at the group of children.) *"Hey friends! Look at this cool plane* (hold up the toy plane)*! Do you think I should show* (wave the toy plane in front of the children) *my plane to my friend Dottie Duck?"* (Nod your head yes and encourage the children to say *"yes."*) *"That's a great idea! Neigh, neigh! But what should I tell Dottie Duck? Hmm..."* (Look confused, scratch head, and pause.) *"Hey friends, I know! Do you think I should tell Dottie Duck to look at my cool plane?"* (Nod your head yes and encourage the children to say *"yes."*) *"That's a great idea! Neigh, neigh! Let's do it!"* (Turn to look at Dottie Duck and smile.) *"Dottie Duck,* (hold up the toy plane) *look at my cool plane!"*
Dottie Duck:	(Look at Harry Horse and the toy plane and smile.) *"Cool plane, Harry Horse! Quack, quack!"*
Harry Horse and Dottie Duck:	(Harry Horse and Dottie Duck play together with the toy planes for a few moments while ***showing and telling***.)
Harry Horse:	(Turn to look at the group of children.) *"Hey friends, did I do a good job showing and telling with Dottie Duck?"* (Nod your head yes and encourage the children to say *"yes."*) *"That's right! Neigh, neigh!"*
Harry Horse and Dottie Duck:	(Say *"good job," give a "horse high-five"* and *"duck high-five,"* clap, cheers, and encourage the children to clap as well. Harry Horse and Dottie Duck each keep their own toy plane. Dottie Duck sits on the other side of the Good Friend Square (i.e., the Good Friend Square is between Harry Horse and Dottie Duck). Harry Horse ***social coaches*** the children as needed while they practice ***showing and telling*** with Dottie Duck.)
Harry Horse:	*"Now let's see _______ (behavioral coach) try! _______ (Behavioral coach), please come sit on the Good Friend Square."*
Behavioral coach:	(Sit on the Good Friend Square.)
Harry Horse:	*"_______ (Behavioral coach), can you show us how to show and tell with Dottie Duck?"*
Behavioral coach:	*"Okay, Harry Horse."*

Harry Horse: (Turn to look at the group of children.) *"Remember to look at Dottie Duck with your* (point to your eyes to prompt the children to say *"eyes"*)*...EYES and smile with your* (point to your mouth to prompt the children to say *"mouth"*)*...MOUTH when you show your toy* (wave the toy plane in front of the children) *and tell Dottie Duck to look at your toy. And don't forget to use* (pause briefly to prompt the children to say *"names"*)*...NAMES."* (Give a toy plane to the behavioral coach.)

Dottie Duck and Behavioral coach: (Dottie Duck and the behavioral coach engage in parallel play with the toy planes for a few moments.)

Behavioral coach: (Turn to look at Dottie Duck and smile.) *"Dottie Duck,* (hold up the toy plane) *look at my cool plane!"*

Dottie Duck: (Look at the behavioral coach and the toy plane and smile.) *"Cool plane, _______ (behavioral coach)! Quack, quack!"*

Dottie Duck and Behavioral coach: (Dottie Duck and the behavioral coach play together with the toy planes for a few moments while ***showing and telling***.)

Harry Horse: *"Great job showing and telling, _______ (behavioral coach)! Neigh, neigh!"*

Harry Horse and Behavioral coach: (Say *"good job," give a "horse high-five"* and *"duck high-five,"* clap, cheer, and encourage the children to clap as well. The behavioral coach returns the toy plane to Harry Horse and leaves the Good Friend Square.)

Behavioral Rehearsal: Show and Tell During Play (Showing Your Toy)

Harry Horse: (Turn to look at the group of children.) *"Okay friends! Now let's see our Making Friends Helper _______ try! _______ (Making Friends Helper), come sit on the Good Friend Square and show us how to show and tell with Dottie Duck."*

(The Making Friends Helper should sit on the Good Friend Square.)

"Remember to look at Dottie Duck with your (point to your eyes to prompt the children to say *"eyes"*)*...EYES and smile with your* (point to your mouth to prompt the children to say *"mouth"*)*...MOUTH when you show your toy* (wave the toy plane in front of the children) *and tell Dottie Duck to look at your toy. And don't forget to use* (pause briefly to prompt the children to say *"names"*)*...NAMES."* (Give a toy plane to the Making Friends Helper.)

(If needed, ***social coach*** the Making Friends Helper to ***look and smile*** at Dottie Duck, ***show*** the toy plane, and ***say, "Dottie Duck, look at my cool plane!"***)

Dottie Duck: (Look at the Making Friends Helper and smile.) *"Cool plane, _______ (Making Friends Helper)! Quack, quack!"*

(Dottie Duck and the Making Friends Helper play together with the toy planes for a few moments while ***showing and telling***.)

Harry Horse: *"Great job showing and telling, _______ (Making Friends Helper)! Neigh, neigh!"*

(Say *"good job," give a "horse high-five"* and *"duck high-five,"* clap, cheer, and encourage the children to clap as well. The Making Friends Helper should return the toy plane to Harry Horse.)

"Okay, Making Friends Helper, choose another friend to sit on the Good Friend Square." (If needed, ***social coach*** the Making Friends Helper to choose another child before returning to their seat.)

Repeat the following with each child:

Harry Horse: (Have each child take turns sitting on the Good Friend Square and practicing ***show and tell*** with Dottie Duck.)

(Turn to look at the group of children.) *"Okay friends! Now let's see _______ (child) try! _______ (Child), come sit on the Good Friend Square and show us how to show and tell with Dottie Duck."*

(The child should sit on the Good Friend Square.) *"Remember to look at Dottie Duck with your* (point to your eyes to prompt the children to say *"eyes"*)*...EYES and smile with your* (point to your mouth to prompt the children to say *"mouth"*)*...MOUTH when you show your toy* (wave the toy plane in front of the children) *and tell Dottie Duck to look at your toy. And don't forget to use* (pause briefly to prompt the children to say *"names"*)*... NAMES."* (Give a toy plane to the child.)

(If needed, ***social coach*** the child to ***look and smile*** at Dottie Duck, ***show*** the toy plane, and ***say, "Dottie Duck, look at my cool plane!"***)

Dottie Duck: (Look at the child and the toy plane and smile.) *"Cool plane, _______ (child)! Quack, quack!"*

(Dottie Duck and the child play together with the toy planes for a few moments while ***showing and telling***.)

Harry Horse: *"Great job showing and telling, _______ (child)! Neigh, neigh!"*

(Say *"good job," give a "horse high-five"* and *"duck high-five,"* clap, cheer, and encourage the children to clap as well. The child should return the toy plane to Harry Horse.)

"Okay, _______ (child), choose another friend to sit on the Good Friend Square." (If needed, ***social coach*** the child to choose another child before returning to their seat.)

Role Play: Show and Tell During Play ("Watch Me!")

Harry Horse: *"Let's keep playing!"* (Turn to look at the group of children.) *"Hey friends, another great way to show and tell is to tell our friends to 'watch me' or 'look at me.'"*

Harry Horse and Dottie Duck: (Harry Horse and Dottie Duck engage in parallel play with the toy cars.)

Harry Horse: (Turn to look at the group of children.) *"Hey friends! Watch me make this cool jump* (demonstrate jumping the toy car high in the air)*! Do you think I should show* (wave the toy car in front of the children) *my cool jump to my friend Dottie Duck?"* (Nod your head yes and encourage the children to say *"yes."*)

"That's a great idea! Neigh, neigh! But what should I tell Dottie Duck? Hmm...." (Look confused, scratch head, and pause.)

"Hey friends, I know! Do you think I should tell Dottie Duck to 'watch me' or 'look at me'?" (Nod your head yes and encourage the children to say *"yes."*)

"That's a great idea! Neigh, neigh! Let's do it!" (Turn to look at Dottie Duck and smile.) *"Dottie Duck, watch me* (jump the toy car through the air)*!"*

Dottie Duck: (Look at Harry Horse and the toy car and smile.) *"Cool jump, Harry Horse! Quack, quack!"*

Harry Horse and Dottie Duck: (Harry Horse and Dottie Duck play together with the toy planes for a few moments while ***showing and telling*** by saying, *"Look at me!"* and *"Watch me!"*)

Harry Horse: (Turn to look at the group of children.) *"Hey friends, did I do a good job showing and telling with Dottie Duck?"* (Nod your head yes and encourage the children to say *"yes."*)

"That's right! Neigh, neigh!"

Harry Horse and Dottie Duck: (Say *"good job," give a "horse high-five"* and *"duck high-five,"* clap, cheer, and encourage the children to clap as well. Harry Horse and Dottie Duck each keep their own toy car. Dottie Duck sits on the other side of the Good Friend Square (i.e., the Good Friend Square is between Harry Horse and Dottie Duck). Harry Horse ***social coaches*** the children as needed while the children practice ***showing and telling*** with Dottie Duck.)

Harry Horse: *"Now let's see _______ (behavioral coach) try! _______ (Behavioral coach), please come sit on the Good Friend Square."*

Behavioral coach: (Sit on the Good Friend Square.)

Harry Horse: *"_______ (Behavioral coach), can you show us how to show and tell with Dottie Duck?"*

Behavioral coach: *"Okay, Harry Horse."*

Harry Horse: (Turn to look at the group of children.) *"Remember to look at Dottie Duck with your* (point to your eyes to prompt the children to say *"eyes"*)*...EYES and smile with your* (point to your mouth to prompt the children to say *"mouth"*)*...MOUTH when you show your toy* (wave the toy plane in front of the children) *and tell Dottie Duck to 'watch me' or 'look at me.' And don't forget to use* (pause briefly to prompt the children to say *"names"*)*...NAMES."*

(Give a toy car to the behavioral coach.)

Behavioral coach: (Turn to look at Dottie Duck and smile.) *"Dottie Duck, watch me* (jump the toy car through the air)*!"*

Dottie Duck: (Look at the behavioral coach and the toy car and smile.) *"Cool jump, _______ (Behavioral coach)! Quack, quack!"*

Dottie Duck and Behavioral coach: (Dottie Duck and behavioral coach play together with the toy planes for a few moments while ***showing and telling*** by ***saying, "Look at me!"*** and ***"Watch me!"***)

Harry Horse: *"Great job showing and telling, _______ (behavioral coach)! Neigh, neigh!"*

Harry Horse and Behavioral coach: (Say *"good job," give a "horse high-five"* and *"duck high-five,"* clap, cheer, and encourage the children to clap as well. The behavioral coach returns the toy car to Harry Horse and leaves the Good Friend Square.)

Dottie Duck: (Place the Dottie Duck puppet to the side.)

Role Play: Show and Tell During Play ("Watch Me!")

Harry Horse: *"Okay friends! Now let's ALL practice showing and telling with each other. Let's take turns saying 'watch me' to the friend sitting next to us. Remember to look at your friend with your* (point to your eyes to prompt the children to say *"eyes"*)*...EYES and smile with your* (point to your mouth to prompt the children to say *"mouth"*)*...MOUTH when you show your toy* (wave the toy car in front of the children) *and when you tell your friend to 'watch me.' And don't forget to use* (pause briefly to prompt the children to say *"names"*)*... NAMES. I'll go first."*

(Turn to look at the behavioral coach that played the role of Dottie Duck and smile.) *"_______ (Behavioral coach), watch me* (jump the toy car through the air)*!"*

Behavioral coach: (Turn to look at Harry Horse and smile.) *"Great job showing and telling, Harry Horse!"*

(Behavioral coaches clap and cheer and encourage the children to clap as well.)

"Hey friends, now it's my turn to show and tell."

(Turn to look at the nearest child to their side and smile.) *"_______ (Child), watch me* (jump the toy car through the air)*!"*

Harry Horse: *"Great job showing and telling, _______ (behavioral coach)! Neigh, neigh!"*

(Behavioral coaches clap and cheer and encourage the children to clap as well.)

Repeat the following with each child:

Harry Horse: (Have each child take turns demonstrating ***show and tell*** from their seat with the person sitting next to them.)

"Hey friends, now it's _______ (child) turn to show and tell with _______ (person sitting next to them)."

Behavioral coach: (The behavioral coach hands the toy car to the child.)

Harry Horse: (If necessary, Harry Horse ***social coaches*** the child to ***look and smile*** at the person next to them, jump the toy car through the air, and ***say, "_______ (Child), watch me!"*** or ***"_______ (Child), look at me!")***

"Great job showing and telling, _______ (child)! Neigh, neigh!"

(Behavioral coaches clap and cheer and encourage the children to clap as well.)

Didactic Lesson Wrap-Up

Group leader: *"Well friends, you all did a great job showing and telling by looking at your friend with your* (point to your eyes to prompt the children to say *"eyes"*)*... EYES and smiling with your* (point to your mouth to prompt the children to say *"mouth"*)*...MOUTH when you showed your toys* (wave the toy plane and car in front of the children) *and told your friend to look at your toy or 'watch me' or 'look at me.' And nice job using* (pause briefly to prompt the children to say *"names"*)*...NAMES!"*

"You each earned ____ (number) stars for showing and telling! Let's start with _______ (child)."

Award each child the same number of stars by repeating the following with each child:

Group leader: *"Where's ____ (child)?"* (Wait until all the children are looking at the child.)

"____ (Child), how many stars did you earn?" (Pause briefly to allow the child to respond.)

"That's right! Let's all count for ____ (child)! One, two, three... (add stars to the Star Chart as they are counted aloud)*! Everybody clap for ____ (child)!"* (All behavioral coaches clap and cheer and encourage the children to clap as well.)

Session 7 Continued

Simon Says

BEHAVIORAL REHEARSAL ACTIVITY 1

Materials Needed

- None.

Room Setup

- Remove or place all carpet squares to the side.
- The group leader stands at the front of the room facing the children.
- The children and behavioral coaches sit in a semi-circle facing the group leader.

Rules: Simon Says

- The group leader reads the script below to explain the rules.
- The group leader provides commands to ONE child at a time. This child is known as the *Simon Says Friend.*
- Before the child acts out the command, they should ***show and tell*** with the group.
  - If needed, behavioral coaches should ***social coach*** the child to ***show and tell*** by saying, "***Look at me, friends!***" or "***Watch me, friends!***"
- After the child has acted out the command, the group leader presents the SAME command to all the children.
- After all the children are demonstrating the command, the group leader says, *"Simon says FREEZE!* (Pause.) *And sit."* and the children should stop moving and sit down.
  - If needed, behavioral coaches should ***social coach*** the children to ***listen and follow directions***.
- The group leader then ***social coaches*** the children to ***be a good sport*** with each other.
  - If needed, behavioral coaches should ***social coach*** the children to ***be a good sport*** by ***saying*** "***good job***" while ***using names*** and ***giving high-fives***.
- Repeat this cycle for each command.
- All commands begin with *"Simon says…"*
  - The purpose of the game is to practice ***show and tell*** rather than to eliminate group members.
- Keep commands simple and fun. Present commands that require some movement.
  - Examples:
    - *"Simon says hop like a kangaroo!"*
    - *"Simon says stomp your feet like a giant!"*
  - The group leader and behavioral coaches may need to model the commands for the children.

- To resume the game, the group leader chooses the next child to demonstrate the command.

Behavioral Rehearsal: Simon Says (15 Minutes)

The group leader leads the activity. The behavioral coaches and children sit nearby as the group leader explains the rules.

Group leader: *"Hey friends, now we're going to play Simon Says! I'm going to tell each of you to do some fun and silly things like 'Simon says walk like a robot'* (demonstrate walking like a robot) *or 'Simon says waddle like a penguin'* (demonstrate waddling like a penguin)*."*

"But before you walk like a robot or waddle like a penguin, you need to show and tell by looking at your friends with your (point to your eyes to prompt the children to say *"eyes")...EYES and smiling with your* (point to your mouth to prompt the children to say *"mouth")...MOUTH when you tell your friends to 'look' or 'watch me.' And don't forget to use* (pause briefly to prompt the children to say *"names")...NAMES."*

"And make sure to listen and follow directions because I'm going to call your name one (hold up your index finger) *at a time to be our Simon Says Friend. The Simon Says Friends will be our first friend to show and tell."*

"Okay, let's have _______ (behavioral coach 1) and _______ (behavioral coach 2) try first!"

Role Play: Simon Says

The group leader leads the role play. The two behavioral coaches demonstrate how to play *Simon Says*.

Group leader: *"Okay _______ (behavioral coach 1) and _______ (behavioral coach 2), let's play Simon Says and practice showing and telling. Our first Simon Says Friend is _______ (behavioral coach 1)."*

"_______ (Behavioral coach 1), Simon says show and tell your friends how to walk like a robot!"

Behavioral coach 1: (Turn to look at behavioral coach and children.) *"Hey friends, watch me!"* (Walk like a robot.) *Look at me!"*

Group leader: *"Great job showing and telling, _______ (behavioral coach 1)! Now Simon says everybody stand up and walk like a robot!"*

(Wait until all the behavioral coaches and children are walking like robots.)

"Simon says FREEZE! (Pause.) And sit." (All behavioral coaches and children should stop moving and sit down.)

"Great job listening and following direction everyone! Now let's practice being a good sport with our friends next to us by saying 'good job' and giving a high-five." (If needed, behavioral coaches should ***social coach*** the children to ***be a good sport***.)

"Great job being good sports everyone! Let's keep playing. Our next Simon Says Friend is_______ (behavioral coach 2). _______ (Behavioral coach 2), Simon says show and tell your friends how to waddle like a penguin."

Behavioral coach 2: (Turn to look at behavioral coach 1 and children.) *"Hey friends, look at me!"* (Waddle like a penguin.) *Look at me!"*

Group leader: *"Great job showing and telling, _______ (behavioral coach 2)!" Now Simon says everybody stand up and waddle like a penguin!"*

(Wait until all the behavioral coaches and children are waddling like penguins.)

"Simon says FREEZE! (Pause.) And sit." (All behavioral coaches and children should stop moving and sit down.)

"Great job listening and following directions everyone! Now let's practice being a good sport with our friends next to us by saying 'good job' and giving a high-five." (If needed, behavioral coaches should ***social coach*** the children to ***be a good sport***.)

"Great job being good sports everyone! Okay friends, let's keep playing! Are we ready?"

Behavioral Rehearsal: Simon Says

Group leader: *"Our next Simon Says Friend is _______ (child). _______ (Child), Simon says show and tell your friends how to _______ (command)!"*

(If needed, behavioral coaches should ***social coach*** the child to ***show and tell*** by saying ***"Look at me, friends!"*** or ***"Watch me, friends!"***)

"Great job showing and telling, _______ (child)! Now Simon says everybody stand up and _______ (command)!"

(Wait until all the children and behavioral coaches are waddling like penguins.)

"Simon says FREEZE! (Pause.) And sit." (All children and behavioral coaches should stop moving and sit down.)

"Great job listening and following directions everyone! Now let's practice being a good sport with our friends next to us by saying 'good job' and giving a high-five." (If needed, behavioral coaches should ***social coach*** the children to ***be a good sport***.)

"Great job being good sports!"

Play *Simon Says* in this manner for several minutes using the *Sample Commands* below. The group leader may need to model the command for the children.

Table 7.1 Simon Says Commands

Peck like a chicken	Gallop like a horse
Stomp your feet like a giant	Walk backward
Shake your hips	Crawl like a baby
Hop like a kangaroo	Give a friend a high-five
Swim like a shark	Chomp like an alligator
Slither like a snake	Act like a monkey
Shake your legs	Dig like a dog
Spin like a top	Shake your whole body
Wiggle like a worm	Walk like a crab
Dance	Hop like a frog
Move slow like a turtle	Fly like a plane

Behavioral Rehearsal Wrap-Up

Group leader: *"Well friends, great job showing and telling and being good sports! Give yourselves a big round of applause!"* (All behavioral coaches clap and cheer and encourage the children to clap as well.)

"Now everyone should come sit in the Listening Circle." (Have children return to the Listening Circle to sit on their carpet squares.)

"Okay friends, you did a great job showing and telling by looking at your friends with your (point to your eyes to prompt the children to say *"eyes")... EYES and smiling with your* (point to your mouth to prompt the children to say *"mouth")...MOUTH when you showed your friends what to do and told your friends to 'look at me' or 'watch me'! And nice job using* (pause briefly to prompt the children to say *"names")...NAMES!"*

"You each earned ____ (number) more stars for being a good sport! Let's start with ____ (child)."

Award each child the same number of stars by repeating the following with each child:

Group leader: *"Where's _____ (child)?"* (Wait until all the children are looking at the child.)

"_____ (Child), how many stars did you earn?" (Pause briefly to allow the child to respond.)

"That's right! Let's all count for _____ (child)! One, two, three... (add stars to the Star Chart as they are counted aloud)*! Everybody clap for _____ (child)!"* (All behavioral coaches clap and cheer and encourage the children to clap as well.)

Break Time (10 Minutes)

- The puppets may be used to lead the children to and from the bathroom during break time.
- To assist with transitions and limit unstructured time, behavioral coaches may review the lesson with the children while waiting for the remaining children to return from the bathroom.
- You may want to award stars for good behavior after returning from the bathroom.

Session 7 Continued

Show Go Lego

BEHAVIORAL REHEARSAL ACTIVITY 2

Materials Needed

- Lego Duplo sets (one set per dyad).
- Tables and chairs (optional).

Room Setup

- Place Lego Duplo sets in separate corners of the room.
- The group leader sits on the floor in front of the room.
- The children and behavioral coaches should sit on the floor in a semi-circle facing the group leader.

Rules: Show Go Lego

- The group leader reads the script below to explain the rules.
- The group leader divides the children into dyads.
  - If there is an odd number of children, pair one child with a behavioral coach.
  - Assign at least one behavioral coach per dyad to provide ***social coaching***.
- Direct each dyad to sit around the Lego Duplo set.
- Behavioral coaches ***social coach*** the children to cooperatively choose the first building theme.
  - Behavioral coaches may need to help children identify a theme.
- The children will then build with the Lego Duplo set based on the chosen theme.
- As the children play, the behavioral coaches ***social coach*** the children to ***show and tell***.
- After approximately two minutes of play, the group leader announces that each dyad will take turns ***showing and telling*** to the entire group in one minute.
- After approximately one additional minute of play (three minutes total), the group leader instructs the dyads to take turns standing up as they ***show and tell*** what they made to the entire group.
- The group leader then ***social coaches*** the children to ***be a good sport*** with a nearby friend.
- Behavioral coaches should model ways to respond to the children's ***showing and telling***.
  - Examples: *"So cool!" "Awesome!" "I want to build that too!"*
- Behavioral coaches should ***praise*** and reinforce the children if they respond to each other's ***showing and telling*** either spontaneously or upon observing behavioral coaches' modeling.

Behavioral Rehearsal: Show Go Lego (15 Minutes)

The group leader explains the activity and leads the group ***show and tell***. The behavioral coaches ***social coach*** the children in dyads to ***show and tell*** during the game playing.

Group leader: *"Hey friends, now we're going to play Show Go Lego. You and your friend will use Legos to build some cool things together.*

While you're building, you should practice showing and telling by looking at your friend with your (point to your eyes to prompt the children to say *"eyes"*)*...EYES and smiling with your* (point to your mouth to prompt the children to say *"mouth"*)*...MOUTH when you show what you made* (hold up the Legos in front of the children) *and tell your friend to look at what you made or to 'watch me' or 'look at me' while using names.*

We'll build Legos with our friend for three minutes and then we'll practice showing and telling and being a good sport with everybody! Okay, let's play Show Go Lego!"

(Create dyads and direct each dyad to sit around a Duplo Lego set with a behavioral coach.)

Behavioral coach: *"Okay friends, what should we build first?"* (Behavioral coaches may need to help children identify a building theme.)

"Let's remember to show and tell with our friend." (As the children play, the behavioral coaches will ***social coach*** the children to ***show and tell*** and ***be good sports*** while building.)

(Continue in this manner for TWO minutes.)

Group leader: *"In one minute we're going to stop building and show and tell with all our friends."* (If needed, behavioral coaches should ***social coach*** the children ***show and tell*** and ***be good sports*** while building.)

(Continue building and ***showing and telling*** for ONE minute.)

(Repeat the following with each dyad.) *"Okay friends, now let's show and tell our friends what we made! _______ (Children) will go first / next. Stand up and show and tell ALL your friends what you built."* (If needed, behavioral coaches should ***social coach*** the children to ***show and tell*** by saying, ***"Look at our _______!"***)

"Great job showing and telling _______ (children)! Let's all practice being good sports by saying 'good job' and giving a high-five with our friends!" (If needed, behavioral coaches should ***social coach*** the children to ***be good sports***.)

(Have each dyad take turns ***showing and telling*** in this manner until every child has shared. Then repeat the cycle by choosing a new building theme. Have children take turns choosing the building theme.)

Table 7.2 Examples of Building Themes

House	Spaceship	Boat
School	Car/racecar	Pirate ship
City	Princess	Castle
Bridge	Truck	Dinosaur
Racetrack	Airplane	Dragon
Animal	Superhero	Wizard

Behavioral Rehearsal Wrap-Up

Group leader: *"Well friends, great job showing and telling and being good sports! Give yourselves a big round of applause!"* (All behavioral coaches clap and cheer and encourage the children to clap as well.)

"Now everyone should come sit in the Listening Circle." (Have children return to the Listening Circle to sit on their carpet squares.)

"Okay friends, you did a great job showing and telling by looking at your friends with your (point to your eyes to prompt the children to say *"eyes")... EYES and smiling with your* (point to your mouth to prompt the children to say *"mouth")...MOUTH when you showed your friends what you made and told your friends to 'look at me' or 'watch me'! And nice job using* (pause briefly to prompt the children to say *"names")...NAMES!"*

"You each earned ____ (number) more stars for showing and telling! Let's start with _______ (child)."

Award each child the same number of stars by repeating the following with each child:

Group leader: *"Where's _______ (child)?"* (Wait until all the children are looking at the child.)

"_______ (Child), how many stars did you earn?" (Pause briefly to allow the child to respond.)

"That's right! Let's all count for _______ (child)! One, two, three... (add stars to the Star Chart as they are counted aloud)*! Everybody clap for _______ (child)!"* (All behavioral coaches clap and cheer and encourage the children to clap as well.)

"Now we're going to play another game with our parents and practice showing and telling some more!"

Session 7 Continued

Show and Tell During Play

PARENT COACHED PLAY: DYADIC PLAYDATES

Materials Needed

- Games brought by children and parents from home.
- Turn-taking games provided by the treatment team.
- Tables and chairs or carpet squares.
- *Parent Coached Play Cards.*

Room Setup

- If available, organize tables in separate corners of the room with four to six chairs per table.
- If tables are not available, place two carpet squares in separate corners of the room to indicate where the children will sit.

Rules: Dyadic Playdates

- The group leader divides the families into groups of two families each.
  - If there are an odd number of children, pair one child with a behavioral coach who will serve as a ***playmate***. In this case, you will need an additional coach to serve as a behavioral coach for the parent.
  - To avoid social exclusion, avoid having children play in triads as much as possible.
- Assign each group to sit at a table or specific play area.
  - Children should sit next to each other.
  - Parents will act as ***social coaches*** by sitting on the other side of their child to minimize interrupting the natural flow of play between the children.
  - One behavioral coach will be assigned to each dyad to provide ***social coaching*** suggestions and feedback to parents.
- Children will take turns playing the games brought from home or games provided by the treatment team.
- Each child will have ten minutes to play their chosen game with their ***playmate*** and will then switch games.
- Parents will choose which child's game will be played first.
- To minimize unstructured periods, parents will help the children set up the game in a cooperative fashion (handing game pieces to each other, offering suggestions, etc.).
- As they play, parents will ***social coach*** the children on previously learned and newly learned skills using the guidelines highlighted on the *Parent Coached Play Cards.*

- Behavioral coaches will provide support to parents in their ***social coaching*** using the ***4 Ps*** (***priming, prompting, praising,*** and ***providing corrective feedback***) and will model appropriate coaching behavior when necessary.
- After approximately nine minutes of play, instruct the parents to prepare the children for the upcoming game swap.
- After approximately one additional minute of play (ten minutes total), instruct the parents to have the children clean up and swap games.
- Repeat the cycle with the second game for the remaining ten minutes before returning to the *Listening Circle*.

Behavioral Coaching: Dyadic Playdates

Behavioral coaches will ***social coach*** parents during dyadic ***playdates*** in the following ways:

- ***Priming***:
  - Begin the play interactions with parents going over the rules for ***show and tell*** BEFORE GAME PLAYING.
    - Example: *"Remember to practice showing and telling by looking at your friend with your* (point to your eyes to prompt the child to say *"eyes"*)*…EYES and smiling with your* (point to your mouth to prompt the child to say *"mouth"*)*…MOUTH when you show your game and tell your friend to look at your game or to 'watch me' or 'look at me.' And don't forget to use* (pause briefly to prompt the child to say *"names"*)*…NAMES!"*
- ***Prompting***:
  - Remind parents to use the buzzwords to ***prompt*** their child to ***show and tell*** IN THE MOMENT.
  - Help parents to identify opportunities to proactively ***prompt*** their child to ***show and tell***.
    - Example: *"Remember to show and tell."*
    - Example: *"Remember to show your toy and tell your friend to 'look.'"*
    - Example: *"What should you say if you want to show and tell?"*
- ***Praising***:
  - Remind parents to ***praise*** and reinforce their child whenever their child ***shows and tells*** CORRECTLY.
    - Example: *"Great job showing and telling!"*
    - Example: *"Great job telling your friend to 'watch me'!"*
    - Example: *"Great job looking at your friend when you showed your toy!"*
- ***Providing corrective feedback using a praise sandwich***:
  - Remind parents to ***praise*** their child's ATTEMPTS to ***show and tell*** and identify what could be done differently next time.
    - Example: *"Good job telling your friend to look at your toy. Remember to show your toy next time, but nice job!"*
    - Example: *"Nice try showing and telling. Don't forget to tell your friend to 'watch me' next time, but good job!"*
    - Example: *"Good job showing and telling. Don't forget to look and smile next time, but good try!"*
- Remind parents to continue to ***social coach*** on previously learned skills:
  - ***Listening and following directions.***
  - ***Meeting and greeting friends.***

- ***Sharing and giving a turn.***
- ***Asking for a turn.***
- ***Keeping cool.***
- ***Being a good sport.***

Parent Coached Play: Dyadic Playdates (20 Minutes)

- Have each child choose a turn-taking game brought from home or provided by the treatment team.
- The group leader sits on the floor at the front of the room.
- The families sit on the floor in a semi-circle facing the group leader.

Group leader: *"Hey friends, we're going to have more playdates and play with the fun games you brought from home. As you play with friends, we want you all to practice showing and telling by looking at your friend with your* (point to your eyes to prompt the children to say *"eyes")...EYES and smiling with your* (point to your mouth to prompt the children to say *"mouth")...MOUTH when you show your game and tell your friend to 'look' at your game or to 'watch me' or 'look at me.' And don't forget to use* (pause briefly to prompt the children to say *"names")...NAMES!"*

"And remember to be a good sport and keep cool and ask for turns and share and give turns! Parents, remember to social coach your children by using your Parent Coached Play Cards. Okay, let's play with our games!"

- Before playing, parents will ***social coach*** their child to ***say*** "***hi***" to one another ***using names***.
- Parents will ***social coach*** their children to ***show and tell, ask for a turn***, ***share and take turns, keep cool,*** and ***be a good sport*** throughout the game playing.
- After approximately nine minutes of play, instruct the parents to prepare the children for the upcoming game swap by saying, *"Parents, tell your children that we'll be swapping games in one minute."*
- After approximately one additional minute of play (ten minutes total), instruct the parents to swap games by saying, *"Parents, it's time to swap games. Social coach the children to ask for a turn and share and give a turn before playing the next game."*
- After approximately nine minutes of playing the second game, instruct the parents to prepare the children for clean up by saying, *"Parents, tell your children that we'll be cleaning up in one minute."*
- After approximately one additional minute of play (ten minutes total), ***prompt*** the parents to instruct their children to clean up by saying, *"Parents, it's time to clean up. Let's social coach the children to listen and follow directions by cleaning up and then say 'bye' to their friend using names before sitting in the Listening Circle."*
- If needed, parents will ***social coach*** their child to ***listen and follow directions*** to clean up.
- Then parents will ***social coach*** their child to ***say*** "***bye***" to their friend ***using names.***

Final Wrap-Up (10 Minutes)

- The group leader sits on the floor at the front of the room.
- The children sit on the carpet squares in a semi-circle facing the group leader, with parents sitting behind their children.

Group leader: *"Okay friends, you all did a great job playing your games and showing and telling. When we're showing and telling, do you think we should LOOK at our friend with our EYES and SMILE with our MOUTH?"* (Pause briefly to allow children to respond *"yes."*)

"That's right, friends! And when we're showing and telling, do you think we should show our friends our toys or games?" (Pause briefly to allow children to respond *"yes."*)

"That's right, friends! And when we're showing and telling, do you think we should tell our friends to 'look at me' or 'watch me' and use our friends' names?" (Pause briefly to allow children to respond *"yes."*)

"You all did such a great job showing and telling today that you each earned ____ (number) more stars! Let's start with ____ (child)."

Award each child the same number of stars by repeating the following with each child:

Group leader: *"Where's _____ (child)?"* (Wait until all the children are looking at the child.)

"_____ (Child), how many stars did you earn?" (Pause briefly to allow the child to respond.)

"That's right! Let's all count for _____ (child)! One, two, three... (add stars to the Star Chart as they are counted aloud)*! Everybody clap for _____ (child)!"* (All behavioral coaches clap and cheer and encourage the children to clap as well.)

"And remember you all earned those stars by showing and telling! Everyone did a great job, and parents you did an excellent job social coaching! Parents, remember your homework assignments this week are for you and your children to practice showing and telling and continue practicing all the other things we've learned to be a good friend using the 4 Ps. And don't forget to have a playdate and go to your playgroups."

"Alright little friends, do you want to count our stars?" (Pause briefly to allow the children to respond.)

"Let's all count together and see how many stars we earned today! One, two, three...(count the number of stars for one child)*!"*

"You each earned ____ (total number) stars today! Round of applause for our friends!" (All behavioral coaches should clap and cheer and encourage the families to clap as well.)

"Great job, friends! Don't forget to choose your reward before you leave. See you all next week!"

Session 7 Continued

Preparing for Playdates and Show and Tell During Play

PEERS® FOR PRESCHOOLERS: PARENT HANDOUT

Planning Playdate Activities

- **Activities should be based on the *common interests* of your child and their *playmate.***
  - ***Common interests* are those games and activities that are fun for BOTH your child and their *playmate.***
    - Choose games or activities your child and their ***playmate*** commonly play at school or daycare or during the ***playgroup,*** if possible.
      - If it is not possible to play these games or activities, you may ask the parent(s) of the ***potential playmate*** what games or activities their child likes and choose from among those that are ***common interests*** for both children.
    - Avoid trying to increase your child's flexibility in play interests by introducing new games or activities during the ***playdate***.
      - This may decrease your child's motivation, increase their frustration, and decrease your child's social engagement with their peer during the ***playdate***.
      - Increasing your child's flexibility in play interests may occur during parent-child play during the week (if this is a goal).

- **Choose a range of indoor and/or outdoor games and activities that:**
  - **Require social interaction between your child and their *potential playmate.***
  - **Provide adult supervision, but do not heavily rely on adult facilitation.**
    - Adult supervision (monitoring play) should be constant during the ***playdate***.
    - Adult facilitation (organizing and intervening in play) will vary according to the needs of your child and should lessen as your child builds their play skills.
      - Constant adult facilitation may interfere with the natural flow of the children's play.
      - At first, you may need to be more active in ***social coaching***.

- **Avoid games and activities that:**
  - Require extensive setup during the ***playdate***.
  - Your child may have difficulty ***sharing or giving a turn***.
  - Your child or their ***playmate*** may have difficulty transitioning away from.
  - May trigger your child's or their ***playmate's*** sensitivities.

Preparing for Playdates

- **Make sure you have practiced playing the games and activities that will be available during the *playdate* with your child before the *playdate*.**
    - Practice as close to the ***playdate*** as possible (e.g., the evening before or the morning of the ***playdate***).
        - Practice allows you to assess what potential problems may arise (challenging behaviors, issues around unstructured time, excessive language demands, etc.).

- **Games and activity materials should be visible but NOT accessible to the children.**
    - Gather all the games and activity materials you'll need for the ***playdate*** in one area that is VISIBLE to the children so they can see what their play options are.
        - This will reduce unstructured or "down time" in between activities.
        - Have "back up" or additional games and activities ready in case the children are not interested in the primary activity, lose interest in the activity, or the activity ends sooner than expected.
    - Be sure games and activity materials are NOT accessible to the children, but easily accessible to YOU during the ***playdate***.

- **Put away toys and items you or your child are unwilling to share, such as:**
    - Highly preferred items that would be difficult for your child to transition away from or ***share*** cooperatively with the ***playmate***.
    - Items you or your child would be upset if lost, broken, or damaged.

- **Be prepared to have snacks for the children and parent(s).**
    - Find out about the ***playmate's*** dietary restrictions and preferences.
    - Snack time can be useful in providing a "break" during the ***playdate***.
    - Create opportunities for cooperative interactions during snack time.
        - For example, children can:
            - Ask each other what they would like to eat or drink.
            - Help each other make snacks.
            - Help each other distribute snacks.
            - Help each other clean up.

- **Remember to keep it short and sweet at first.**
    - Initial ***playdates*** should be no more than 1–1.5 hours.
    - Longer ***playdates*** run the risk of children getting tired or bored.
    - Leave the ***playmate*** and your child wanting more.
    - The best time to end a ***playdate*** is when everyone is having fun.
    - You may choose to pick-up and drop-off the other child if you are concerned the other parent will be late (if not present)
    - Be prepared with a reason for ending the ***playdate***.
        - Example: *"Well it's getting late, and we need to make dinner soon."*
        - Example: *"It's almost nap time, so I guess we need to wrap things up."*
        - Example: *"We have some afternoon plans, so we're going to have to wrap things up soon."*

Snapshot of the Lesson: Show and Tell During Play

The objective of this lesson is to teach children how to ***show and tell during play.*** There are two ways that children can ***show and tell during play***. Steps for ***showing and telling*** include:

A. ***Showing your toy***:
   1. ***Look at your friend with your eyes*** (point to your eyes).
   2. ***Smile with your mouth*** (point to your mouth and smile).
   3. ***Show your toy to your friend*** (wave your toy in front of your friend).
   4. ***Tell your friend to look*** at your toy by saying, ***"Look at my (cool toy)!"*** while ***using names.***

B. ***"Watch me!"*** **or** ***"Look at me!"***:
   1. ***Look at your friend with your eyes*** (point to your eyes).
   2. ***Smile with your mouth*** (point to your mouth and smile).
   3. ***Tell your friend to look*** at you by saying, ***"Watch me!"*** or ***"Look at me!"*** while ***using names.***
   4. ***Do something fun with your toy*** (e.g., fly a toy plane through the air).

Homework Assignments

1. **Playdates.**
   - Schedule and have a ***playdate*** with a ***playmate***.
   - Prepare for the ***playdate*** using the ***5 Ws***.
     - ***WHO: Playdates*** should be one-on-one.
     - ***WHAT: Playdates*** should be activity-based.
     - ***WHERE:*** Schedule initial ***playdates*** to take place in your home or somewhere you can provide ***social coaching.***
     - ***WHEN:*** Try to keep initial ***playdates*** to no more than 1–1.5 hours.
     - ***HOW:*** Coordinate how the children will get to and from the ***playdate.***
   - Do a final practice with your child of the games and activities that will be available during the ***playdate.***
   - Gather all the games and activity materials for the ***playdate*** in one area that is VISIBLE and easily accessible to YOU but not the children.
   - Provide ***social coaching*** during the ***playdate*** and assess if this is a good ***playmate*** for your child.

2. **Practice show and tell during play.**
   - Practice having your child ***showing and telling*** this week during preferred and highly motivating activities while providing ***social coaching*** using the ***4 Ps***.
     - ***Priming:*** Review the rules for ***show and tell*** with your child BEFORE PRACTICING.
     - ***Prompting:*** Remind your child IN THE MOMENT to ***show and tell*** whenever the opportunities present.

- ***Praising: Praise*** your child using the buzzwords whenever they are ***showing and telling*** CORRECTLY.
- ***Providing corrective feedback: Provide corrective feedback*** in the form of a ***praise sandwich*** whenever your child ATTEMPTS to ***show and tell***.
- Please send us a 30–60-second video of ***social coaching*** for ***showing and telling*** with your child to be viewed during homework review.
  - Please include:
    - Skills your child did well.
    - Skills you would like to work on with your child.

3. **Provide social coaching on previously learned skills.**
   - Continue providing ***social coaching*** to your child throughout the week using the ***4 Ps.***
   - Previous skills include:
     - ***Listening and following directions.***
     - ***Meeting and greeting friends.***
     - ***Sharing and giving a turn.***
     - ***Asking for a turn.***
     - ***Keeping cool.***
     - ***Being a good sport.***

4. **Bring a turn-taking game.**
   - Bring a turn-taking game that your child enjoys playing and can be played with the other children.

Session 7 Continued

Show and Tell During Play

PEERS® FOR PRESCHOOLERS: PARENT COACHED PLAY CARD

Snapshot of the Lesson: Show and Tell During Play

A. ***Showing your toy*:**
  1. ***Look at your friend with your eyes*** (point to your eyes).
  2. ***Smile with your mouth*** (point to your mouth and smile).
  3. ***Show your toy to your friend*** (wave your toy in front of your friend).
  4. ***Tell your friend to look*** at your toy by saying, ***"Look at my (cool toy)!"*** while ***using names.***

B. ***"Watch me!"* or *"Look at me!"*:**
  1. ***Look at your friend with your eyes*** (point to your eyes).
  2. ***Smile with your mouth*** (point to your mouth and smile).
  3. ***Tell your friend to look*** at you by saying, ***"Watch me!"*** or ***"Look at me!"*** while ***using names.***
  4. ***Do something fun with your toy*** (e.g., fly a toy plane through the air).

Priming BEFORE Game Playing:

- Example: *"Remember to practice showing and telling by looking at your friend with your* (point to your eyes to prompt the child to say *"eyes"*)...*EYES and smiling with your* (point to your mouth to prompt the child to say *"mouth"*)...*MOUTH when you show your game and tell your friend to 'look' at your game or to 'watch me' or 'look at me.' And don't forget to use* (pause briefly to prompt the child to say *"names"*)...*NAMES!"*

Prompting IN THE MOMENT

- Example: *"Remember to show and tell by saying 'Watch me'!"*
- Example: *"Remember to show your toy and tell your friend to 'Look at me'!"*
- Example: *"What should you say if you want to show and tell?"*

Praising for CORRECT Use of Skills

- Example: *"Great job showing and telling!"*
- Example: *"Great job telling your friend to 'watch me'!"*
- Example: *"Great job looking at your friend when you showed your toy!"*

Providing Corrective Feedback for ATTEMPTS Using a Praise Sandwich

- Example: *"Good job showing your toy. Remember to tell your friend 'Watch me' next time, but nice job!"*
- Example: *"Nice try showing and telling. Don't forget to use names next time, but good job!"*
- Example: *"Great job showing and telling. Remember to look and smile next time, but good job!"*

- Continue to provide ***social coaching*** on previously learned skills:
  - ***Listening and following directions.***
  - ***Meeting and greeting friends.***
  - ***Sharing and giving a turn.***
  - ***Asking for a turn.***
  - ***Keeping cool.***
  - ***Being a good sport.***

Session 7 Continued

Preparing for Playdates and Show and Tell During Play

PEERS® FOR PRESCHOOLERS: PARENT HOMEWORK WORKSHEET

Child's Name:	*Parent's Name:*		*Date:*	
HOMEWORK ASSIGNMENTS	PRIMING (REVIEWING RULES BEFORE PRACTICE)	PROMPTING (IN THE MOMENT)	PRAISING (USING BUZZWORDS)	PROVIDING CORRECTIVE FEEDBACK (USING A PRAISE SANDWICH)
Show and tell during play				
Practice previous skills: • **Being a good sport** • **Keeping cool** • **Asking for a turn** • **Sharing and giving turns** • **Meeting and greeting friends** • **Listening and following directions**				
Playdate: • **Plan a playdate using the 5 Ws** • **Prime your child before the playdate** • **Provide social coaching during the playdate using the 4 Ps**				
Bring a turn-taking game	Did you bring a turn-taking game? YES or NO (Circle)		Which game did you bring?	

Please fill out this worksheet by describing what you did to complete the homework assignments. Worksheets will be collected during Homework Review at the next session of PEERS® for Preschoolers.

Session 8

Coaching During Playdates and Don't Be Bossy

PARENT SESSION THERAPIST GUIDE

Parent Session Agenda

- Homework Review (40 minutes).
- Didactic Lessons (20 minutes).
- Parent Coached Play (20 minutes).
- Final Wrap-Up (10 minutes).

Materials Needed

- Conference room with a large table and enough chairs for the parent group leader and all parents to sit comfortably around the table.
  - Avoid sitting in a circle without a table as this creates the atmosphere of group therapy.
- Name tags for parents and treatment team.
- *Parent Handouts* (for the current week and the previous weeks).
- *Parent Homework Worksheets* (for the current week and the previous weeks).
- *Parent Coached Play Cards* (for the current week and the previous weeks).
- *Attendance and Homework Compliance Sheets* for parent group leader.
- Pens for note taking (consider having extra pens for parents who need them).

Homework Review (40 Minutes)

1. **Playdates.**
   - Have parents report on the ***playdate*** and confirm that they planned using the ***5 Ws.***
   - Review what parents did to ***social coach*** their child BEFORE, DURING, and AFTER the ***playdate***.
   - Identify what skills their child did well and what skills they need to work on.
     - Confirm that parents ***praised*** skills that were done well and provided ***priming, prompting,*** and/or ***corrective feedback*** for emerging skills.
   - Have parents assess if this is a good ***playmate*** for their child.
   - Have parents identify who their child might have a ***playdate*** with in the coming week (does not have to be a different ***playmate***).

DOI: 10.4324/9781003502968-9

2. **Practice show and tell during play.**
    - Review the 30–60-second video of ***social coaching*** for ***show and tell during play*** for each family. (For larger groups, you may need to review video recordings in two smaller groups with two different parent group leaders).
        - Have parents identify:
            - Skills their child did well.
            - Skills they would like to work on with their child.
        - Provide ***social coaching*** tips as appropriate for each family.
    - If parents did not send a video of ***social coaching***, confirm the following:
        - Parents practiced having their child ***show and tell*** during preferred and highly motivating activities while providing ***social coaching*** using the ***4 Ps.***
            - ***Priming:*** Reviewed the rules for ***show and tell*** with their child BEFORE PRACTICING.
            - ***Prompting:*** Reminded their child IN THE MOMENT to ***show and tell*** whenever the opportunity presented.
            - ***Praising: Praised*** their child using the buzzwords whenever they were ***showing and telling*** CORRECTLY.
            - ***Providing corrective feedback: Provided corrective feedback*** in the form of a ***praise sandwich*** whenever their child ATTEMPTED to ***show and tell***.

3. **Provide social coaching on previously learned skills.**
    - Confirm parents continued to provide ***social coaching*** to their child throughout the week using the ***4 Ps*** for previously learned skills:
        - ***Listening and following directions.***
        - ***Meeting and greeting friends.***
        - ***Sharing and giving turns.***
        - ***Asking for a turn.***
        - ***Keeping cool.***
        - ***Being a good sport.***

4. **Bring a turn-taking game.**
    - Confirm the following:
        - Brought a turn-taking game that their child enjoys playing and can be played with the other children. (To avoid distractions, these games should be left with the parents until *Parent Coached Play*.)

Didactic Lessons (20 Minutes)

PEERS® Neuroaffirming Pledge:

- We value neurodiversity, acceptance, and authenticity.
- We honor the diverse ways people experience the world.
- We respect each person's unique perspectives and communication styles.
- We recognize there is no one right way to connect with others.
- If using the strategies taught in PEERS® feels like camouflaging or masking and/or they don't align with your goals or the goals of your family, then you do not have to use them.
- Learning and using the skills taught in PEERS® is a PERSONAL CHOICE.

Didactic Lesson: Coaching During Playdates

- Distribute *Parent Handouts.*
  - Sections in **bold print** come directly from the *Parent Handout.*
  - Terms that are ***bold and italicized*** are buzzwords and represent important concepts from the didactic lesson.
- Explain, *"The past few weeks we've discussed how to plan, suggest, and prepare for playdates. Today, we're going to review a few additional social coaching strategies beyond the 4 Ps to use when social coaching your child during their playdates."*

Social Coaching Strategies During Playdates

- **Avoid parallel play between your child and their *playmate* during activities.**
  - **Parallel play is when children are sitting side by side but play is independent and not interactive.**
  - **Replacement behaviors for parallel play include:**
    - ***Asking for a turn.***
    - ***Sharing and giving turns.***
    - ***Being a good sport.***
    - ***Showing and telling during play.***
  - **If you notice your child is not interacting with their *playmate* during play, provide *prompting* or *corrective feedback using a praise sandwich.***
    - ***Prompting* examples:**
      - ***"Maybe your friend would like to play with your toy cars."***
      - ***"I think your friend likes Legos, too."***
      - ***"I wonder if your friend also likes building blocks."***
    - ***Providing corrective feedback (praise sandwich)* examples:**
      - ***"Good job playing nicely. Let's make sure to give your friend a turn too, but nice job!"***
      - ***"Nice job sharing your toys. Let's make sure to show and tell with your friend while you're playing, but good job!"***
      - ***"Great job giving your friend a turn. Let's make sure to also be a good sport, but good job!"***

- **Create cooperative play interactions during activities.**
  - **Distribute important play or activity items equally between the children rather than placing all the items in between the children (e.g., not a "free for all").**
    - **This will encourage ongoing social interaction between the children.**
      - **If we place all the materials in between the children, they may end up playing side by side (parallel play) with little or no social interaction.**
      - **By distributing important materials equally to each child, the children will need to interact with each other, which will make it more likely they will be socially engaged throughout the activity.**
  - **Examples of cooperative play interactions during activities:**

- **Art project: Distribute different colored markers to each child, distribute glue to one child and scissors to another child, etc.**
- **Baking/making a snack: Distribute different ingredients to each child, assign tasks (one child is responsible for mixing and another child is responsible for measuring, etc).**
- **Blocks/building sets: Distribute blocks to each child equally, distribute different types of blocks to each child, etc.**

- **Encourage the children to direct comments, ideas, and questions to each other rather than to you.**
  - **If the children ask you a question or ask you for help, redirect them to each other FIRST to see if they're able to work together to solve the problem.**
  - **Examples of redirecting:**
    - ***"Why don't you ask _______(child) for help?"***
    - ***"See if _______(child) knows how to do it."***
    - ***"_______(Child) can help you. Ask them for help."***
  - **This is also an example of how practicing and/or previewing the activity with your child BEFORE the *playdate* may be especially helpful.**
    - **Your child may be able to be an "expert" in that game or activity, which may lead to more balanced, equal interactions between the children.**

- **Provide structure when presenting games and activities.**
  - **If the game or activity does not have structure, try to create structure.**
    - **This will help your child and their *playmate* know what behaviors are expected.**
  - **Examples of providing structure to unstructured games and activities:**
    - ***"Why don't you build a racetrack with the blocks?"***
    - ***"Let's have you each take turns deciding what to draw!"***
    - ***"How about building a tower with the Legos?"***

- **Creatively incorporate your child's specialized interests into the games or activities, especially if this is a *common interest* with their *playmate*.**
  - **It can be helpful to include specialized interests in play if:**
    - **The *playmate* has a *common interest* in the activity.**
    - **Your child does not become overly preoccupied with the specialized interest to the point they ignore their *playmate*.**
  - **Avoid including specialized interests in play if:**
    - **The *playmate* does not have a *common interest* in the activity.**
    - **Your child will have significant difficulty *sharing and giving a turn* or transitioning away from the activity.**
  - **Examples of incorporating specialized interests into play:**
    - **Pretending to be a superhero while playing hide and seek.**
    - **Building a Disney castle when playing with block or Legos.**
    - **Making dinosaur cookies when baking.**
  - **Incorporating specialized interests and *common interests* into play may make the play interactions more exciting and rewarding for your child and their *playmate*.**
  - **Limit the amount of time spent engaging in specialized interests if they become boring for the *playmate*.**

Didactic Lesson: Don't Be Bossy

Explain, *"Last week we introduced how to show and tell during play. Today's child lesson will focus on how to not be bossy during play. Another way of saying this is to "be flexible." This lesson does not apply to prosocial behaviors like nicely explaining the rules or helping friends during playtime. Instead, this lesson is focused on helping children reduce insistencies on telling others what to do at the expense of friendship. The goal of this lesson is to avoid conflict and increase reciprocity and cooperation during play."*

> **Snapshot of the Lesson: Don't Be Bossy**
>
> **The objective of this lesson is to teach children how to *not be bossy.* Another way of saying this is to *"be flexible."* Steps for *not being bossy* include:**
>
> 1. ***Keep cool.***
> 2. ***Take deep breaths* (demonstrate taking two *deep breaths*).**
> 3. ***Nicely say "okay."***
> 4. ***Let your friend have a turn choosing what to do.***
> 5. ***Keep playing nicely.***

Say, *"So those are the steps for not being bossy. It's important to note that this strategy is not intended to make our children submissive to others. Instead, it is meant to help children make space for their friend's ideas and to encourage more cooperative and equal play interactions. If you find that your child's friend rarely wants to do what your child suggests, or vice versa, then this may not be a good choice for a friend."*

Parent Coached Play

- Distribute the *Parent Coached Play Cards.*
- Review the examples of the ***4 Ps*** provided on the *Parent Coached Play Card.*
- Remind parents that in a few moments we will be joining the children for *Parent Coached Play* in the context of mock dyadic ***playdates***.
- Parents should keep the *Parent Coached Play Card* in front of them during the dyadic ***playdate*** for recommendations on how to ***social coach*** children on ***not being bossy.***

Homework Assignments

(Briefly review the homework assignments and troubleshoot any potential problems with parents.)

1. **Playdates.**
   - **Schedule and have a *playdate* with a *playmate.***
   - **Prepare for the *playdate* using the *5 Ws.***
     - ***WHO: Playdates* should be one-on-one.**
     - ***WHAT: Playdates* should be activity-based.**

  - ***WHERE:*** **Schedule initial *playdates* to take place in your home or somewhere you can provide *social coaching.***
  - ***WHEN:*** **Try to keep initial *playdates* to no more than 1–1.5 hours.**
  - ***HOW:*** **Coordinate how the children will get to and from the *playdate.***
- **Do a final practice with your child of the games and activities that will be available during the *playdate.***
- **Gather all the games and activity materials for the *playdate* in one area that is VISIBLE and easily accessible to YOU but not the children.**
- **Provide *social coaching* during the *playdate* and assess if this is a good *playmate* for your child.**

2. **Practice not being bossy.**
   - **Practice having your child *not be bossy* this week during preferred and highly motivating activities while providing *social coaching* using the *4 Ps.***
     - ***Priming:*** **Review the rules for *not being bossy* with your child BEFORE PRACTICING.**
     - ***Prompting:*** **Remind your child IN THE MOMENT to *not be bossy* whenever the opportunities present.**
     - ***Praising: Praise*** **your child using the buzzwords whenever they are *not being bossy* CORRECTLY.**
     - ***Providing corrective feedback: Provide corrective feedback*** **in the form of a *praise sandwich* whenever your child ATTEMPTS to *not be bossy.***
   - **Please send us a 30–60-second video of *social coaching* for *not being bossy* with your child to be viewed during homework review.**
     - **Please include:**
       - **Skills your child did well.**
       - **Skills you would like to work on with your child.**

3. **Provide social coaching on previously learned skills.**
   - **Continue providing *social coaching* to your child throughout the week using the *4 Ps.***
   - **Previous skills include:**
     - ***Listening and following directions.***
     - ***Meeting and greeting friends.***
     - ***Sharing and giving a turn.***
     - ***Asking for a turn.***
     - ***Keeping cool.***
     - ***Being a good sport.***
     - ***Showing and telling.***

4. **Bring a turn-taking game.**
   - **Bring a turn-taking game that your child enjoys playing and can be played with the other children.**

Session 8 Continued

Don't Be Bossy

CHILD SESSION THERAPIST GUIDE

Child Session Agenda

- Didactic Lesson: *Don't Be Bossy* (20 minutes).
- Group Behavioral Rehearsal Activity 1: *Hot or Cold* (15 minutes).
- Break Time (10 minutes).
- Group Behavioral Rehearsal Activity 2: *Swap Draw* (15 minutes).
- Parent Coached Play: *Dyadic Playdates* (20 minutes).
- Final Wrap-Up (10 minutes).

Snapshot of the Lesson: Don't Be Bossy

The objective of this lesson is to teach children how to ***not be bossy***. Another way of saying this is to ***"be flexible."*** Steps for ***not being bossy*** include:

1. ***Keep cool.***
2. ***Take deep breaths*** (demonstrate taking two ***deep breaths***).
3. ***Nicely say "okay."***
4. ***Let your friend have a turn choosing what to do.***
5. ***Keep playing nicely.***

Materials Needed

- Elephant puppet.
- Monkey puppet.
- Building blocks.
- Carpet squares or chairs.
- "Making Friends Helper" badge.
- Star chart with names of children.
- Marker for star chart.
- Name tags for families and treatment team.
- Prize bins with prizes.

Preparing for the Lesson

- Use the script below with the group leader using an elephant puppet to play the part of "Ellie Elephant."

- A behavioral coach uses a monkey puppet to play the part of "Mikey Monkey."
- An additional behavioral coach assists in the behavioral rehearsal and provides encouragement and feedback to the group.
- A child is chosen at the beginning of the lesson as the "Making Friends Helper."
  - The "Making Friends Helper" wears a special badge and is the first child to practice the skill.
- The group leader and the behavioral coach sit on the floor at the front of the room.
- A special-colored carpet square (e.g., red) is placed at the front of the room next to the group leader to be used as the "Good Friend Square."
- For the children, additional carpet squares of the same color (e.g., green) are placed in a semi-circle facing the group leader and the "Good Friend Square."
- Note: If carpet squares are unavailable, the children and behavioral coaches may sit on chairs.
- The material in *italics* should be read by the indicated person.
- The material in ***bold and italics*** represents buzzwords and should be emphasized when read.
- The material in CAPITAL LETTERS within the script should be given extra emphasis while the group is encouraged to say the words in unison.

Behavioral Coaching Techniques

Behavioral coaches should use the following coaching techniques described below throughout the lesson and the behavioral rehearsal activities. (Note: ***priming*** occurs during the introduction to the activity.)

- ***Prompting***:
  - Use the buzzwords to ***prompt*** the children to ***not be bossy***.
    - Example: *"Remember to not be bossy."*
    - Example: *"Remember to keep cool and let them have a turn choosing what to do."*
    - Example: *"What should you do if your friend doesn't want to use your idea?"*
- ***Praising***:
  - Reinforce ***not being bossy*** by ***praising*** the children when they use the skills.
    - Example: *"Great job not being bossy!"*
    - Example: *"Great job nicely saying 'okay'!"*
    - Example: *"Good job letting them have a turn choosing what to do!"*
- ***Providing corrective feedback using a praise sandwich***:
  - Reinforce ATTEMPTS to ***not be bossy*** by ***praising*** the children and identifying what could be done differently next time.
    - Example: *"Good job not being bossy. Remember to nicely say 'okay' next time, but nice try!"*
    - Example: *"Nice try not being bossy. Remember to let them have a turn choosing what to do next time, but good job!"*
    - Example: *"Nice try not being bossy. Don't forget to keep playing nicely next time, but great job!"*
- Continue to provide ***social coaching*** on previously learned skills:
  - ***Listening and following directions.***
  - ***Meeting and greeting friends.***
  - ***Sharing and giving a turn.***
  - ***Asking for a turn.***

- ***Keeping cool.***
- ***Being a good sport.***
- ***Showing and telling.***

Didactic Lesson: Don't Be Bossy (20 Minutes)

Have the children sit in a semi-circle on the carpet squares facing the group leader.

Ellie Elephant: (Sit at the front of the room and choose a Making Friends Helper.) *"Who wants to be our Making Friends Helper?"*

(Choose from among the children raising their hands and place the "Making Friends Helper" badge on the child. The child stays in their seat for now.)

"Hi friends! I'm Ellie Elephant. (Trumpet, Trumpet)! Today we're going to practice not (shake your head to indicate no) *being bossy. Not* (shake your head to indicate no) *being bossy is a great way to be nice to our friends!"*

"Who should we not (shake your head to indicate no) *be bossy with? We should not* (shake your head to indicate no) *be bossy with our FRIENDS, TEACHERS, MOMMIES, DADDIES, BROTHERS, AND SISTERS."*

"When should we not (shake your head to indicate no) *be bossy? We should not* (shake your head to indicate no) *be bossy when we're playing with our friends or our family."*

"How should we not (shake your head to indicate no) *be bossy? We should not* (shake your head to indicate no) *be bossy by being flexible. That means we can offer to help our friends or give ideas to our friends. But if our friends say no, then we should keep cool, take deep breaths* (demonstrate taking two **deep breaths**), *nicely say 'okay,' then let them have a turn choosing what to do, and keep playing nicely."*

"Remember, even though it can be hard, it's important to not (shake your head to indicate no) *be bossy if we want to be a good friend! (Trumpet, Trumpet)!"*

Role Play: Don't Be Bossy

Mikey Monkey: *(Build a short tower with blocks while commenting to self. Have blocks scattered around on the floor in front of you and Ellie Elephant.)*

Ellie Elephant: (Watch Mikey Monkey build for a few moments.)

Mikey Monkey: (Turn to look at Ellie Elephant and smile.) *"Ellie Elephant, do you want to play with me?"*

Ellie Elephant: *"Okay, Mikey Monkey!"* (Join Mikey Monkey and build together for a few moments.)

(Turn to the group of children.) *"Hey friends! I'm having fun playing with Mikey Monkey, but this tower is small. I'm going to show him how to make a bigger tower."*

(Look at Mikey Monkey and smile.) *"Mikey Monkey, let's build a bigger tower like this."* (Rearrange several blocks on the tower to make it taller.)

Mikey Monkey: (Look at Ellie Elephant and frown.) *"No thanks. I don't want a big tower."*

Ellie Elephant: (Turn to look at the group of children.) *"Hey friends, it looks like Mikey Monkey doesn't want to make a big tower. Do you think I should get mad or sad?"* (Shake your head no and encourage the children to say *"no."*)

"That's right, friends! And do you think I should be bossy and make Mikey Monkey build a big tower?" (Shake your head no and encourage the children to say *"no."*)

"That's right, friends! (Trumpet, Trumpet)! I should not (shake your head to indicate no) *be bossy! Instead, I should be flexible! Do you think I should keep cool, take deep breaths* (demonstrate taking two ***deep breaths***), *nicely say 'okay,' then let Mikey Monkey have a turn choosing what to do, and keep playing nicely?"* (Nod your head yes and encourage the children to say *"yes."*)

"That's a great idea! (Trumpet, Trumpet)! Let's do it!" (Look at Mikey Monkey and smile.) *"Okay, Mikey Monkey. We don't have to build a big tower."* (Rearrange the blocks to make a short tower.)

Mikey Monkey: *"Thanks, Ellie Elephant! Let's keep playing!"*

Ellie Elephant: *"Okay, Mikey Monkey!"*

Ellie Elephant and Mikey Monkey: (Continue to build a short tower together while ***showing and telling*** with each other.)

Ellie Elephant: *"Hey friends, did I do a good job not* (shake your head to indicate no) *being bossy?"* (Nod your head yes and encourage the children to say *"yes."*) *"That's right, friends! (Trumpet, Trumpet)!"*

Ellie Elephant and Mikey Monkey: (Say *"good job," give an "elephant high-five"* and *"monkey high-five,"* clap, cheer, and encourage the children to clap as well. Mikey Monkey sits on the other side of the Good Friend Square (i.e., the Good Friend Square is between Ellie Elephant and Mikey Monkey). Ellie Elephant ***social coaches*** the children as needed while they practice ***not being bossy*** with Mikey Monkey.)

Mikey Monkey: (Return the blocks to their original small structure, with a few blocks scattered on the floor.)

Ellie Elephant: *"Now let's see _____ (behavioral coach) try! _____ (Behavioral coach), please come sit on the Good Friend Square."*

Behavioral coach: (Sit on the Good Friend Square.)

Ellie Elephant: *"_____ (Behavioral coach), can you show us how to not* (shake your head to indicate no) *be bossy with Mikey Monkey?"*

Behavioral coach: *"Okay, Ellie Elephant."*

Ellie Elephant: (Turn to look at the group of children.) *"Remember, if Mikey Monkey says no when you try to help or give ideas, then you should not* (shake your head to indicate no) *be bossy. Instead, you should be flexible by keeping cool, taking deep breaths* (demonstrate taking two ***deep breaths***), *nicely saying 'okay,' letting Mikey Monkey have a turn choosing what to do, and keep playing nicely."*

Mikey Monkey: (Build a short tower with blocks while commenting to yourself.)

Behavioral coach: (Watch Mikey Monkey build for a few moments.)

Mikey Monkey: (Turn to look at the behavioral coach member and smile.) *"_____ (Behavioral coach), do you want to play with me?"*

Behavioral coach: *"Okay, Mikey Monkey!"*

(Join Mikey Monkey and build together for a few moments.)

(Turn to the group of children.) *"Hey friends! I'm having fun playing with Mikey Monkey, but this tower is small. I'm going to show him how to make a bigger tower."*

(Look at Mikey Monkey and smile.) *"Mikey Monkey, let's build a bigger tower like this."* (Rearrange several blocks on the tower to make it taller.)

Mikey Monkey: (After the behavioral coach places a few blocks on the tower, look at them and frown, then remove one of the blocks that they placed to make the tower taller.) *"No thanks. I don't want a big tower."*

Ellie Elephant: (Look at the behavioral coach member.) *"_____ (Behavioral coach), Mikey Monkey doesn't want to build a big tower. Remember to not* (shake your head to indicate no) *be bossy. Instead, you should be flexible by keeping cool, taking deep breaths* (demonstrate taking two ***deep breaths***), *nicely saying 'okay,' then letting Mikey Monkey have a turn choosing what to do, and keep playing nicely."*

Behavioral coach: (Look at Mikey Monkey.) *"Okay, Mikey Monkey. We don't have to build a big tower."* (Rearrange the blocks to make a short tower.)

Mikey Monkey: (Look at the behavioral coach member and smile.) *"Thanks, ____ (behavioral coach)! Let's keep playing!"*

Behavioral coach: *"Okay, Mikey Monkey!"*

Mikey Monkey and Behavioral coach: (Continue to build a short tower together while commenting to each other.)

Ellie Elephant: *"Great job not* (shake your head to indicate no) *being bossy, ____ (behavioral coach)! (Trumpet, Trumpet)!"*

Ellie Elephant and Behavioral coach: (Say *"good job," give an "elephant high-five"* and *"monkey high-five,"* clap, cheer, and encourage the children to clap as well. The behavioral leaves the Good Friend Square.)

Mikey Monkey: (Return the blocks to their original small structure, with a few blocks scattered on the floor.)

Behavioral Rehearsal: Don't Be Bossy

Ellie Elephant: (Turn to look at the group of children.) *"Okay friends! Now let's see our Making Friends Helper _____ try! _____ (Making Friends Helper), come sit on the Good Friend Square and show us how to not* (shake your head to indicate no) *be bossy with Mikey Monkey."*

(The Making Friends Helper should sit on the Good Friend Square.)

"Remember if Mikey Monkey says no when you try to help or give ideas, then you should not (shake your head to indicate no) *be bossy. Instead, you should be flexible by keeping cool, taking deep breaths* (demonstrate taking two ***deep breaths***), *nicely saying 'okay,' then letting Mikey Monkey take a turn choosing what to do, and keep playing nicely."*

Mikey Monkey: (Build a short tower with blocks while commenting to yourself.)

(Turn to look at the Making Friends Helper and smile.) *"____ (Making Friends Helper), do you want to play with me?"*

Ellie Elephant: (If needed, ***social coach*** the Making Friends Helper to ***look, smile,*** say ***"Okay, Mikey Monkey,"*** and join Mikey Monkey in building a tower.)

Mikey Monkey: (After the Making Friends Helper places a few blocks on the tower, remove one of the blocks that they placed to make the tower taller.) *"I don't want a big tower."*

Ellie Elephant: (If needed, ***social coach*** the Making Friends Helper to ***not be bossy***.)

"Great job not (shake your head to indicate no) *being bossy, _____ (Making Friends Helper)! (Trumpet, Trumpet)!"*

(Say *"good job," give an "elephant high-five"* and *"monkey high-five,"* clap, cheer, and encourage the children to clap as well.)

"Okay, Making Friends Helper, choose another friend to sit on the Good Friend Square." (If needed, ***social coach*** the Making Friends Helper to choose another child before returning to their seat.)

Mikey Monkey: (Return the blocks to their original small structure, with a few blocks scattered on the floor.)

Repeat the following with each child:

Ellie Elephant: (Have each child take turns sitting on the Good Friend Square and practicing ***not being bossy*** with Mikey Monkey.)

(Turn to look at the group of children.) *"Okay friends! Now let's see ____ (child) try! ____ (Child), come sit on the Good Friend Square and show us how to not* (shake your head to indicate no) *be bossy with Mikey Monkey."*

(The child should sit on the Good Friend Square.)

"Remember if Mikey Monkey says "no" when you try to help or give ideas, then you should not (shake your head to indicate no) *be bossy. Instead, you should be flexible by keeping cool, taking deep breaths* (demonstrate taking two ***deep breaths***), *nicely saying 'okay,' then let Mikey Monkey have a turn choosing what to do, and keep playing nicely."*

Mikey Monkey: (Build a short tower with blocks while commenting to yourself.)

(Turn to look at the child and smile.) *"____ (Child), do you want to play with me?"*

Ellie Elephant: (If needed, ***social coach*** the child to ***look, smile,*** say ***"Okay, Mikey Monkey,"*** and join Mikey Monkey in building a tower.)

Mikey Monkey: (After the child places a few blocks on the tower, remove one of the blocks that they placed to make the tower taller.) *"I don't want a big tower."*

Ellie Elephant: (If needed, ***social coach*** the child to ***not be bossy***.)

"Great job not (shake your head to indicate no) *being bossy, _____ (child)! (Trumpet, Trumpet)!"*

(Say *"good job," give an "elephant high-five"* and *"monkey high-five,"* clap, cheer, and encourage the children to clap as well.)

"Okay, ____ (child), choose another friend to sit on the Good Friend Square." (If needed, **social coach** the child to choose another child before returning to their seat.)

Mikey Monkey: (Return the blocks to their original small structure, with a few blocks scattered on the floor.)

Didactic Lesson Wrap-Up

Group leader: *"Well friends, you all did a great job not* (shake your head to indicate no) *being bossy when Mikey Monkey didn't want to use your ideas. Instead, you were flexible by keeping cool, taking deep breaths* (demonstrate taking two **deep breaths**)*, nicely saying 'okay,' then letting Mikey Monkey have a turn choosing what to do while playing nicely."*

"You each earned ____ (number) stars for not being bossy! Let's start with ____ (child)."

Award each child the same number of stars by repeating the following with each child:

Group leader: *"Where's ____ (child)?"* (Wait until all the children are looking at the child.)

"____ (Child), how many stars did you earn?" (Pause briefly to allow the child to respond.)

"That's right! Let's all count for ____ (child)! One, two, three... (add stars to the Star Chart as they are counted aloud)*! Everybody clap for ____ (child)!"* (All behavioral coaches clap and cheer and encourage the children to clap as well.)

Session 8 Continued

Hot or Cold

BEHAVIORAL REHEARSAL ACTIVITY 1

Materials Needed

- A small object to be hidden.

Room Setup

- Remove or place all carpet squares to the side.
- The group leader stands at the front of the room facing the children.
- The children and behavioral coaches sit in a semi-circle facing the group leader.

Rules: Hot or Cold

- The group leader reads the script below to explain the rules.
- A behavioral coach is chosen to be the *"finding friend."* This will be the person who looks for the hidden object.
  - Do NOT allow children to be the *finding friend*.
- The children are the "*helping friends*" and direct the *finding friend* to find the hidden object.
- Instruct the *finding friend* to wait outside of the room while the object is hidden.
- Hide the object somewhere in the room with suggestions from the *helping friends*.
  - Prior to beginning the lesson, the group leader and behavioral coaches should brainstorm several hiding places.
- Call the *finding friend* back into the room and instruct them to stand at the front of the room.
- The *finding friend* asks a *helping friend* individually if they are *"hot or cold"* (i.e., standing close or far away from the hidden object) and if they should take steps in a specific manner (forward or back, one or two steps, etc.).
  - Asking ONE *helping friend* at a time ensures that each child gets an opportunity to practice ***not being bossy***.
  - The *helping friend* says *"hot"* if the *finding friend* is standing close to the hidden object or "cold" if the *finding friend* is standing far away from the hidden object.
- The *finding friend* randomly chooses to either follow or not follow the *helping friend's* instructions.
- If the *helping friend's* instructions are not followed, then the *helping friend* should practice ***not being bossy***.
- Once the object is found, ***praise*** the children for ***not being bossy*** and continue the game by hiding another object.

Behavioral Rehearsal: Hot or Cold (15 Minutes)

The group leader leads the activity. The behavioral coaches and children sit nearby as the group leader explains the rules.

Group leader: *"Hey friends, we're going to play a game called Hot or Cold. ____ (Behavioral coach) is the 'finding friend' and you will each take turns being the 'helping friend.' The 'finding friend' will wait outside while we hide the ____ (small object)* (hold up the small object) *somewhere in the room."*

"When the 'finding friend' comes back into the room, they will ask the 'helping friend' TWO questions. The first question is if they are hot or cold. The second question is which way they should move, like if they should take one step (take one step) *or two steps* (take two steps) *or move this way* (demonstrate moving to the right) *or move that way* (demonstrate moving to the left)*."*

"But friends, there's a secret! The 'helping friend' can't (shake your head no) *tell the 'finding friend' where the toy is. The 'helping friend' can only say 'hot' or 'cold' and tell the 'finding friend' how or where to move."*

(Put the toy down on the floor.) *"So if our 'finding friend' is close to the toy* (take a few steps toward the toy)*, we say, 'Hot!' But, if they are far from the toy* (take a few steps away from the toy)*, then we say, 'Cold'! So friends, if I'm close to the toy* (take a few steps toward the toy)*, what do you say?* (Pause briefly to allow the children to say, *"hot"*). *That's right, friends! And if I'm far from the toy* (take a few steps away from the toy)*, what do you say?* (Pause briefly to allow the children to say, *"cold"*). *That's right, friends!"*

"And friends, sometimes the finding friend may not listen to your ideas. Remember to not (shake your head to indicate no) *be bossy. Instead, you should be flexible by keeping cool, taking deep breaths* (demonstrate taking two ***deep breaths***)*, nicely saying 'okay,' then letting the finding friend have a turn choosing what to do, and keep playing nicely."*

"Okay, _____ (behavioral coach 1) and _____ (behavioral coach 2) will go first!"

Role Play: Hot or Cold

The group leader leads the role play. The two behavioral coaches demonstrate how to play *Hot or Cold*. Behavioral coach 1 is the *finding friend*, and behavioral coach 2 is the *helping friend*. The other behavioral coaches and children sit nearby watching the role play.

Group leader: (Turn to look at behavioral coach 1.) *"____ (Behavioral coach 1), please stand outside so that we can hide the ____ (small object)."*

Behavioral coach 1: *"Okay, ____ (group leader)."* (Leave the room.)

Group leader:	(Hide the small object. Loudly call out so that behavioral coach 1 can hear from outside.) *"____ (Behavioral coach 1), we're ready. Come back in!"*
Behavioral coach 1:	(Enter the room.)
Group leader:	(Turn to look at behavioral coach 1.) *"____ (Behavioral coach 1), ask the helping friend ____ (behavioral coach 2) if you're hot or cold and how you should move."*
Behavioral coach 1:	(Turn to look and smile at behavioral coach 2.) *"____ (Behavioral coach 2), am I hot or cold?"*
Behavioral coach 2:	(Turn to look and smile at behavioral coach 1.) *"You're ____ (hot/cold)."*
Behavioral coach 1:	(Turn to look and smile at behavioral coach 2.) *"Should I take one or two steps forward?"*
Behavioral coach 2:	(Turn to look and smile at behavioral coach 1.) *"Take one step forward."*
Behavioral coach 1:	*"Okay, ____ (behavioral coach 2)."* (Take one step forward.) *"____ (Behavioral coach 2), am I hot or cold?"*
Behavioral coach 2:	*"You're ____ (hot/cold)."*
Behavioral coach 1:	*"Should I take one or two steps forward?"*
Behavioral coach 2:	*"Take one small step forward."*
Behavioral coach 1:	*"No thanks. This time I'll take two big steps."* (Take two big steps.)
Behavioral coach 2:	*"Okay, ____ (behavioral coach 1)."*
Group leader:	*"Great job not being bossy, ____ (behavioral coach 2) when ____ (behavioral coach 1) didn't listen to your idea! Let's keep playing. It's your turn ____ (behavioral coach 1)."*

Repeat these steps until the hidden object is found.

Group leader:	*"Great job not being bossy, ____ (behavioral coach 2)!"* (Turn to look at the group of children and smile.) *"Okay friends, now it's everybody's turn to play Hot or Cold! Are we ready?"*

Behavioral Rehearsal: Hot or Cold

Group leader:	*"____ (Behavioral coach), wait outside the room again while we hide the ____ (object)."*
Behavioral coach:	*"Okay, ____ (group leader)."* (Leave the room.)
Group leader:	(Hide the small object with suggestions from the children.) (Loudly call out so that the behavioral coach can hear from outside.) *"____ (Behavioral coach), we're ready. Come back in!"*
Behavioral coach:	(Enter the room.)
Group leader:	*"Our first helping friend is ____ (child). ____ (Behavioral coach), ask the helping friend ____ (child) if you're hot or cold and how you should move."*
Behavioral coach:	(Turn to look and smile at the child.) *"____ (Child), am I hot or cold?"* (If needed, ***social coach*** the child to say, *"You're ____ (hot/cold).")* (Turn to look and smile at the child.) *"Should I take one or two steps forward?"* (If needed, ***social coach*** the child to say how many steps (big or small), and in which direction.) (The behavioral coach will alternate randomly between saying, *"Okay, ____ (child)"* and following the instructions, or saying, *"No thanks. This time I'll ____"* and doing something different.)
Group leader:	(When the behavioral coach does not follow the child's instruction say, *"____ (Child), ____ (behavioral coach) didn't listen to your idea. Remember to not be bossy. Instead, you should be flexible by keeping cool, taking deep breaths* (demonstrate taking two ***deep breaths***), *saying 'okay,' then let ____ (behavioral coach) have a turn choosing what to do, and keep playing nicely."* (If needed, ***social coach*** the child to ***not be bossy***.) *"Great job not being bossy, ____ (child)! Let's keep playing. Now it's ____ (new child) turn to be the helping friend. ____ (Behavioral coach), ask our new helping friend ____ (new child) if you're hot or cold and how you should move."*

Repeat the sequence above until the hidden object is found. Continue to play in this manner while finding new hiding places for the hidden object, ensuring that each child has multiple opportunities to practice ***not being bossy*** when their instructions are not followed.

Behavioral Rehearsal Wrap-Up

Group leader: *"Well friends, great job not being bossy! Give yourselves a big round of applause!"* (All behavioral coaches clap and cheer and encourage the children to clap as well.)

"Now everyone should come sit in the Listening Circle." (Have children return to the Listening Circle to sit on their carpet squares.)

"Okay friends, you did a great job not (shake your head to indicate no) *being bossy when ____ (behavioral coach) didn't use your ideas. Instead, you were flexible by keeping cool, taking deep breaths* (demonstrate taking two ***deep breaths***), *nicely saying 'okay,' then letting ____ (behavioral coach) have a turn choosing what to do while playing nicely."*

"You each earned ____ (number) more stars for not being bossy! Let's start with ____ (child)."

Award each child the same number of stars by repeating the following with each child:

Group leader: *"Where's _____ (child)?"* (Wait until all the children are looking at the child.)

"_____ (Child), how many stars did you earn?" (Pause briefly to allow the child to respond.)

"That's right! Let's all count for _____ (child)! One, two, three... (add stars to the Star Chart as they are counted aloud)*! Everybody clap for _____ (child)!"* (All behavioral coaches clap and cheer and encourage the children to clap as well.)

Break Time (10 Minutes)

- The puppets may be used to lead the children to and from the bathroom during break time.
- To assist with transitions and limit unstructured time, behavioral coaches may review the lesson with the children while waiting for the remaining children to return from the bathroom.
- You may want to award stars for good behavior after returning from the bathroom.

Swap Draw

BEHAVIORAL REHEARSAL ACTIVITY 2

Materials Needed

- Drawing paper (approximately four to five sheets per group).
- Coloring tools (approximately three to four per group).
  - Examples: washable markers, crayons, colored pencils.
- Tables or hard, flat surfaces to draw on.
  - Chairs (when using tables).

Room Setup

- Organize tables and chairs or drawing surfaces around the room.
- Place sets of paper and coloring tools on the tables or drawing surfaces, providing enough space for children and behavioral coaches to sit around the materials.
- The group leader sits on the floor at the front of the room while explaining the rules.
- The children and behavioral coaches sit on the floor in a semi-circle facing the group leader.

Rules: Swap Draw

- The group leader reads the script below to explain the rules.
- The group leader divides the children into dyads.
  - If there are an odd number of children, pair one child with a behavioral coach.
  - Assign at least one behavioral coach per dyad to ***social coach***.
- Direct each dyad to sit in a circle around a set of materials.
- The behavioral coach will pick one child to be the first *"drawing friend."*
- The other child will be the *"choosing friend"* and will choose a theme for the *drawing friend* to draw.
  - Behavioral coaches may need to help the *choosing friend* identify a theme.
- The behavioral coach places one piece of paper and the coloring tools in front of the *drawing friend* and instructs the child to begin drawing.
- The *drawing friend* may or may not choose to draw the theme chosen by the *choosing friend.*
- While waiting for their turn, the *choosing friend* should practice ***not being bossy*** as they watch the other child add to the drawing.
- The behavioral coach helps facilitate positive play interactions by asking questions and making comments (e.g., *"What do you think _______ (child) is drawing?"* or *"That's so cool!").)*
- Every 10–20 seconds, the behavioral coach instructs the children to swap the drawing materials and the *choosing friend* will become the *drawing friend* and vice versa.

- The new *choosing friend* will choose something new to add to the drawing.
  - The behavioral coach may need to help the *choosing friend* identify something new to add.
- The *drawing friend* may or may not choose to draw what the *choosing friend* suggests.
- While waiting for their turn, the *choosing friend* should practice ***not being bossy*** as they watch the other child add to the drawing.
- Behavioral coaches may provide new paper to the children as needed.

Behavioral Rehearsal: Swap Draw (15 Minutes)

The group leader explains the activity. The behavioral coaches and children sit nearby as the group leader explains the rules. The behavioral coaches ***social coach*** the children in dyads to ***not be bossy*** during the game playing.

Group leader: *"Hey friends, now we're going to play Swap Draw. You'll get to draw a fun picture with your friend, like robots or outer space."*

"But only one friend (hold up one finger) *will draw at a time. If you're the 'drawing friend' that means you get to draw. But if you're the 'choosing friend' that means you get to pick what the 'drawing friend' is supposed to draw."*

"Sometimes the 'drawing friend' may not draw what the 'choosing friend' wants, so if that happens to you, you'll need to practice not being bossy. Remember to not (shake your head to indicate no) *be bossy by keeping cool, taking deep breaths* (demonstrate taking two ***deep breaths***), *nicely saying 'okay,' then let your friend have a turn choosing what to do, and keep playing nicely."*

"When you're the 'drawing friend' and you hear the word 'swap,' you'll give your friend the drawing paper and coloring tools and then you get to be the 'choosing friend.' Okay, let's play Swap Draw!"

Behavioral Rehearsal: Swap Draw

The children and the behavioral coaches move to their drawing stations.

Behavioral coach: (The behavioral coach places ONE piece of paper and the coloring tools in front of the *drawing friend*.)

"Okay friends, let's practice sharing and giving a turn by letting ____ (child) be the first 'drawing friend' and letting ____ (child) be the first 'choosing friend.'" (If needed, ***social coach*** the children to ***share and give a turn***.)

"____ (Child), what should our drawing friend draw first?" (If needed, ***social coach*** the *choosing friend* to choose a theme.)

(If the *drawing friend* chooses to draw something different, help the *choosing friend* practice ***not being bossy*** by saying, *"Our drawing friend wants to draw something different. Let's practice not being bossy and taking deep breaths to keep cool."*)

(If the *drawing friend* draws what the *choosing friend* chose, ***praise*** the *drawing friends* by saying, *"Great job sharing and taking turns, _______ (child)."*)

(The behavioral coach helps facilitate positive play interactions by asking questions and making comments (e.g., *"What do you think _______ (child) is drawing?"* or *"That's so cool!"*).)

Every 10–20 seconds, the behavioral coach instructs the children to swap the drawing materials and the *choosing friend* will become the *drawing friend* and vice versa.

Behavioral coach: *"And...swap! Now we're going to practice sharing and giving a turn by letting ____ (child) be the next 'drawing friend' and letting ____ (child) be the next 'choosing friend.'"* (Have the children swap the drawing paper and coloring tools.)

"____ (Child), what should our drawing friend draw next?" (If needed, ***social coach*** the *choosing friend* to choose something new to add to the drawing, and practice ***not being bossy*** if the *drawing friend* chooses to draw something different. The behavioral coach helps facilitate positive play interactions by asking questions and making comments (e.g., *"What do you think _______ (child) is drawing?"* or *"That's so cool!"*).)

Repeat the pattern above for the remainder of the playtime. Provide new drawing paper as needed.

Table 8.1 Drawing Theme Examples

House	Outer space	Beach
School	Trains	Underwater world
Park	Forest	Castle
Friends	Jungle	Dinosaurs
Family	Airplanes	Dragons
Cars	Superheroes	Wizards
Animals	Witches	Princesses

Behavioral Rehearsal Wrap-Up

Group leader: *"Well friends, great job not being bossy! Give yourselves a big round of applause!"* (All behavioral coaches clap and cheer and encourage the children to clap as well.)

"Now everyone should come sit in the Listening Circle." (Have children return to the Listening Circle to sit on their carpet squares.)

"Okay friends, you did a great job not (shake your head to indicate no) *being bossy. Instead, you were flexible by keeping cool, taking deep breaths* (demonstrate taking two ***deep breaths***), *nicely saying 'okay,' then letting your friend have a turn choosing what to do while playing nicely."*

"You each earned ____ (number) more stars for not being bossy! Let's start with ____ (child)."

Award each child the same number of stars by repeating the following with each child:

Group leader: *"Where's _____ (child)?"* (Wait until all the children are looking at the child.)

"_____ (Child), how many stars did you earn?" (Pause briefly to allow the child to respond.)

"That's right! Let's all count for _____ (child)! One, two, three... (add stars to the Star Chart as they are counted aloud)*! Everybody clap for _____ (child)!"* (All behavioral coaches clap and cheer and encourage the children to clap as well.)

"Now we're going to play another game with our parents and practice not being bossy some more!"

Session 8 Continued

Don't Be Bossy

PARENT COACHED PLAY: DYADIC PLAYDATES

Materials Needed

- Games brought by children and parents from home.
- Turn-taking games provided by the treatment team.
- Tables and chairs or carpet squares.
- *Parent Coached Play Cards*.

Room Setup

- If available, organize tables in separate corners of the room with four to six chairs per table.
- If tables are not available, place two carpet squares in separate corners of the room to indicate where the children will sit.
- The group leader sits on the floor at the front of the room.
- The families sit on the floor in a semi-circle facing the group leader.

Rules: Dyadic Playdates

- The group leader divides the families into groups of two families each.
  - If there are an odd number of children, pair one child with a behavioral coach who will serve as a ***playmate***. In this case, you will need an additional coach to serve as a behavioral coach for the parent.
  - To avoid social exclusion, avoid having children play in triads as much as possible.
- Assign each group to sit at a table or specific play area.
  - Children should sit next to each other.
  - Parents will act as ***social coaches*** by sitting on the other side of their child to minimize interrupting the natural flow of play between the children.
  - One behavioral coach will be assigned to each dyad to provide ***social coaching*** suggestions and feedback to parents.
- Children will take turns playing the games brought from home or games provided by the treatment team.
- Each child will have ten minutes to play their chosen game with their ***playmate*** and will then switch games.
- Parents will choose which child's game will be played first.
- To minimize unstructured periods, parents will help the children set up the game in a cooperative fashion (handing game pieces to each other, offering suggestions, etc.).

- As they play, parents will ***social coach*** the children on previously learned and newly learned skills using the guidelines highlighted on the *Parent Coached Play Cards*.
- Behavioral coaches will provide support to parents in their ***social coaching*** using the ***4 Ps*** (***priming, prompting, praising,*** and ***providing corrective feedback***) and will model appropriate coaching behavior when necessary.
- After approximately nine minutes of play, instruct the parents to prepare the children for the upcoming game swap.
- After approximately one additional minute of play (ten minutes total), instruct the parents to have the children clean up and swap games.
- Repeat the cycle with the second game for the remaining ten minutes before returning to the *Listening Circle*.

Behavioral Coaching: Dyadic Playdates

Behavioral coaches will ***social coach*** parents during dyadic ***playdates*** in the following ways:

- ***Priming***:
  - Begin the play interactions with parents going over the rules for ***not being bossy*** BEFORE GAME PLAYING.
    - Example: *"Remember to practice not* (shake your head to indicate no) *being bossy. Instead, you should be flexible by keeping cool, taking deep breaths* (demonstrate taking two ***deep breaths***)*, nicely saying 'okay,' then let your friend have a turn choosing what to do while playing nicely."*
- ***Prompting***:
  - Remind parents to use the buzzwords to ***prompt*** their child to ***not be bossy*** IN THE MOMENT.
  - Help parents to identify opportunities to proactively ***prompt*** their child to ***not be bossy***.
    - Example: *"Remember to not be bossy."*
    - Example: *"Remember to keep cool and let your friend have a turn choosing what to do."*
    - Example: *"What should you do if your friend doesn't want to use your idea?"*
- ***Praising***:
  - Remind parents to ***praise*** and reinforce their child whenever their child is ***not being bossy***.
    - Example: *"Great job not being bossy!"*
    - Example: *"Great job nicely saying 'okay'!"*
    - Example: *"Good job letting your friend have a turn choosing what to do!"*
- ***Providing corrective feedback using a praise sandwich***:
  - Remind parents to ***praise*** their child's ATTEMPTS to ***not be bossy*** and identify what could be done differently next time.
    - Example: *"Good job not being bossy. Remember to nicely say 'okay' next time, but nice try!"*
    - Example: *"Nice try not being bossy. Remember to let your friend have a turn choosing what to do next time, but good job!"*
    - Example: *"Nice try not being bossy. Don't forget to keep playing nicely next time, but great job!"*
- Remind parents to continue to ***social coach*** on previously learned skills:
  - ***Listening and following directions.***
  - ***Meeting and greeting friends.***
  - ***Sharing and giving a turn.***
  - ***Asking for a turn.***

- ***Keeping cool.***
- ***Being a good sport.***
- ***Showing and telling.***

Parent Coached Play: Dyadic Playdates (20 Minutes)

- Have each child choose a turn-taking game brought from home or provided by the treatment team.
- The group leader sits on the floor at the front of the room.
- The families sit on the floor in a semi-circle facing the group leader.

Group leader: *"Hey friends, we're going to have more playdates and play with the cool games you brought from home. While you're playing, we want you to practice not* (shake your head to indicate no) *being bossy if your friend says no when you try to help or give ideas. Instead, we can be flexible by keeping cool, taking deep breaths* (demonstrate taking two ***deep breaths***), *saying 'okay,' then let your friend have a turn choosing what they want to do while playing nicely."*

"And don't forget to ask for a turn, share and give turns and be good sports while playing. Parents, remember to social coach your children by using your Parent Coached Play Cards. Okay, let's play with our games!"

- Before playing, parents will ***social coach*** their child to ***say "hi"*** to one another ***using names***.
- Parents will ***social coach*** their children to ***not be bossy, show and tell, ask for a turn***, ***share and take turns, keep cool,*** and ***be a good sport*** throughout the game playing.
- After approximately nine minutes of play, instruct the parents to prepare the children for the upcoming game swap by saying, *"Parents, tell your children that we'll be swapping games in one minute."*
- After approximately one additional minute of play (ten minutes total), instruct the parents to swap games by saying, *"Parents, it's time to swap games. Social coach the children to ask for a turn and share and give a turn before playing the next game."*
- After approximately nine minutes of playing the second game, instruct the parents to prepare the children for clean up by saying, *"Parents, tell your children that we'll be cleaning up in one minute."*
- After approximately one additional minute of play (ten minutes total), ***prompt*** the parents to instruct their children to clean up by saying, *"Parents, it's time to clean up. Let's social coach the children to listen and follow directions by cleaning up and then say 'bye' to their friend using names before sitting in the Listening Circle."*
- If needed, parents will ***social coach*** their child to ***listen and follow directions*** to clean up.
- Then parents will ***social coach*** their child to ***say "bye"*** to their friend ***using names.***

Final Wrap-Up (10 minutes)

- The group leader sits on the floor at the front of the room.
- The children sit on the carpet squares in a semi-circle facing the group leader, with parents sitting behind their children.

Group leader: *"Okay friends, you all did a great job playing your games and not* (shake your head to indicate no) *being bossy. When we're not* (shake your head to indicate no) *being bossy, do you think we should get mad or sad if our friends don't want our help?"* (Pause briefly to allow children to respond *"no."*)

"That's right, friends! And when we're not (shake your head to indicate no) *being bossy, do you think we should keep telling our friends what to do if they don't try our ideas?"* (Pause briefly to allow children to respond *"no."*)

"That's right, friends! Instead, do you think we should be flexible by keeping cool, taking deep breaths, saying 'okay,' then letting our friends have a turn choosing what to do while playing nicely?" (Pause briefly to allow the children to say *"yes."*)

"That's right, friends! You all did such a great job not being bossy today that you each earned ____ (number) more stars! Let's start with ____ (child)."

Award each child the same number of stars by repeating the following with each child:

Group leader: *"Where's _____ (child)?"* (Wait all the children are looking at the child.)

"_____ (Child), how many stars did you earn?" (Pause briefly to allow the child to respond.)

"That's right! Let's all count for _____ (child)! One, two, three... (add stars to the Star Chart as they are counted aloud)*! Everybody clap for _____ (child)!"* (All behavioral coaches clap and cheer and encourage the children to clap as well.)

"And remember you all earned those stars by not being bossy! Everyone did a great job, and parents you did an excellent job social coaching! Parents, remember your homework assignments this week are for your children to practice not being bossy and continue practicing all the other things we've learned to be a good friend using the 4 Ps. And don't forget to have a playdate and go to your playgroups."

"Alright little friends, do you want to count our stars?" (Pause briefly to allow the children to respond.)

"Let's all count together and see how many stars we earned today! One, two, three…(count the number of stars for one child)*!"*

"You each earned ____ (total number) stars today! Round of applause for our friends!" (All behavioral coaches should clap and cheer and encourage the families to clap as well.)

"Great job, friends! Don't forget to choose your reward before you leave. See you all next week!"

Session 8 Continued

Coaching During Playdates and Don't Be Bossy

PEERS® FOR PRESCHOOLERS: PARENT HANDOUT

Social Coaching Strategies During Playdates

- **Avoid parallel play between your child and their *playmate* during activities.**
  - Parallel play is when children are sitting side by side but play is independent and not interactive.
  - Replacement behaviors for parallel play include:
    - ***Asking for a turn.***
    - ***Sharing and giving turns.***
    - ***Being a good sport.***
    - ***Showing and telling during play.***
  - If you notice your child is not interacting with their ***playmate*** during play, provide ***prompting*** or ***corrective feedback using a praise sandwich***.
    - ***Prompting*** examples:
      - *"Maybe your friend would like to play with your toy cars."*
      - *"I think your friend likes Legos, too."*
      - *"I wonder if your friend also likes building blocks."*
    - ***Providing corrective feedback (praise sandwich)*** examples:
      - *"Good job playing nicely. Let's make sure to give your friend a turn too, but nice job!"*
      - *"Nice job sharing your toys. Let's make sure to show and tell with your friend while you're playing, but good job!"*
      - *"Great job giving your friend a turn. Let's make sure to also be a good sport, but good job!"*

- **Create cooperative play interactions during activities.**
  - Distribute important play or activity items equally between the children rather than placing all the items in between the children (e.g., not a "free for all").
    - This will encourage ongoing social interaction between the children.
      - If we place all the materials in between the children, they may end up playing side by side (parallel play) with little or no social interaction.
      - By distributing important materials equally to each child, the children will need to interact with each other, which will make it more likely they will be socially engaged throughout the activity.

- Examples of cooperative play interactions during activities:
  - Art project: Distribute different colored markers to each child, distribute glue to one child and scissors to another child, etc.
  - Baking/making a snack: Distribute different ingredients to each child, assign tasks (one child is responsible for mixing and another child is responsible for measuring, etc.).
  - Blocks/building sets: Distribute blocks to each child equally, distribute different types of blocks to each child, etc.
- Encourage the children to direct comments, ideas, and questions to each other rather than to you.
  - If the children ask you a question or ask you for help, redirect them to each other FIRST to see if they're able to work together to solve the problem.
  - Examples or redirecting:
    - *"Why don't you ask _______(child) for help?"*
    - *"See if _______(child) knows how to do it."*
    - *"_______(Child) can help you. Ask them for help."*
  - This is also an example of how practicing and/or previewing the activity with your child BEFORE the ***playdate*** may be especially helpful.
    - Your child may be able to be an "expert" in that game or activity, which may lead to more balanced, equal interactions between the children.

- **Provide structure when presenting games and activities.**
  - If the game or activity does not have structure, try to create structure.
    - This will help your child and their ***playmate*** know what behaviors are expected.
  - Examples of providing structure to unstructured games and activities:
    - *"Why don't you build a racetrack with the blocks?"*
    - *"Let's have you each take turns deciding what to draw!"*
    - *"How about building a tower with the Legos?"*

- **Creatively incorporate your child's specialized interests into the games or activities, especially if this is a *common interest* with their *playmate*.**
  - It can be helpful to include specialized interests in play if:
    - The ***playmate*** has a ***common interest*** in the activity.
    - Your child does not become overly preoccupied with the **specialized interest** to the point they ignore their ***playmate.***
  - Avoid including specialized interests in play if:
    - The ***playmate*** does not have a ***common interest*** in the activity.
    - Your child will have significant difficulty ***sharing and giving a turn*** or transitioning away from the activity.
  - Examples of incorporating specialized interests into play:
    - Pretending to be a superhero while playing hide and seek.
    - Building a Disney castle when playing with blocks or Legos.
    - Making dinosaur cookies when baking.
  - Incorporating specialized interests and ***common interests*** into play may make the play interactions more exciting and rewarding for your child and their ***playmate***.

◦ Limit the amount of time spent engaging in specialized interests if they become boring for the ***playmate***.

Snapshot of the Lesson: Don't Be Bossy

The objective of this lesson is to teach children how to ***not be bossy.*** Another way of saying this is to ***"be flexible."*** Steps for ***not being bossy*** include:

1. ***Keep cool.***
2. ***Take deep breaths*** (demonstrate taking two ***deep breaths***).
3. ***Nicely say "okay."***
4. ***Let your friend have a turn choosing what to do.***
5. ***Keep playing nicely.***

Homework Assignments

1. **Playdates.**
   - Schedule and have a ***playdate*** with a ***playmate***.
   - Prepare for the ***playdate*** using the ***5 Ws***.
     - ***WHO: Playdates*** should be one-on-one**.**
     - ***WHAT: Playdates*** should be activity-based**.**
     - ***WHERE:*** Schedule initial ***playdates*** to take place in your home or somewhere you can provide ***social coaching.***
     - ***WHEN:*** Try to keep initial ***playdates*** to no more than 1–1.5 hours.
     - ***HOW:*** Coordinate how the children will get to and from the ***playdate.***
   - Do a final practice with your child of the games and activities that will be available during the ***playdate.***
   - Gather all the games and activity materials for the ***playdate*** in one area that is VISIBLE and easily accessible to YOU but not the children.
   - Provide ***social coaching*** during the ***playdate*** and assess if this is a good ***playmate*** for your child.

2. **Practice not being bossy.**
   - Practice having your child ***not be bossy*** this week during preferred and highly motivating activities while providing ***social coaching*** using the ***4 Ps***.
     - ***Priming:*** Review the rules for ***not being bossy*** with your child BEFORE PRACTICING.
     - ***Prompting:*** Remind your child IN THE MOMENT to ***not be bossy*** whenever the opportunities present.
     - ***Praising: Praise*** your child using the buzzwords whenever they are ***not being bossy*** CORRECTLY.

- ***Providing corrective feedback: Provide corrective feedback*** in the form of a ***praise sandwich*** whenever your child ATTEMPTS to ***not be bossy.***
- Please send us a 30–60-second video of ***social coaching*** for ***not being bossy*** with your child to be viewed during homework review.
  - Please include:
    - Skills your child did well.
    - Skills you would like to work on with your child.

3. **Provide social coaching on previously learned skills.**
   - Continue providing ***social coaching*** to your child throughout the week using the ***4 Ps.***
   - Previous skills include:
     - ***Listening and following directions.***
     - ***Meeting and greeting friends.***
     - ***Sharing and giving a turn.***
     - ***Asking for a turn.***
     - ***Keeping cool.***
     - ***Being a good sport.***
     - ***Showing and telling.***

4. **Bring a turn-taking game.**
   - Bring a turn-taking game that your child enjoys playing and can be played with the other children.

Session 8 Continued

Don't Be Bossy

PEERS® FOR PRESCHOOLERS: PARENT COACHED PLAY CARD

Snapshot of the Lesson: Don't Be Bossy

1. ***Keep cool.***
2. ***Take deep breaths*** (demonstrate taking two ***deep breaths***).
3. ***Nicely say "okay."***
4. ***Let your friend have a turn choosing what to do.***
5. ***Keep playing nicely.***

Priming BEFORE Game Playing:

- Example: *"Remember to practice not* (shake your head to indicate no) *being bossy. Instead, you should be flexible by keeping cool, taking deep breaths* (demonstrate taking two ***deep breaths***), *nicely saying 'okay,' then letting your friend have a turn choosing what to do while playing nicely."*

Prompting IN THE MOMENT

- Example: *"Remember to not be bossy."*
- Example: *"Remember to keep cool and let your friend have a turn choosing what to do."*
- Example: *"What should you do if your friend doesn't want to use your idea?"*

Praising for CORRECT Use of Skills

- Example: *"Great job not being bossy!"*
- Example: *"Great job nicely saying 'okay'!"*
- Example: *"Good job letting your friend have a turn choosing what to do!"*

Providing Corrective Feedback for ATTEMPTS Using a Praise Sandwich

- Example: *"Good job not being bossy. Remember to nicely say 'okay' next time, but nice try!"*
- Example: *"Nice try not being bossy. Remember to let your friend have a turn choosing what to do next time, but good job!"*
- Example: *"Nice try not being bossy. Don't forget to keep playing nicely next time, but great job!"*

- Continue to provide ***social coaching*** on previously learned skills:
  - ***Listening and following directions.***
  - ***Meeting and greeting friends.***
  - ***Sharing and giving a turn.***
  - ***Asking for a turn.***
  - ***Keeping cool.***
  - ***Being a good sport.***
  - ***Showing and telling.***

Session 8 Continued

Coaching During Playdates and Don't Be Bossy

PEERS® FOR PRESCHOOLERS: PARENT HOMEWORK WORKSHEET

Child's Name:	*Parent's Name:*		*Date:*	
HOMEWORK ASSIGNMENTS	PRIMING (REVIEWING RULES BEFORE PRACTICE)	PROMPTING (IN THE MOMENT)	PRAISING (USING BUZZWORDS)	PROVIDING CORRECTIVE FEEDBACK (USING A PRAISE SANDWICH)
Don't be bossy				
Practice previous skills: • **Show and tell during play** • **Being a good sport** • **Keeping cool** • **Asking for a turn** • **Sharing and giving turns** • **Meeting and greeting friends** • **Listening and following directions**				

<table>
<tr><td>Child's Name:</td><td colspan="2">Parent's Name:</td><td colspan="2">Date:</td></tr>
<tr><td>HOMEWORK ASSIGNMENTS</td><td>PRIMING (REVIEWING RULES BEFORE PRACTICE)</td><td>PROMPTING (IN THE MOMENT)</td><td>PRAISING (USING BUZZWORDS)</td><td>PROVIDING CORRECTIVE FEEDBACK (USING A PRAISE SANDWICH)</td></tr>
<tr><td>Playdate:
• Plan a playdate using the 5 Ws
• Prime your child before the playdate
• Provide social coaching during the playdate using the 4 Ps</td><td colspan="4"></td></tr>
<tr><td>Bring a turn-taking game</td><td colspan="2">Did you bring a turn-taking game?
YES or NO
(Circle)</td><td colspan="2">Which game did you bring?</td></tr>
</table>

Please fill out this worksheet by describing what you did to complete the homework assignments.
Worksheets will be collected during Homework Review at the next session of PEERS® for Preschoolers.

Session 9

Social Coaching Strategies and Asking a Friend to Play

PARENT SESSION THERAPIST GUIDE

Parent Session Agenda

- Homework Review (40 minutes).
- Didactic Lessons (20 minutes).
- Parent Coached Play (20 minutes).
- Final Wrap-Up (10 minutes).

Materials Needed

- Conference room with a large table and enough chairs for the parent group leader and all parents to sit comfortably around the table.
    - Avoid sitting in a circle without a table as this creates the atmosphere of group therapy.
- Name tags for parents and treatment team.
- *Parent Handout*s (for the current week and the previous weeks).
- *Parent Homework Worksheets* (for the current week and the previous week).
- *Parent Coached Play Cards* (for the current week and the previous week).
- *Attendance and Homework Compliance Sheets* for parent group leader.
- Pens for note-taking (consider having extra pens for parents who need them).

Homework Review (40 Minutes)

1. **Playdates.**
    - Have parents report on the ***playdate*** and confirm that they planned using the ***5 Ws.***
    - Review what parents did to ***social coach*** their child BEFORE, DURING, and AFTER the ***playdate***.
    - Identify what skills their child did well and what skills they need to work on.
        - Confirm that parents ***praised*** skills that were done well and provided ***priming, prompting,*** and/or ***corrective feedback*** for emerging skills.
    - Have parents assess if this is a good ***playmate*** for their child.
    - Have parents identify who their child might have a ***playdate*** with in the coming week (does not have to be a different ***playmate***).

DOI: 10.4324/9781003502968-10

2. **Practice not being bossy.**
   - Review the 30–60-second video of ***social coaching*** for ***not being bossy*** for each family. (For larger groups, you may need to review video recordings in two smaller groups with two different parent group leaders).
     - Have parents identify:
       - Skills their child did well.
       - Skills they would like to work on with their child.
     - Provide ***social coaching*** tips as appropriate for each family.
   - If parents did not send a video of ***social coaching***, confirm the following:
     - Parents practiced having their child ***not be bossy*** during preferred and highly motivating activities while providing ***social coaching*** using the ***4 Ps.***
       - ***Priming:*** Reviewed the rules for ***not being bossy*** with their child BEFORE PRACTICING.
       - ***Prompting:*** Reminded their child IN THE MOMENT to ***not be bossy*** whenever the opportunity presented.
       - ***Praising: Praised*** their child using the buzzwords whenever they were ***not being bossy*** CORRECTLY.
       - ***Providing corrective feedback**: **Provided corrective feedback*** in the form of a ***praise sandwich*** whenever their child ATTEMPTED to ***not be bossy***.

3. **Provide social coaching on previously learned skills.**
   - Confirm parents continued to provide ***social coaching*** to their child throughout the week using the ***4 Ps*** for previously learned skills:
     - ***Listening and following directions.***
     - ***Meeting and greeting friends.***
     - ***Sharing and giving turns.***
     - ***Asking for a turn.***
     - ***Keeping cool.***
     - ***Being a good sport.***
     - ***Showing and telling.***

4. **Bring a turn-taking game.**
   - Confirm the following:
     - Brought a turn-taking game that their child enjoys playing and can be played with the other children. (To avoid distractions, these games should be left with the parents until *Parent Coached Play*.)

Didactic Lessons (20 Minutes)

PEERS® Neuroaffirming Pledge:

- We value neurodiversity, acceptance, and authenticity.
- We honor the diverse ways people experience the world.
- We respect each person's unique perspectives and communication styles.
- We recognize there is no one right way to connect with others.

- If using the strategies taught in PEERS® feels like camouflaging or masking and/or they don't align with your goals or the goals of your family, then you do not have to use them.
- Learning and using the skills taught in PEERS® is a PERSONAL CHOICE.

- **Didactic Lesson: Different Praising Strategies When Social Coaching**
- Distribute *Parent Handouts*.
  - Sections in **bold print** come directly from the *Parent Handout*.
  - Terms that are bold and italicized are buzzwords and represent important concepts from the didactic lesson.
- Explain, "Last week we talked about social coaching strategies during playdates. Today, we're going to review a few additional social coaching strategies related to PRAISING and PROMPTING that you can use when social coaching your child."

- **There are different ways you can *praise* and reinforce your child:**
  - ***Verbal praise.***
  - ***Physical praise.***
  - ***Gestural praise.***

- ***Verbal praise* (*praising* with words):**
  - **Steps for giving *verbal labeled praise*:**
    1. **Get your child's attention by:**
       - **Using their name.**
       - **Making eye contact with your child.**
       - **Gently touching your child's arm.**
    2. **Give simple *praise*:**
       - ***"Good job…"***
       - ***"Nice job…"***
       - ***"Nice try…"***
    3. **Use the PEERS® buzzwords to label the specific behavior you are *praising*:**
       - ***"…showing and telling!"***
       - ***"…keeping cool!"***
       - ***"…sharing and giving a turn!"***
  - **If you use general *praise* (e.g., *"Good job."*), your child may not know what behavior they are being *praised* for.**

- ***Physical praise* (*praise* with physical contact):**
  - **Examples of *physical praise*:**
    - **High-five.**
    - **Pound.**
    - **Fist bump.**
    - **Hug.**
    - **Pat on the back.**
  - **You may combine *physical praise* with *verbal praise.***
  - ***Physical praise* is useful when you cannot speak to your child (e.g., silence is required).**

- ***Gestural praise*** **(*praise* with gestures):**
    - **Examples of *gestural praise*:**
        - **Smiling.**
        - **Thumbs up.**
        - **Clapping.**
    - **You may combine *gestural praise* with *verbal praise* and/or *physical praise.***
    - ***Gestural praise* is useful when you cannot speak to your child (e.g., you are across a room).**

- **How you *praise* or reinforce your child will vary depending on:**
    - **Your child's preferences:**
        - **If your child is uncomfortable with physical touch, you may want to avoid *physical praise.***
    - **The setting:**
        - **The situation or place where the *social coaching* is occurring may warrant certain types of *praise* (home, school, *playdate*, *playgroup*, in the community, etc.).**
        - **You may need to use more *gestural praise* (e.g., smiling or giving a thumbs up across the room) during a *playgroup.***

- **Try to *praise* or reinforce your child as soon as they demonstrate the appropriate skill(s) or behavior(s).**

- ***Praising* appropriate use of skills will likely strengthen the value of the *praise* and reinforcement.**

- **When *social coaching* new skills or behaviors, *praise* and reinforce your child frequently.**

- ***Praise* your child's ATTEMPTS to use the social skills.**
    - **This will likely help your child learn the new skill or behavior faster.**
    - **This will help keep your child's motivation high and frustration low.**

- **If your child uses a skill spontaneously (e.g., without *prompting* or *social coaching* from you) or upon being *prompted*:**
    - ***Praise* and reinforce both spontaneous and *prompted* occurrences.**
    - **Provide EXTRA *praise* and reinforcement for spontaneous occurrences.**

- **As your child improves in their social skills, you can begin gradually fading out your *praise* and reinforcement (i.e., provide less *praising*).**
    - **At that point, it is likely the social interactions with their peers are becoming more intrinsically motivating for your child.**
    - **If your child starts to use the social skill(s) less over time, you may need to reintroduce more frequent *praise.***

Didactic Lesson: Different Prompting Strategies When Social Coaching

- **Make sure to have your child's attention BEFORE *prompting*.**
    - **This will help avoid a pattern of interaction where your attempts to *social coach* or *prompt* go unnoticed or even ignored by your child.**
        - **You do not want to indirectly reinforce nonresponsive behavior.**
    - **Having your child's attention before *prompting* will help you be consistent and contingent with your *prompting*.**
    - **You can gain your child's attention by:**
        - **Using their name before *prompting*.**
        - **A light touch on the arm before *prompting*.**
        - **Ask them if you have their attention before *prompting*.**
        - **Request their attention before *prompting*.**

- **Use the PEERS® for Preschoolers buzzwords to *prompt* your child.**
    - **Buzzwords are short, targeted phrases that come directly from the PEERS® for Preschoolers lessons.**
    - **The use of short buzzwords and buzzphrases will minimize the stimulus overload that too many words can create.**
    - **Using buzzwords across settings will help you and other caregivers to be consistent in your *social coaching*, which is better for learning.**
        - **Consider sharing the *Parent Handouts* with your child's teachers and caregivers so they can also use the buzzwords when *prompting* and providing other forms of *social coaching*.**
    - **The use of buzzwords when *prompting* will make it more likely that your child will:**
        - **Understand your *social coaching*.**
        - **Pay attention to your *social coaching*.**
        - **Respond appropriately to your *prompts*.**

- **Consider which type of *prompting* is the most effective and appropriate for your child according to the specific skill and the situation.**
    - **Types of *prompting* (from most to least intrusive):**
        - ***Physical prompts* ("hand over hand"):**
            - ***Physical prompts* involve providing physical assistance to your child in using a specific skill.**
                - **Example: Physically guiding your child's hand to *share* a toy with their friend.**
        - ***Verbal prompts*:**
            - ***Verbal prompts* involve providing verbal instruction for your child to use a specific skill by:**
                - **Making a request:**
                    - **Example: *"Remember to share and give a turn."***
                - **Asking a question:**
                    - **Example: *"Your friend wants a turn, what should we do?"***

- ***Gestural prompts*:**
  - ***Gestural prompts* involve providing some type of gesture as a "sign" for your child to use the specific skill.**
    - **Example: Pointing to a toy and then to a *playmate* to *prompt* your child to *share and give a turn* to their friend.**
    - **Example: Looking at your child expectantly and raising your eyebrows and shoulders to *prompt* your child to *share and give a turn* in response to their friend *asking for a turn*.**

- **The frequency of *prompting* will be determined by the environment and how familiar your child is with the skill.**
  - **You may need to provide more *prompting* when *social coaching* on emerging skills.**
    - **As your child improves in the skill, your *social coaching* will change by:**
      - **Presenting fewer *prompts*.**
      - **Increasing the time before presenting *prompts*.**
      - **Increasing the time between *prompts*.**
      - **Using less intrusive *prompts* (e.g., *physical prompts*).**
  - **During *playdates*, monitor *social coaching* to avoid significantly disrupting the natural flow of children's play and social interaction.**
    - **Limit the frequency of *prompts*.**
    - **Limit the rate of *prompting* (this will depend on the child, their *playmate*, the activity, and the skill).**
  - **Remember, the goal is to eventually fade out *prompting* altogether.**

Didactic Lesson: Asking a Friend to Play

Explain, *"In previous lessons we've talked about how to help your children maintain and sustain play by doing things like sharing and giving a turn, asking for a turn, being a good sport, and showing and telling during play. Today's child lesson will focus on how to appropriately initiate play interactions with friends and potential playmates by asking a friend to play."*

Snapshot of the Lesson: Asking a Friend to Play

The objective of this lesson is to teach children how to *ask a friend to play.* Steps for *asking a friend to play* include:

1. ***Look at your friends with your eyes*** (point to your eyes).
2. ***Smile with your mouth*** (point to your mouth and smile).
3. ***Say, "Do you want to play?" while using names***.
4. If your friend says yes, ***think of something fun to play***.
5. ***Say, "Let's play _____ (activity/game)!"*** **while** ***using names***.

Parent Coached Play

- Distribute the *Parent Coached Play Cards.*
- Review the examples of the ***4 Ps*** provided on the *Parent Coached Play Card.*
- Remind parents that in a few moments we will be joining the children for *Parent Coached Play* in the context of mock dyadic ***playdates***.
- Parents should keep the *Parent Coached Play Card* in front of them during the dyadic ***playdate*** for recommendations on how to ***social coach*** children on ***asking a friend to play.***

Homework Assignments

(Briefly review the homework assignments and troubleshoot any potential problems with parents.)

1. **Playdates.**
   - **Schedule and have a *playdate* with a *playmate.***
   - **Prepare for the *playdate* using the *5 Ws.***
     - ***WHO: Playdates* should be one-on-one.**
     - ***WHAT: Playdates* should be activity-based.**
     - ***WHERE:* Schedule initial *playdates* to take place in your home or somewhere you can provide *social coaching.***
     - ***WHEN:* Try to keep initial *playdates* to no more than 1–1.5 hours.**
     - ***HOW:* Coordinate how the children will get to and from the *playdate.***
   - **Do a final practice with your child of the games and activities that will be available during the *playdate.***
   - **Gather all the games and activity materials for the *playdate* in one area that is VISIBLE and easily accessible to YOU but not the children.**
   - **Provide *social coaching* during the *playdate* and assess if this is a good *playmate* for your child.**

2. **Practice asking a friend to play.**
   - **Practice having your child *ask a friend to play* this week during preferred and highly motivating activities while providing *social coaching* using the *4 Ps.***
     - ***Priming:* Review the rules for *asking a friend to play* with your child BEFORE PRACTICING.**
     - ***Prompting:* Remind your child IN THE MOMENT to *ask a friend to play* whenever the opportunities present.**
     - ***Praising: Praise* your child using the buzzwords whenever they *ask a friend to play* CORRECTLY.**
     - ***Providing corrective feedback: Provide corrective feedback* in the form of a *praise sandwich* whenever your child ATTEMPTS to *ask a friend to play.***
   - **Please send us a 30–60-second video of *social coaching* for *asking a friend to play* with your child to be viewed during homework review.**

  - **Please include:**
    - **Skills your child did well.**
    - **Skills you would like to work on with your child.**

3. **Provide social coaching on previously learned skills.**
   - **Continue providing *social coaching* to your child throughout the week using the *4 Ps.***
   - **Previous skills include:**
     - ***Listening and following directions.***
     - ***Meeting and greeting friends.***
     - ***Sharing and giving a turn.***
     - ***Asking for a turn.***
     - ***Keeping cool.***
     - ***Being a good sport.***
     - ***Showing and telling.***
     - ***Don't be bossy.***

4. **Bring a turn-taking game.**
   - **Bring a turn-taking game that your child enjoys playing and can be played with the other children.**

Session 9 Continued

Asking a Friend to Play

CHILD SESSION THERAPIST GUIDE

Child Session Agenda

- Didactic Lesson: *Asking a Friend to Play* (20 minutes).
- Group Behavioral Rehearsal Activity 1: *Red Rover* (15 minutes).
- Break Time (10 minutes).
- Group Behavioral Rehearsal Activity 2: *Swap and Play* (15 minutes).
- Parent Coached Play: *Dyadic Playdates* (20 minutes).
- Final Wrap-Up (10 minutes).

Snapshot of the Lesson: Asking a Friend to Play

The objective of this lesson is to teach children how to ***ask a friend to play***. Steps for ***asking a friend to play*** include:

1. ***Look at your friend with your eyes*** (point to your eyes).
2. ***Smile with your mouth*** (point to your mouth and smile).
3. ***Say "Do you want to play?" using names***.
4. If your friend says yes, **think of something fun to play**.
5. **Say "Let's play _____ (activity/game)!" using names**.

Materials Needed

- Lion puppet.
- Cow puppet.
- Small ball.
- Carpet squares or chairs.
- "Making Friends Helper" badge.
- Star chart with names of children.
- Marker for star chart.
- Name tags for families and treatment team.
- Prize bins with prizes.

Preparing for the Lesson

- Use the script below with the group leader using a lion puppet to play the part of "Larry Lion."
- A behavioral coach uses a cow puppet to play the part of "Kelly Cow."
- An additional behavioral coach assists in the behavioral rehearsal and provides encouragement and feedback to the group.

- A child is chosen at the beginning of the lesson as the "Making Friends Helper."
  - The "Making Friends Helper" wears a special badge and is the first child to practice the skill.
- The group leader and the behavioral coach sit on the floor at the front of the room.
- A special-colored carpet square (e.g., red) is placed at the front of the room next to the group leader to be used as the "Good Friend Square."
- For the children, additional carpet squares of the same color (e.g., green) are placed in a semi-circle facing the child group leader and the "Good Friend Square."
- Note: If carpet squares are unavailable, the children and behavioral coaches may sit on chairs.
- The material in *italics* should be read by the indicated person.
- The material in ***bold and italics*** represents buzzwords and should be emphasized when read.
- The material in CAPITAL LETTERS within the script should be given extra emphasis while the group is encouraged to say the words in unison.

Behavioral Coaching Techniques

Behavioral coaches should use the following coaching techniques described below throughout the lesson and the behavioral rehearsal activities. (Note: ***priming*** occurs during the introduction to the activity.)

- ***Prompting*:**
  - Use the buzzwords to ***prompt*** the children to ***ask a friend to play***.
    - Example: *"Remember to ask your friend to play."*
    - Example: *"Remember to think of something fun to play."*
    - Example: *"What should you do if your friend says yes?"*
- ***Praising*:**
  - Reinforce ***asking a friend to play*** by ***praising*** the children.
    - Example: *"Nice job asking your friend to play!"*
    - Example: *"Great job saying, 'Do you want to play with me?'"*
    - Example: *"Good job thinking of something fun to play!"*
- ***Providing corrective feedback using a praise sandwich*:**
  - Reinforce ATTEMPTS to ***ask a friend to play*** by ***praising*** the children and identifying what could be done differently next time.
    - Example: *"Good job asking a friend to play. Remember to use names next time, but nice try!"*
    - Example: *"Nice try asking a friend to play! Don't forget to say, 'Do you want to play with me?' but good job!"*
    - Example: *"Nice try asking a friend to play! Don't forget to think of something fun to play next time, but great job!"*
- Continue to provide ***social coaching*** on previously learned skills:
  - ***Listening and following directions.***
  - ***Meeting and greeting friends.***
  - ***Sharing and giving a turn.***
  - ***Asking for a turn.***
  - ***Keeping cool.***
  - ***Being a good sport.***
  - ***Showing and telling.***
  - ***Don't be bossy.***

Didactic Lesson: Asking a Friend to Play (20 minutes)

Have the children sit in a semi-circle on the carpet squares facing the group leader.

Larry Lion: (Sit at the front of the room and choose a Making Friends Helper.) *"Who wants to be our Making Friends Helper?"*

(Choose from among the children raising their hands and place the "Making Friends Helper" badge on the child. The child stays in their seat for now.)

"Hi friends! I'm Larry Lion. Grrr, Grrr! Today we're going to practice asking a friend to play. Asking a friend to play is a great way to be nice to our friends!"

"Why should we ask our friends to play? We should ask our friends to play because it's more fun!"

"Who should we ask to play? We should ask to play with our FRIENDS, TEACHERS, MOMMIES, DADDIES, BROTHERS, AND SISTERS."

"How should we ask our friends to play? We should ask our friends to play by looking at our friend with our (point to your eyes and then to Larry Lion's eyes)*...EYES, smiling with our* (point to your mouth and smile)*...MOUTH, and saying, 'Do you want to play?' If our friends say yes, then we need to think of something fun to play. We could say, 'Let's play chase' or "Let's play catch!' And don't forget to use* (pause briefly to prompt the children to say *"names"*)*...NAMES!"*

"Remember, asking a friend to play is a nice way to be a good friend! Grrr, Grrr!"

Role Play: Asking a Friend to Play

Larry Lion and Kelly Cow: (Larry Lion looks bored while playing with the small ball. Kelly Cow is nearby and does not have a toy.)

Larry Lion: (Turn to look at the group of children.) *"Hey friends! Grrr, Grrr! It's NO FUN playing with this ball all by myself. Do you think I should ask my friend Kelly Cow to play?"* (Nod your head yes and encourage the children to say *"yes."*)

"That's a great idea! Let's do it! Grrr, Grrr!" (Turn to look at Kelly Cow and smile.) *"Kelly Cow, do you want to play?"*

Kelly Cow: (Turn to look at Larry Lion and smile.) *"Sure, Larry Lion! Moo, moo!"*

Larry Lion: (Turn to look at the group of children.) *"Hey friends, Kelly Cow said yes.*

	Now do you think I should think of something fun to play?" (Nod your head yes and encourage the children to say *"yes."*)
	"That's a great idea! Grrr, Grrr! But what should we play? Hmm…" (Look confused, scratch your head, and pause.)
	"Hey friends, I know! I have this ball (hold up the small ball). *Should I ask Kelly Cow to play catch?"* (Nod your head yes and encourage the children to say *"yes."*)
	"That's a great idea! Grrr, Grrr! Let's do it!" (Turn to look at Kelly Cow and smile.) *"Kelly Cow,* (hold up the small ball) *let's play catch!"*
Kelly Cow:	*"Okay, Larry Lion! Moo, moo!"*
Larry Lion:	*"Here, Kelly Cow!"* (Throw the small ball to Kelly Cow.)
Kelly Cow:	(Catch the small ball.) *"Nice throw! Catch, Larry Lion!"* (Throw the small ball to Larry Lion.)
Larry Lion:	(Catch the small ball.)
Larry Lion and Kelly Cow:	(Look at each other and smile.) *"That was fun!"*
Larry Lion:	(Turn to look at the group of children.) *"Hey friends, did I do a good job of asking my friend Kelly Cow to play?"* (Nod your head yes and encourage the children to say *"yes."*)
	"That's right! Grrr, grrr!"
Larry Lion and Kelly Cow:	(Say *"good job," give a "lion high-five"* and *"cow high-five,"* clap, cheer, and encourage the children to clap as well. Larry Lion keeps the small ball. Kelly Cow sits on the other side of the Good Friend Square (i.e., the Good Friend Square is between Larry Lion and Kelly Cow). Larry Lion ***social coaches*** the children as needed while they practice ***asking a friend to play*** with Kelly Cow.)
Larry Lion:	*"Now let's see _____ (behavioral coach) try! _____ (Behavioral coach), please come sit on the Good Friend Square."*
Behavioral coach:	(Sit on the Good Friend Square.)
Larry Lion:	*"_____ (Behavioral coach), can you show us how to ask Kelly Cow to play?"*
Behavioral coach:	*"Okay, Larry Lion."*

Larry Lion:	(Turn to look at the group of children.) *"Remember to look at Kelly Cow with your* (point to your eyes to prompt the children to say *"eyes"*)*...EYES and smile with your* (point to your mouth to prompt the children to say *"mouth"*)*...MOUTH when you say, 'Kelly Cow, do you want to play?' If Kelly Cow says yes, then think of something fun to play. And don't forget to use* (pause briefly to prompt the children to say *"names"*)*...NAMES."* (Hand the small ball to the behavioral coach.)
Behavioral coach:	(Turn to look at Kelly Cow and smile.) *"Kelly Cow, do you want to play?"*
Kelly Cow:	(Look at the behavioral coach and smile.) *"Sure, _____ (behavioral coach)! Moo, moo!"*
Larry Lion:	(Turn to look at the behavioral coach.) *"_____ (Behavioral coach), Kelly Cow said yes. Now think of something fun to play!"*
Behavioral coach:	(Look at Kelly Cow and smile.) *"Kelly Cow, let's play catch*!" (Hold up the small ball.)
Kelly Cow:	*"Okay, _____ (behavioral coach)! Moo, moo!"*
Behavioral coach:	*"Here, Kelly Cow* (throw the small ball to Kelly Cow)*!"*
Kelly Cow:	(Catch the small ball.) *"Nice throw! Catch, _____ (behavioral coach)!"* (Throw the small ball to the behavioral coach.)
Behavioral coach:	(Catch the small ball.)
Larry Lion:	*"That looked so fun! Great job asking a friend to play, _____ (behavioral coach)! Grrr, grrr!"*
Larry Lion and Behavioral coach:	(Say *"good job," give a "lion high-five"* and *"cow high-five,"* clap, cheer, and encourage the children to clap as well. The behavioral coach gives the ball back to Larry Lion and leaves the Good Friend Square.)

Behavioral Rehearsal: Asking a Friend to Play

Larry Lion:	(Turn to look at the group of children.) *"Okay friends! Now let's see our Making Friends Helper ____ try! ____ (Making Friends Helper), come sit on the Good Friend Square and show us how to ask Kelly Cow to play."* (The Making Friends Helper should sit on the Good Friend Square.)

"Remember to look at Kelly Cow with your (point to your eyes to prompt the children to say *"eyes")...EYES and smile with your* (point to your mouth to prompt the children to say *"mouth")...MOUTH when you say, 'Kelly Cow, do you want to play?' If Kelly Cow says yes, then think of something fun to play. And don't forget to use* (pause briefly to prompt the children to say *"names")...NAMES."*

(Hand the small ball to the Making Friends Helper.)

(If needed, ***social coach*** the Making Friends Helper to ***look, smile,*** and ***say, "Kelly Cow, do you want to play?"***)

Kelly Cow: (Look at the Making Friends Helper and smile.) *"Sure, _____ (Making Friends Helper)! Moo, moo!"*

Larry Lion: (If needed, ***social coach*** the Making Friends Helper to ***look, smile,*** and ***say, "Kelly Cow, let's play catch!"***)

Kelly Cow: *"Okay, _____ (Making Friends Helper)! Moo, moo!"*

Larry Lion: (If needed, ***social coach*** the Making Friends Helper to throw the small ball to Kelly Cow.)

Kelly Cow: (Catch the ball.) *"Nice throw! Catch, _____ (Making Friends Helper)!"*

(Throw the small ball to the Making Friends Helper.)

Larry Lion: *"Great job asking a friend to play, _____ (Making Friends Helper)! Grrr, grrr!"*

(Say *"good job," give a "lion high-five"* and *"cow high-five,"* clap, cheer, and encourage the children to clap as well.)

(The Making Friends Helper should return the small ball to Larry Lion.)

"Okay, Making Friends Helper, choose another friend to sit on the Good Friend Square." (If needed, ***social coach*** the Making Friends Helper to choose another child before returning to their seat.)

Repeat the following with each child:

Larry Lion: (Have each child take turns sitting on the Good Friend Square and practicing ***asking a friend to play*** with Kelly Cow.)

(Turn to look at the group of children.) *"Okay friends! Now let's see ____ (child) try! ____ (Child), come sit on the Good Friend Square and show us how to ask Kelly Cow to play."*

(The child should sit on the Good Friend Square.)

"Remember to look at Kelly Cow with your (point to your eyes to prompt the children to say *"eyes")...EYES and smile with your* (point to your mouth to prompt the children to say *"mouth")...MOUTH when you say, 'Kelly Cow, do you want to play?' If Kelly Cow says yes, then think of something fun to play. And don't forget to use* (pause briefly to prompt the children to say *"names")...NAMES."*

(Hand the small ball to the child.)

(If needed, ***social coach*** the child to ***look, smile,*** and ***say, "Kelly Cow, do you want to play?"***)

Kelly Cow: (Look at the child and smile.) *"Sure, ____ (child)! Moo, moo!"*

Larry Lion: (If needed, ***social coach*** the child ***look, smile,*** and ***say, "Kelly Cow, let's play catch!"***)

Kelly Cow: *"Okay, ____ (child)! Moo, moo!"*

Larry Lion: (If needed, ***social coach*** the child to throw the small ball to Kelly Cow.)

Kelly Cow: (Catch the ball.) *"Nice throw! Catch, ____ (child)!"* (Throw the small ball to the child.)

Larry Lion: *"Great job asking a friend to play, ____ (child)! Grrr, grrr!"*

(Say *"good job," give a "lion high-five"* and *"cow high-five,"* clap, cheer, and encourage the children to clap as well.)

(The child should return the small ball to Larry Lion.)

"Okay, ____ (Child), choose another friend to sit on the Good Friend Square." (If needed, ***social coach*** the child to choose another child before returning to their seat.)

Didactic Lesson Wrap-Up

Group leader: *"Well friends, you all did a great job asking a friend to play by looking at your friend with your* (point to your eyes to prompt the children to say *"eyes")...EYES and smiling with your* (point to your mouth to prompt the children to say *"mouth")...MOUTH when you said, 'Kelly Cow, do you want to play?' And great job thinking of something fun to play when Kelly Cow said yes. And nice job using* (pause briefly to prompt the children to say *"names")...NAMES!"*

"You each earned ____ (number) stars for asking a friend to play! Let's start with ____ (child)."

Award each child the same number of stars by repeating the following with each child:

Group leader: *"Where's ____ (child)?"* (Wait until all the children are looking at the child.)

"____ (Child), how many stars did you earn?" (Pause briefly to allow the child to respond.)

"That's right! Let's all count for ____ (child)! One, two, three... (add stars to the Star Chart as they are counted aloud)*! Everybody clap for ____ (child)!"* (All behavioral coaches clap and cheer and encourage the children to clap as well.)

Session 9 Continued

Red Rover

BEHAVIORAL REHEARSAL ACTIVITY 1

Materials Needed

- None.

Room Setup

- Remove or place all carpet squares to the side.
- The group leader stands at the front of the room facing the children.
- Children and behavioral coaches sit in a semi-circle facing the group leader as the rules are explained.

Rules: Red Rover

- The group leader reads the script below to explain the rules.
- Divide the children into two teams.
  - Assign a behavioral coach to each team to act as team leader.
- The two teams should stand approximately 10–15 feet apart and face each other.
  - Intersperse remaining behavioral coaches among the children to ***social coach***.
- Children should hold the hand of the child or behavioral coach next to them to form a chain.
- Throughout the game, help the teams choose which child from the opposing team they want to "call over" (i.e., walk over and join their team) based on various attributes.
  - Examples:
    - *"Call over somebody wearing a blue shirt. Who's wearing a blue shirt?"*
    - *"Call over a friend wearing a hat. Which friend is wearing a hat?"*
    - *"Call over someone with brown hair. Which friend has brown hair?"*
- Before the identified child can walk over, a *calling friend* from the opposing team should ***ask a friend to play*** by saying, "_______ *(Child), do you want to play Red Rover?"*
- The child should respond to the *calling friend* by saying, *"yes"* or *"okay."*
- All behavioral coaches and children should then sing the *Red Rover* song:
  - *"Red rover, red rover, let _______ (child from the opposing team) walk over!"*
- Repeat the cycle EACH time a child is "called over" to the opposing team.
- Once a child is "called over" they will be the new *calling friend.*
- Make sure all children have a turn being "called over" and being the *calling friend.*

Behavioral Rehearsal: Red Rover (15 Minutes)

The group leader leads the activity. The behavioral coaches and children sit nearby as the group leader explains the rules.

Group leader: *"Hey friends, now we're going to play a game called Red Rover! We will have two teams that will take turns calling friends over by singing the Red Rover Song. Each of you will take turns being a 'calling friend.' The calling friend will ask a friend to play from the other team by looking at your friends with your* (point to your eyes to prompt the children to say *"eyes")... EYES and smiling with your* (point to your mouth to prompt the children to say *"mouth")...MOUTH when you say, 'Do you want to play Red Rover?' And don't forget to use...*(pause briefly to prompt the children to say *"names")...NAMES!"*

"If your friends say yes, then we'll all sing the Red Rover song that goes like this: 'Red rover, red rover, let ____ (behavioral coach 1) walk over!"

"Remember to listen because when your name is called, you'll walk over to join the other team and then YOU will become the calling friend!"

"Okay, let's have ____ (behavioral coach 1), ____ (behavioral coach 2) and ____ (behavioral coach 3) try first!"

Role Play: Red Rover

The group leader leads the role play. The three behavioral coaches demonstrate how to play *Red Rover*. Behavioral coach 1 is on one team, and behavioral coaches 2 and 3 are on the opposing team. The children and other behavioral coaches are interspersed equally across the two groups and stand ten to 15 feet apart from each other. Each team holds hands with one another to keep the children from wandering during game playing.

Group leader: *"Okay, let's have ____ (behavioral coach 1)'s team go first. ____ (Behavioral coach 1) will be our first calling friend. ____ (Behavioral coach 1), call over somebody ____ (attribute to describe behavioral coach 2). Who's ____ (attribute to describe behavioral coach 2)?"*

Behavioral coach 1: *"____ (Behavioral coach 2)."*

Group leader *"Great job, ____ (behavioral coach 1)! Now ask ____ (behavioral coach 2) to play and think of something fun to play like Red Rover."*

Behavioral coach 1: (Turn to look and smile at behavioral coach 2.) *"____ (Behavioral coach 2), do you want to play Red Rover?"*

Behavioral coach 2: (Look and smile at behavioral coach 1.) *"Okay, ____ (behavioral coach 1)."*

Behavioral coach 1: *"Red rover, red rover, let ____ (behavioral coach 2) walk over!"*

Behavioral coach 2: (***Say "Bye!"*** to behavioral coach 3 ***using names*** and then walk over to the other team and ***say "Hi!"*** to behavioral coach 1 ***using names***.)

Group leader: *"Great job asking your friend to play and thinking of something fun to play! ____ (Behavioral coach 3), now it's your turn to be the calling friend and ask a friend to play. ____ (Behavioral coach 3), call over somebody ____ (attribute to describe behavioral coach 1). Who's ____ (attribute to describe behavioral coach 1)?"*

Behavioral coach 3: *"____ (Behavioral coach 1)."*

Group leader: *"Great job, ____ (behavioral coach 3)! Now ask ____ (behavioral coach 1) to play and think of something fun to play like Red Rover."*

Behavioral coach 3: (Turn to look and smile at behavioral coach 1.) *"____ (Behavioral coach 1), do you want to play Red Rover?"*

Behavioral coach 1: (Look and smile at behavioral coach 3.) *"Okay, ____ (behavioral coach 3)."*

Behavioral coach 3: *"Red rover, red rover, let ____ (behavioral coach 1) walk over!"*

Behavioral coach 1: (***Say "Bye!"*** to behavioral coach 2 ***using names*** and then walk over to the other team and ***say "Hi!"*** to behavioral coach 3 ***using names***.)

Group leader: *"Great job asking your friend to play and saying 'hi' and 'bye' using names! Okay friends, now it's everybody's turn to play Red Rover. Are we ready?"*

Behavioral Rehearsal: Red Rover

Group leader: *"Okay, let's have ____ (child) be the next calling friend to ask a friend to play. ____ (Child), call over somebody ____ (attribute to describe a child from the opposing team). Who's ____ (attribute to describe a child from the opposing team)?"*

(If needed, behavioral coaches should ***social coach*** the children to identify the correct child.)

"Great job, ____ (child)! Now ask ____ (child from the opposing team) to play and think of something fun to play like Red Rover."

(If needed, behavioral coaches should ***social coach*** the children to ***ask a friend to play*** Red Rover.)

Behavioral coaches and children: *"Red rover, red rover, let ____ (child from the opposing team) walk over!"*

(If needed, behavioral coaches should ***social coach*** the children to ***listen and follow directions*** and say ***"hi" and "bye"*** to teammates using names.)

Group leader: *"Great job asking your friend to play and saying 'hi' and 'bye' using names! Let's keep on playing. Are we ready?"*

Repeat the sequence above until all the children have had at least one turn being the *calling friend* and have had the opportunity to practice ***asking a friend to play***.

Behavioral Rehearsal Wrap-Up

Group leader: *"Well friends, great job asking a friend to play! Give yourselves a big round of applause!"* (All behavioral coaches clap and cheer and encourage the children to clap as well.)

"Now everyone should come sit in the Listening Circle." (Have children return to the Listening Circle to sit on their carpet squares.)

"Okay friends, you did a great job asking a friend to play and thinking of something fun to play by looking at your friends with your (point to your eyes to prompt the children to say *"eyes"*)*...EYES and smiling with your* (point to your mouth to prompt the children to say *"mouth"*)*...MOUTH when you said, 'Do you want to play Red Rover?' And nice job using* (pause briefly to prompt the children to say *"names"*)*...NAMES!"*

"You each earned ____ (number) more stars for asking a friend to play! Let's start with ____ (Child)."

Award each child the same number of stars by repeating the following with each child:

Group leader: *"Where's _____ (child)?"* (Wait until all the children are looking at the child.)

"_____ (Child), how many stars did you earn?" (Pause briefly to allow the child to respond.)

"That's right! Let's all count for _____ (child)! One, two, three... (add stars to the Star Chart as they are counted aloud)*! Everybody clap for _____ (child)!"* (All behavioral coaches clap and cheer and encourage the children to clap as well.)

Break Time (10 Minutes)

- The puppets may be used to lead the children to and from the bathroom during break time.
- To assist with transitions and limit unstructured time, behavioral coaches may review the lesson with the children while waiting for the remaining children to return from the bathroom.
- You may want to award stars for good behavior after returning from the bathroom.

Session 9 Continued

Swap and Play

BEHAVIORAL REHEARSAL ACTIVITY 2

Materials Needed

- A range of activities or sets of toys (one per dyad/triad).
  - Examples: blocks, drawing materials, toy vehicles, etc.
  - Note: Substitute games/toys as appropriate to match the interests of the children.
  - A bean bag for *Hot Potato* at each table.
- Tables and chairs (each table should be large enough to fit two to three children and one behavioral coach).

Room Setup

- Remove or place all carpet squares to the side.
- If tables are available, position tables in different corners of the room with three to four chairs around each table to create an activity area.
- Place one activity or one set of toys on each table but out of reach of the children.
- The group leader sits on the floor in front of the room while explaining the rules.
- The children and behavioral coaches sit on the floor in a semi-circle facing the group leader.

Rules: Swap and Play

- The group leader reads the script below to explain the rules.
- Divide the children into dyads and assign each group to an activity area.
  - If there are an odd number of children, create one triad.
  - Assign one behavioral coach per activity area to ***social coach***.
- Before the children go to their activity areas, the behavioral coach will choose ONE child from each dyad/triad to be the *"asking friend"* who will practice ***asking a friend to play***.
- After approximately two minutes of play, the behavioral coaches will identify ONE child from each group to swap groups and become the *"joining friend."*
- Before *joining friends* can start playing in their new activity areas, the behavioral coaches should ***social coach*** the children who did NOT swap groups to ***ask a friend to play*** (i.e., ask the child joining the game to play).
- Repeat the cycle, ensuring each child ***asks a friend to play*** and has a turn to play at each activity area.

Behavioral Rehearsal: Swap and Play (15 Minutes)

The group leader explains the activity. The behavioral coaches and children sit nearby as the group leader explains the rules.

Group leader: *"Hey friends, now we're going to play a game called Swap and Play. You'll play in groups. Some friends will play with the blocks* (point to the blocks activity area), *other friends will draw* (point to the drawing activity area), *and other friends will play with cars* (point to the toy car activity area). *"*

"Everyone will get a turn to play with all the games and toys because your friends are going to be asking you to play! Each group will have a 'joining friend' and an 'asking friend.' The 'joining friend' will switch tables after two minutes of playing. But before the 'joining friends' can join the game, the 'asking friend' will ask to play by looking at your friends with your (point to your eyes to prompt the children to say *"eyes")...EYES and smiling with your* (point to your mouth to prompt the children to say *"mouth"*)... *MOUTH when you say, 'Do you want to play?' Then think of something fun to play by saying, 'Let's play blocks!' or 'Let's draw!' or 'Let's play with cars!' And don't forget to use* (pause briefly to prompt the children to say *"names"*)...*NAMES."*

"After a few minutes, I'm going to tell you to FREEZE (demonstrate freezing in place) *and one friend from each group will swap groups and become the new 'joining friend'."*

"Okay, let's have ____ (behavioral coach 1), ____ (behavioral coach 2), and ____ (behavioral coach 3) try first!"

Role Play: Swap and Play

The group leader leads the role play. The three behavioral coaches demonstrate how to play *Swap and Play*. Behavioral coaches 1 and 2 are standing near the activity area with blocks. Behavioral coach 3 is sitting in the activity area with drawing.

Group leader: *"Okay, ____ (behavioral coach 1) and ____ (behavioral coach 2), you'll play with the blocks first. ____ (Behavioral coach 1) will be the 'asking friend' and ____ (behavioral coach 2) will be the 'joining friend.' Before you can play, ____ (behavioral coach 1), ask your friend to play and think of something fun to play."*

Behavioral coach 1: (Turn to look at behavioral coach 2 and smile.) *"____ (Behavioral coach 2), do you want to play?"*

Behavioral coach 2: (Look and smile at behavioral coach 1.) *"Okay, ____ (behavioral coach 1)!"*

Behavioral coach 1: *"____ (Behavioral coach 2), let's play blocks and build a tower!"*

Behavioral coach 2:	*"Okay, ____ (behavioral coach 1)!"*
Behavioral coaches 1 and 2:	(Build a tower with the blocks while ***showing and telling*** and ***being good sports***.)
Group leader:	*"Great job asking your friend to play and thinking of something fun to play, ____ (behavioral coach 1)!"*
Behavioral coaches 1 and 2:	(Continue to play cooperatively with the blocks while ***showing and telling*** and ***being good sports*** for a few moments.)
Group leader:	*"Okay, FREEZE! ____ (Behavioral coach 2), get ready to swap groups. Ready? And…SWAP!"*
Behavioral coach 2:	(Stand up and walk to the drawing area where behavioral coach 3 is waiting. Do not join the drawing activity.)
Group leader:	*"____ (Behavioral coach 3) is now the 'asking friend' and ____ (behavioral coach 2) is the 'joining friend.' Before you can play, ____ (behavioral coach 3), ask your friend to play and think of something fun to play."*
Behavioral coach 3:	(Turn to look at behavioral coach 2 and smile.) *"____ (Behavioral coach 2), do you want to play?"*
Behavioral coach 2:	(Look and smile at behavioral coach 3.) *"Okay, ____ (behavioral coach 3)!"*
Behavioral coach 3:	*"____ (Behavioral coach 2), let's draw a spaceship!"*
Behavioral coach 2:	*"Okay, ____ (behavioral coach 3)!"*
Behavioral coaches 2 and 3:	(Begin drawing together while ***showing and telling*** and ***being good sports***.)
Group leader:	*"Great job asking your friend to play and thinking of something fun to play, ____ (behavioral coach 3)!"* *"Okay friends, now it's everybody's turn to play Swap and Play. Are we ready?"*

Behavioral Rehearsal: Swap and Play

Children are directed to activity areas. The behavioral coaches ***social coach*** the children in dyads or triads to ***ask a friend to play*** during the game playing.

Behavioral coach:	*"Before you can play, let's practice asking a friend to play and thinking of something fun to play. ____ (Child 1) will be the 'asking friend' and ____*

(child 2) will be the 'joining friend.' ____ (Child 1), ask your friend to play and think of something fun to play."

(If needed, the behavioral coach should ***social coach*** the *asking child* to ***ask a friend to play*** and help the *joining child* to accept the invitation.)

"Great job asking your friend to play! Let's play!"

After two minutes of play, the group leader will instruct everyone to swap groups:

Group leader: *"Everyone FREEZE! And...SWAP!"*

Behavioral coach: *"Everyone FREEZE! ____ (Child), it's time to swap groups.*

(Each behavioral coach assigns a child from their activity area to be a *joining friend* and directs (or briefly escorts) the *joining friend* to the new activity area. Each behavioral coach will remain in their own activity area to assist the *asking friend* with ***asking a friend to play***.)

When the *joining friend* joins the new activity area, the behavioral coach will ***social coach*** the *asking friend* to ***ask a friend to play***:

Behavioral coach: *"Before you can play again, let's have our 'asking friend' ____ (child) practice asking a friend to play and thinking of something fun to play."*

(If needed, the behavioral coach should ***social coach*** the *asking friend* to ***ask a friend to play*** and help the *joining friend* to accept the invitation.)

"Great job asking your friend to play! Let's play!"

Repeat the above cycle every two minutes, ensuring that every child has at least one turn being the *asking friend* by practicing ***asking a friend to play***.

Behavioral Rehearsal Wrap-Up

Group leader: *"Well friends, great job asking a friend to play! Give yourselves a big round of applause!"* (All behavioral coaches clap and cheer and encourage the children to clap as well.)

"Now everyone should come sit in the Listening Circle." (Have children return to the Listening Circle to sit on their carpet squares.)

"Okay friends, you did a great job asking your friends to play by looking at your friends with your (point to your eyes to prompt the children to say *"eyes")...EYES and smiling with your* (point to your mouth to prompt the children to say *"mouth"*)*...MOUTH when you said, 'Do you want to play?'*

And nice job thinking of something fun to play when you said, 'Let's play blocks!' or 'Let's draw!' or 'Let's play with cars!'"

"You each earned ____ (number) more stars for asking a friend to play!

Let's start with ____ (child)."

Award each child the same number of stars by repeating the following with each child:

Group leader: *"Where's ____ (child)?"* (Wait until all the children are looking at the child.)

"____ (Child), how many stars did you earn?" (Pause briefly to allow the child to respond.)

"That's right! Let's all count for ____ (child)! One, two, three... (add stars to the Star Chart as they are counted aloud)*! Everybody clap for ____ (child)!"* (All behavioral coaches clap and cheer and encourage the children to clap as well.)

"Now we're going to play another game with our parents and practice asking a friend to play some more!"

Session 9 Continued

Asking a Friend to Play

PARENT COACHED PLAY: DYADIC PLAYDATES

Materials Needed

- Games brought by children and parents from home.
- Turn-taking games provided by the treatment team.
- Tables and chairs or carpet squares.
- *Parent Coached Play Cards*.

Room Setup

- If available, organize tables in separate corners of the room with four to six chairs per table.
- If tables are not available, place two carpet squares in separate corners of the room to indicate where the children will sit.

Rules: Dyadic Playdates

- The child group leader divides the families into groups of two families each.
    - If there are an odd number of children, pair one child with a behavioral coach who will serve as a ***playmate***. In this case, you will need an additional coach to serve as a behavioral coach for the parent.
    - To avoid social exclusion, avoid having children play in triads as much as possible.
- Assign each group to sit at a table or specific play area.
    - Children should sit next to each other.
    - Parents will act as ***social coaches*** by sitting on the other side of their child to minimize interrupting the natural flow of play between the children.
    - One behavioral coach will be assigned to each dyad to provide ***social coaching*** suggestions and feedback to parents.
- Children will take turns playing the games brought from home or games provided by the treatment team.
- Each child will have ten minutes to play their chosen game with their ***playmate*** and will then switch games.
- Parents will choose which child's game will be played first.
- To minimize unstructured periods, parents will help the children set up the game in a cooperative fashion (handing game pieces to each other, offering suggestions, etc.).
- Before playing each game, parents will ***social coach*** the children to ***ask a friend to play***.

- As they play, parents will ***social coach*** the children on previously learned and newly learned skills using the guidelines highlighted on the *Parent Coached Play Cards.*
- Behavioral coaches will provide support to parents in their ***social coaching*** using the ***4 Ps*** (***priming, prompting, praising,*** and ***providing corrective feedback***) and will model appropriate coaching behavior when necessary.
- After approximately nine minutes of play, instruct the parents to prepare the children for the upcoming game swap.
- After approximately one additional minute of play (ten minutes total), instruct the parents to have the children clean up and swap games.
- Repeat the cycle with the second game for the remaining ten minutes before returning to the *Listening Circle*.

Behavioral Coaching: Dyadic Playdates

Behavioral coaches will ***social coach*** parents during dyadic ***playdates*** in the following ways:

- ***Priming***:
  - Begin the play interactions with parents going over the rules for ***asking a friend to play*** BEFORE GAME PLAYING.
    - Example: *"Remember to ask to play by looking at your friend with your* (point to your eyes to prompt the child to say *"eyes"*)*...EYES and smile with your* (point to your mouth to prompt the child to say *"mouth"*)*...MOUTH when you say, 'Do you want to play?' If your friend says 'yes,' then think of something fun to play. And don't forget to use* (pause briefly to prompt the child to say *"names"*)*...NAMES."*
- ***Prompting***:
  - Remind parents to use the buzzwords to ***prompt*** their child to ***ask a friend to play*** IN THE MOMENT.
  - Help parents to identify opportunities to proactively ***prompt*** their child to ***ask a friend to play.***
    - Example: *"Remember to ask your friend to play."*
    - Example: *"Remember to think of something fun to play."*
    - Example: *"What should you do if your friend says yes?"*
- ***Praising***:
  - Remind parents to ***praise*** and reinforce their child whenever their child ***asks a friend to play*** CORRECTLY.
    - Example: *"Nice job asking your friend to play!"*
    - Example: *"Great job saying, 'Do you want to play with me?'"*
    - Example: *"Good job thinking of something fun to play!"*
- ***Providing corrective feedback using a praise sandwich***:
  - Remind parents to ***praise*** their child's ATTEMPTS to ***ask a friend to play*** and identify what could be done differently next time.
    - Example: *"Good job asking a friend to play. Remember to use names next time, but nice try!"*
    - Example: *"Nice try asking a friend to play! Don't forget to say, 'Do you want to play with me?' but good job!"*

  - Example: *"Nice try asking a friend to play! Don't forget to think of something fun to play next time, but great job!"*
- Remind parents to continue to ***social coach*** on previously learned skills:
  - ***Listening and following directions.***
  - ***Meeting and greeting friends.***
  - ***Sharing and giving a turn.***
  - ***Asking for a turn.***
  - ***Keeping cool.***
  - ***Being a good sport.***
  - ***Showing and telling.***
  - ***Don't be bossy.***

Parent Coached Play: Dyadic Playdates (20 Minutes)

- Have each child choose a turn-taking game brought from home or provided by the treatment team.
- The group leader sits on the floor at the front of the room.
- The families sit on the floor in a semi-circle facing the group leader.

Group leader: *"Hey friends, we're going to have more playdates and play with the fun games you brought from home. This time, we're practicing how to ask a friend to play. Each of you will ask a friend to play by looking at your friend with your* (point to your eyes to prompt the children to say *"eyes"*)*...EYES and smiling with your* (point to your mouth to prompt the children to say *"mouth"*)*...MOUTH when you say, 'Do you want to play?'"*

"And if your friend says yes, then you should think of something fun to play by saying, 'Let's play _______ (game brought in by a child)!' (point to the game brought in by a child) *or 'Let's play _______ (another game brought in by a child)!'* (point to the game brought in by a child)*."*

"You'll play the game for a few minutes before you'll swap games. Then the other person will ask a friend to play. Parents, remember to social coach your children by using your Parent Coached Play Cards. Okay, let's play with our games!"

- Before playing, parents will ***social coach*** their child to ***say "hi"*** to one another ***using names.***
- At the beginning of each new game, parents will have children practice ***asking a friend to play***.
- Parents will ***social coach*** their children to ***not be bossy, show and tell, ask for a turn***, ***share and take turns, keep cool,*** and ***be a good sport*** throughout the game playing.
- After approximately nine minutes of play, instruct the parents to prepare the children for the upcoming game swap by saying, *"Parents, tell your children that we'll be swapping games in one minute."*
- After approximately one additional minute of play (ten minutes total), instruct the parents to swap games by saying, *"Parents, it's time to swap games. Social coach the children to ask a friend to play before playing the next game."*
- After approximately nine minutes of playing the second game, instruct the parents to prepare the children for clean up by saying, *"Parents, tell your children that we'll be cleaning up in one minute."*

- After approximately one additional minute of play (ten minutes total), ***prompt*** the parents to instruct their children to clean up by saying, *"Parents, it's time to clean up. Let's social coach the children to listen and follow directions by cleaning up and then say 'bye' to their friend using names before sitting in the Listening Circle."*
- If needed, parents will ***social coach*** their child to ***listen and follow directions*** to clean up.
- Then parents will ***social coach*** their child to ***say "bye"*** to their friend ***using names***.

Final Wrap-Up (10 minutes)

- The group leader sits on the floor at the front of the room.
- The children sit on the carpet squares in a semi-circle facing the group leader, with parents sitting behind their children.

Group leader: *"Okay friends, you all did a great job playing your games and asking a friend to play. When we're asking a friend to play, do you think we should LOOK at our friend with our EYES and SMILE with our MOUTH?"* (Pause briefly to allow children to respond *"yes."*)

"That's right, friends! And when we're asking a friend to play, do you think we should say, 'Do you want to play?' and use names?" (Pause briefly to allow children to respond *"yes."*)

"That's right, friends! And if our friend says yes, do you think we should think of something fun to play by saying, 'Let's play blocks!' or 'Let's play tag!' and use names?" (Pause briefly to allow children to respond *"yes."*)

"That's right, friends! You all did such a great job asking a friend to play today that you each earned ____ (number) more stars! Let's start with ____ (child)."

Award each child the same number of stars by repeating the following with each child:

Group leader: *"Where's _____ (child)?"* (Wait until all the children are looking at the child.)

"_____ (Child), how many stars did you earn?" (Pause briefly to allow the child to respond.)

"That's right! Let's all count for _____ (child)! One, two, three... (add stars to the Star Chart as they are counted aloud)*! Everybody clap for _____ (child)!"* (All behavioral coaches clap and cheer and encourage the children to clap as well.)

"And remember you all earned those stars by asking a friend to play! Everyone did a great job, and parents you did an excellent job social coaching! Parents, remember your homework assignments this week are for you and your children to practice asking a friend to play and for you to continue practicing all the other things we've learned to be a good friend using the 4 Ps. And don't forget to have a playdate and go to your playgroups."

"Alright little friends, do you want to count our stars?" (Pause briefly to allow the children to respond.)

"Let's all count together and see how many stars we earned today! One, two, three...(count the number of stars for one child)*!"*

"You each earned ____ (total number) stars today! Round of applause for our friends!" (All behavioral coaches should clap and cheer and encourage the families to clap as well.)

"Great job, friends! Don't forget to choose your reward before you leave. See you all next week!"

Session 9 Continued

Coaching During Playdates and Asking a Friend to Play

PEERS® FOR PRESCHOOLERS: PARENT HANDOUT

Different Praising Strategies

- There are different ways you can ***praise*** and reinforce your child:
  - ***Verbal praise.***
  - ***Physical praise.***
  - ***Gestural praise.***

- ***Verbal praise*** (***praising*** with words):
  - Steps for giving ***verbal labeled praise***:
    1. Get your child's attention by:
       - Using their name.
       - Making eye contact with your child.
       - Gently touching your child's arm.
    2. Give simple ***praise***:
       - *"Good job…"*
       - *"Nice job…"*
       - *"Nice try…"*
    3. Use the PEERS® buzzwords to label the specific behavior you are ***praising***:
       - *"…showing and telling!"*
       - *"…keeping cool!"*
       - *"…sharing and giving a turn!"*
  - If you use general ***praise*** (e.g., *"Good job."*), your child may not know what behavior they are being ***praised*** for.

- ***Physical praise*** (***praise*** with physical contact):
  - Examples of ***physical praise***:
    - High-five.
    - Pound.
    - Fist bump.
    - Hug.
    - Pat on the back.

- You may combine ***physical praise*** with ***verbal praise.***
- ***Physical praise*** is useful when you cannot speak to your child (e.g., silence is required).

- ***Gestural praise*** (***praise*** with gestures):
  - Examples of ***gestural praise***:
    - Smiling.
    - Thumbs up.
    - Clapping.
  - You may combine ***gestural praise*** with ***verbal praise*** and/or ***physical praise***.
  - ***Gestural praise*** is useful when you cannot speak to your child (e.g., you are across a room).

- How you ***praise*** or reinforce your child will vary depending on:
  - Your child's preferences:
    - If your child is uncomfortable with physical touch, you may want to avoid ***physical praise***.
  - The setting:
    - The situation or place where the ***social coaching*** is occurring may warrant certain types of ***praise*** (home, school, ***playdate***, ***playgroup***, in the community, etc.).
    - You may need to use more ***gestural praise*** (e.g., smiling or giving a thumbs up across the room) during a ***playgroup***.

- Try to ***praise*** or reinforce your child as soon as they demonstrate the appropriate skill(s) or behavior(s).

- ***Praising*** appropriate use of skills will likely strengthen the value of the ***praise*** and reinforcement.

- When ***social coaching*** new skills or behaviors, ***praise*** and reinforce your child frequently.

- ***Praise*** your child's ATTEMPTS to use the social skills.
  - This will likely help your child learn the new skill or behavior faster.
  - This will help keep your child's motivation high and frustration low.

- If your child uses a skill spontaneously (e.g., without ***prompting*** or ***social coaching*** from you) or upon being ***prompted***:
  - ***Praise*** and reinforce both spontaneous and ***prompted*** occurrences.
  - Provide EXTRA ***praise*** and reinforcement for spontaneous occurrences.

- As your child improves in their social skills, you can begin gradually fading out your ***praise*** and reinforcement (i.e., provide less ***praising***).
  - At that point, it is likely the social interactions with their peers are becoming more intrinsically motivating for your child.
  - If your child starts to use the social skill(s) less over time, you may need to reintroduce more frequent ***praise***.

Different Prompting Strategies When Social Coaching

- **Make sure to have your child's attention BEFORE *prompting*.**
  - This will help avoid a pattern of interaction where your attempts to ***social coach*** or ***prompt*** go unnoticed or even ignored by your child.
    - You do not want to indirectly reinforce nonresponsive behavior.
  - Having your child's attention before ***prompting*** will help you be consistent and contingent with your ***prompting***.
  - You can gain your child's attention by:
    - Using their name before ***prompting***.
    - A light touch on the arm before ***prompting***.
    - Ask them if you have their attention before ***prompting***.
    - Request their attention before ***prompting***.

- **Use the PEERS® for Preschoolers buzzwords to *prompt* your child.**
  - Buzzwords are short, targeted phrases that come directly from the PEERS® for Preschoolers lessons.
  - The use of short buzzwords and buzzphrases will minimize the stimulus overload that too many words can create.
  - Using buzzwords across settings will help you and other caregivers to be consistent in your ***social coaching***, which is better for learning.
    - Consider sharing the *Parent Handouts* with your child's teachers and caregivers so they can also use the buzzwords when ***prompting*** and providing other forms of ***social coaching***.
  - The use of buzzwords when ***prompting*** will make it more likely that your child will:
    - Understand your ***social coaching***.
    - Pay attention to your ***social coaching***.
    - Respond appropriately to your ***prompts***.

- **Consider which type of *prompting* is the most effective and appropriate for your child according to the specific skill and situation.**
  - Types of ***prompting*** (from most to least intrusive):
    - ***Physical prompts*** ("hand over hand"):
      - ***Physical prompts*** involve providing physical assistance to your child in using a specific skill.
        - Example: Physically guiding your child's hand to ***share*** a toy with their friend.
    - ***Verbal prompts***:
      - ***Verbal prompts*** involve providing verbal instruction for your child to use a specific skill by:
        - Making a request:
          - Example: *"Remember to share and give a turn."*
        - Asking a question:
          - Example: "*Your friend wants a turn, what should we do?*"
    - ***Gestural prompts***:
      - ***Gestural prompts*** involve providing some type of gesture as a "sign" for your child to use the specific skill.

- Example: Pointing to a toy and then to a ***playmate*** to ***prompt*** your child to ***share and give a turn*** to their friend.
- Example: Looking at your child expectantly and raising your eyebrows and shoulders to ***prompt*** your child to ***share and give a turn*** in response to their friend ***asking for a turn***.

- **The frequency of *prompting* will be determined by the environment and how familiar your child is with the skill.**
  - You may need to provide more ***prompting*** when ***social coaching*** on emerging skills.
    - As your child improves in the skill, your ***social coaching*** will change by:
      - Presenting fewer ***prompts***.
      - Increasing the time before presenting ***prompts.***
      - Increasing the time between ***prompts***.
      - Using less intrusive ***prompts*** (e.g., ***physical prompts***).
  - During ***playdates***, monitor ***social coaching*** to avoid significantly disrupting the natural flow of children's play and social interaction.
    - Limit the frequency of ***prompts***.
    - Limit the rate of ***prompting*** (this will depend on the child, their ***playmate***, the activity, and the skill).
  - Remember, the goal is to eventually fade out ***prompting*** altogether.

Snapshot of the Lesson: Asking a Friend to Play

The objective of this lesson is to teach children how to ***ask a friend to play.*** Steps for ***asking a friend to play*** include:

1. ***Look at your friends with your eyes*** (point to your eyes).
2. ***Smile with your mouth*** (point to your mouth and smile).
3. ***Say, "Do you want to play?" while using names***.
4. If your friend says yes, ***think of something fun to play***.
5. ***Say, "Let's play _____ (activity/game)!"*** **while** ***using names***.

Homework Assignments

1. **Playdates.**
   - Schedule and have a ***playdate*** with a ***playmate***.
   - Prepare for the ***playdate*** using the ***5 Ws***.
     - ***WHO: Playdates*** should be one-on-one.
     - ***WHAT: Playdates*** should be activity-based.
     - ***WHERE:*** Schedule initial ***playdates*** to take place in your home or somewhere you can provide ***social coaching***.

- *WHEN:* Try to keep initial *playdates* to no more than 1–1.5 hours.
- *HOW:* Coordinate how the children will get to and from the *playdate*.

- Do a final practice with your child of the games and activities that will be available during the *playdate*.
- Gather all the games and activity materials for the *playdate* in one area that is VISIBLE and easily accessible to YOU but not the children.
- Provide *social coaching* during the *playdate* and assess if this is a good *playmate* for your child.

2. **Practice asking a friend to play.**
   - Practice having your child *ask a friend to play* this week during preferred and highly motivating activities while providing *social coaching* using the *4 Ps*.
     - *Priming:* Review the rules for *asking a friend to play* with your child BEFORE PRACTICING.
     - *Prompting:* Remind your child IN THE MOMENT to *ask a friend to play* whenever the opportunities present.
     - *Praising: Praise* your child using the buzzwords whenever they *ask a friend to play* CORRECTLY.
     - *Providing corrective feedback: Provide corrective feedback* in the form of a *praise sandwich* whenever your child ATTEMPTS to *ask a friend to play*.
   - Please send us a 30–60-second video of *social coaching* for *asking a friend to play* with your child to be viewed during homework review.
     - Please include:
       - Skills your child did well.
       - Skills you would like to work on with your child.

3. **Provide social coaching on previously learned skills.**
   - Continue providing *social coaching* to your child throughout the week using the *4 Ps.*
   - Previous skills include:
     - *Listening and following directions.*
     - *Meeting and greeting friends.*
     - *Sharing and giving a turn.*
     - *Asking for a turn.*
     - *Keeping cool.*
     - *Being a good sport.*
     - *Showing and telling.*
     - *Don't be bossy.*

4. **Bring a turn-taking game.**
   - Bring a turn-taking game that your child enjoys playing and can be played with the other children.

Session 9 Continued

Asking a Friend to Play

PEERS® FOR PRESCHOOLERS: PARENT COACHED PLAY CARD

Snapshot of the Lesson: Asking a Friend to Play

1. ***Look at your friends with your eyes*** (point to your eyes).
2. ***Smile with your mouth*** (point to your mouth and smile).
3. ***Say, "Do you want to play?" while using names.***
4. If your friend says yes, ***think of something fun to play.***
5. ***Say, "Let's play _____ (activity/game)!"*** **while** ***using names.***

Priming BEFORE Game Playing

- Example: *"Remember to ask to play by looking at your friend with your* (point to your eyes to prompt the child to say *"eyes"*)*...EYES and smile with your* (point to your mouth to prompt the child to say *"mouth"*)*...MOUTH when you say, 'Do you want to play?' If your friend says 'yes,' then think of something fun to play. And don't forget to use* (pause briefly to prompt the child to say *"names"*)*...NAMES."*

Prompting IN THE MOMENT

- Example: *"Remember to ask your friend to play."*
- Example: *"Remember to think of something fun to play."*
- Example: *"What should you do if your friend says yes?"*

Praising for CORRECT Use of Skills

- Example: *"Nice job asking your friend to play!"*
- Example: *"Great job saying, 'Do you want to play with me?'"*
- Example: *"Good job thinking of something fun to play!"*

Providing Corrective Feedback for ATTEMPTS Using a Praise Sandwich

- Example: *"Good job asking a friend to play. Remember to use names next time, but nice try!"*
- Example: *"Nice try asking a friend to play! Don't forget to say, 'Do you want to play with me?' but good job!"*

- Example: *"Nice try asking a friend to play! Don't forget to think of something fun to play next time, but great job!"*

- Continue to provide ***social coaching*** on previously learned skills:
  - ***Listening and following directions.***
  - ***Meeting and greeting friends.***
  - ***Sharing and giving a turn.***
  - ***Asking for a turn.***
  - ***Keeping cool.***
  - ***Being a good sport.***
  - ***Showing and telling.***
  - ***Don't be bossy.***

Session 9 Continued

Coaching During Playdates and Asking a Friend to Play

PEERS® FOR PRESCHOOLERS: PARENT HOMEWORK WORKSHEET

Child's Name:	Parent's Name:		Date:	
HOMEWORK ASSIGNMENTS	PRIMING (REVIEWING RULES BEFORE PRACTICE)	PROMPTING (IN THE MOMENT)	PRAISING (USING BUZZWORDS)	PROVIDING CORRECTIVE FEEDBACK (USING A PRAISE SANDWICH)
Asking a friend to play				
Practice previous skills: • **Don't be bossy** • **Show and tell during play** • **Being a good sport** • **Keeping cool** • **Asking for a turn** • **Sharing and giving turns** • **Meeting and greeting friends** • **Listening and following directions**				

Child's Name:	Parent's Name:		Date:	
HOMEWORK ASSIGNMENTS	PRIMING (REVIEWING RULES BEFORE PRACTICE)	PROMPTING (IN THE MOMENT)	PRAISING (USING BUZZWORDS)	PROVIDING CORRECTIVE FEEDBACK (USING A PRAISE SANDWICH)
Playdate: • **Plan a playdate using the 5 Ws** • **Prime your child before the playdate** • **Provide social coaching during the playdate using the 4 Ps**				
Bring a turn-taking game	Did you bring a turn-taking game? YES or NO (Circle)		Which game did you bring?	

Please fill out this worksheet by describing what you did to complete the homework assignments. Worksheets will be collected during Homework Review at the next session of PEERS® for Preschoolers.

Session 10

Joining a Game

PARENT SESSION THERAPIST GUIDE

Parent Session Agenda

- Homework Review (40 minutes).
- Didactic Lessons (20 minutes).
- Parent Coached Play (20 minutes).
- Final Wrap-Up (10 minutes).

Materials Needed

- Conference room with a large table and enough chairs for the parent group leader and all parents to sit comfortably around the table.
  - Avoid sitting in a circle without a table as this creates the atmosphere of group therapy.
- Name tags for parents and treatment team.
- *Parent Handouts* (for the current week and the previous week).
- *Parent Homework Worksheets* (for the current week and the previous week).
- *Parent Coached Play Cards* (for the current week and the previous week).
- *Attendance and Homework Compliance Sheets* for parent group leader.
- Pens for note taking (consider having extra pens for parents who need them).

Homework Review (40 Minutes)

1. **Playdates.**
   - Have parents report on the ***playdate*** and confirm that they planned using the ***5 Ws.***
   - Review what parents did to ***social coach*** their child BEFORE, DURING, and AFTER the ***playdate***.
   - Identify what skills their child did well and what skills they need to work on.
     - Confirm that parents ***praised*** skills that were done well and provided ***priming, prompting,*** and/or ***corrective feedback*** for emerging skills.
   - Have parents assess if this is a good ***playmate*** for their child.
   - Have parents identify who their child might have a ***playdate*** with in the coming week (does not have to be a different ***playmate***).

2. **Practice asking a friend to play.**
   - Review the 30–60-second video of ***social coaching*** for ***asking a friend to play*** for each family. (For larger groups, you may need to review video recordings in two smaller groups with two different parent group leaders).

DOI: 10.4324/9781003502968-11

- Have parents identify:
  - Skills their child did well.
  - Skills they would like to work on with their child.
- Provide ***social coaching*** tips as appropriate for each family.

- If parents did not send a video of ***social coaching***, confirm the following:
  - Parents practiced having their child ***ask a friend to play*** during preferred and highly motivating activities while providing ***social coaching*** using the ***4 Ps.***
    - ***Priming:*** Reviewed the rules for ***asking a friend to play*** with their child BEFORE PRACTICING.
    - ***Prompting:*** Reminded their child IN THE MOMENT to ***ask a friend to play*** whenever the opportunity presented.
    - ***Praising: Praised*** their child using the buzzwords whenever they ***asked a friend to play*** CORRECTLY.
    - ***Providing corrective feedback***: ***Provided corrective feedback*** in the form of a ***praise sandwich*** whenever their child ATTEMPTED to ***ask a friend to play***.

3. **Provide social coaching on previously learned skills.**
   - Confirm parents continued to provide ***social coaching*** to their child throughout the week using the ***4 Ps*** for previously learned skills:
     - ***Listening and following directions.***
     - ***Meeting and greeting friends.***
     - ***Sharing and giving a turn.***
     - ***Asking for a turn.***
     - ***Keeping cool.***
     - ***Being a good sport.***
     - ***Showing and telling.***
     - ***Don't be bossy.***

4. **Bring a turn-taking game.**
   - Confirm the following:
     - Brought a turn-taking game that their child enjoys playing and can be played with the other children. (To avoid distractions, these games should be left with the parents until *Parent Coached Play*.)

Didactic Lessons (20 Minutes)

PEERS® Neuroaffirming Pledge:

- We value neurodiversity, acceptance, and authenticity.
- We honor the diverse ways people experience the world.
- We respect each person's unique perspectives and communication styles.
- We recognize there is no one right way to connect with others.
- If using the strategies taught in PEERS® feels like camouflaging or masking and/or they don't align with your goals or the goals of your family, then you do not have to use them.
- Learning and using the skills taught in PEERS® is a PERSONAL CHOICE.

Didactic Lesson: Joining a Game

- Distribute *Parent Handouts*.
  - Sections in **bold print** come directly from the *Parent Handout*.

  - Terms that are ***bold and italicized*** are buzzwords and represent important concepts from the didactic lesson.
- Explain, *"Last week in the child lesson we talked about how to initiate play interactions by asking a friend to play. Today we're going to review some social coaching strategies that relate to this week's child didactic lesson on joining a game. Joining game playing is a great way for your children to make new friends and to enhance existing friendships or acquaintances. Before we go over the social coaching strategies you can use to support your child's attempts to join games, we should begin with going over the child didactic lesson to give you some context."*

Snapshot of the Lesson: Joining a Game

The objective of this lesson is to teach children how to *join a game.* Steps for *joining a game* include:

1. ***Watch the game* (point to your eyes).**
2. ***Know the rules* (point to your head).**
3. ***Move closer* (demonstrate moving closer with your body).**
4. ***Look at your friends with your eyes* (point to your eyes).**
5. ***Smile with your mouth* (point to your mouth and smile).**
6. **Say, "Can I play?" using names.**
   - **If your friends say yes, *join the game.***
   - **If your friends say no, *keep cool* and *find something else to do.***

Parent Social Coaching Strategies for Joining a Game

Explain, *"So now that we know the steps for joining a game, we need to talk about how you can provide social coaching to your child when they attempt to join games with their peers."*

- **Create opportunities for your child to *join games* while you are present.**
  - ***Joining games* with *playmates* often occurs in settings like school or daycare, outside the presence of parents.**
  - **Create opportunities for your child to practice *joining a game* where you can *social coach* using the *4 Ps.***
    - **Example: Practicing at home with siblings or other family members.**
    - **Example: Visiting a local playground where your child can *join games* with other children while you are present.**
  - **Practicing *joining a game* with a parent present to provide *social coaching* will:**
    - **Enhance your child's mastery of the skills.**
    - **Make it more likely they will use the skills appropriately when parents are not present.**

- **Identify opportunities during your child's daily routine to practice *joining a game* with familiar people in familiar places.**

- It may be easier for you to *social coach* your child when *joining a game* if the practice is part of your normal routine.
    - Example: Practice at school/daycare drop-off or pick-up when you are present.
    - Example: Practice at *playgroups* during unstructured time when you are present.
- Using your child's daily routine to practice *joining games* with familiar people in familiar places will:
    - Decrease your child's anxiety when practicing.
    - Increase their comfort in following the steps.
    - Make it more likely that others will accept your child's attempts to join.

- Remember to *prime* your child before the practice by going over the rules for *joining a game.*
  - The best time to *prime* your child is moments (not minutes or hours) before attempting to *join a game.*
  - Be sure to use the buzzwords when going over the steps.
  - Encourage your child to help you generate the steps.
    - Example: Say *"Look at your friends with your…* (point to your eyes)" and wait for your child to say "eyes."
    - Example: Say, *"Smile with your…* (point to your mouth and smile)" and allow your child to say "mouth."
  - *Praise* your child when they remember the steps for *joining a game.*

- *Prompt* your child to follow the steps by asking them questions about the game they are attempting to join.
  - Example: *"Do you know what they're playing?"*
    - Make sure they know the game before attempting to join.
    - Joining an unfamiliar game will slow down the play and may frustrate the players.
  - Example: *"Do you know the rules?"*
    - Have them explain the rules before joining.
    - Children sometimes change the rules to familiar games, so your child may need to watch for a while before understanding the rules.
    - Consider helping your child understand the rules by watching together and pointing out what you observe about the game playing.
  - Example: *"Who could you ask to join the game?"*
    - Children are more likely to allow familiar *playmates* to join play (if they don't have a bad reputation with the group).
    - When possible, helping your child identify someone they know may increase their chances of being accepted.

- *Prompt* your child to wait for a pause in the game before joining when relevant.
  - As children get older, their social interactions become more sophisticated, including the timing of entering play.
  - The rules for entering play will eventually include the added step of waiting for a pause in the game before joining.

- Younger children will often interrupt game playing when attempting to *join a game*, which may not be seen as intrusive at earlier stages of development.
- Parents can help children judge when the best time is to join.
- Typically, the ideal time to *join a game* is when there is a pause in the activities (e.g., someone just scored, the ball went out of bounds, the players are figuring out the rules).
- Parents should be prepared to add this step to your *social coaching* as your children mature.

- *Prompt* your child to use their *playmate's* name when *joining a game.*
  - *Using names* when *joining games* will:
    - Get the *playmate's* attention.
    - Demonstrate that your child already knows the player(s).
    - May create a natural pause by directing the attention to your child.

- If your child is unfamiliar with the players, *prompt* them to ask the leader if they can *join the game.*
  - While observing the group, you may recognize that one or two players appear to be more dominant in the game playing.
    - These may be the kids who are calling the plays and enforcing the rules.
  - *Prompting* your child to ask the leader of the game if they can join may make it more likely that they will be accepted by the whole group.
  - When relevant, *prompting* your child to ask the player in possession of the ball if they can *join the game* may increase their chance of being accepted because:
    - The person with the ball is in control at that moment and in a position of leadership.
    - Asking the person who is holding the ball may create a natural pause in the game.

- If your child does not know the game or the rules of the game:
  - They should NOT attempt to *join the game* at that moment.
    - It may be challenging for your child to meaningfully participate in the game.
    - They may be less likely to be accepted by their *playmates* during the game.
    - It may be overwhelming and frustrating for your child to attempt to learn the rules of the game while simultaneously attempting to socialize with their peers.
  - Parents may *social coach* in the moment by teaching your child the rules of the game if they are simple.
    - Help your child to become familiar with the rules of the game BEFORE *joining the game* to increase the likelihood that your child will experience positive peer interactions.
    - Model for your child how to figure out the rules of the game so they may be more likely to use those developing skills in the future.
    - Make sure that you are not targeting too many new behaviors or skills at once.
    - Keep in mind that the rules of games vary by playground, school, park, etc.

- If the rules of the game cannot be easily taught in the moment:
  - *Social coach* your child to *keep cool* and *find something else to do.*
  - Redirect your child to other *playmates* when possible.

- **Have your child wait until the children play a game familiar to your child.**
- **Parents should *social coach* by providing practice opportunities at home during the week to teach and familiarize your child with the rules of the game.**
- **Preview the game with your child BEFORE they attempt to *join the game* again with their *playmates.***

- **If the *playmates* do not allow your child to *join the game*:**
  - ***Social coach* your child to *keep cool* and *find something else to do.***
  - **Redirect your child to other *playmates* when possible.**
  - ***Praise* your child for their efforts to *join the game.***
  - **Normalize the fact that we don't get to join every game (the same is true for parents).**

- **Create practice opportunities to accept being turned down when attempting to *join a game.***
  - **When practicing *joining a game* with your child during the week, parents should say "no" periodically (e.g., *"Next time"* or *"Maybe later"*) and have your child practice *keeping cool* and *finding something else to do.***
    - ***Prompt* your child BEFORE by saying, *"Okay, let's practice keeping cool if I say no. Remember to keep cool and find something else to do."***

Parent Coached Play

- Distribute the *Parent Coached Play Cards.*
- Review the examples of the ***4 Ps*** provided on the *Parent Coached Play Card.*
- Remind parents that in a few moments we will be joining the children for *Parent Coached Play* in the context of mock dyadic ***playdates***.
- Parents should keep the *Parent Coached Play Card* in front of them during the dyadic ***playdate*** for recommendations on how to ***social coach*** children on ***joining a game***.

Homework Assignments

(Briefly review the homework assignments and troubleshoot any potential problems with parents.)

1. **Playdates.**
   - **Schedule and have a *playdate* with a *playmate.***
   - **Prepare for the *playdate* using the *5 Ws.***
     - ***WHO: Playdates* should be one-on-one.**
     - ***WHAT: Playdates* should be activity-based.**
     - ***WHERE:* Schedule initial *playdates* to take place in your home or somewhere you can provide *social coaching.***
     - ***WHEN:* Try to keep initial *playdates* to no more than 1–1.5 hours.**
     - ***HOW:* Coordinate how the children will get to and from the *playdate.***
   - **Do a final practice with your child of the games and activities that will be available during the *playdate.***

- **Gather all the games and activity materials for the *playdate* in one area that is VISIBLE and easily accessible to YOU but not the children.**
- **Provide *social coaching* during the *playdate* and assess if this is a good *playmate* for your child.**

2. **Practice joining a game.**
    - **Practice having your child *join a game* this week during preferred and highly motivating activities while providing *social coaching* using the *4 Ps*.**
        - ***Priming:* Review the rules for *joining a game* with your child BEFORE PRACTICING.**
        - ***Prompting:* Remind your child IN THE MOMENT to *join a game* whenever the opportunities present.**
        - ***Praising: Praise* your child using the buzzwords whenever they *join a game* CORRECTLY.**
        - ***Providing corrective feedback: Provide corrective feedback* in the form of a *praise sandwich* whenever your child ATTEMPTS to *join a game*.**
    - **Please send us a 30–60-second video of *social coaching* your child to *join a game* to be viewed during homework review.**
        - **Please include:**
            - **Skills your child did well.**
            - **Skills you would like to work on with your child.**

3. **Provide social coaching on previously learned skills.**
    - **Continue providing *social coaching* to your child throughout the week using the *4 Ps*.**
    - **Previous skills include:**
        - ***Listening and following directions.***
        - ***Meeting and greeting friends.***
        - ***Sharing and giving a turn.***
        - ***Asking for a turn.***
        - ***Keeping cool.***
        - ***Being a good sport.***
        - ***Showing and telling.***
        - ***Don't be bossy.***
        - ***Asking a friend to play.***

4. **Bring a turn-taking game.**
    - **Bring a turn-taking game that your child enjoys playing and can be played with the other children.**

Session 10 Continued

Joining a Game

CHILD SESSION THERAPIST GUIDE

Child Session Agenda

- Didactic Lesson: *Joining a Game* (20 minutes).
- Group Behavioral Rehearsal Activity 1: *What Time Is It, Friend?* (15 minutes).
- Break Time (10 minutes).
- Group Behavioral Rehearsal Activity 2: *Ring Around the Rosie* (15 minutes).
- Parent Coached Play: *Dyadic Playdates* (20 minutes).
- Final Wrap-Up (10 minutes).

Snapshot of the Lesson: Joining a Game

The objective of this lesson is to teach children how to ***join a game***. Steps for ***joining a game*** include:

1. ***Watch the game*** (point to your eyes).
2. ***Know the rules*** (point to your head).
3. ***Move closer*** (demonstrate moving closer with your body).
4. ***Look at your friends with your eyes*** (point to your eyes).
5. ***Smile with your mouth*** (point to your mouth and smile).
6. ***Say, "Can I play?" using names***.
   - If your friends say yes, ***join the game***.
   - If your friends say no, ***keep cool*** and ***find something else to do.***

Materials Needed

- Pig puppet.
- Horse puppet.
- Mouse puppet.
- Hacky sack.
- Carpet squares or chairs.
- "Making Friends Helper" badge.
- Star chart with names of children.
- Marker for star chart.
- Name tags for families and treatment team.
- Prize bins with prizes.

Preparing for the Lesson

- Use the script below with the group leader using a pig puppet to play the part of "Penny Pig."
- A behavioral coach uses a horse puppet to play the part of "Harry Horse."
- A second behavioral coach uses a mouse puppet to play the part of "Marty Mouse."
- A third behavioral coach assists with the behavioral rehearsal and provides encouragement and feedback to the group.
- A child is chosen at the beginning of the lesson as the "Making Friends Helper."
  - The "Making Friends Helper" wears a special badge and is the first child to practice the skill.
- The group leader and the behavioral coaches sit on the floor at the front of the room.
- A special-colored carpet square (e.g., red) is placed at the front of the room next to the child group leader to be used as the "Good Friend Square."
- For the children, additional carpet squares of the same color (e.g., green) are placed in a semi-circle facing the child group leader and the "Good Friend Square."
- Note: If carpet squares are unavailable, the children and behavioral coach may sit on chairs.
- The material in *italics* should be read by the indicated person.
- The material in ***bold and italics*** represents buzzwords and should be emphasized when read.
- The material in CAPITAL LETTERS within the script should be given extra emphasis while the group is encouraged to say the words in unison.

Behavioral Coaching Techniques

Behavioral coaches should use the following coaching techniques described below throughout the lesson and the behavioral rehearsal activities. (Note: ***priming*** occurs during the introduction to the activity.)

- ***Prompting:***
  - Use the buzzwords to ***prompt*** the children to ***join a game***.
    - Example: *"Remember to join the game."*
    - Example: *"Don't forget to join the game if your friends say yes."*
    - Example: *"Remember to move closer when you ask to play."*
- ***Praising:***
  - Reinforce ***joining a game*** by ***praising*** the children.
    - Example: *"Great job joining the game!"*
    - Example: *"Great job joining the game by saying, 'Can I play?'"*
    - Example: *"Good job watching the game first!"*
- ***Providing corrective feedback using a praise sandwich:***
  - Reinforce ATTEMPTS to ***join a game*** by ***praising*** the children and identifying what could be done differently next time.
    - Example: *"Good job joining the game. Next time remember to watch the game first, but nice try!"*
    - Example: *"Nice try joining the game. Don't forget to keep cool if your friends say no, but good job!"*
    - Example: *"Good job joining the game. Remember to use names next time, but great job!"*

- Continue to provide ***social coaching*** on previously learned skills:
  - ***Listening and following directions.***
  - ***Meeting and greeting friends.***
  - ***Sharing and giving a turn.***
  - ***Asking for a turn.***
  - ***Keeping cool.***
  - ***Being a good sport.***
  - ***Showing and telling.***
  - ***Don't be bossy.***
  - ***Asking a friend to play.***

Didactic Lesson: Joining a Game

Have the children sit in a semi-circle on the carpet squares facing the group leader.

Penny Pig: (Sit at the front of the room and choose a Making Friends Helper.) *"Who wants to be our Making Friends Helper?"*

(Choose from among the children raising their hands and place the "Making Friends Helper" badge on the child. The child stays in their seat for now.)

"Hi friends! I'm Penny Pig. Oink, oink! Today we're going to practice joining a game. Joining a game is a great way to be nice to our friends!"

"Who should we join a game with? We should join a game with our FRIENDS, TEACHERS, MOMMIES, DADDIES, BROTHERS, AND SISTERS."

"When should we join a game? We should join a game when our friends are playing a game and we want to play, too."

"How should we join a game? First, we should join a game by watching the game (point to your eyes and then to Penny Pig's eyes) *and knowing the rules* (point to your head)*."*

"Then, if we know the rules, we should move closer (move your body closer), *look at our friend with our* (point to your eyes and then to Harry Horse's eyes)*...EYES, smile with our* (point to your mouth and smile)*...MOUTH,* and *say, 'Can I play?' And don't forget to use* (pause briefly to prompt the children to say *"names"*)*...NAMES!"*

"If our friends say yes, join the game. If our friends say no, keep cool and find something else to do."

"Remember, joining a game is a nice way to be a good friend! Oink, oink!"

Role Play: Joining a Game

Marty Mouse:	(Turn to look at Harry Horse and smile.) *"Hey Harry Horse, let's play Hot Potato! Squeak, squeak!"*
Harry Horse:	(Turn to look at Marty Mouse and smile.) *"Okay, Marty Mouse! Neigh, neigh!"*
Penny Pig, Marty Mouse, and Harry Horse:	(Play Hot Potato with the hacky sack while ***showing and telling*** and ***being good sports***. Penny Pig is watching nearby.)
Penny Pig:	(Turn to look at the group of children and smile.) *"Hey friends! Marty Mouse and Harry Horse are having so much fun playing together! I wish I could play too. Hmmm...."* (Look confused, scratch your head, and pause.) *"Hey friends, I know! Do you think I should join the game?"* (Nod your head yes and encourage the children to say *"yes."*) *"That's a great idea! Oink, oink! Let's do it!"* *"First I'll watch the game* (point to your eyes and then to Penny Pig's eyes) *and make sure I know the rules* (tap your head with your index finger)*."* (Turn to watch Marty Mouse and Harry Horse playing Hot Potato. Tap your head with your index finger to demonstrate that you are thinking about the rules of the game.) (Turn to look at the group of children and smile.) *"Hey friends, Marty Mouse and Harry Horse are playing Hot Potato! I know the rules! Now should I move closer* (move your body closer) *and say, 'Marty Mouse and Harry Horse, can I play?'"* (Nod your head yes and encourage the children to say *"yes."*) *"That's a great idea! Oink, oink! Let's do it!"* (Move closer, look at Marty Mouse and Harry Horse and smile.) *"Marty Mouse and Harry Horse, can I play?"*
Marty Mouse and Harry Horse:	(Turn to look at Penny Pig and smile.) *"Okay, Penny Pig!"*
Penny Pig:	*"Thanks, Marty Mouse and Harry Horse! Oink, oink!"*
Penny Pig, Marty Mouse, and Harry Horse:	(Penny Pig joins Marty Mouse and Harry Horse. Play Hot Potato while ***showing and telling*** and ***being good sports*** for a few moments.)

Penny Pig: (Turn to look at the group of children and smile.) *"Hey friends, did I do a good job of joining the game?"* (Nod your head yes and encourage the children to say *"yes."*)

"That's right! Oink, oink!"

Penny Pig, Marty Mouse, and Harry Horse: (Say *"good job," give a "pig high-five," "mouse high-five,"* and *"horse high-five,"* clap, cheer, and encourage the children to clap as well. Marty Mouse and Harry Horse sit on the other side of the Good Friend Square (i.e., the Good Friend Square is between Penny Pig on one side and Marty Mouse and Harry Horse on the other side). Penny Pig ***social coaches*** the children as needed while they practice ***joining a game*** with Marty Mouse and Harry Horse.)

Marty Mouse: (Hold onto the hacky sack.)

Penny Pig: *"Now let's see _____ (behavioral coach) try! _____ (Behavioral coach), please come sit on the Good Friend Square."*

Behavioral coach: (Sit on the Good Friend Square.)

Penny Pig: *"_____ (Behavioral coach), can you show us how to join a game with Marty Mouse and Harry Horse?"*

Behavioral coach: *"Okay, Penny Pig."*

Penny Pig: (Turn to look at the group of children.) *"Remember to first watch the game* (point to your eyes) *and make sure you know the rules* (tap your head with your index finger). *If you know the rules, then remember to move closer* (move your body closer), *look at your friends with your* (point to your eyes to prompt the children to say *"eyes"*)*...EYES and smile with your* (point to your mouth to prompt the children to say *"mouth"*)*...MOUTH when you say, 'Marty Mouse and Harry Horse, can I play?' And don't forget to use* (pause briefly to prompt the children to say *"names"*)*...NAMES."*

Marty Mouse: (Turn to look at Harry Horse and smile.) *"Hey Harry Horse, let's play Hot Potato! Squeak, squeak!"*

Harry Horse: (Turn to look at Marty Mouse and smile.) *"Okay, Marty Mouse! Neigh, neigh!"*

Marty Mouse and Harry Horse: (Play Hot Potato with the hacky sack while ***showing and telling*** and ***being good sports***.)

Penny Pig:	(Turn to look at the behavioral coach.) *"First watch the game* (point to your eyes)*."*
Behavioral coach:	(Turn to look at Marty Mouse and Harry Horse playing Hot Potato.)
Penny Pig:	(Look at the behavioral coach.) *"Do you know the rules* (tap your head with your index finger)*?"*
Behavioral coach:	(Turn to look at Penny Pig and smile.) *"Yes! They're playing Hot Potato. You pass the hot potato back and forth as fast as you can, but you can't drop it!"*
Penny Pig:	(Look at the behavioral coach.) *"Great job! Now join the game by moving closer* (move your body closer), *and saying, 'Marty Mouse and Harry Horse, can I play?'"*
Behavioral coach:	(Move closer, look at Marty Mouse and Harry Horse and smile.) *"Marty Mouse and Harry Horse, can I play?"*
Marty Mouse and Harry Horse:	(Turn to look at the behavioral coach and smile.) *"Okay, _____ (behavioral coach)!"*
Behavioral coach, Marty Mouse, and Harry Horse:	(The behavioral coach joins Marty Mouse and Harry Horse. Play Hot Potato while ***showing and telling*** and ***being good sports*** for a few moments.)
Penny Pig:	*"Great job joining the game, _____ (behavioral coach)! Oink, oink!"*
	(Say *"good job," give a "pig high-five," "mouse high-five,"* and *"horse high-five,"* clap, cheer, and encourage the children to clap as well. The behavioral coach should return the hacky sack to Marty Mouse and leave the Good Friend Square.)

Behavioral Rehearsal: Joining a Game

Penny Pig:	(Turn to look at the group of children and smile.) *"Okay friends! Now let's see our Making Friends Helper ____ try! ____ (Making Friends Helper), come sit on the Good Friend Square and show us how to join a game with Marty Mouse and Harry Horse."*
	(The Making Friends Helper should sit on the Good Friend Square.)
	"Remember to first watch the game (point to your eyes) *and make sure you know the rules* (tap your head with your index finger). *If you know the rules, then remember to move closer* (move your body closer), *look at your friends with your* (point to your eyes to prompt the children to say *"eyes"*)*...EYES*

and smile with your (point to your mouth to prompt the children to say *"mouth"*)*...MOUTH when you say, 'Marty Mouse and Harry Horse, can I play?' And don't forget to use* (pause briefly to prompt the children to say *"names"*)*...NAMES."*

Marty Mouse: (Turn to look at Harry Horse and smile.) *"Hey Harry Horse, let's play Hot Potato! Squeak, squeak!"*

Harry Horse: (Turn to look at Marty Mouse and smile.) "Okay, Marty Mouse! Neig*h, neigh!"*

Marty Mouse and Harry Horse: (Play Hot Potato with the hacky sack while ***showing and telling and being good sports***.)

Penny Pig: (Turn to look at the Making Friends Helper.) *"First watch the game* (point to your eyes)*."*

(If needed, ***social coach*** the Making Friends Helper to ***watch*** Marty Mouse and Harry Horse playing Hot Potato.)

(Look at the Making Friends Helper.) *"Do you know the rules* (tap your head with your index finger)*?"*

(If needed, ***social coach*** the Making Friends Helper by explaining the rules of the game.)

(Look at the Making Friends Helper.) *"Great job! Now join the game by moving closer* (move your body closer), *and saying, 'Marty Mouse and Harry Horse, can I play?'"*

(If needed, ***social coach*** the Making Friends Helper to ***move closer, look, smile,*** and ***say, "Marty Mouse and Harry Horse, can I play?"***)

Marty Mouse and Harry Horse: (Turn to look at the Making Friends Helper and smile.) *"Okay, _____ (Making Friends Helper)!"*

(The Making Friends Helper joins Marty Mouse and Harry Horse. Play Hot Potato while ***showing and telling*** and ***being good sports*** for a few moments.)

Penny Pig: *"Great job joining the game, _____ (Making Friends Helper)! Oink, oink!"*

(Say *"good job," give a "pig high-five," "mouse high-five,"* and *"horse high-five,"* clap, cheer, and encourage the children to clap as well. The Making Friends Helper should return the hacky sack to Marty Mouse.)

"Okay, Making Friends Helper, choose another friend to sit on the Good Friend Square." (If needed, ***social coach*** the Making Friends Helper to choose another child before returning to their seat.)

Repeat the following with each child:

Penny Pig: (Have each child take turns sitting on the Good Friend Square and practicing ***joining a game*** with Marty Mouse and Harry Horse.)

(Turn to look at the group of children.) *"Okay friends! Now let's see ____ (child) try! ____ (Child), come sit on the Good Friend Square and show us how to join a game with Marty Mouse and Harry Horse."*

(The child should sit on the Good Friend Square.)

"Remember to first watch the game (point to your eyes) *and make sure you know the rules* (tap your head with your index finger). *If you know the rules, then remember to move closer* (move your body closer), *look at your friends with your* (point to your eyes to prompt the children to say *"eyes"*)*...EYES and smile with your* (point to your mouth to prompt the children to say *"mouth"*)*...MOUTH when you say, 'Marty Mouse and Harry Horse, can I play?' And don't forget to use* (pause briefly to prompt the children to say *"names"*)*...NAMES."*

Marty Mouse: (Turn to look at Harry Horse and smile.) *"Hey Harry Horse, let's play Hot Potato! Squeak, squeak!"*

Harry Horse: (Turn to look at Marty Mouse and smile.) *"Okay, Marty Mouse! Neigh, neigh!"*

Marty Mouse and Harry Horse: (Play Hot Potato with the hacky sack while ***showing and telling and being good sports***.)

Penny Pig: (Turn to look at the child.) *"First watch the game* (point to your eyes)*."*

(If needed, ***social coach*** the child to ***watch*** Marty Mouse and Harry Horse playing Hot Potato.)

(Look at the child.) *"Do you know the rules* (tap your head with your index finger)*?"*

(If needed, ***social coach*** the child by explaining the rules of the game.)

(Look at the child.) *"Great job! Now join the game by moving closer* (move your body closer), *and saying, 'Marty Mouse and Harry Horse, can I play?'"*

(If needed, ***social coach*** the child to ***move closer, look, smile,*** and ***say, "Marty Mouse and Harry Horse, can I play?"***)

Marty Mouse and Harry Horse: (Turn to look at the child and smile.) *"Okay, _____ (child)!"*

Marty Mouse and Harry Horse: (The child joins Marty Mouse and Harry Horse. Play Hot Potato while ***showing and telling*** and ***being good sports*** for a few moments.)

Penny Pig: *"Great job joining the game, _____ (child)! Oink, oink!"*

(Say *"good job," give a "pig high-five," "mouse high-five,"* and *"horse high-five,"* clap, cheer, and encourage the children to clap as well. The child should return the hacky sack to Marty Mouse.)

"Okay, ____ (child), choose another friend to sit on the Good Friend Square." (If needed, ***social coach*** the child to choose another child before returning to their seat.)

Didactic Lesson Wrap-Up

Group leader: *"Well friends, you all did a great job joining a game by first watching the game* (point to your eyes) *and making sure you knew the rules* (tap your head with your index finger). *Then you moved closer* (move your body closer), *looked at your friends with your* (point to your eyes to prompt the children to say *"eyes"*)*...EYES and smiled with your* (point to your mouth to prompt the children to say *"mouth"*)*...MOUTH and said, 'Marty Mouse and Harry Horse, can I play?' And nice job using* (pause briefly to prompt the children to say *"names"*)*...NAMES!"*

"You each earned ____ (number) stars for joining a game! Let's start with ____ (child)."

Award each child the same number of stars by repeating the following with each child:

Group leader: *"Where's ____ (child)?"* (Wait until all the children are looking at the child.)

"____ (Child), how many stars did you earn?" (Pause briefly to allow the child to respond.)

"That's right! Let's all count for ____ (child)! One, two, three... (add stars to the Star Chart as they are counted aloud)*! Everybody clap for ____ (child)!"* (All behavioral coaches clap and cheer and encourage the children to clap as well.)

Session 10 Continued

What Time Is It, Friend?

BEHAVIORAL REHEARSAL ACTIVITY 1

Materials Needed

- Safety cones or masking tape.

Room Setup

- Remove or place all carpet squares to the side.
- Use the safety cones or masking tape to delineate a *"friend zone"* at one end of the room and a *"safe zone"* at the opposite end of the room.
- The group leader stands in the *friend zone* at the front of the room.
- Children and behavioral coaches stand in the *safe zone* facing the group leader.

Rules: What Time Is It, Friend?

- The group leader reads the script below to explain the rules, which are based on the popular game, *What Time Is It, Mr. Fox?*
- Pick a child to be the first *"friend."*
  - The *friend* should stand next to the group leader in the *friend zone.*
- The children and behavioral coaches are standing next to each other while holding hands in the *safe zone.*
- Pick one child from the *safe zone* to be the *"joining friend."*
  - The *joining friend* stands outside of the *safe zone* with a behavioral coach and practices ***joining a game.***
  - The behavioral coach ***social coaches*** the *joining friend* in ***joining the game.***
  - If there is a large group, you can pick two children to be *joining friends* at the same time.
- To begin the game, the children should call out in unison, *"What time is it, ____ (child)?"*
- The *friend* should respond by calling out a time (e.g., *"It's 2 o'clock"* or *"It's 4 o'clock"*).
- The children and behavioral coaches should take the specified number of steps forward (e.g., two steps or four steps) while counting aloud.
- Then briefly pause the game to allow the *joining friend* to ***join the game.***
- The behavioral coach in the *safe zone* ***social coaches*** the children to ***listen*** to the *joining friends* as they practice ***joining a game.***
- Then resume the game.
- After a few repetitions, the *friend* should say, *"It's tag time!"* and chase the children back to the *safe zone.*

- If the *friend* tags a child, then that child will be the new *friend.*
  - The *friend* cannot tag a child once a child is behind the *safe zone*.
- If the *friend* is unable to tag a child, then ask the current *friend* to choose the next *friend.*
- Repeat this cycle until all children have had at least one turn being the *friend* and *joining friend.*

Behavioral Rehearsal: What Time Is It, Friend? (15 Minutes)

The group leader explains the activity. The behavioral coaches and children sit nearby as the group leader explains the rules.

Group leader *"Hey friends, now we're going to play What Time Is It, Friend? It's like the game called What Time Is It, Mr. Fox?"*

"I'll pick the first friend to stand next to me in the friend zone. Everyone else will stand in the safe zone (point to the *safe zone*) *and hold hands. Then I'll pick one* (hold up one finger) *friend to be the joining friend. The joining friend will practice joining the game. Then all of you will ask the friend, 'What time is it?' using the friend's name."*

"If the friend says '2 o'clock' then you all take two steps forward (demonstrate taking two steps forward while counting aloud). *If the friend says '4 o'clock' then you all take four steps forward* (demonstrate taking four steps forward while counting aloud). *If the friend says, 'It's tag time!' run back to the safe zone before you're tagged. If you get tagged, then you're the new friend."*

"As we play, the joining friend will watch us. The joining friend will then join the game by first watching the game (point to your eyes) *and knowing the rules* (tap your head with your finger). *If they know the rules, they'll move closer* (move your body closer), *look at their friends with their* (point to your eyes to prompt the children to say *"eyes"*)*...EYES and smile with their* (point to your mouth to prompt the children to say *"mouth"*)*...MOUTH when they say, 'Can I play?' And don't forget to use* (pause briefly to prompt the children to say *"names"*)*...NAMES."*

"Okay, let's have _____ (behavioral coach 1) and _____ (behavioral coach 2) try first!"

Role Play: What Time Is It, Friend?

The group leader is the first *friend.* The two behavioral coaches stand on the sidelines of the play area and demonstrate how to ***join a game***. The other behavioral coaches and children stand in the *safe zone* holding hands while they play *What Time Is It, Friend?*

Group leader: *"Okay _____ (behavioral coaches 1 and 2), let's play What Time Is It, Friend? and practice joining a game. I'll be the first friend, and _____ (behavioral coach 1) will be our joining friend."*

Behavioral coach 2:	(Turn to look at behavioral coach 1.) *"Let's first watch the game and make sure you know the rules."*
Group leader:	(Turn to look at the children and smile.) *"Okay friends, let's play. Remember to ask, 'What time is it, _____ (group leader)?' And don't forget to hold hands when you step forward."*
Behavioral coaches and children:	*"What time is it, _____ (group leader)?"*
Group leader:	*"It's 2 o'clock, friends."*
Behavioral coaches and children:	(Take two steps forward while counting aloud and holding hands.) *"What time is it, _____ (group leader)?"*
Group leader:	*"It's 4 o'clock, friends."*
Behavioral coaches and children:	(Take four steps forward while counting aloud and holding hands.)
Group leader:	*"Now it's time for our joining friend to join the game. Let's see how _____ (behavioral coach 1) joins the game."*
Behavioral coach 2:	(Turn to look at behavioral coach 1.) *"Great job watching the game. Do you know the rules?"*
Behavioral coach 1:	*"Yes! They're playing 'What time is it, Friend?'"*
Behavioral coach 2:	*"Great! Now you can join the game by moving closer, looking at your friends with your eyes, smiling with your mouth, and saying, 'Friends, can I play?' If your friends say, 'yes,' then you can join the game!"*
Behavioral coach 1:	(Turn to look at the behavioral coaches and children in the *safe zone*.) *"Friends, can I play?"*
Behavioral coaches and children:	*"Okay, _____ (behavioral coach 1)!"*
Behavioral coach 1:	*"Thanks, friends!"*
Behavioral coaches 1 and 2:	(Join the behavioral coach and children in the play area.)
Group leader:	*"Great job joining the game, _____ (behavioral coach 1)! Okay friends, let's keep playing!"*
Behavioral coaches and children:	*"What time is it, _____ (group leader)?"*

Group leader:	*"It's 1 o'clock, friends."*
Behavioral coaches and children:	(Take one step forward while counting aloud and holding hands.) *"What time is it, _____ (group leader)?"*
Group leader:	*"It's tag time!"* (Chase the behavioral coaches and children back toward the *safe zone*.)
Behavioral coaches and children:	(Run toward the *safe zone* to avoid being tagged.)
Group leader:	(Return to the *friend zone* and face the children.) *"Great job playing!"*
Behavioral coach 2:	(Return to your original position outside of the *safe zone* to ***social coach*** the *joining friends*.)
Group leader:	*"Okay friends, now it's everybody's turn to practice joining the game while we play What Time Is It, Friend?*

Behavioral Rehearsal: What Time Is It, Friend?

Group leader:	*"Our next friend is _____ (child). Come stand next to me in the friend zone. And our next joining friend is _____ (child). Go stand next to _____ (behavioral coach 2). Are we ready? All together now."*
Behavioral coaches	(If needed, behavioral coaches should ***social coach*** the children in the *safe zone* to call out in unison, *"What time is it, ____ (child)?"* while holding hands.)
Group leader:	(If needed, the group leader should ***social coach*** the *friend* to respond.)
Behavioral coaches and children:	(If needed, behavioral coaches should ***social coach*** the children to take the specified number of steps forward while holding hands.)
Group leader:	*"Great job using names and following directions! Are we ready? All together now. Remember to hold hands."*
Behavioral coaches and children:	(If needed, behavioral coaches should ***social coach*** the children to call out in unison, *"What time is it, ____ (child)?"* while holding hands.)
Group leader:	*"Okay friends, now it's time for our joining friend to join the game. Let's see how they join the game."*
Behavioral coach 2:	(If needed, behavioral coach 2 should ***social coach*** the *joining friend* to ***join the game***.)
Behavioral coaches	(If needed, behavioral coaches should ***social coach*** the children to

and children: accept the *joining friend's* request to ***join the game***.)

Group leader: *"Great job joining the game! Let's keep playing!"*

Repeat the sequence above until all the children have had at least one turn being the *friend* and the *joining friend* and have had the opportunity to practice ***joining a game***.

Behavioral Rehearsal Wrap-Up

Group leader: *"Well friends, great job joining the game! Give yourselves a big round of applause!"* (All behavioral coaches clap and cheer and encourage the children to clap as well.)

"Now everyone should come sit in the Listening Circle." (Have children return to the Listening Circle to sit on their carpet squares.)

"Okay friends, you did such a great job joining the game by first watching the game (point to your eyes) *and making sure you knew the rules* (tap your head with your index finger). *Then you moved closer* (move your body closer), *looked at your friends with your* (point to your eyes to prompt the children to say *"eyes"*)...*EYES and smiled with your* (point to your mouth to prompt the children to say *"mouth"*)...*MOUTH and said, 'Can I play?' And nice job using* (pause briefly to prompt the children to say *"names"*)...*NAMES!"*

"You each earned ____ (number) more stars for joining a game! Let's start with ____ (child)."

Award each child the same number of stars by repeating the following with each child:

Group leader: *"Where's _____ (child)?"* (Wait until all the children are looking at the child.)

"_____ (Child), how many stars did you earn?" (Pause briefly to allow the child to respond.)

"That's right! Let's all count for _____ (child)! One, two, three... (add stars to the Star Chart as they are counted aloud)*! Everybody clap for _____ (child)!"* (All behavioral coaches clap and cheer and encourage the children to clap as well.)

Break Time (10 Minutes)

- The puppets may be used to lead the children to and from the bathroom during break time.
- To assist with transitions and limit unstructured time, behavioral coaches may review the lesson with the children while waiting for the remaining children to return from the bathroom.
- You may want to award stars for good behavior after returning from the bathroom.

Session 10 Continued

Ring Around the Rosie

BEHAVIORAL REHEARSAL ACTIVITY 2

Materials Needed

- None.

Room Setup

- Remove or place all carpet squares to the side.
- The group leader sits on the floor in front of the room.
- Children and behavioral coaches sit on the floor in a semi-circle facing the group leader.

Rules: Ring Around the Rosie

- The group leader reads the script below to explain the rules.
- Instruct the children and behavioral coaches to hold hands and walk in a circle as they sing the *Ring Around the Rosie* song:
  - *Ring Around the Rosie* song:
    *"Ring around the rosie,
    A pocket full of posies,
    Ashes, ashes,
    We all fall down!"*
- The children and behavioral coaches should act out the last line of the song (*"We all fall down!"*) by sitting down on the floor.
- Once the children are familiar with the game, pick a child to be the *"joining friend"* to practice ***joining the game***.
  - The *joining friend* stands next to the child group leader.
- Instruct the remaining children and behavioral coaches to resume playing the game.
- Then briefly pause the game to allow the *joining friend* to ***join the game***.
- The behavioral coaches ***social coach*** the children to ***listen*** to and accept the *joining friend* as they practice ***joining the game***.
- Then resume the game.
- New commands may be introduced in the last line of the song, *"We all ________."*
  - Examples: *"We all spin around," "We all stand still," "We all kneel down,"* etc.
- Before introducing a new command, the group leader demonstrates the new command with the children and behavioral coaches. Repeat this cycle until all children have had at least one turn being the *joining friend.*

Behavioral Rehearsal: Ring Around the Rosie (15 Minutes)

The group leader explains the activity. The behavioral coaches and children sit in a circle nearby as the group leader explains the rules.

Group leader: *"Hey friends, now we're going to play a game called 'Ring Around the Rosie.' I'll pick a joining friend to stand next to me. Everyone else will stand in a circle holding hands. Then you'll walk in a circle singing the 'Ring Around the Rosie' song. The song goes like this: 'Ring around the rosie, a pocket full of posies, ashes ashes, we all fall down!' And when we say, 'We all fall down,' we'll all sit on the floor like this* (sit on the floor).*"*

"As we play, the joining friend will watch us. The joining friend will then join the game by first watching the game (point to your eyes) *and knowing the rules* (tap your head with your finger). *When they know the rules, they'll move closer* (move your body closer), *look at their friends with their* (point to your eyes to prompt the children to say *"eyes"*)*...EYES and smile with their* (point to your mouth to prompt the children to say *"mouth"*)*...MOUTH when they say, 'Can I play?' And don't forget to use* (pause briefly to prompt the children to say *"names"*)*...NAMES."*

"Okay, let's have ____ (behavioral coach) try first!"

Role Play: Ring Around the Rosie

The group leader will lead the role play. A behavioral coach is the first *joining friend* and stands next to the group leader outside of the circle. The remaining behavioral coaches and children demonstrate how to play *Ring Around the Rosie.*

Group leader: *"Okay friends, let's play Ring Around the Rosie. ____ (Behavioral coach 1) will be our joining friend and will practice joining the game. ____ (Behavioral coach 1), let's start by watching the game and knowing the rules. Are we ready? All together now."*

Behavioral coaches and children: *"Ring around the rosie, a pocket full of posies, ashes, ashes, we all fall down!"* (Behavioral coaches and the children sit down.)

Group leader: (Turn to look at the behavioral coaches and children.) *"Let's see what ____ (behavioral coach 1) does next to join the game."*

(Turn to look at behavioral coach 1.) *"Great job watching the game ____ (behavioral coach 1). Do you know the rules?"*

Behavioral coach 1: *"Yes! They're playing 'Ring Around the Rosie'"*

Group leader: *"That's right! Now you can join the game by moving closer* (move your body closer), *looking at your friends with your eyes* (point to your eyes), *smiling with your mouth* (point to your mouth), *and saying, 'Friends, can I play?' And if your friends say, 'yes,' then you can join the game!"*

Behavioral coach 1:	(Turn to look at the behavioral coaches and children.) *"Friends, can I play?"*
Behavioral coach and children:	*"Okay, ____ (behavioral coach 1)!"*
Behavioral coach 1:	*"Thanks, friends!"* (Join the behavioral coaches and children.)
Group leader:	*"Great job joining the game, ____ (behavioral coach 1)!"*

Behavioral Rehearsal: Ring Around the Rosie

Group leader:	*"Okay friends, let's keep on playing. Our next joining friend is ____ (child). ____ (Child), come stand next to me and practice joining the game.* (Have the *joining friend* stand next to the group leader outside of the circle.) *"____ (Child), let's start by watching the game and knowing the rules. Are we ready? All together now."* (If needed, ***social coach*** the children to sing the *Ring Around the Rosie* song.) *"Okay friends, now it's time for our joining friend to join the game. Let's see how they join the game."* (If needed, the group leader should ***social coach*** the *joining friend* to ***join the game***.)
Behavioral coaches:	(If needed, behavioral coaches should ***social coach*** the children to accept the *joining friend's* request to ***join the game***.)
Group leader:	*"Great job joining the game ____ (child)! Our next joining friend is ____ (child). ____ (Child), come stand next to me and practice joining the game.* (Have the *joining friend* stand next to the group leader.) *"Okay friends, now make sure to listen and follow directions because we're not going to fall down anymore. We're going to do some other fun things! For example, if I say, 'We all spin around!' we should all spin around like this* (demonstrate spinning around). *Can you me how to spin around?* (Pause briefly to allow the children to demonstrate spinning around.) *That's right, friends!"* *"Are we ready? All together now."*
Behavioral coaches and children:	*"Ring around the rosie, a pocket full of posies, ashes, ashes, we all spin around!"*
Group leader:	(After a few moments say, "*FREEZE!* (Pause.) *And sit!*")

Table 10.1 Sample Commands

Spin around	Touch the floor	Touch our toes
Kneel down	Tap our nose	Hop on one foot
Rub our tummies	Tap our heads	Stand on our tip-toes
Stand on one foot	Touch our knees	Swim like an octopus
Hop on two feet	Fly like a bird	Slither like a snake

Group leader: Repeat the above cycle using new commands after each turn by saying, *"This time we're going ______ (action)!* (Demonstrate the action). *Can you all show me how to ______ (action)?"*

Ensure that every child has at least one turn being the *joining friend* and practicing ***joining the game***.

Behavioral Rehearsal Wrap-Up

Group leader: *"Well friends, great job joining a game! Give yourselves a big round of applause!"* (All behavioral coaches clap and cheer and encourage the children to clap as well.)

"Now everyone should come sit in the Listening Circle." (Have children return to the Listening Circle to sit on their carpet squares.)

"Okay friends, you did such a great job joining the game by first watching the game (point to your eyes) *and making sure you knew the rules* (tap your head with your index finger). *Then you moved closer* (move your body closer), *looked at your friends with your* (point to your eyes to prompt the children to say *"eyes"*)*...EYES and smiled with your* (point to your mouth to prompt the children to say *"mouth"*)*...MOUTH when you said, 'Can I play?' And nice job using* (pause briefly to prompt the children to say *"names"*)*...NAMES!"*

"You each earned ____ (number) more stars for joining a game! Let's start with ____ (child)."

Award each child the same number of stars by repeating the following with each child:

Group leader: *"Where's ____ (child)?"* (Wait until all the children are looking at the child.)

"____ (Child), how many stars did you earn?" (Pause briefly to allow the child to respond.)

"That's right! Let's all count for ____ (child)! One, two, three... (add stars to the Star Chart as they are counted aloud)*! Everybody clap for ____ (child)!"* (All behavioral coaches clap and cheer and encourage the children to clap as well.)

"Now we're going to play another game with our parents and practice joining more games!"

Session 10 Continued

Joining a Game

PARENT COACHED PLAY: DYADIC PLAYDATES

Materials Needed

- Games brought by children and parents from home.
- Turn-taking games provided by the treatment team.
- Tables and chairs or carpet squares.
- *Parent Coached Play Cards.*

Room Setup

- If available, organize tables in separate corners of the room with four to six chairs per table.
- If tables are not available, place two carpet squares in separate corners of the room to indicate where the children will sit.

Rules: Dyadic Playdates

- The group leader divides the families into groups of two families each.
  - If there are an odd number of children, pair one child with a behavioral coach who will serve as a ***playmate***. In this case, you will need an additional coach to serve as a behavioral coach for the parent.
- Assign each group to sit at a table or specific play area.
  - Children should sit next to each other.
  - Parents will act as ***social coaches*** by sitting on the other side of their child to minimize interrupting the natural flow of play between the children.
  - One behavioral coach will be assigned to each dyad to provide ***social coaching*** suggestions and feedback to parents.
- Children will take turns playing the games brought from home or games provided by the treatment team.
- Each child will have ten minutes to play their chosen game with their ***playmate*** (including the other child ***joining a game***) and will then switch games.
- Parents will choose which child's game will be played first.
- Families will take turns practicing ***joining a game***.
  - One family will sit down at the play area.
  - The remaining family will stand near the play area.
    - The standing child will be the ***joining friend*** and will practice ***joining a game***.
- Parents of the child in the play area will help set up the activity.

- As the child in the play area is setting up the activity, the parent of the ***joining child*** will ***social coach*** their child to ***join the game***.
- The parents of the child setting up the game will ***social coach*** their child to accept their friend's request to ***join the game***.
  - The children should NOT be allowed to reject the child from ***joining the game***.
- After approximately seven minutes of play, instruct the parents to prepare the children for the upcoming game swap (this allows two minutes for ***joining the game***).
- After approximately one additional minute of play (eight minutes of game playing in total), instruct the parents to swap games.
- Repeat the cycle with the second game, having the other child practice ***joining the game***.

Behavioral Coaching: Dyadic Playdates

Behavioral coaches will ***social coach*** parents during dyadic ***playdates*** in the following ways:

- ***Priming*:**
  - Begin the play interactions with parents going over the rules for ***joining a game*** BEFORE GAME PLAYING.
    - Example: *"Remember when you join a game you need to first watch the* game (point to your eyes) *and make sure you know the rules* (tap your head with your index finger). *If you know the rules, then remember to move closer* (move your body closer), *look at your friends with your* (point to your eyes to prompt the child to say *"eyes"*)*...EYES and smile with your* (point to your mouth to prompt the child to say *"mouth"*)*...MOUTH when you say, 'Can I play?' And don't forget to use* (pause briefly to prompt the child to say *"names"*)*...NAMES."*
- ***Prompting*:**
  - Remind parents to use the buzzwords to ***prompt*** their child to ***join a game*** IN THE MOMENT.
    - Example: *"Remember to join the game."*
    - Example: *"Don't forget to join the game if your friends say yes."*
    - Example: *"Remember to move closer when you ask to play."*
- ***Praising*:**
  - Remind parents to ***praise*** and reinforce their child whenever their child ***joins a game*** CORRECTLY.
    - Example: *"Great job joining the game!"*
    - Example: *"Great job joining the game by saying, 'Can I play?'"*
    - Example: *"Good job watching the game first!"*
- ***Providing corrective feedback using a praise sandwich*:**
  - Remind parents to ***praise*** their child's ATTEMPTS to ***join a game*** and identify what could be done differently next time.
    - Example: *"Good job joining the game. Next time remember to watch the game first, but nice try!"*
    - Example: *"Nice try joining the game. Don't forget to keep cool if your friends say no, but good job!"*
    - Example: *"Good job joining the game. Remember to use names next time, but great job!"*
- Remind parents to continue to ***social coach*** on previously learned skills:

- ***Listening and following directions.***
- ***Meeting and greeting friends.***
- ***Sharing and giving a turn.***
- ***Asking for a turn.***
- ***Keeping cool.***
- ***Being a good sport.***
- ***Showing and telling.***
- ***Don't be bossy.***
- ***Asking a friend to play.***

Parent Coached Play: Dyadic Playdates (20 Minutes)

- Have each child choose a turn-taking game brought from home or provided by the treatment team.
- The group leader sits on the floor at the front of the room.
- The families sit on the floor in a semi-circle facing the group leader.

Group leader: *"Hey friends, we're going to have more playdates and play with the fun games you brought from home. This time, we're going to practice joining a game. You'll take turns joining a game by first watching the game* (point to your eyes) *and making sure you know the rules* (tap your head with your index finger). *When you know the rules, you should then join the game by moving closer* (move your body closer), *looking at your friends with your* (point to your eyes to prompt the children to say *"eyes"*)*...EYES and smiling with your* (point to your mouth to prompt the children to say *"mouth"*)*... MOUTH when you say, 'Can I play?' while using NAMES."*

"And if your friends say yes, then you should join the game. You'll play the game for a few minutes before we tell you to swap games. Parents, remember to social coach your children by using your Parent Coached Play Cards. Okay, let's play with our games!"

- At the beginning of each game, parents will have children practice ***joining the game***.
  - One child will sit in the play area while their parent helps set up the game.
  - The remaining family will stand near the play area and will practice ***joining the game***.
- As the family in the play area is setting up the game, the parent of the *joining child* will ***social coach*** their child to ***join the game***.
- The parent of the child setting up the game will ***social coach*** their child to accept their friend's request to ***join the game***.
- After approximately seven minutes of play, ***prompt*** parents to prepare the children for the upcoming game swap by saying, *"Parents, tell your children that we'll be swapping games in one minute."*
- After approximately one additional minute of play (eight minutes of game playing in total), instruct the parents to swap games by saying, *"Parents, it's time to swap games. After cleaning up, parents will social coach their child to join the new game before playing."*
- As the family in the play area is setting up the new game, the parent of the *joining child* will ***social coach*** their child to ***join the game***.
- The parent of the child setting up the new game will ***social coach*** their child to accept their friend's request to ***join the game***.

- After approximately seven minutes of playing the second game, instruct the parents to prepare the children for clean up by saying, *"Parents, tell your children that we'll be cleaning up in one minute."*
- After approximately one additional minute of play (eight minutes of game playing in total), ***prompt*** the parents to instruct their children to clean up by saying, *"Parents, it's time to clean up. Let's social coach the children to listen and follow directions by cleaning up and then say 'bye' to their friend using names before sitting in the Listening Circle."*
- If needed, parents will ***social coach*** their child to ***listen and follow directions*** to clean up.
- Then parents will ***social coach*** their child to ***say*** "***bye***" to their friend ***using names.***

Final Wrap-Up (10 minutes)

- The group leader sits on the floor at the front of the room.
- The children sit on the carpet squares in a semi-circle facing the group leader, with parents sitting behind their children.

Group leader: *"Okay friends, you all did a great job playing nicely and joining the games. When we're joining a game, do you think we should first watch the game* (point to your eyes) *and make sure we know the rules* (tap your head with your index finger)*?"* (Pause briefly to allow children to respond *"yes."*)

"That's right, friends! And if we know the rules, do you think we should move closer and LOOK at our friend with our EYES and SMILE with our MOUTH?" (Pause briefly to allow children to respond *"yes."*)

"That's right, friends! And when we're joining a game, do you think we should say, 'Can I play?' and use names?" (Pause briefly to allow children to respond *"yes."*)

"That's right, friends! But remember, we should only join the game if our friends say yes. If our friends say no, we should keep cool and find something else to do."

"You all did such a great job joining a game today that you each earned ____ (number) more stars! Let's start with ____ (child)."

Award each child the same number of stars by repeating the following with each child:

Group leader: *"Where's _____ (child)?"* (Wait until all the children are looking at the child.)

"_____ (Child), how many stars did you earn?" (Pause briefly to allow the child to respond.)

"That's right! Let's all count for _____ (child)! One, two, three... (add stars to the Star Chart as they are counted aloud)*! Everybody clap for _____*

(child)!" (All behavioral coaches clap and cheer and encourage the children to clap as well.)

"And remember you all earned those stars by joining a game! Everyone did a great job, and parents you did an excellent job social coaching! Parents, remember your homework assignments this week are for you and your children to practice joining a game and for you to continue practicing all the other things we've learned to be a good friend using the 4 Ps. And don't forget to have a playdate and go to your playgroups."

"Alright little friends, do you want to count our stars?" (Pause briefly to allow the children to respond.)

"Let's all count together and see how many stars we earned today! One, two, three…(count the number of stars for one child)*!"*

"You each earned ____ (total number) stars today! Round of applause for our friends!" (All behavioral coaches should clap and cheer and encourage the families to clap as well.)

"Great job, friends! Don't forget to choose your reward before you leave. See you all next week!"

Session 10 Continued

Joining a Game

PEERS® FOR PRESCHOOLERS: PARENT HANDOUT

Snapshot of the Lesson: Joining a Game

The objective of this lesson is to teach children how to ***join a game.*** Steps for ***joining a game*** include:

1. ***Watch the game*** (point to your eyes).
2. ***Know the rules*** (point to your head).
3. ***Move closer*** (demonstrate moving closer with your body).
4. ***Look at your friends with your eyes*** (point to your eyes).
5. ***Smile with your mouth*** (point to your mouth and smile).
6. ***Say, "Can I play?" using names.***
   - If your friends say yes, ***join the game***.
   - If your friends say no, ***keep cool*** and ***find something else to do***.

Parent Social Coaching Strategies for Joining a Game

- **Create opportunities for your child to *join games* while you are present.**
  - ***Joining games*** with ***playmates*** often occurs in settings like school or daycare, outside the presence of parents.
  - Create opportunities for your child to practice ***joining a game*** where you can ***social coach*** using the ***4 Ps.***
    - Example: Practicing at home with siblings or other family members.
    - Example: Visiting a local playground where your child can ***join games*** with other children while you are present.
  - Practicing ***joining a game*** with a parent present to provide ***social coaching*** will:
    - Enhance your child's mastery of the skills.
    - Make it more likely they will use the skills appropriately when parents are not present.
- **Identify opportunities during your child's daily routine to practice *joining a game* with familiar people in familiar places.**
  - It may be easier for you to ***social coach*** your child when ***joining a game*** if the practice is part of your normal routine.
    - Example: Practice at school/daycare drop-off or pick-up when you are present.

- Example: Practice at ***playgroups*** during unstructured time when you are present.
  - Using your child's daily routine to practice ***joining games*** with familiar people in familiar places will:
    - Decrease your child's anxiety when practicing.
    - Increase their comfort in following the steps.
    - Make it more likely that others will accept your child's attempts to join.

- **Remember to *prime* your child before the practice by going over the rules for *joining a game.***
  - The best time to ***prime*** your child is moments (not minutes or hours) before attempting to ***join a game***.
  - Be sure to use the buzzwords when going over the steps.
  - Encourage your child to help you generate the steps.
    - Example: Say "*Look at your friends with your...* (point to your eyes)" and wait for your child to say "eyes."
    - Example: Say, *"Smile with your...* (point to your mouth and smile)" and allow your child to say "mouth."
  - ***Praise*** your child when they remember the steps for ***joining a game***.

- ***Prompt* your child to follow the steps by asking them questions about the game they are attempting to join.**
  - Example: *"Do you know what they're playing?"*
    - Make sure they know the game before attempting to join.
    - Joining an unfamiliar game will slow down the play and may frustrate the players.
  - Example: *"Do you know the rules?"*
    - Have them explain the rules before joining.
    - Children sometimes change the rules to familiar games, so your child may need to watch for a while before understanding the rules.
    - Consider helping your child understand the rules by watching together and pointing out what you observe about the game playing.
  - Example: *"Who could you ask to join the game?"*
    - Children are more likely to allow familiar ***playmates*** to join play (if they don't have a bad reputation with the group).
    - When possible, helping your child identify someone they know may increase their chances of being accepted.

- ***Prompt* your child to wait for a pause in the game before joining when relevant.**
  - As children get older, their social interactions become more sophisticated, including the timing of entering play.
  - The rules for entering play will eventually include the added step of waiting for a pause in the game before joining.
  - Younger children will often interrupt game playing when attempting to ***join a game***, which may not be seen as intrusive at earlier stages of development.
  - Parents can help children judge when the best time is to join.
  - Typically, the ideal time to ***join a game*** is when there is a pause in the activities (e.g., someone just scored, the ball went out of bounds, the players are figuring out the rules).

- Parents should be prepared to add this step to your ***social coaching*** as your children mature.

- ***Prompt*** **your child to use their *playmate's* name when *joining a game.***
  - ***Using names*** when ***joining games*** will:
    - Get the ***playmate's*** attention.
    - Demonstrate that your child already knows the player(s).
    - May create a natural pause by directing the attention to your child.

- **If your child is unfamiliar with the players, *prompt* them to ask the leader if they can *join the game.***
  - While observing the group, you may recognize that one or two players appear to be more dominant in the game playing.
    - These may be the kids who are calling the plays and enforcing the rules.
  - ***Prompting*** your child to ask the leader of the game if they can join may make it more likely that they will be accepted by the whole group.
  - When relevant, ***prompting*** your child to ask the player in possession of the ball if they can ***join the game*** may increase their chance of being accepted because:
    - The person with the ball is in control at that moment and in a position of leadership.
    - Asking the person who is holding the ball may create a natural pause in the game.

- **If your child does not know the game or the rules of the game:**
  - **They should NOT attempt to *join the game* at that moment.**
    - It may be challenging for your child to meaningfully participate in the game.
    - They may be less likely to be accepted by their ***playmates*** during the game.
    - It may be overwhelming and frustrating for your child to attempt to learn the rules of the game while simultaneously attempting to socialize with their peers.
  - **Parents may *social coach* in the moment by teaching your child the rules of the game if they are simple.**
    - Help your child to become familiar with the rules of the game BEFORE ***joining the game*** to increase the likelihood that your child will experience positive peer interactions.
    - Model for your child how to figure out the rules of the game so they may be more likely to use those developing skills in the future.
    - Make sure that you are not targeting too many new behaviors or skills at once.
    - Keep in mind that the rules of games vary by playground, school, park, etc.

- **If the rules of the game cannot be easily taught in the moment:**
  - ***Social coach*** your child to ***keep cool*** and ***find something else to do.***
  - Redirect your child to other ***playmates*** when possible.
  - Have your child wait until the children play a game familiar to your child.
  - Parents should ***social coach*** by providing practice opportunities at home during the week to teach and familiarize your child with the rules of the game.
  - Preview the game with your child BEFORE they attempt to ***join the game*** again with their ***playmates***.

- **If the *playmates* do not allow your child to *join the game*:**
  - ***Social coach*** your child to ***keep cool*** and ***find something else to do***.
  - Redirect your child to other ***playmates*** when possible.
  - ***Praise*** your child for their efforts to ***join the game***.
  - Normalize the fact that we don't get to join every game (the same is true for parents).
- **Create practice opportunities to accept being turned down when attempting to *join a game.***
  - When practicing ***joining a game*** with your child during the week, parents should say no periodically (e.g., *"Next time"* or *"Maybe later"*) and have your child practice ***keeping cool*** and ***finding something else to do***.
    - ***Prompt*** your child BEFORE by saying, *"Okay, let's practice keeping cool if I say no. Remember to keep cool and find something else to do."*

Homework Assignments

1. **Playdates.**
   - Schedule and have a ***playdate*** with a ***playmate***.
   - Prepare for the ***playdate*** using the ***5 Ws***.
     - ***WHO: Playdates*** should be **one-on-one.**
     - ***WHAT: Playdates*** should be **activity-based.**
     - ***WHERE:*** Schedule initial ***playdates*** to take place in your home or somewhere you can provide ***social coaching***.
     - ***WHEN:*** Try to keep initial ***playdates*** to no more than 1–1.5 hours.
     - ***HOW:*** Coordinate how the children will get to and from the ***playdate.***
   - Do a final practice with your child of the games and activities that will be available during the ***playdate***.
   - Gather all the games and activity materials for the ***playdate*** in one area that is VISIBLE and easily accessible to YOU but not the children.
   - Provide ***social coaching*** during the ***playdate*** and assess if this is a good ***playmate*** for your child.
2. **Practice joining a game.**
   - Practice having your child ***join a game*** this week during preferred and highly motivating activities while providing ***social coaching*** using the ***4 Ps***.
     - ***Priming:*** Review the rules for ***joining a game*** with your child BEFORE PRACTICING.
     - ***Prompting:*** Remind your child IN THE MOMENT to ***join a game*** whenever the opportunities present.
     - ***Praising: Praise*** your child using the buzzwords whenever they ***join a game*** CORRECTLY.
     - ***Providing corrective feedback: Provide corrective feedback*** in the form of a ***praise sandwich*** whenever your child ATTEMPTS to ***join a game.***

- Please send us a 30–60-second video of ***social coaching*** your child to ***join a game*** to be viewed during homework review.
  - Please include:
    - Skills your child did well.
    - Skills you would like to work on with your child.

3. **Provide *social coaching* on previously learned skills.**
   - Continue providing ***social coaching*** to your child throughout the week using the ***4 Ps.***
   - Previous skills include:
     - ***Listening and following directions.***
     - ***Meeting and greeting friends.***
     - ***Sharing and giving a turn.***
     - ***Asking for a turn.***
     - ***Keeping cool.***
     - ***Being a good sport.***
     - ***Showing and telling.***
     - ***Don't be bossy.***
     - ***Asking a friend to play.***

4. **Bring a turn-taking game.**
   - Bring a turn-taking game that your child enjoys playing and can be played with the other children.

Session 10 Continued

Joining a Game

PEERS® FOR PRESCHOOLERS: PARENT COACHED PLAY CARDS

Snapshot of the Lesson: Joining a Game

1. ***Watch the game*** (point to your eyes).
2. ***Know the rules*** (point to your head).
3. ***Move closer*** (demonstrate moving closer with your body).
4. ***Look at your friends with your eyes*** (point to your eyes).
5. ***Smile with your mouth*** (point to your mouth and smile).
6. ***Say, "Can I play?" using names.***
    - If your friends say yes, ***join the game***.
    - If your friends say no, ***keep cool*** and ***find something else to do***.

Priming BEFORE Game Playing

- Example: *"Remember when you join a game you need to first watch the* game (point to your eyes) *and make sure you know the rules* (tap your head with your index finger). *If you know the rules, then remember to move closer* (move your body closer), *look at your friends with your* (point to your eyes to prompt the child to say *"eyes"*)...*EYES and smile with your* (point to your mouth to prompt the child to say *"mouth"*)...*MOUTH when you say, 'Can I play?' And don't forget to use* (pause briefly to prompt the child to say *"names"*)...*NAMES."*

Prompting IN THE MOMENT

- Example: *"Remember to join the game."*
- Example: *"Don't forget to join the game if your friends say yes."*
- Example: *"Remember to move closer when you ask to play."*

Praising for CORRECT Use of Skills

- Example: *"Great job joining the game!"*
- Example: *"Great job joining the game by saying, 'Can I play?'"*
- Example: *"Good job watching the game first!"*

Providing Corrective Feedback for ATTEMPTS Using a Praise Sandwich

- Example: *"Good job joining the game. Next time remember to watch the game first, but nice try!"*
- Example: *"Nice try joining the game. Don't forget to keep cool if your friends say no, but good job!"*
- Example: *"Good job joining the game. Remember to use names next time, but great job!"*

- Continue to provide ***social coaching*** on previously learned skills:
  - ***Listening and following directions.***
  - ***Meeting and greeting friends.***
  - ***Sharing and giving a turn.***
  - ***Asking for a turn.***
  - ***Keeping cool.***
  - ***Being a good sport.***
  - ***Showing and telling.***
  - ***Don't be bossy.***
  - ***Asking a friend to play.***

Session 10 Continued

Joining a Game

PEERS® FOR PRESCHOOLERS: PARENT HOMEWORK WORKSHEET

Child's Name:	Parent's Name:		Date:	
HOMEWORK ASSIGNMENTS	PRIMING (REVIEWING RULES BEFORE PRACTICE)	PROMPTING (IN THE MOMENT)	PRAISING (USING BUZZWORDS)	PROVIDING CORRECTIVE FEEDBACK (USING A PRAISE SANDWICH)
Joining a game				
Practice previous skills: • **Asking a friend to play** • **Don't be bossy** • **Show and tell during play** • **Being a good sport** • **Keeping cool** • **Asking for a turn** • **Sharing and giving turns** • **Meeting and greeting friends** • **Listening and following directions**				

Child's Name:	Parent's Name:		Date:	
HOMEWORK ASSIGNMENTS	PRIMING (REVIEWING RULES BEFORE PRACTICE)	PROMPTING (IN THE MOMENT)	PRAISING (USING BUZZWORDS)	PROVIDING CORRECTIVE FEEDBACK (USING A PRAISE SANDWICH)
Playdate: • **Plan a playdate using the 5 Ws** • **Prime your child before the playdate** • **Provide social coaching during the playdate using the 4 Ps**				
Bring a turn-taking game	Did you bring a turn-taking game? YES or NO (Circle)		Which game did you bring?	

Please fill out this worksheet by describing what you did to complete the homework assignments. Worksheets will be collected during Homework Review at the next session of PEERS® for Preschoolers.

Session 11

Asking to Play Something Different

PARENT SESSION THERAPIST GUIDE

Parent Session Agenda

- Homework Review (40 minutes).
- Didactic Lessons (20 minutes).
- Parent Coached Play (20 minutes).
- Final Wrap-Up (10 minutes).

Materials Needed

- Conference room with a large table and enough chairs for the parent group leader and all parents to sit comfortably around the table.
  - Avoid sitting in a circle without a table as this creates the atmosphere of group therapy.
- Name tags for parents and treatment team.
- *Parent Handouts* (for the current week and the previous week).
- *Parent Homework Worksheets* (for the current week and the previous week).
- *Parent Coached Play Cards* (for the current week and the previous week).
- *Attendance and Homework Compliance Sheets* for parent group leader.
- Pens for note-taking (consider having extra pens for parents who need them).

Homework Review (40 Minutes)

1. **Playdates.**
   - Have parents report on the ***playdate*** and confirm that they planned using the ***5 Ws.***
   - Review what parents did to ***social coach*** their child BEFORE, DURING, and AFTER the ***playdate***.
   - Identify what skills their child did well and what skills they need to work on.
     - Confirm that parents ***praised*** skills that were done well and provided ***priming, prompting***, and/or ***corrective feedback*** for emerging skills.
   - Have parents assess if this is a good ***playmate*** for their child.
   - Have parents identify who their child might have a ***playdate*** with in the coming week (does not have to be a different ***playmate***).

2. **Practice joining a game.**
   - Review the 30–60-second video of ***social coaching*** for ***joining a game*** for each family. (For larger groups, you may need to review video recordings in two smaller groups with two different parent group leaders).

DOI: 10.4324/9781003502968-12

  - Have parents identify:
    - Skills their child did well.
    - Skills they would like to work on with their child.
  - Provide ***social coaching*** tips as appropriate for each family.
- If parents did not send a video of ***social coaching***, confirm the following:
  - Parents practiced having their child ***join a game*** during preferred and highly motivating activities while providing ***social coaching*** using the ***4 Ps.***
    - ***Priming:*** Reviewed the rules for ***joining a game*** with their child BEFORE PRACTICING.
    - ***Prompting:*** Reminded their child IN THE MOMENT to ***join a game*** whenever the opportunity presented.
    - ***Praising: Praised*** their child using the buzzwords whenever they ***joined a game*** CORRECTLY.
    - ***Providing corrective feedback: Provided corrective feedback*** in the form of a ***praise sandwich*** whenever their child ATTEMPTED to ***join a game***.

3. **Provide social coaching on previously learned skills.**
   - Confirm parents continued to provide ***social coaching*** to their child throughout the week using the ***4 Ps*** for previously learned skills:
     - ***Listening and following directions.***
     - ***Meeting and greeting friends.***
     - ***Sharing and giving a turn.***
     - ***Asking for a turn.***
     - ***Keeping cool.***
     - ***Being a good sport.***
     - ***Showing and telling.***
     - ***Don't be bossy.***
     - ***Asking a friend to play.***

4. **Bring a turn-taking game.**
   - Confirm the following:
     - Brought a turn-taking game that their child enjoys playing and can be played with the other children. (To avoid distractions, these games should be left with the parents until *Parent Coached Play*.)

Didactic Lessons (20 Minutes)

PEERS® Neuroaffirming Pledge:

- We value neurodiversity, acceptance, and authenticity.
- We honor the diverse ways people experience the world.
- We respect each person's unique perspectives and communication styles.
- We recognize there is no one right way to connect with others.
- If using the strategies taught in PEERS® feels like camouflaging or masking and/or they don't align with your goals or the goals of your family, then you do not have to use them.
- Learning and using the skills taught in PEERS® is a PERSONAL CHOICE.

Didactic Lesson: Asking to Play Something Different

- Distribute *Parent Handouts.*
  - Sections in **bold print** come directly from the *Parent Handout.*
  - Terms that are ***bold and italicized*** are buzzwords and represent important concepts from the didactic lesson.
- Explain, *"The last two lessons we've focused on teaching the children how to initiate social interactions by asking a friend to play or joining a game that their friends are already playing. Today's lesson will focus on helping children sustain positive play interactions by helping them transition to new play activities, or what we call 'asking to play something different.' Before we go over the social coaching strategies you can use to support your child's attempts to ask to play something different, we should begin with going over the child didactic lesson to give you some context."*

Snapshot of the Lesson: Asking to Play Something Different

The objective of this lesson is to teach children how to *ask to play something different.* Steps for *asking to play something different* include:

1. ***Think of something fun to play* (point to your head).**
2. ***Look at your friends with your eyes* (point to your eyes).**
3. ***Smile with your mouth* (point to your mouth and smile).**
4. ***Ask to play something different using names* (e.g., *"(Friend), let's play _____!"*).**

If your friend says no:

1. ***Keep cool and play nicely.***
2. ***Look at your friends with your eyes* (point to your eyes).**
3. ***Smile with your mouth* (point to your mouth and smile).**
4. ***Say "okay" using names.***
5. ***Play nicely with your friends.***
6. **If you're still upset, then *take deep breaths to keep cool* (take two slow *deep breaths*).**

Parent Social Coaching Strategies for Asking to Play Something Different

- **Help your child *think of something fun to play.***
  - **When practicing *asking to play something different,* parents may need to *social coach* your child to *think of something fun to play.***
  - **When practicing during the week, at first parents may need to provide choices for other fun toys or games your child can play with.**
    - **Example: *"If you want to play something different, we have trains or Bingo."***
    - **Make sure that the available choices are preferred and fun for your child.**
    - **This will increase the chances that they will want to use the skills.**

- **If your goal is to target flexibility, then that skill should be targeted separately – not when practicing *asking to play something different.***
  - **Remember, it is important not to target too many new skills at once as this can be frustrating and less motivating for your child.**

- **Help your child to identify alternative games prior to *playdates.***
  - **When planning *playdates* using the *5 Ws*, we often have an idea of what the activity will be in advance (i.e., the "*what*" in the *5 Ws*).**
  - **Be prepared that your child and/or their *playmate* may get bored and want to *play something different.***
  - **Prior to the *playdate*, help your child come up with a list of possible alternative activities that your child and their *playmate* might play.**
  - **You may need to *social coach* your child to choose activities that are fun for BOTH your child and their *playmate.***
    - **If you are unsure what games and toys the *playmate* likes, consider asking the parents of the *playmate* for some ideas.**
  - **Be sure to let your child know in advance that they may not be able to play ALL these activities during the *playdate.***

- **Have alternative activities visible but not accessible during *playdates.***
  - **In the moment, parents should have a range of activities that are visible but NOT accessible to your child to help your child *think of something fun to play* that is a *common interest* with their *playmate.***
    - **These items should be from the list of alternative activities discussed with your child prior to the *playdate.***
  - **By choosing activities and toys that are *common interests,* the *playmate* may be more open to *playing something different.***
    - **A *playmate's* agreement to *play something different* will naturally reinforce your child's use of the skill and increases the chances that your child will use the skills in the future.**
  - **If your child or their *playmate* do not agree on what to play differently, you might suggest taking turns playing both activities.**
    - **Allow your child's *playmate* to have the first turn since they are the guest.**
    - **Be sure to give a one-minute alert when switching activities as this will promote an easier transition.**
  - **If your child or their *playmate* becomes upset that there is not enough time to play with ALL the toys and games, you might suggest that they have another *playdate* to play with the other games and toys.**

- **Help your child to *keep cool* if the *playmate* doesn't want to *play something different.***
  - **If your child's friend does not want to *play something different*, then parents may need to *social coach* your child to *keep cool.***
    - **Parents may need to *social coach* your child to *take deep breaths* to *keep cool.***
    - **Parents may even want to demonstrate *taking deep breaths* with your child to encourage them to use the skills.**
    - ***Praise* them immediately when they use the skills for *keeping cool.***

- **Have your child practice taking "no" for an answer.**
  - **When practicing *asking to play something different* with your child during the week, parents may want to practice saying "no" (e.g., *"Next time"* or *"Maybe later"* or *"No thanks"* or *"Not now"*) and have your child *keep cool.***
  - **Parents should *prompt* your child BEFORE practicing taking "no" for an answer.**
    - **Example: *"Okay, let's practice keeping cool if I say no. Remember to keep cool and play nicely."***
    - **Remember to *praise* them when they use the skills for *keeping cool.***

- **Practice playing less preferred activities and games if your child has difficulty *keeping cool* when taking "no" for an answer.**
  - **Some children will initially get upset if their attempts to *ask to play something different* are turned down for highly preferred activities.**
  - **In initially helping your child to *keep cool*, parents should practice having your child suggest new activities that are neutral or less preferred by your child.**
    - **This is likely to make it easier for your child to initially practice the skills for *keeping cool* when hearing "no."**
    - **As your child improves in *keeping cool*, parents may gradually have the child *keep cool* when suggesting new activities that are more preferred or fun for your child.**

- **Practice *playing nicely* when offers to *play something different* are turned down.**
  - **Parents may need to *social coach* your child to not only *keep cool* but also continue *playing nicely* with their friend.**
  - **If your child has difficulty continuing to *play nicely*, explain that they are simply *taking turns* with game playing (e.g., friends *take turns* choosing games and toys to play with).**
    - **Example: *"Remember to play nicely by giving a turn to your friend in choosing the game."***
  - **If you discover that your child's *playmate* rarely allows your child to choose the games or toys, and this bothers your child, then consider whether this is a good choice in *playmate* for your child moving forward.**

Parent Coached Play

- Distribute the *Parent Coached Play Cards*.
- Review the examples of the ***4 Ps*** provided on the *Parent Coached Play Card.*
- Remind parents that in a few moments we will be joining the children for *Parent Coached Play* in the context of mock dyadic ***playdates***.
- Parents should keep the *Parent Coached Play Card* in front of them during the dyadic ***playdate*** for recommendations on how to ***social coach*** children on ***asking a friend to play***.

Homework Assignments

(Briefly review the homework assignments and troubleshoot any potential problems with parents.)

1. **Playdates.**
   - **Schedule and have a *playdate* with a *playmate.***
   - **Prepare for the *playdate* using the *5 Ws.***

- ◦ ***WHO: Playdates*** **should be one-on-one.**
  - ◦ ***WHAT: Playdates*** **should be activity-based.**
  - ◦ ***WHERE:*** **Schedule initial *playdates* to take place in your home or somewhere you can provide *social coaching.***
  - ◦ ***WHEN:*** **Try to keep initial *playdates* to no more than 1–1.5 hours.**
  - ◦ ***HOW:*** **Coordinate how the children will get to and from the *playdate.***
- **Do a final practice with your child of the games and activities that will be available during the *playdate.***
- **Gather all the games and activity materials for the *playdate* in one area that is VISIBLE and easily accessible to YOU but not the children.**
- **Provide *social coaching* during the *playdate* and assess if this is a good *playmate* for your child.**

2. **Practice asking to play something different.**
   - **Practice having your child *ask to play something different* this week while providing *social coaching* using the *4 Ps.***
     - ◦ ***Priming:*** **Review the rules for *asking to play something different* with your child BEFORE PRACTICING.**
     - ◦ ***Prompting:*** **Remind your child IN THE MOMENT to *ask to play something different* whenever the opportunities present.**
     - ◦ ***Praising: Praise*** **your child using the buzzwords whenever they *ask to play something different* CORRECTLY.**
     - ◦ ***Providing corrective feedback: Provide corrective feedback*** **in the form of a *praise sandwich* whenever your child ATTEMPTS to *ask to play something different.***
   - **Please send us a 30–60-second video of *social coaching* your child to *ask to play something different* to be viewed during homework review.**
     - ◦ **Please include:**
       - ▪ **Skills your child did well.**
       - ▪ **Skills you would like to work on with your child.**

3. **Provide social coaching on previously learned skills.**
   - **Continue providing *social coaching* to your child throughout the week using the *4 Ps.***
   - **Previous skills include:**
     - ◦ ***Listening and following directions.***
     - ◦ ***Meeting and greeting friends.***
     - ◦ ***Sharing and giving a turn.***
     - ◦ ***Asking for a turn.***
     - ◦ ***Keeping cool.***
     - ◦ ***Being a good sport.***
     - ◦ ***Showing and telling.***
     - ◦ ***Don't be bossy.***
     - ◦ ***Asking a friend to play.***
     - ◦ ***Joining a game.***

4. **Bring a turn-taking game.**
   - **Bring a turn-taking game that your child enjoys playing and can be played with the other children.**

Session 11 Continued

Asking to Play Something Different

CHILD SESSION THERAPIST GUIDE

Child Session Agenda

- Didactic Lesson: *Asking to Play Something Different* (20 minutes).
- Group Behavioral Rehearsal Activity 1: *Elbow to Elbow* (15 minutes).
- Break Time (10 minutes).
- Group Behavioral Rehearsal Activity 2: *Swap and Play* (15 minutes).
- Parent Coached Play: *Dyadic Playdates* (20 minutes).
- Final Wrap-Up (10 minutes).

Snapshot of the Lesson: Asking to Play Something Different

The objective of this lesson is to teach children how to ***ask to play something different.*** Steps for ***asking to play something different*** include:

1. ***Think of something fun to play*** (point to your head).
2. ***Look at your friends with your eyes*** (point to your eyes).
3. ***Smile with your mouth*** (point to your mouth and smile).
4. ***Ask to play something different using names*** (e.g., ***"(Friend), let's play _____!"***).

If your friend says no:

1. ***Keep cool and play nicely.***
2. ***Look at your friends with your eyes*** (point to your eyes).
3. ***Smile with your mouth*** (point to your mouth and smile).
4. ***Say "okay" using names***.
5. ***Play nicely with your friends***.
6. If you're still upset, then ***take deep breaths to keep cool*** (take two slow ***deep breaths***).

Materials Needed

- Tiger puppet.
- Elephant puppet.
- Small ball.
- Two toy cars.
- Carpet squares or chairs.
- Making Friends Helper" badge.
- Star chart with names of children.
- Marker for star chart.
- Name tags for families and treatment team.
- Prize bins with prizes.

Preparing for the Lesson

- Use the script below with the group leader using a tiger puppet to play the part of "Timmy Tiger."
- A behavioral coach uses an elephant puppet to play the part of "Ellie Elephant."
- An additional behavioral coach assists with the behavioral rehearsal and provides encouragement and feedback to the group.
- A child is chosen at the beginning of the lesson as the "Making Friends Helper."
  - The "Making Friends Helper" wears a special badge and is the first child to practice the skill.
- The group leader and the behavioral coach sit on the floor at the front of the room.
- A special-colored carpet square (e.g., red) is placed at the front of the room next to the child group leader to be used as the "Good Friend Square."
- For the children, additional carpet squares of the same color (e.g., green) are placed in a semicircle facing the child group leader and the "Good Friend Square."
- Note: If carpet squares are unavailable, the children and behavioral coach may sit on chairs.
- The material in *italics* should be read by the indicated person.
- The material in ***bold and italics*** represents buzzwords and should be emphasized when read.
- The material in CAPITAL LETTERS within the script should be given extra emphasis while the group is encouraged to say the words in unison.

Behavioral Coaching Techniques

Behavioral coaches should use the following coaching techniques described below throughout the lesson and the behavioral rehearsal activities. (Note: ***priming*** occurs during the introduction to the activity.)

- ***Prompting***:
  - Use the buzzwords to ***prompt*** the children to ***ask to play something different***.
    - Example: *"Remember to ask to play something different if you get bored."*
    - Example: *"Don't forget to think of something fun to play."*
    - Example: *"Should you keep cool if your friend says no?"*
- ***Praising***:
  - Reinforce ***asking to play something different*** by ***praising*** the children.
    - Example: *"Great job asking to play something different!"*
    - Example: *"Great job thinking of something fun to play!'"*
    - Example: *"Good job keeping cool and playing nicely when your friend said no!"*
- ***Providing corrective feedback using a praise sandwich***:
  - Reinforce ATTEMPTS to ***ask to play something different*** by ***praising*** the children and identifying what could be done differently next time.
    - Example: *"Nice try asking to play something different. Remember to think of something fun to play next time, but good job!"*
    - Example: *"Good job asking to play something different. Remember to look and smile next time, but nice try!"*
    - Example: *"Nice try thinking of something fun to play. Don't forget to keep cool and play nicely next time if your friend says no, but great job!"*
- Continue to provide ***social coaching*** on previously learned skills:

- ***Listening and following directions.***
- ***Meeting and greeting friends.***
- ***Sharing and giving a turn.***
- ***Asking for a turn.***
- ***Keeping cool.***
- ***Being a good sport.***
- ***Showing and telling.***
- ***Don't be bossy.***
- ***Asking a friend to play.***
- ***Joining a game.***

Didactic Lesson: Asking to Play Something Different (20 minutes)

Have the children sit in a semi-circle on the carpet squares facing the group leader.

Timmy Tiger: (Sit at the front of the room and choose a Making Friends Helper.) *"Who wants to be our Making Friends Helper?"*

(Choose from among the children raising their hands and place the "Making Friends Helper" badge on the child. The child stays in their seat for now.)

"Hi friends! I'm Timmy Tiger. Grrr, grrr! Today we're going to practice asking to play something different. Asking to play something different is a great way to be nice to our friends!"

"Who should we ask to play something different with? We should ask to play something different with our FRIENDS, TEACHERS, MOMMIES, DADDIES, BROTHERS, AND SISTERS."

"When should we ask to play something different? We should ask to play something different when we get bored, or when we want to play another game, or when we want to play with another toy."

"How should we ask to play something different? We should ask to play something different by looking at our friend with our (point to your eyes and then to Timmy Tiger's eyes)*...EYES, smiling with our* (point to your mouth and smile)*...MOUTH, then thinking of something fun to play and asking our friend to play something different. And don't forget to use...NAMES."*

"But friends, sometimes our friends might say 'no.' Do you think we should cry or yell or hit if our friends don't want to play something different?" (Shake your head no and encourage the children to say *"no."*)

"That's right, friends! Do you think we should keep cool by taking deep breaths and keep playing nicely?" (Nod your head yes and encourage the children to say *"yes."*)

"That's right, friends! Remember, asking to play something different is a nice way to be a good friend! Grrr, grrr!"

Role Play: Asking to Play Something Different

Timmy Tiger and Ellie Elephant: (Throw the small ball to one another while ***showing and telling*** and ***being good sports***. The toy cars are nearby.)

Timmy Tiger: (Turn to look at the group of children.) *"Hey friends! I'm having fun playing with my friend Ellie Elephant, but I want to play something different. Do you think I should think of something fun to play?"* (Nod your head yes and encourage the children to say *"yes."*)

"That's a great idea! Grrr, grrr! Hmm...but what should we play?"

(Look confused, scratch your head, and pause.)

"Hey friends, I know! I want to play with those cool cars over there (point to the two toy cars nearby). *Do you think I should ask my friend Ellie Elephant to play cars with me?"* (Nod your head yes and encourage the children to say *"yes."*)

"That's a great idea! Grrr, grrr! Let's do it!" (Turn to look at Ellie Elephant and smile.) *"Ellie Elephant,* (point to the toy cars) *let's play cars!"*

(Turn to look at the group of children.) *"Hey friends, did I do a good job of asking to play something different with Ellie Elephant?"* (Nod your head yes and encourage the children to say *"yes."*)

"That's right! Let's see what Ellie Elephant says." (Turn to look at Ellie Elephant and smile.) *"Ellie Elephant,* (point to the toy cars) *let's play cars!"*

Ellie Elephant: (Look at Timmy Tiger and the toy cars.) *"No, maybe later. I want to play catch."*

Timmy Tiger: (Turn to look at the group of children.) *"Hey friends, Ellie Elephant said no. Do you think I should keep cool and play nicely by saying, 'Okay, Ellie Elephant' and take some deep breaths?"* (Nod your head yes and encourage the children to say *"yes."*)

"That's right, friends!" (Turn to look at Ellie Elephant and smile.) *"Let's keep playing! Okay, Ellie Elephant."* (Take two ***deep breaths***.)

Timmy Tiger and Ellie Elephant: (Resume playing with the small ball for a few moments while ***showing and telling*** and ***being good sports***.)

Timmy Tiger: (Turn to look at the group of children.) *"Hey friends, did I do a good job of asking to play something different and then keeping cool and playing nicely when Ellie Elephant said no?"* (Nod your head yes and encourage the children to say *"yes."*) *"That's right! Grrr, grrr!"*

Timmy Tiger and Ellie Elephant:	(Say *"good job," give a "tiger high-five," and "elephant high-five,"* clap, cheer, and encourage the children to clap as well. Ellie Elephant sits on the other side of the Good Friend Square (i.e., the Good Friend Square is between Timmy Tiger and Ellie Elephant). ***Social coach*** the children as needed while they practice ***asking to play something different*** with Ellie Elephant.)
Ellie Elephant:	(Hold onto the small ball.)
Timmy Tiger:	*"Now let's see _____ (behavioral coach) try! _____ (Behavioral coach), please come sit on the Good Friend Square."*
Behavioral coach:	(Sit on the Good Friend Square.)
Timmy Tiger:	*"____ (Behavioral coach), can you show us how to ask to play something different with Ellie Elephant?"*
Behavioral coach:	*"Okay, Timmy Tiger."*
Timmy Tiger:	(Turn to look at the group of children.) *"Remember to look at Ellie Elephant with your* (point to your eyes to prompt the children to say *"eyes"*)*...EYES and smile with your* (point to your mouth to prompt the children to say *"mouth"*)*...MOUTH when you ask to play something different. And if Ellie Elephant says no, remember to keep cool and play nicely by saying, 'Okay, Ellie Elephant.' And don't forget to use* (pause briefly to prompt the children to say *"names"*)*...NAMES."*
Ellie Elephant:	(Look at the behavioral coach and smile.) *"____ (Behavioral coach), let's play catch!"*
Behavioral coach:	(Turn to look at Ellie Elephant and smile.) *"Okay, Ellie Elephant!"*
Ellie Elephant:	*"Catch, _____ (behavioral coach)!"* (Throw the small ball to the behavioral coach).
Ellie Elephant and Behavioral coach:	(Throw the small ball to one another while ***showing and telling*** and ***beinggood sports***. The toy cars are nearby.)
	(Turn to look at the group of children.) *"Hey friends, I'm having fun playing with Ellie Elephant, but I'm bored playing catch. I'm going to practice asking to play something different and thinking of something fun to play with my friend Ellie Elephant."*
	(Turn to look at Ellie Elephant and smile.) *"Ellie Elephant,* (point to the toy cars) *let's play cars!"*
Ellie Elephant:	(Look at the behavioral coach and the toy cars.) *"No, maybe later. I want to play catch."*

Timmy Tiger: (Turn to look at the behavioral coach.) *"____ (Behavioral coach), Ellie Elephant said no. Don't forget to keep cool and play nicely by saying, 'Okay, Ellie Elephant.' And remember to take deep breaths if you need to keep cool."*

Behavioral coach: (Take two ***deep breaths***) *"Okay, Ellie Elephant."*

Ellie Elephant: *"Okay. Ready? Catch!"*

Ellie Elephant and Behavioral coach: (Resume playing with the small ball for a few moments while ***showing and telling*** and ***being good sports***.)

Timmy Tiger: *"Great job asking to play something different and keeping cool when Ellie Elephant said no, _____ (behavioral coach)! Grrr, grrr!"*

Timmy Tiger and Behavioral coach: (Say *"good job," give a "tiger high-five," and "elephant high-five,"* clap, cheer, and encourage the children to clap as well. The behavioral coach returns the small ball to Ellie Elephant and leaves the Good Friend Square.)

Behavioral Rehearsal: Asking to Play Something Different

Timmy Tiger: (Turn to look at the group of children and smile.) *"Okay friends! Now let's see our Making Friends Helper _____ try! _____ (Making Friends Helper), come sit on the Good Friend Square and show us how to ask to play something different with Ellie Elephant."*

(The Making Friends Helper should sit on the Good Friend Square.)

"Remember to look at Ellie Elephant with your (point to your eyes to prompt the children to say *"eyes")...EYES and smile with your* (point to your mouth to prompt the children to say *"mouth")...MOUTH when you ask to play something different. And if Ellie Elephant says no, remember to keep cool and play nicely by saying, 'Okay, Ellie Elephant.' And don't forget to use* (pause briefly to prompt the children to say *names")... NAMES."*

Ellie Elephant: (Look at the Making Friends Helper and smile.) *"____ (Making Friends Helper), let's play catch!"*

Timmy Tiger: (If needed, ***social coach*** the Making Friends Helper to respond by saying, *"Okay, Ellie Elephant!"*).

Ellie Elephant: *"Catch, _____ (Making Friends Helper)!"* (Throw the small ball to the Making Friends Helper).

Timmy Tiger: (If needed, ***social coach*** the Making Friends Helper to throw the small ball back and forth with Ellie Elephant. The toy cars are nearby.)

"Okay, _____ (Making Friends Helper), pretend you're having fun playing with Ellie Elephant, but now you want to play with the toy cars instead. What should you do?"

(If needed, ***social coach*** the Making Friends Helper to ***look, smile,*** and ***ask to play something different*** by ***saying, "Ellie Elephant, let's play cars!"***)

Ellie Elephant: (Look at the Making Friends Helper and the toy cars.) *"No, maybe later."*

Timmy Tiger: (If needed, ***social coach*** the Making Friends Helper to ***look, smile, keep cool***, and ***play nicely by saying "Okay, Ellie Elephant."***)

Ellie Elephant: (Ellie Elephant and the Making Friends Helper continue to play with the small ball for a few moments while ***showing and telling*** and ***being good sports***.)

Timmy Tiger: *"Great job asking to play something different and keeping cool when Ellie Elephant said no, _____ (Making Friends Helper)! Grrr, grrr!"*

(Say *"good job," give a "tiger high-five," and "elephant high-five,"* clap, cheer, and encourage the children to clap as well. The Making Friends Helper should return the small ball to Ellie Elephant.)

"Okay, Making Friends Helper, choose another friend to sit on the Good Friend Square." (If needed, ***social coach*** the Making Friends Helper to choose another child before returning to their seat.)

Repeat the following with each child:

Timmy Tiger: (Have each child take turns sitting on the Good Friend Square and practicing ***asking to play something different*** with Ellie Elephant.)

(Turn to look at the group of children.) *"Okay friends! Now let's see _____ (child) try! _____ (Child), come sit on the Good Friend Square and show us how to ask to play something different with Ellie Elephant."*

(The child should sit on the Good Friend Square.)

"Remember to look at Ellie Elephant with your (point to your eyes to prompt the children to say *"eyes"*)*...EYES and smile with your* (point to your mouth to prompt the children to say *"mouth"*)*...MOUTH when you ask to play something different. And if Ellie Elephant says no, remember to keep cool and play nicely by saying, 'Okay, Ellie Elephant.' And don't forget to use* (pause briefly to prompt the children to say *"names"*)*... NAMES."*

Ellie Elephant: (Ellie Elephant looks at the child and smiles.) *"____ (Child), let's play catch!"*

Timmy Tiger: (If needed, ***social coach*** the child to respond by saying, *"Okay, Ellie Elephant!"*).

Ellie Elephant: *"Catch, _____ (child)!"* (Throw the small ball to the child).

Timmy Tiger: (If needed, ***social coach*** the child to throw the small ball back and forth with Ellie Elephant. The toy cars are nearby.)

"Okay, _____ (child), pretend you're having fun playing with Ellie Elephant, but now you want to play with the toy cars instead. What should you do?"

(If needed, ***social coach*** the child to ***look, smile,*** and ***ask to play something different*** by ***saying, "Ellie Elephant, let's play cars!"***)

Ellie Elephant: (Look at the child and the toy cars.) *"No, maybe later."*

Timmy Tiger: (If needed, ***social coach*** the child to ***look, smile, keep cool***, and ***play nicely by saying "Okay, Ellie Elephant."***)

Ellie Elephant: (Ellie Elephant and the child continue to play with the small ball for a few moments while ***showing and telling*** and ***being good sports***.)

Timmy Tiger: *"Great job asking to play something different and keeping cool when Ellie Elephant said no, _____ (child)! Grrr, grrr!"*

(Say *"good job," give a "tiger high-five," and "elephant high-five,"* clap, cheer, and encourage the children to clap as well. The child should return the small ball to Ellie Elephant.)

"Okay, _____ (child), choose another friend to sit on the Good FriendSquare." (If needed, ***social coach*** the child to choose another child before returning to their seat.)

Didactic Lesson Wrap-Up

Group leader: *"Well friends, you all did a great job asking to play something different by looking at Ellie Elephant with your* (point to your eyes to prompt the children to say *"eyes")...EYES and smiling with your* (point to your mouth to prompt the children to say *"mouth")...MOUTH when you asked to play something different. And great job keeping cool and playing nicely when your friends said no. And nice job using* (pause briefly to prompt the children to say *"names")...NAMES!"*

"You each earned ____ (number) stars for asking to play something different! Let's start with ____ (Child)."

Award each child the same number of stars by repeating the following with each child:

Group leader: *"Where's ____ (child)?"* (Wait until all the children are looking at the child.)

"____ (Child), how many stars did you earn?" (Pause briefly to allow the child to respond.)

"That's right! Let's all count for ____ (child)! One, two, three... (add stars to the Star Chart as they are counted aloud)*! Everybody clap for ____ (Child)!"* (All behavioral coaches clap and cheer and encourage the children to clap as well.)

Session 11 Continued

Elbow to Elbow

BEHAVIORAL REHEARSAL ACTIVITY 1

Materials Needed

- Music and music player.
- Safety cones or masking tape.

Room Setup

- Remove or place all carpet squares to the side.
- Use the safety cones or masking tape to designate a large play area called the *dancing zone*.
- The group leader stands at the front of the room.
- The children and behavioral coaches stand in the *dancing zone* facing the group leader.

Rules: Elbow to Elbow

- The group leader reads the script below to explain the rules.
- Play the music and cue the children to begin to dance.
- Pause the music every ten seconds and instruct the children to stop dancing when the music stops by saying, "*FREEZE!*"
- Present a command, and the children will practice ***listening and following directions***.
  - Present one command per pause.
  - Avoid commands involving the face.
  - Examples: Elbow to elbow, foot to foot, thumb to thumb, etc.
- The children quickly look for a friend and ***follow directions*** by acting out the command.
  - Example commands:
    - For *"elbow to elbow,"* the children touch elbows.
    - For *"finger to finger,"* the children touch fingers.
  - If there is an odd number of children, the children form a triad.
- Once all the children are demonstrating the command, restart the music and the children resume dancing.
- Once the children are familiar with the game, ***social coach*** the children to ***ask to play something different*** by having them choose different body parts or articles of clothing.
  - Choose children one at a time to practice ***asking to play something different***.
- Examples: Hand to wrist, toe to ankle, knee to foot, etc. Rotate between accepting or declining the children's requests.

- Repeat the cycle, making sure all children have at least two chances to practice ***asking to play something different*** and ***keeping cool*** when their request is not accepted.

Behavioral Rehearsal: Elbow to Elbow (15 Minutes)

The group leader leads the activity. The behavioral coaches and children sit on the floor in the *dancing zone* while the group leader explains the rules.

Group leader:	*"Hey friends, now we're going to play a game called Elbow to Elbow. We'll play some music, and you'll dance with your friends in the dancing zone* (point to the *dancing zone*). *When the music stops, we'll say "FREEZE!" and you will all freeze in place* (demonstrate freezing in place) *and then listen to what I say next."*
	"I'm going to tell you to do silly things. If I say, 'Stand elbow to elbow,' then find a little friend and touch your elbows together like this (stand elbow to elbow with a nearby behavioral coach). *Or if I say, 'Stand toe to toe,' then find a little friend and touch your toes together like this* (stand toe to toe with a nearby behavioral coach)*."*
	"Then you'll practice asking to play something different. You'll each ask me to play something different by looking at me with your (point to your eyes to prompt the children to say *"eyes"*)*...EYES and smiling with your* (point to your mouth to prompt the children to say *"mouth"*)*...MOUTH when you think of something fun to play by choosing different body parts like 'shoulder to shoulder' like this* (stand with shoulders touching with a nearby behavioral coach) *or 'thumb to thumb' like this* (stand with thumbs touching with a nearby behavioral coach). *You can ask to play something different by saying, 'Let's play shoulder to shoulder!' or 'Let's play thumb to thumb!' And remember to use* (pause briefly to prompt the children to say *"names"*)*...NAMES."*
	"And if I say no, remember to keep cool by taking two deep breaths (demonstrate taking two ***deep breaths***) *and keep playing nicely. Okay, _____ (behavioral coach 1) and _____ (behavioral coach 2) go first!"*

Role Play: Elbow to Elbow

The group leader will lead the role play. Two behavioral coaches demonstrate how to play *Elbow to Elbow* while the children sit and watch in the *dancing zone.*

Group leader:	(Start playing the music.) *"The music is playing. _____ (Behavioral coaches 1 and 2) begin dancing!"*
Behavioral coaches 1 and 2:	(Dance in the *dancing zone.*)

Group leader:	(Pause the music after ten seconds). *"The music stopped. Everybody FREEZE!"*
Behavioral coaches 1 and 2:	(Freeze in place.)
Group leader:	*"Great job listening and following directions! Ready? Find a friend and stand elbow to elbow!"*
Behavioral coaches 1 and 2:	(Stand elbow to elbow.)
Group leader:	*"Great job listening and following directions! _____ (Behavioral coach 1), now pretend you want to play something different. Think of something fun to play by using different body parts like your hands or feet. And don't forget to keep cool by taking two deep breaths and play nicely if I say 'no' or 'maybe later.'"*
Behavioral coach 1:	*"Let's play shoulder to shoulder, _____ (group leader)!"*
Group leader:	*"Great job asking to play something different, _____ (behavioral coach 1)! The music is playing again. ____ (Behavioral coaches 1 and 2) begin dancing!"*
Behavioral coaches 1 and 2:	(Dance in the *dancing zone*.)
Group leader:	(Pause the music after ten seconds). *"The music stopped. Everybody FREEZE!"*
Behavioral coaches 1 and 2:	(Freeze in place.)
Group leader:	*"Great job listening and following directions! Now find a friend and stand shoulder to shoulder!"*
Behavioral coaches 1 and 2:	(Stand shoulder to shoulder.)
Group leader:	*"Great job listening and following directions! _____ (Behavioral coach 2), now pretend you want to play something different. Think of something fun to play by using different body parts like your hands or feet. And don't forget to keep cool by taking two deep breaths and play nicely if I say 'no' or 'maybe later.'"*
Behavioral coach 2:	*"Let's play toe to toe, _____ (group leader)!"*
Group leader:	*"No, maybe later. I want to play shoulder to shoulder."*
Behavioral coach 2:	*"Okay, _____ (group leader)."* (***Keep cool*** by taking ***two deep breaths***.)

Group leader:	*"Great job asking to play something different and keeping cool, _____ (behavioral coach 2)! The music is playing again. ____ (Behavioral coaches 1 and 2) begin dancing!"*
	(Pause the music after ten seconds) *"The music stopped. Everybody FREEZE!"*
Behavioral coaches 1 and 2:	(Freeze in place.)
Group leader:	*"Great job listening and following directions! Now find a friend and stand shoulder to shoulder!"*
Behavioral coaches 1 and 2:	(Stand shoulder to shoulder.)
Group leader:	*"Nice job, ____ (behavioral coaches 1 and 2)! Okay friends, now it's everyone's turn to play. Are we ready?"*

Behavioral Rehearsal: Elbow to Elbow

Group leader:	(Once the children and behavioral coaches are all standing in the *dancing zone*, begin to play the music.) *"The music is playing. Everybody begin dancing!"*
	(Pause the music after ten seconds.) *"The music stopped. Everybody FREEZE!"* (If needed, behavioral coaches should ***social coach*** the children to ***listen and follow directions***.)
	"Great job listening and following directions! Now find a little friend and stand elbow to elbow!" (Wait for children and behavioral coaches to stand elbow to elbow. Encourage children to play with one another.)
	"Great job listening and following directions! _____ (Child), now pretend you want to play something different. Think of something fun to play by using different body parts like your hands or feet. And don't forget to keep cool by taking two deep breaths and play nicely if I say 'no' or 'maybe later.'"

Table 11.1 Simple Sample Commands

Elbow to elbow	Back to back	Toe to toe
Knee to knee	Hand to hand	Heel to heel
Finger to finger	Foot to foot	Shoulder to shoulder
Thumb to thumb	Arm to arm	Ankle to ankle

Table 11.2 Complex Sample Commands

Hand to wrist	Shoulder to elbow	Toe to ankle
Ankle to foot	Hand to shoulder	Knee to pinky finger
Hand to thumb	Thumb to shoulder	Wrist to knee
Elbow to knee	Elbow to pinky finger	Back to hand
Knee to foot	Shoulder to wrist	Back to thumb

Group leader: (Randomly alternate between AGREEING to ***play something different*** and DECLINING to ***play something different***.)

AGREEING to *play something different*:

"Good idea, _____ (child)! And great job asking to play something different! Let's keep playing. Are we ready?"

DECLINING to *play something different:*

"No, maybe later. I want to play _____ (current command)." (Wait a moment to allow the child to demonstrate ***keeping cool***, taking ***deep breaths***, and **saying *"Okay, _____ (group leader)."***)

"Great job asking to play something different and keeping cool when I said no, _____ (child)! Let's keep playing. Are we ready?"

Repeat the cycle above, making sure all children have at least two chances to practice ***asking to play something different*** and ***keeping cool*** when their request is not accepted.

Behavioral Rehearsal Wrap-Up

Group leader: *"Well friends, great job asking to play something different! Give yourselves a big round of applause!"* (All behavioral coaches clap and cheer and encourage the children to clap as well.)

"Now everyone should come sit in the Listening Circle." (Have children return to the Listening Circle to sit on their carpet squares.)

"*Okay friends, you did such a great job asking to play something different by looking at your friends with your* (point to your eyes to prompt the children to say *"eyes"*)*...EYES and smiling with your* (point to your mouth to prompt the children to say *"mouth"*)*...MOUTH when you asked to play something different. And nice job using* (pause briefly to prompt the children to say *"names"*)*...NAMES!*"

"You each earned ____ (number) more stars for asking to play something different! Let's start with ____ (child)."

Award each child the same number of stars by repeating the following with each child:

Group leader: *"Where's ____ (child)?"* (Wait until all the children are looking at the child.)

"____ (Child), how many stars did you earn?" (Pause briefly to allow the child to respond.)

"That's right! Let's all count for ____ (child)! One, two, three... (add stars to the Star Chart as they are counted aloud)*! Everybody clap for ____ (child)!"* (All behavioral coaches clap and cheer and encourage the children to clap as well.)

Break Time (10 Minutes)

- The puppets may be used to lead the children to and from the bathroom during break time.
- To assist with transitions and limit unstructured time, behavioral coaches may review the lesson with the children while waiting for the remaining children to return from the bathroom.
- You may want to award stars for good behavior after returning from the bathroom.

Session 11 Continued

Swap and Play

BEHAVIORAL REHEARSAL ACTIVITY 2

Materials Needed

- A range of activities or sets of toys (one per dyad/triad).
  - Examples: blocks, drawing materials, toy vehicles, etc.
  - Note: Substitute games/toys as appropriate to match the interests of the children.
- A bean bag for *Hot Potato* at each table.
- Tables and chairs (each table should be large enough to fit two to three children and one behavioral coach).

Room Setup

- Remove or place all carpet squares to the side.
- If tables are available, position tables in different corners of the room with three to four chairs around each table to create an activity area.
  - Two to three children and one behavioral coach will sit at each table.
- Place one activity or one set of toys on each table but out of reach of the children.
- The group leader sits on the floor in front of the room.
- The children and behavioral coaches sit on the floor in a semi-circle facing the group leader.

Rules: Swap and Play

- The group leader reads the script below to explain the rules.
- Divide the children into dyads and assign each group to a table.
  - If there are an odd number of children, create one triad.
  - Assign one behavioral coach per group to ***social coach***.
- Instruct the children to begin playing with the activity or toys available in their play areas.
- After approximately two minutes of play, the group leader will announce, *"FREEZE! And swap!"*
- The behavioral coach at each table will then pick one child to practice ***asking to play something different*** by playing *Hot Potato* using the beanbag.
  - The children should NOT be allowed to reject the other children's bids to ***ask to play something different***.
  - Note: *Hot Potato* was chosen as this is often a favorite game of the children. If *Hot Potato* is not a preferred game, a different highly preferred activity can be chosen for ***asking to play something different***.

- The children should then begin to play *Hot Potato*.
  - Behavioral coaches may need to role play how to play *Hot Potato* (i.e., quickly passing the small beanbag back and forth to one another, acting as if the *Hot Potato* is too hot to hold for more than a second while ***showing and telling*** and ***being good sports***).
- After approximately two minutes of playing *Hot Potato*, the group leader will announce, *"FREEZE! And swap!"*
- Behavioral coaches will then rotate the children to a new table with new activities and toys where they will practice the next cycle of ***asking to play something different***.
- Repeat the cycle, making sure that each child has multiple turns ***asking to play something different.***

Behavioral Rehearsal: Swap and Play (15 Minutes)

The group leader explains the activity. The behavioral coaches and children sit nearby as the group leader explains the rules.

Group leader: *"Hey friends, now we're going to play a game called Swap and Play."*

"You'll each start by playing with the toys at your table, like ____ (list out activities and toys). Then after a few minutes, we'll say, "FREEZE! And swap!" Can everyone show me how to freeze?" (Demonstrate how to freeze in place along with the children and behavioral coaches.)

"Nice job freezing, friends! Next, you'll practice asking to play something different with a friend, like Hot Potato! (Demonstrate playing *Hot Potato* with a nearby behavioral coach for a few turns.)

"When you practice asking to play something different, you can think of something fun to play by looking at your friend with your (point to your eyes to prompt the children to say *"eyes"*)*...EYES and smiling with your* (point to your mouth to prompt the children to say *"mouth"*)*...MOUTH when you say, 'Let's play Hot Potato!' And don't forget to use* (pause briefly to prompt the children to say *"names"*)*...NAMES."*

"After a few more minutes, we'll freeze and swap games again by moving to a new table with new games and toys, and you'll practice asking to play something different some more."

"Okay, let's have ____ (behavioral coach 1) and ____ (behavioral coach 2) try first!"

Role Play: Swap and Play

The group leader will lead the role play. The two behavioral coaches demonstrate how to ***ask to play something different***. (Note: In the role play, the behavioral coaches will always accept the other coach's bid to ***play something different*** to discourage children from rejecting each other's bids during their play.)

Behavioral coaches 1 and 2:	(Sit at one of the play areas and play cooperatively while ***showing and telling*** and ***being good sports*** for a few moments.)
Group leader:	*"Okay ____ (behavioral coaches 1 and 2), FREEZE! And swap!"*
Behavioral coaches 1 and 2:	(Stop playing, freeze in place, and listen to the group leader.)
Group leader:	*"It's time to ask to play something different. ____ (Behavioral coach 1), you go first. Pretend you want to play Hot Potato instead. What should you do?"*
Behavioral coach 1:	(Turn to look at behavioral coach 2 and smile.) *"____ (Behavioral coach 2), let's play Hot Potato!"*
Behavioral coach 2:	*"Okay, ____ (behavioral coach 1)!"*
Group leader:	*"Great job asking to play something different, ____ (behavioral coach 1)!"*
Behavioral coaches 1 and 2:	(Pick up the beanbag and play *Hot Potato* for a few moments while ***showing and telling*** and ***being good sports***.)
Group leader:	*"Okay, FREEZE! And swap! Now you're going to move to the table with ____ (activity at the table) and ____ (behavioral coach 2) is going to ask to play something different."*
	(Behavioral coaches 1 and 2 move tables.)
Behavioral coach 2:	*"____ (Behavioral coach 1), let's play____ (activity at the table)!"*
Behavioral coach 1:	*"Okay, ____ (behavioral coach 2)!"*
Group leader:	*"Great job asking to play something different, ____ (behavioral coach 2)!"*
Behavioral coaches 1 and 2:	(Play cooperatively while ***showing and telling*** and ***being good sports*** for a few moments.)
Group leader:	*"Okay ____ (behavioral coach 1 and 2), FREEZE! And swap!"*
Behavioral coaches 1 and 2:	(Stop playing, freeze in place, and listen to the group leader.)
Group leader:	*"It's time to ask to play something different. ____ (Behavioral coach 1), it's your turn. Pretend you want to play Hot Potato instead. What should you do?"*

Behavioral coach 1:	(Turn to look at behavioral coach 2 and smile.) *"____ (Behavioral coach 2), let's play Hot Potato!"*
Behavioral coach 2:	*"Okay, ____ (behavioral coach 1)!"*
Behavioral coaches 1 and 2	(Pick up the beanbag and play *Hot Potato* for a few moments while ***showing and telling*** and ***being good sports***.)
Group leader:	*"Great job asking to play something different, ____ (behavioral coaches 1 and 2)! Okay friends, now it's everybody's turn to play Swap and Play. Are we ready?"*

Behavioral Rehearsal: Swap and Play

Children are directed to activity areas. The behavioral coaches ***social coach*** the children in dyads or triads to ***ask to play something different*** during the game playing.

Behavioral coach:	*"Okay friends, we're going to start by playing ____ (activity). In a few minutes we're going to swap games and practice asking to play something different so be ready!"* (Children will play with the games and toys at their table for approximately TWO MINUTES. If needed, behavioral coachcs should ***social coach*** the children to ***show and tell, share and take turns***, and ***be good sports***.)
Group leader:	*"Okay friends, FREEZE! And swap! It's time to practice asking to play something different."*
Behavioral coach:	(Pick the first child to practice ***asking to play something different***.) *"____ (Child), pretend you want to play Hot Potato instead. Show us how to ask to play something different and think of something fun to play like Hot Potato."* (If needed, behavioral coaches should ***social coach*** the children to ***ask to play something different***.) (If needed, behavioral coaches should ***social coach*** the children to accept the play request.) (Children will play *Hot Potato* for approximately TWO MINUTES. If needed, behavioral coaches should ***social coach*** the children ***to show and tell, share and take turns and be good sports***.)
Group leader:	*"Okay friends, FREEZE! And swap! Great job asking to play something different! Let's swap games again!"*

Behavioral coaches: (Rotate the children to a new table with new activities and toys where they will practice the next cycle of ***asking to play something different***. Behavioral coaches will move tables with the children.)

Repeat the sequence above making sure that each child has multiple turns ***asking to play something different.***

Behavioral Rehearsal Wrap-Up

Group leader: *"Well friends, great job asking to play something different! Give yourselves a big round of applause!"* (All behavioral coaches clap and cheer and encourage the children to clap as well.)

"Now everyone should come sit in the Listening Circle." (Have children return to the Listening Circle to sit on their carpet squares.)

"Okay friends, you did such a great job asking to play something different by looking at your friend with your (point to your eyes to prompt the children to say *"eyes"*)*...EYES and smiling with your* (point to your mouth to prompt the children to say *"mouth"*)*...MOUTH when you asked to play something different like Hot Potato. And nice job using* (pause briefly to prompt the children to say *"names"*)*...NAMES!*"

"You each earned ____ (number) more stars for asking to play something different! Let's start with ____ (child)."

Award each child the same number of stars by repeating the following with each child:

Group leader: *"Where's _____ (child)?"* (Wait until all the children are looking at the child.)

"_____ (Child), how many stars did you earn?" (Pause briefly to allow the child to respond.)

"That's right! Let's all count for _____ (child)! One, two, three... (add stars to the Star Chart as they are counted aloud)*! Everybody clap for _____ (child)!"* (All behavioral coaches clap and cheer and encourage the children to clap as well.)

Session 11 Continued

Asking to Play Something Different

PARENT COACHED PLAY: DYADIC PLAYDATES

Materials Needed

- Games brought by children and parents from home.
- Turn-taking games provided by the treatment team.
- Set of toys provided by the treatment team (e.g., blocks, Legos, drawing materials, toy vehicles, toy animals).
- Tables and chairs or carpet squares.
- *Parent Coached Play Cards*.

Room Setup

- If available, organize tables in separate corners of the room with four to six chairs per table.
- If tables are not available, place two carpet squares in separate corners of the room to indicate where the children will sit.

Rules: Dyadic Playdates

- The group leader divides the families into groups of two families each.
    - If there are an odd number of children, pair one child with a behavioral coach who will serve as a ***playmate***. In this case, you will need an additional coach to serve as a behavioral coach for the parent.
- Assign each group to sit at a table or specific play area.
    - Children should sit next to each other.
    - Parents will act as ***social coaches*** by sitting on the other side of their child to minimize interrupting the natural flow of play between the children.
    - One behavioral coach will be assigned to each dyad to provide ***social coaching*** suggestions and feedback to parents.
- Children will begin by playing with the sets of toys provided by the treatment team (e.g., blocks, Legos, drawing materials, toy vehicles, toy animals).
- Parents help the children set up the activity in a cooperative fashion (handing each other the toys, offering suggestions, etc.).
- After approximately one minute of play, instruct the parents to prepare the children for the upcoming game swap.

- After approximately one additional minute of play (two minutes total of game playing), the group leader will instruct the parents to swap games and to ***social coach*** their children to ***ask to play something different***.
- The parent of the child whose game is chosen first should ***social coach*** their child to ***ask to play something different***.
- If needed, parents will ***social coach*** the children to accept each other's requests.
  - The children should NOT be allowed to reject the other children's bid to ***play something different***.
- After approximately six minutes of play, instruct the parents to prepare the children for the upcoming game swap.
- After approximately one additional minute of play (seven minutes total of game playing), the group leader will instruct the parents to swap games and to ***social coach*** their children to ***ask to play something different***.
- The parent of the child whose game was NOT chosen first should ***social coach*** their child to ***ask to play something different***.
- If needed, parents will ***social coach*** the children to accept each other's requests.
  - The children should NOT be allowed to reject the other children's bid to ***play something different***.
- After approximately six minutes of play, instruct the parents to prepare the children for clean up.
- After approximately one additional minute of play (seven minutes total of game playing), parents will ***social coach*** the children to clean up and return to the Listening Circle.

Behavioral Coaching: Dyadic Playdates

Behavioral coaches will ***social coach*** parents during dyadic ***playdates*** in the following ways:

- ***Priming*:**
  - Begin the play interactions with parents going over the rules for ***asking a friend to play*** BEFORE GAME PLAYING.
    - Example: *"Remember to ask to play something different by looking with your* (point to your eyes to prompt the child to say *"eyes"*)*...EYES and smiling with your* (point to your mouth to prompt the child to say *"mouth"*)*...MOUTH when you ask to play something different. And if your friend says no, remember to keep cool and play nicely by saying, 'Okay' using names."*
- ***Prompting*:**
  - Remind parents to use the buzzwords to ***prompt*** their child to ***ask to play something different*** IN THE MOMENT.
    - Example: *"Remember to ask to play something different if you get bored."*
    - Example: *"Don't forget to think of something fun to play."*
    - Example: *"Should you keep cool if your friend says no?"*
- ***Praising*:**
  - Remind parents to ***praise*** and reinforce their child when their child ***asks to play something different*** CORRECTLY.
    - Example: *"Great job asking to play something different!"*
    - Example: *"Great job thinking of something fun to play!'"*

    - Example: *"Good job keeping cool and playing nicely!"*
- ***Providing corrective feedback using a praise sandwich***:
  - Remind parents to ***praise*** their child's ATTEMPTS to ***ask to play something different*** and identify what could be done differently next time.
    - Example: *"Nice try asking to play something different. Remember to think of something fun to play next time, but good job!"*
    - Example: *"Good job asking to play something different. Remember to look and smile next time, but nice try!"*
    - Example: *"Nice try thinking of something fun to play. Don't forget to keep cool and play nicely next time, but great job!"*
- Reminding parents to continue to ***social coach*** on previously learned skills:
  - ***Listening and following directions.***
  - ***Meeting and greeting friends.***
  - ***Sharing and giving a turn.***
  - ***Asking for a turn.***
  - ***Keeping cool.***
  - ***Being a good sport.***
  - ***Showing and telling.***
  - ***Don't be bossy.***
  - ***Asking a friend to play.***
  - ***Joining a game***

Parent Coached Play: Dyadic Playdates (20 Minutes)

- Have each child choose a turn-taking game brought from home or provided by the treatment team.
- The group leader sits on the floor at the front of the room.
- The families sit on the floor in a semi-circle facing the group leader.

Group leader: *"Hey friends, we're going to have more playdates and play with the fun games you brought from home. First you'll play with the toys we provided in your play area. After a few minutes, you'll practice asking to play something different by looking at your friend with your* (point to your eyes to prompt the children to say *"eyes"*)*...EYES and smiling with your* (point to your mouth to prompt the children to say *"mouth"*)*...MOUTH and thinking of something fun to play by saying, 'Let's play ____ (game brought in by a child)!'* (point to the game brought in by a child) *or 'Let's play ____ (another game brought in by a child)!'* (point to the game brought in by a child). *And don't forget to use (pause briefly to prompt the children to say "names")...NAMES."*

"You'll play for a few more minutes before you'll practice asking to play something different again. Parents, remember to social coach your children by using your Parent Coached Play Cards. Okay, let's play with our games!"

- Before playing, parents will ***social coach*** their child to ***say*** "***hi***" to one another ***using names***.
- Children begin by playing with the sets of toys provided by the treatment team.
- Parents help the children set up the activity in a cooperative fashion.

- After approximately one minute of play, the behavioral coach will instruct the parents to prepare the children for the upcoming game swap by saying, *"Parents, tell your children that we'll be swapping games and asking to play something different in one minute."*
- After approximately one additional minute of play (two minutes total of game playing), the behavioral coach will instruct the parents to swap games by saying, *"Parents, it's time to swap games. Social coach the children to ask to play something different and keep cool by cleaning up and playing the next game."*
  - The parent of the child whose game was chosen first should ***social coach*** their child to ***ask to play something different***.
  - The children should NOT be allowed to reject the other children's bid to ***play something different***.
- After approximately six minutes of play, the behavioral coach will instruct the parents to prepare the children for the upcoming game swap by saying, *"Parents, tell your children that we'll be swapping games and asking to play something different in one minute."*
- After approximately one additional minute of play (seven minutes total of game playing), the behavioral coach will instruct the parents to swap games by saying, *"Parents, it's time to swap games. Social coach the children to ask to play something different and keep cool by cleaning up and playing the next game."*
  - The parent of the child whose game was NOT chosen first should ***social coach*** their child to ***ask to play something different***.
  - The children should NOT be allowed to reject the other children's bid to ***play something different***.
- After approximately six minutes of play, instruct the parents to prepare the children for clean up by saying, *"Parents, tell your children that we'll be cleaning up in one minute."*
- After approximately one additional minute of play (seven minutes total of game playing), ***prompt*** the parents to instruct their children to clean up by saying, *"Parents, it's time to clean up. Let's social coach the children to listen and follow directions by cleaning up and then say 'bye' to their friend using names before sitting in the Listening Circle."*
- If needed, parents will ***social coach*** their child to ***listen and follow directions*** to clean up.
- Then parents will ***social coach*** their child to ***say*** "***bye***" to their friend ***using names.***

Final Wrap-Up (10 minutes)

- The group leader sits on the floor at the front of the room.
- The children sit on the carpet squares in a semi-circle facing the group leader, with parents sitting behind their children.

Group leader: *"Okay friends, you all did a great job playing your games and asking to play something different. When we want to play something different, do you think we should LOOK at our friend with our EYES and SMILE with our MOUTH?"* (Pause briefly to allow children to respond *"yes."*)

"That's right, friends! And when we think of something fun to play, do you think we should ask to play something different by saying, "Let's play cars" or "Let's play blocks" and use names?" (Pause briefly to allow children to respond *"yes."*)

"That's right, friends! But sometimes our friends will say no or maybe later. Do you think we should keep cool and play nicely with our friends? (Pause briefly to allow children to respond *"yes."*)

"That's right, friends! You all did such a great job asking to play something different today that you each earned ____ (number) more stars! Let's start with ____ (child)."

Award each child the same number of stars by repeating the following with each child:

Group leader: *"Where's _____ (child)?" (Wait until all the children are looking at the child.)*

"_____ (Child), how many stars did you earn?" (Pause briefly to allow the child to respond.)

"That's right! Let's all count for _____ (child)! One, two, three... (add stars to the Star Chart as they are counted aloud)*! Everybody clap for _____ (child)!"* (All behavioral coaches clap and cheer and encourage the children to clap as well.)

"And remember you all earned those stars by asking to play something different! Everyone did a great job, and parents you did an excellent job social coaching! Parents, remember your homework assignments this week are for you and your children to practice asking to play something different and for you to continue practicing all the other things we've learned to be a good friend using the 4 Ps. And don't forget to have a playdate and go to your playgroups."

"Alright little friends, do you want to count our stars?" (Pause briefly to allow the children to respond.)

"Let's all count together and see how many stars we earned today! One, two, three...(count the number of stars for one child)*!"*

"You each earned ____ (total number) stars today! Round of applause for our friends!" (All behavioral coaches should clap and cheer and encourage the families to clap as well.)

"Great job, friends! Don't forget to choose your reward before you leave. See you all next week!"

Session 11 Continued

Asking to Play Something Different

PEERS® FOR PRESCHOOLERS: PARENT HANDOUT

Snapshot of the Lesson: Asking to Play Something Different

The objective of this lesson is to teach children how to ***ask to play something different.*** Steps for ***asking to play something different*** include:

1. ***Think of something fun to play*** (point to your head).
2. ***Look at your friends with your eyes*** (point to your eyes).
3. ***Smile with your mouth*** (point to your mouth and smile).
4. ***Ask to play something different using names*** (e.g., ***"(Friend), let's play _____!"***).

If your friend says no:

1. ***Keep cool and play nicely.***
2. ***Look at your friends with your eyes*** (point to your eyes).
3. ***Smile with your mouth*** (point to your mouth and smile).
4. ***Say "okay" using names.***
5. ***Play nicely with your friends.***
6. If you're still upset, then ***take deep breaths to keep cool*** (take two slow ***deep breaths***).

Parent Social Coaching Strategies for Asking to Play Something Different

- **Help your child *think of something fun to play.***
  - When practicing ***asking to play something different***, parents may need to ***social coach*** their child to ***think of something fun to play***.
  - When practicing during the week, at first parents may need to provide choices for other fun toys or games their child can play with.
    - Example: *"If you want to play something different, we have trains or Bingo."*
    - Make sure that the available choices are preferred and fun for your child.
    - This will increase the chances that they will want to use the skills.
    - If your goal is to target flexibility, then that skill should be targeted separately – not when practicing ***asking to play something different***.

- Remember, it is important not to target too many new skills at once as this can be frustrating and less motivating for your child.

- **Help your child to identify alternative games prior to *playdates*.**
  - When planning ***playdates*** using the ***5 Ws***, we often have an idea of what the activity will be in advance (i.e., the "***what***" in the ***5 Ws***).
  - Be prepared that your child and/or their ***playmate*** may get bored and want to ***play something different***.
  - Prior to the ***playdate***, help your child come up with a list of possible alternative activities that your child and their ***playmate*** might play.
  - You may need to ***social coach*** your child to choose activities that are fun for BOTH your child and their ***playmate***.
    - If you are unsure what games and toys the ***playmate*** likes, consider asking the parents of the ***playmate*** for some ideas.
  - Be sure to let your child know in advance that they may not be able to play ALL these activities during the ***playdate***.

- **Have alternative activities visible but not accessible during *playdates*.**
  - In the moment, parents should have a range of activities that are visible but NOT accessible to your child to help your child ***think of something fun to play*** that is a ***common interest*** with their ***playmate***.
    - These items should be from the list of alternative activities discussed with your child prior to the ***playdate***.
  - By choosing activities and toys that are ***common interests,*** the ***playmate*** may be more open to ***playing something different***.
    - A ***playmate's*** agreement to ***play something different*** will naturally reinforce your child's use of the skill and increases the chances that your child will use the skills in the future.
  - If your child or their ***playmate*** do not agree on what to play differently, you might suggest taking turns playing both activities.
    - Allow your child's ***playmate*** to have the first turn since they are the guest.
    - Be sure to give a one-minute alert when switching activities as this will promote an easier transition.
  - If your child or their ***playmate*** becomes upset that there is not enough time to play with ALL the toys and games, you might suggest that they have another ***playdate*** to play with the other games and toys.

- **Help your child to *keep cool* if the *playmate* doesn't want to *play something different.***
  - If your child's friend does not want to ***play something different***, then parents may need to ***social coach*** their child to ***keep cool***.
    - Parents may need to ***social coach*** their child to ***take deep breaths*** to ***keep cool***.
    - Parents may even want to demonstrate ***taking deep breaths*** with their child to encourage them to use the skills.
    - ***Praise*** them immediately when they use the skills for ***keeping cool***.

- **Have your child practice taking "no" for an answer.**
  - When practicing ***asking to play something different*** with your child during the week, parents may want to practice saying "no" (e.g., *"Next time"* or *"Maybe later"* or *"No thanks"* or *"Not now"*) and have your child ***keep cool***.
  - Parents should ***prompt*** their child BEFORE practicing ***taking "no" for an answer***.
    - Example: *"Okay, let's practice keeping cool if I say no. Remember to keep cool and play nicely."*
    - Remember to ***praise*** them when they use the skills for ***keeping cool***.

- **Practice playing less preferred activities and games if your child has difficulty *keeping cool* when taking "no" for an answer.**
  - Some children will initially get upset if their attempts to ***ask to play something different*** are turned down for highly preferred activities.
  - In initially helping your child to ***keep cool***, parents should practice having their child suggest new activities that are neutral or less preferred by your child.
    - This is likely to make it easier for your child to initially practice the skills for ***keeping cool*** when hearing "no."
    - As your child improves in ***keeping cool***, parents may gradually have the child ***keep cool*** when suggesting new activities that are more preferred or fun for your child.

- **Practice *playing nicely* when offers to *play something different* are turned down.**
  - Parents may need to ***social coach*** their child to not only ***keep cool*** but also continue ***playing nicely*** with their friend.
  - If your child has difficulty continuing to ***play nicely***, explain that they are simply ***taking turns*** with game playing (e.g., friends take turns choosing games and toys to play with).
    - Example: *"Remember to play nicely by giving a turn to your friend in choosing the game."*
  - If you discover that your child's ***playmate*** rarely allows your child to choose the games or toys, and this bothers your child, then consider whether this is a good choice in ***playmate*** for your child moving forward.

Homework Assignments

1. **Playdates.**
   - Schedule and have a ***playdate*** with a ***playmate***.
   - Prepare for the ***playdate*** using the ***5 Ws***.
     - ***WHO: Playdates*** should be one-on-one.
     - ***WHAT: Playdates*** should be activity-based.
     - ***WHERE:*** Schedule initial ***playdates*** to take place in your home or somewhere you can provide ***social coaching***.
     - ***WHEN:*** Try to keep initial ***playdates*** to no more than 1–1.5 hours.
     - ***HOW:*** Coordinate how the children will get to and from the ***playdate***.
   - Do a final practice with your child of the games and activities that will be available during the ***playdate***.

- Gather all the games and activity materials for the ***playdate*** in one area that is VISIBLE and easily accessible to YOU but not the children.
- Provide ***social coaching*** during the ***playdate*** and assess if this is a good ***playmate*** for your child.

2. **Practice asking to play something different.**
   - Practice having your child ***ask to play something different*** this week while providing ***social coaching*** using the ***4 Ps***.
     - ***Priming:*** Review the rules for ***asking to play something different*** with your child BEFORE PRACTICING.
     - ***Prompting:*** Remind your child IN THE MOMENT to ***ask to play something different*** whenever the opportunities present.
     - ***Praising: Praise*** your child using the buzzwords whenever they ***ask to play something different*** CORRECTLY.
     - ***Providing corrective feedback: Provide corrective feedback*** in the form of a ***praise sandwich*** whenever your child ATTEMPTS to ***ask to play something different.***
   - Please send us a 30–60-second video of ***social coaching*** your child to ***ask to play something different*** to be viewed during homework review.
     - Please include:
       - Skills your child did well.
       - Skills you would like to work on with your child.

3. **Provide social coaching on previously learned skills.**
   - Continue providing ***social coaching*** to your child throughout the week using the ***4 Ps.***
   - Previous skills include:
     - ***Listening and following directions.***
     - ***Meeting and greeting friends.***
     - ***Sharing and giving a turn.***
     - ***Asking for a turn.***
     - ***Keeping cool.***
     - ***Being a good sport.***
     - ***Showing and telling.***
     - ***Don't be bossy.***
     - ***Asking a friend to play.***
     - ***Joining a game.***

4. **Bring a turn-taking game.**
   - Bring a turn-taking game that your child enjoys playing and can be played with the other children.

Session 11 Continued

Asking to Play Something Different

PEERS® FOR PRESCHOOLERS: PARENT COACHED PLAY CARDS

Snapshot of the Lesson: Asking to Play Something Different

1. ***Think of something fun to play*** (point to your head).
2. ***Look at your friends with your eyes*** (point to your eyes).
3. ***Smile with your mouth*** (point to your mouth and smile).
4. ***Ask to play something different using names*** (e.g., ***"(Friend), let's play _____!"***).

If your friend says "no":

1. ***Keep cool and play nicely.***
2. ***Look at your friends with your eyes*** (point to your eyes).
3. ***Smile with your mouth*** (point to your mouth and smile).
4. ***Say "okay" using names.***
5. ***Play nicely with your friends***.
6. If you're still upset, then ***take deep breaths to keep cool*** (take two slow ***deep breaths***).

Priming BEFORE Game Playing

- Example: *"Remember to ask to play something different by looking with your* (point to your eyes to prompt the child to say *"eyes"*)*...EYES and smiling with your* (point to your mouth to prompt the child to say *"mouth"*)*...MOUTH when you ask to play something different. And if your friend says no, remember to keep cool and play nicely by saying, 'Okay' using names."*

Prompting IN THE MOMENT

- Example: *"Remember to ask to play something different if you get bored."*
- Example: *"Don't forget to think of something fun to play."*
- Example: *"Should you keep cool if your friend says no?"*

Praising for CORRECT Use of Skills

- Example: *"Great job asking to play something different!"*
- Example: *"Great job thinking of something fun to play!'"*
- Example: *"Good job keeping cool and playing nicely!"*

Providing Corrective Feedback for ATTEMPTS Using a Praise Sandwich

- Example: *"Nice try asking to play something different. Remember to think of something fun to play next time, but good job!"*
- Example: *"Good job asking to play something different. Remember to look and smile next time, but great job!"*
- Example: *"Nice try thinking of something fun to play. Don't forget to keep cool and play nicely next time, but good try!"*

- Continue to provide ***social coaching*** on previously learned skills:
  - ***Listening and following directions.***
  - ***Meeting and greeting friends.***
  - ***Sharing and giving a turn.***
  - ***Asking for a turn.***
  - ***Keeping cool.***
  - ***Being a good sport.***
  - ***Showing and telling.***
  - ***Don't be bossy.***
  - ***Asking a friend to play.***
  - ***Joining a game.***

Session 11 Continued

Asking to Play Something Different

PEERS® FOR PRESCHOOLERS: PARENT HOMEWORK WORKSHEET

Child's Name:	Parent's Name:		Date:	
HOMEWORK ASSIGNMENTS	PRIMING (REVIEWING RULES BEFORE PRACTICE)	PROMPTING (IN THE MOMENT)	PRAISING (USING BUZZWORDS)	PROVIDING CORRECTIVE FEEDBACK (USING A PRAISE SANDWICH)
Asking to play something different				
Practice previous skills: • **Joining a game** • **Asking a friend to play** • **Don't be bossy** • **Show and tell during play** • **Being a good sport** • **Keeping cool** • **Asking for a turn** • **Sharing and giving turns** • **Meeting and greeting friends** • **Listening and following directions**				

Child's Name:	Parent's Name:		Date:	
HOMEWORK ASSIGNMENTS	PRIMING (REVIEWING RULES BEFORE PRACTICE)	PROMPTING (IN THE MOMENT)	PRAISING (USING BUZZWORDS)	PROVIDING CORRECTIVE FEEDBACK (USING A PRAISE SANDWICH)
Playdate: • **Plan a playdate using the 5 Ws** • **Prime your child before the playdate** • **Provide social coaching during the playdate using the 4 Ps**				
Bring a turn-taking game	Did you bring a turn-taking game? YES or NO (Circle)		Which game did you bring?	

Please fill out this worksheet by describing what you did to complete the homework assignments. Worksheets will be collected during Homework Review at the next session of PEERS® for Preschoolers.

Session 12

Asking and Giving Help

PARENT SESSION THERAPIST GUIDE

Parent Session Agenda

- Homework Review (40 minutes).
- Didactic Lessons (20 minutes).
- Parent Coached Play (20 minutes).
- Final Wrap-Up (10 minutes).

Materials Needed

- Conference room with a large table and enough chairs for the parent group leader and all parents to sit comfortably around the table.
  - Avoid sitting in a circle without a table as this creates the atmosphere of group therapy.
- Name tags for parents and treatment team.
- *Parent Handouts* (for the current week and the previous week).
- *Parent Homework Worksheets* (for the current week and the previous week).
- *Parent Coached Play Cards* (for the current week and the previous week).
- *Attendance and Homework Compliance Sheets* for parent group leader.
- Pens for note-taking (consider having extra pens for parents who need them).

Homework Review (40 Minutes)

1. **Playdates.**
   - Have parents report on the ***playdate*** and confirm that they planned using the ***5 Ws.***
   - Review what parents did to ***social coach*** their child BEFORE, DURING, and AFTER the ***playdate***.
   - Identify what skills their child did well and what skills they need to work on.
     - Confirm that parents ***praised*** skills that were done well and provided ***priming, prompting***, and/or ***corrective feedback*** for emerging skills.
   - Have parents assess if this is a good ***playmate*** for their child.
   - Have parents identify who their child might have a ***playdate*** with in the coming week (does not have to be a different ***playmate***).

2. **Practice asking to play something different.**
   - Review the 30–60-second video of ***social coaching*** for ***asking to play something different*** for each family. (For larger groups, you may need to review video recordings in two smaller groups with two different parent group leaders).

DOI: 10.4324/9781003502968-13

- Have parents identify:
  - Skills their child did well.
  - Skills they would like to work on with their child.
- Provide ***social coaching*** tips as appropriate for each family.

- If parents did not send a video of ***social coaching***, confirm the following:
  - Parents practiced having their child ***ask to play something different*** while providing ***social coaching*** using the ***4 Ps.***
    - ***Priming:*** Reviewed the rules for ***asking to play something different*** with their child BEFORE PRACTICING.
    - ***Prompting:*** Reminded their child IN THE MOMENT to ***ask to play something different*** whenever the opportunity presented.
    - ***Praising: Praised*** their child using the buzzwords whenever they ***asked to play something different*** CORRECTLY.
    - ***Providing corrective feedback: Provided corrective feedback*** in the form of a ***praise sandwich*** whenever their child ATTEMPTED to ***ask to play something different.***

3. **Provide social coaching on previously learned skills.**
   - Confirm parents continued to provide ***social coaching*** to their child throughout the week using the ***4 Ps*** for previously learned skills:
     - ***Listening and following directions.***
     - ***Meeting and greeting friends.***
     - ***Sharing and giving a turn.***
     - ***Asking for a turn.***
     - ***Keeping cool.***
     - ***Being a good sport.***
     - ***Showing and telling.***
     - ***Don't be bossy.***
     - ***Asking a friend to play.***
     - ***Joining a game.***

4. **Bring a turn-taking game.**
   - Confirm the following:
     - Brought a turn-taking game that their child enjoys playing and can be played with the other children. (To avoid distractions, these games should be left with the parents until *Parent Coached Play*.)

Didactic Lessons (20 Minutes)

PEERS® Neuroaffirming Pledge:

- We value neurodiversity, acceptance, and authenticity.
- We honor the diverse ways people experience the world.
- We respect each person's unique perspectives and communication styles.
- We recognize there is no one right way to connect with others.
- If using the strategies taught in PEERS® feels like camouflaging or masking and/or they don't align with your goals or the goals of your family, then you do not have to use them.
- Learning and using the skills taught in PEERS® is a PERSONAL CHOICE.

Didactic Lesson: Asking and Giving Help

- Distribute *Parent Handouts*.
  - Sections in **bold print** come directly from the *Parent Handout*.
  - Terms that are ***bold and italicized*** are buzzwords and represent important concepts from the didactic lesson.
- Explain, *"Today's lesson will focus on helping your children learn to ask and give help. While knowing how to ask and give help is important to friendships, these skills are also transferable and can be used in different settings with different people, like at home or in school. Before we go over how you can support your child's attempts to ask and give help, we will begin with going over the child didactic lesson to give you a framework on which to think about social coaching strategies."*

Snapshot of the Lesson: Asking and Giving Help

The objective of this lesson is to teach children how to *ask and give help.* The steps for *asking and giving help* include:

Asking for Help

1. ***Look at your friends with your eyes*** **(point to your eyes).**
2. ***Smile with your mouth*** **(point to your mouth and smile).**
3. ***Say, "Can you help me?" using names.***

Giving Help

1. ***Look at your friends with your eyes*** **(point to your eyes).**
2. ***Smile with your mouth*** **(point to your mouth and smile).**
3. ***Say "okay" using names.***
4. ***Give help to your friend.***

Parent Social Coaching Strategies for Asking and Giving Help

- **Provide opportunities to practice *asking and giving help* during games and activities that are highly motivating for your child.**
  - ***Prime*** **your child that they will be practicing *asking and giving help* by going over the rules and steps first.**
  - **Make the practice more rewarding by pairing it with a highly preferred activity.**
  - **Do not surprise your child in the middle of playing a highly preferred activity by suggesting that they practice *asking and giving help.***
    - **The rehearsal will distract from the preferred activity and they will be less motivated to practice.**

- **Playing the highly preferred activity should be contingent on practicing *asking and giving help.***

- ***Praise* and relabel natural instances of your child *asking and giving help* using the buzzwords.**
  - **Your child will naturally *ask and give help* throughout the week.**
  - **Be on the lookout for these naturally occurring behaviors and *praise* them using the buzzwords.**
    - **Example: "Great job *asking for help* to put your shoes on!"**
    - **Example: "Nice job *giving me help* with the snacks!"**
  - **By reframing and labeling their behavior using *praise*, your child will be more motivated to *ask and give help* in the future.**

- **Use opportunities that naturally occur throughout the day to have your child practice *asking and giving help.***
  - **Examples of opportunities for your child to *ask and give help*:**
    - **Setting up and cleaning up games or play activities.**
    - **Getting dressed, putting on shoes, etc.**
    - **Preparing snacks and meals.**
    - **Opening doors for family members.**
    - **Helping to carry things.**
    - **Holding their own backpacks.**
    - **Helping to find items in the grocery store.**

- **When practicing *asking and giving help*, keep initial practice opportunities short.**
  - **This is likely to help your child feel more successful and less frustrated.**
  - **Remember to immediately *praise* their efforts at *asking and giving help.***
  - **In the context of games and activities, it may also help the children to learn that *asking and giving help*:**
    - **Will not take away from being able to play the game or activity.**
    - **Will make it easier to play the game or activity.**
    - **Will increase the time spent having fun playing the game or activity.**

- **Create opportunities to *ask and give help* by completing most of the steps of a game or fun activity and having your child complete the last one or two steps.**
  - **By having your child help in completing the last few steps, they will be reinforced and rewarded for *asking and giving help.***
  - **By pairing *asking and giving help* with a reward (e.g., game playing), we create an immediate reinforcement for using the skills with natural reinforcement contingencies.**
    - Example: When playing the game *Memory*, you might position most of the cards and then hand your child the remaining cards while ***social coaching*** them to ***give help*** by saying, *"Can you help me put down the rest of the cards?"* Once your child lays down the remaining cards, ***praise*** them by saying, *"Great job giving help!"*
  - **As *asking and giving help* becomes easier, parents may want to gradually increase the number of steps completed by their child.**

- **Practice *asking and giving help* by having your child take turns with siblings and *playmates.***

- **Consider having your child's sibling or *playmate* complete a few steps of some action, then *social coach* your child to *give help* by completing the remaining steps.**
  - Example: When playing the game *Jenga*, your child's sibling or ***playmate*** might lay down several blocks to build a tower, then ask your child to ***give help*** by completing the tower.
- **Have your child initiate some action and before completing the sequence of steps, *social coach* your child to *ask for help* from a sibling or *playmate* to complete the remaining steps.**
  - Example: When playing the game *Jenga*, your child might lay down several blocks to build a tower, then ***social coach*** your child to ***ask for help*** by asking their sibling or ***playmate*** to help complete the tower.
- **If your child observes that they are sharing the responsibility of *helping* with siblings and *playmates*, they are less likely to feel frustrated by the practice.**

- **During *playdates* and *playgroups*, redirect your child and their *playmates* to *ask and give help* to each other rather than first relying on adult assistance.**
  - ***Playdates* and *playgroups* offer natural social opportunities to *ask and give help.***
  - **Children will often seek help from adults to complete certain tasks during *playdates* and *playgroups.***
  - **If the task is not too difficult, consider having your child *ask and give help* by saying, *"How about asking your friend for help"* or *"Why don't you help your friend."***
    - Example: If your child or their ***playmate asks for help*** in building something using blocks or Legos, ***social coach*** them to ***ask for help*** by saying, *"Why don't you ask _______ (child) for help? They might know how to do it."*
  - **The collateral gains of *social coaching* your child and their *playmates* to *ask and give help* during *playdates* and *playgroups* include:**
    - **The children assuming an "expert role" during that game or activity.**
    - **Encouraging and reinforcing more cooperative, reciprocal play interactions.**

Parent Coached Play

- Distribute the *Parent Coached Play Cards.*
- Review the examples of the ***4 Ps*** provided on the *Parent Coached Play Card.*
- Remind parents that in a few moments we will be joining the children for *Parent Coached Play* in the context of mock dyadic ***playdates***.
- Parents should keep the *Parent Coached Play Card* in front of them during the dyadic ***playdate*** for recommendations on how to ***social coach*** children on ***asking and giving help***.

Homework Assignments

(Briefly review the homework assignments and troubleshoot any potential problems with parents.)

1. **Playdates.**
   - **Schedule and have a *playdate* with a *playmate*.**
   - **Prepare for the *playdate* using the *5 Ws*.**
     - ***WHO: Playdates* should be one-on-one.**

- ◦ ***WHAT: Playdates* should be activity-based.**
- ◦ ***WHERE:* Schedule initial *playdates* to take place in your home or somewhere you can provide *social coaching.***
- ◦ ***WHEN:* Try to keep initial *playdates* to no more than 1–1.5 hours.**
- ◦ ***HOW:* Coordinate how the children will get to and from the *playdate.***

- **Do a final practice with your child of the games and activities that will be available during the *playdate.***
- **Gather all the games and activity materials for the *playdate* in one area that is VISIBLE and easily accessible to YOU but not the children.**
- **Provide *social coaching* during the *playdate* and assess if this is a good *playmate* for your child.**

2. **Practice asking and giving help.**
   - **Practice having your child *ask and give help* this week while providing *social coaching* using the *4 Ps.***
     - ◦ ***Priming:* Review the rules for *asking and giving help* with your child BEFORE PRACTICING.**
     - ◦ ***Prompting:* Remind your child IN THE MOMENT to *ask and give help* whenever the opportunities present.**
     - ◦ ***Praising: Praise* your child using the buzzwords whenever they *ask and give help* CORRECTLY.**
     - ◦ ***Providing corrective feedback: Provide corrective feedback* in the form of a *praise sandwich* whenever your child ATTEMPTS to *ask and give help.***
   - **Please send us a 30–60-second video of *social coaching* your child to *ask and give help* to be viewed during homework review.**
     - ◦ **Please include:**
       - ▪ **Skills your child did well.**
       - ▪ **Skills you would like to work on with your child.**

3. **Provide social coaching on previously learned skills.**
   - **Continue providing *social coaching* to your child throughout the week using the *4 Ps.***
   - **Previous skills include:**
     - ◦ ***Listening and following directions.***
     - ◦ ***Meeting and greeting friends.***
     - ◦ ***Sharing and giving a turn.***
     - ◦ ***Asking for a turn.***
     - ◦ ***Keeping cool.***
     - ◦ ***Being a good sport.***
     - ◦ ***Showing and telling.***
     - ◦ ***Don't be bossy.***
     - ◦ ***Asking a friend to play.***
     - ◦ ***Joining a game.***
     - ◦ ***Asking to play something different.***

4. **Bring a turn-taking game.**
   - **Bring a turn-taking game that your child enjoys playing and can be played with the other children.**

Session 12 Continued

Asking and Giving Help

CHILD SESSION THERAPIST GUIDE

Child Session Agenda

- Didactic Lesson: *Asking and Giving Help* (20 minutes).
- Group Behavioral Rehearsal Activity 1: *Tinker Toy Town* (15 minutes).
- Break Time (10 minutes).
- Group Behavioral Rehearsal Activity 2: *Hot or Cold* (15 minutes).
- Parent Coached Play: *Dyadic Playdates* (20 minutes).
- Final Wrap-Up (10 minutes).

Snapshot of the Lesson: Asking and Giving Help

The objective of this lesson is to teach children how to ***ask and give help.*** The steps for ***asking and giving help*** include:

Asking for Help

1. ***Look at your friends with your eyes*** (point to your eyes).
2. ***Smile with your mouth*** (point to your mouth and smile).
3. ***Say, "Can you help me?" using names***.

Giving Help

1. ***Look at your friends with your eyes*** (point to your eyes).
2. ***Smile with your mouth*** (point to your mouth and smile).
3. ***Say "okay" using names***.
4. ***Give help to your friend***.

Materials Needed

- Monkey puppet.
- Lion puppet.
- Building blocks or Legos.
- A toy box with a lid for building blocks and Legos.
- Carpet squares or chairs.
- Making Friends Helper" badge.
- Star chart with names of children.
- Marker for star chart.
- Name tags for families and treatment team.
- Prize bins with prizes.

Preparing for the Lesson

- Use the script below with the group leader using a monkey puppet to play the part of "Mikey Monkey."
- A behavioral coach uses a lion puppet to play the part of "Larry Lion."
- An additional behavioral coach assists in behavioral rehearsal and provides encouragement and feedback to the group.
- A child is chosen at the beginning of the lesson as the "Making Friends Helper."
  - The "Making Friends Helper" wears a special badge and is the first child to practice the skill.
- The group leader and the behavioral coach sit on the floor at the front of the room.
- A special-colored carpet square (e.g., red) is placed at the front of the room next to the child group leader to be used as the "Good Friend Square."
- For the children, additional carpet squares of the same color (e.g., green) are placed in a semi-circle facing the child group leader and the "Good Friend Square."
- Note: If carpet squares are unavailable, the children and behavioral coach may sit on chairs.
- The material in *italics* should be read by the indicated person.
- The material in ***bold and italics*** represents buzzwords and should be emphasized when read.
- The material in CAPITAL LETTERS within the script should be given extra emphasis while the group is encouraged to say the words in unison.

Behavioral Coaching Techniques

Behavioral coaches should use the following coaching techniques described below throughout the lesson and the behavioral rehearsal activities. (Note: ***priming*** occurs during the introduction to the activity.)

- ***Prompting***:
  - Use the buzzwords to ***prompt*** the children to ***ask and give help***.
    - Example: *"Remember to ask for help."*
    - Example: *"Remember to give help if your friend needs help."*
    - Example: *"What should you say to ask for help?"*
- ***Praising***:
  - Reinforce ***asking and giving help*** by ***praising*** the children.
    - Example: *"Great job asking for help!"*
    - Example: *"Good job looking and smiling when you gave your friend help!"*
    - Example: *"Good job saying, 'Can you help me?'"*
- ***Providing corrective feedback using a praise sandwich***:
  - Reinforce ATTEMPTS to ***ask and give help*** by ***praising*** the children and identifying what could be done differently next time.
    - Example: *"Good job giving your friend help. Remember to say 'okay' next time, but nice job!"*
    - Example: *"Nice job asking for help. Don't forget to look at me, but good job!"*
    - Example: *"Nice try asking for help. Next time, don't forget to use names, but good try!"*
- Behavioral coach should continue to ***social coach*** on previously learned skills:
  - ***Listening and following directions.***
  - ***Meeting and greeting friends.***
  - ***Sharing and giving a turn.***
  - ***Asking for a turn.***
  - ***Keeping cool.***
  - ***Being a good sport.***

- ***Showing and telling.***
- ***Don't be bossy.***
- ***Asking a friend to play.***
- ***Joining a game.***
- ***Asking to play something different.***

Didactic Lesson: Asking and Giving Help

Have the children sit in a semi-circle on the carpet squares facing the group leader.

Mikey Monkey: (Sit at the front of the room and choose a Making Friends Helper.) *"Who wants to be our Making Friends Helper?"*

(Choose from among the children raising their hands and place the "Making Friends Helper" badge on the child. The child stays in their seat for now.)

"Hi friends! I'm Mikey Monkey. Ooh, ooh! Today we're going to practice asking and giving help. Asking and giving help are great ways to be nice to our friends!"

"Who should we ask and give help with? We should ask and give help with our FRIENDS, TEACHERS, MOMMIES, DADDIES, BROTHERS, AND SISTERS."

"*When should we ask and give help? We should ask and give help when our friends need help or when we need help, like when we clean up our toys."*

"How should we ask and give help? We should ask for help by looking at our friends with our (point to your eyes and then Larry Lion's eyes to prompt the children to say *"eyes"*)...*EYES, smiling with our* (point to your mouth and smile to prompt the children to say *"mouth"*)...*MOUTH, and then saying, 'Can you help me?' And when our friends need to help, we should give help by saying 'okay.' And don't forget to use* (pause briefly to prompt the children to say *"names"*)...*NAMES!"*

"Remember, asking and giving help are nice ways to be a good friend! Ooh, ooh!"

Role Play: Asking and Giving Help

Mikey Monkey and Larry Lion: (Play with a large pile of blocks for a few moments while ***showing and telling*** and ***being good sports***. The empty toy box with a lid is sitting nearby.)

Behavioral coach: *"Mikey Monkey, it's time to clean up your toys."*

Mikey Monkey:	(Turn to look at the group of children.) *"Hey friends! It's time to clean up but there are so many blocks that I need help. Should I ask my friend Larry Lion for help?"* (Nod your head yes and encourage the children to say *"yes."*) *"That's a great idea! Ooh, ooh! Let's do it!"* (Turn to look at Larry Lion and smile.) *"Larry Lion, can you help me clean up?"*
Larry Lion:	(Turn to look at Mikey Monkey and smile.) *"Okay, Mikey Monkey.* *Grrr, Grrr!"* (Unsuccessfully attempt to open the lid to the empty toy box.) *"Mikey Monkey, I can't open the box. Can you help me?"*
Mikey Monkey:	(Turn to look at the group of children.) *"Hey friends! My friend Larry Lion needs help opening the box. Do you think I should give help to my friend Larry Lion?"* (Nod your head yes and encourage the children to say *"yes."*) *"That's a great idea! Ooh, ooh! Let's do it!"* (Turn to look at Larry Lion and smile.) *"Okay, Larry Lion."*
Larry Lion:	*"Thanks Mikey Monkey! Grrr, grrr!"*
Mikey Monkey and Larry Lion:	(Help Larry Lion open the lid to the toy box. Working together, put the blocks in the toy box.)
Mikey Monkey:	(Turn to look at the group of children.) *"Hey friends, did we do a good job asking and giving help?"* (Nod your head yes and encourage the children to say *"yes."*) *"That's right! Ooh, ooh!"*
Mikey Monkey and Larry Lion:	(Say *"good job," give a "monkey high-five," and "lion high-five,"* clap, cheer, and encourage the children to clap as well. Larry Lion sits on the other side of the Good Friend Square (i.e., the Good Friend Square is between Mikey Monkey and Larry Lion). ***Social coach*** the children as needed while they practice ***asking and giving help*** with Larry Lion.) (Remove the blocks from the toy box. Re-position the pile of blocks and the toy box in between Larry Lion and the Good Friend Square. Place the lid back on the toy box.)
Mikey Monkey:	*"Now let's see _____ (behavioral coach) try! _____ (Behavioral coach), please come sit on the Good Friend Square."*
Behavioral coach:	(Sit on the Good Friend Square.)
Mikey Monkey:	*"_____ (Behavioral coach), can you show us how to ask and give help with Larry Lion?"*
Behavioral coach:	*"Okay, Mikey Monkey."*

Mikey Monkey:	(Turn to look at the group of children.) *"Remember to ask for help by looking at Larry Lion with your* (point to your eyes to prompt the children to say *"eyes"*)*...EYES and smiling with your* (point to your mouth to prompt the children to say *"mouth"*)*...MOUTH when you say, 'Can you help me?' And if Larry Lion needs help, you should give help by saying 'okay.' And don't forget to use* (pause briefly to prompt the children to say *"names"*)*...NAMES!"*
Larry Lion:	(Turn to look at the behavioral coach member and smile.) *"Hey _____ (behavioral coach), let's play blocks!"*
Behavioral coach:	(Turn to look at Larry Lion and smile.) *"Okay, Larry Lion!"*
Larry Lion and Behavioral coach:	(Play with the large pile of blocks for a few moments while ***showing and telling*** and **being good sports**. The empty toy box with a lid is sitting nearby.)
Mikey Monkey:	*"_____ (Behavioral coach), it's time to clean up your toys."*
Behavioral coach:	(Look at the large pile of blocks and act frustrated.) *"Hmm ... there are too many blocks!"*
Mikey Monkey:	*"_____ (Behavioral coach), remember you can ask Larry Lion for help if there are too many blocks to clean up."*
Behavioral coach:	(Turn to look at Larry Lion and smile.) *"Larry Lion, can you help me clean up?"*
Larry Lion:	(Turn to look at the behavioral coach member and smile.) *"Okay, _____ (behavioral coach). Grrr, Grrr!"*
	(Unsuccessfully attempt to open the lid to the empty toy box.) *"_____ (Behavioral coach), I can't open the box. Can you help me?"*
Behavioral coach:	*"Okay, Larry Lion."*
Larry Lion:	*"Thanks, _____ (behavioral coach)! Grrr, Grrr!"*
Behavioral coach and Larry Lion:	(Help Larry Lion open the lid to the toy box. Working together, put the blocks in the toy box.)
Mikey Monkey:	(Turn to look at the behavioral coach member and smile.) *"Great job asking and giving help, _____ (behavioral coach)! Ooh, ooh!"*
Mikey Monkey and Behavioral coach:	(Say *"good job," give a "monkey high-five," and "lion high-five,"* clap, cheer, and encourage the children to clap as well. The behavioral coach leaves the Good Friend Square.)

Behavioral Rehearsal: Asking and Giving Help

Remove the blocks from the toy box. Re-position the pile of blocks and the toy box in between Larry Lion and the Good Friend Square. Place the lid back on the toy box.

Mikey Monkey: (Turn to look at the group of children and smile.) *"Okay friends! Now let's see our Making Friends Helper _____ try! _____ (Making Friends Helper), come sit on the Good Friend Square and show us how to ask and give help with Larry Lion."*

(The Making Friends Helper should sit on the Good Friend Square.)

"Remember to ask for help by looking at Larry Lion with your (point to your eyes to prompt the children to say *"eyes"*)*...EYES and smiling with your* (point to your mouth to prompt the children to say *"mouth"*)*... MOUTH when you say, 'Can you help me?' And if Larry Lion needs help, you should give help by saying 'okay.' And don't forget to use* (pause briefly to prompt the children to say *"names"*)*...NAMES!"*

Larry Lion: (Turn to look at the Making Friends Helper and smile.) *"Hey _____ (Making Friends Helper), let's play blocks! Grrr, grrr!"*

Mikey Monkey: (If needed, ***social coach*** the Making Friends Helper to look, smile, and *say, "Okay, Larry Lion."*)

Larry Lion: (Larry Lion and the Making Friends Helper play with the large pile of blocks for a few moments while ***showing and telling*** and ***being good sports***. The empty toy box with a lid is sitting nearby.)

Mikey Monkey: *"_____ (Making Friends Helper), it's time to clean up your toys. Remember you can ask Larry Lion for help if there are too many blocks to clean up."*

(If needed, ***social coach*** the Making Friends Helper to ***look, smile,*** and **say, *"Larry Lion, can you help me?"***)

Larry Lion: *"Okay, _____ (Making Friends Helper). Grrr, Grrr!"*

(Unsuccessfully attempt to open the lid to the empty toy box.) *"_____ (Making Friends Helper), I can't open the box. Can you help me?"*

Mikey Monkey: (If needed, ***social coach*** the Making Friends Helper to ***look, smile, say, "Okay, Larry Lion,"*** and ***help*** Larry Lion open the lid to the toy box and put the blocks in the toy box.)

(Turn to look at the Making Friends Helper and smile.) *"Great job asking and giving help, _____ (Making Friends Helper)! Ooh, ooh!"*

(Say *"good job," give a "monkey high-five," and "lion high-five,"* clap, cheer, and encourage the children to clap as well.)

"Okay, Making Friends Helper, choose another friend to sit on the Good Friend Square." (If needed, ***social coach*** the Making Friends Helper to choose another child before returning to their seat.)

Repeat the following with each child:

Remove the blocks from the toy box. Re-position the pile of blocks and the toy box in between Larry Lion and the Good Friend Square. Place the lid back on the toy box.

Mikey Monkey: (Have each child take turns sitting on the Good Friend Square and practicing ***asking and giving help*** with Larry Lion.)

(Turn to look at the group of children.) *"Okay friends! Now let's see _____ (child) try! _____ (Child), come sit on the Good Friend Square and show us how to ask and give help with Larry Lion."*

(The child should sit on the Good Friend Square.)

"Remember to ask for help by looking at Larry Lion with your (point to your eyes to prompt the children to say *"eyes"*)*...EYES and smiling with your* (point to your mouth to prompt the children to say *"mouth"*)*... MOUTH when you say, 'Can you help me?' And if Larry Lion needs help, you should give help by saying 'okay.' And don't forget to use* (pause briefly to prompt the children to say *"names"*)*...NAMES!"*

Larry Lion: (Turn to look at the child and smile.) *"Hey _____ (child), let's play blocks! Grrr, grrr!"*

Mikey Monkey: (If needed, ***social coach*** the child to look, smile, and *say, "Okay, Larry Lion."*)

Larry Lion: (Larry Lion and the child play with the large pile of blocks for a few moments while ***showing and telling*** and ***being good sports***. The empty toy box with a lid is nearby.)

Mikey Monkey: *"_____ (Child), it's time to clean up your toys. Remember you can ask Larry Lion for help if there are too many blocks to clean up."*

(If needed, ***social coach*** the child to ***look, smile,*** and ***say, "Larry Lion, can you help me?"***)

Larry Lion: *"Okay, _____ (child). Grrr, Grrr!"*

(Unsuccessfully attempt to open the lid to the empty toy box.) *"_____ (Child), I can't open the box. Can you help me?"*

Mikey Monkey: (If needed, ***social coach*** the child to ***look, smile, say, "Okay, Larry Lion,"*** and ***help*** Larry Lion open the lid to the toy box and put the blocks in the toy box.)

(Turn to look at the child and smile.) *"Great job asking and giving help, _____ (child)! Ooh, ooh!"*

(Say *"good job," give a "monkey high-five," and "lion high-five,"* clap, cheer, and encourage the children to clap as well.)

"Okay, _____ (child), choose another friend to sit on the Good Friend Square." (If needed, ***social coach*** the child to choose another child before returning to their seat.)

Didactic Lesson Wrap-Up

Group leader: *"Well friends, you all did a great job asking and giving help by looking at Larry Lion with your* (point to your eyes to prompt the children to say *"eyes"*)*...EYES and smiling with your* (point to your mouth to prompt the children to say *"mouth"*)*...MOUTH when you said, 'Can you help me?' And good job saying, 'Okay, Larry Lion' when you gave help. And nice job using* (pause briefly to prompt the children to say *"names"*)*...NAMES!"*

"You each earned ____ (number) stars for asking and giving help! Let's start with ____ (child)."

Award each child the same number of stars by repeating the following with each child:

Group leader: *"Where's ____ (child)?"* (Wait until all the children are looking at the child.)

"____ (Child), how many stars did you earn?" (Pause briefly to allow the child to respond.)

"That's right! Let's all count for ____ (child)! One, two, three... (add stars to the Star Chart as they are counted aloud)*! Everybody clap for ____ (child)!"* (All behavioral coaches clap and cheer and encourage the children to clap as well.)

Session 12 Continued

Tinker Toy Town

BEHAVIORAL REHEARSAL ACTIVITY 1

Materials Needed

- Sets of Tinker Toys (one set per dyad).

Room Setup

- Place sets of Tinker Toys in separate corners of the room, separating each set into two piles.
  - One pile should ONLY include rods.
  - The other pile should ONLY include spools.
- The group leader sits on the floor in front of the room.
- The children and behavioral coach sit on the floor in a semi-circle facing the group leader.

Rules: Tinker Toy Town

- The group leader reads the script below to explain the rules.
- Divide the children into dyads.
  - If there are an odd number of children, pair one child with a behavioral coach.
  - Assign one behavioral coach per dyad to ***social coach***.
- Direct each dyad to sit around the Tinker Toys, with each child sitting next to a pile.
  - One child should ONLY have a pile of rods.
  - The other child should ONLY have a pile of spools.
  - Separating the piles will ensure that children must ask and give help to build the *Tinker Toy Town*.
- Behavioral coaches should ***social coach*** the children to cooperatively choose the first building theme.
  - Behavioral coaches may need to help the children identify a theme for the Tinker Toy Town.
- The children then build cooperatively with the Tinker Toys following the theme of the town; however, the children can only use the Tinker Toys in their own pile to build.
- The children will practice ***asking and giving help*** by asking each other to place desired Tinker Toys on the structure and acting accordingly.

Behavioral Rehearsal: Tinker Toy Town (15 Minutes)

The group leader explains the activity. The behavioral coaches and children sit nearby as the group leader explains the rules.

Group leader: *"Hey friends, now we're going to play a game called Tinker Toy Town. You and your friend will use Tinker Toys to build a town and any other cool things you like. Some of you will have rods* (show rods), *and some of you will have spools* (show spools). *But you can only build with the Tinker Toys that are in front of you. If you need a different Tinker Toy, then you'll practice asking for help by looking at your friend with your* (point to your eyes to prompt the children to say *"eyes"*)*...EYES and smiling with your* (point to your mouth to prompt the children to say *"mouth"*)*...MOUTH when you say, 'Can you help me? Can I have a spool?' or 'Can you help me? Can I have a rod? And remember to give help by saying, 'okay' while using names."*

"Okay, let's play 'Tinker Toy Town!'" (Direct the dyads to sit around a set of Tinker Toys.)

Behavioral Rehearsal: Tinker Toy Town

The behavioral coaches will lead the activity within each dyad.

Behavioral coach: *"Okay friends, what kind of town should we build?"*

(If needed, behavioral coaches should ***social coach*** the children to ***keep cool*** and ***share and give a turn*** when choosing a building theme.)

(Behavioral coaches should ***social coach*** the children to ***ask and give help*** by saying, *"Remember to ask for help if your friend has a Tinker Toy that you want."* Or *"____ (Child) asked for help. Let's remember to listen and give help."*)

(If needed, behavioral coaches should ***social coach*** the children to ***show and tell, be good sports,*** and ***ask and give help*** when sharing their rods and spools for building.)

Table 12.1 Examples of Building Themes

House	Space station	School
City	Spaceship	Castle
Airport	Bridge	Fort
Racetrack	Airplane	Dragon
Animal	Helicopter	Wizard
Windmill	Superhero	Swing set
Merry-go-round	Ferris wheel	Spinning flower

Behavioral Rehearsal Wrap-Up

Group leader: *"Well friends, great job asking and giving help! Give yourselves a big round of applause!"* (All behavioral coaches clap and cheer and encourage the children to clap as well.)

"Now everyone should come sit in the Listening Circle." (Have children return to the Listening Circle to sit on their carpet squares.)

"Okay friends, you did such a great job asking and giving help by looking at your friend with your (point to your eyes to prompt the children to say *"eyes"*)*...EYES and smiling with your* (point to your mouth to prompt the children to say *"mouth"*)*...MOUTH when you said, 'Can you help me?' And good job saying, 'okay' when you gave help. And nice job using* (pause briefly to prompt the children to say *"names"*)*...NAMES!"*

"You each earned ____ (number) more stars for asking and giving help! Let's start with ____ (child)."

Award each child the same number of stars by repeating the following with each child:

Group leader: *"Where's _____ (child)?"* (Wait until all the children are looking at the child.)

"_____ (Child), how many stars did you earn?" (Pause briefly to allow the child to respond.)

"That's right! Let's all count for _____ (child)! One, two, three... (add stars to the Star Chart as they are counted aloud)*! Everybody clap for _____ (child)!"* (All behavioral coaches clap and cheer and encourage the children to clap as well.)

Break Time (10 Minutes)

- The puppets may be used to lead the children to and from the bathroom during break time.
- To assist with transitions and limit unstructured time, behavioral coaches may review the lesson with the children while waiting for the remaining children to return from the bathroom.
- You may want to award stars for good behavior after returning from the bathroom.

Session 12 Continued

Hot or Cold

BEHAVIORAL REHEARSAL ACTIVITY 2

Materials Needed

- A small object to be hidden.

Room Setup

- Remove or place all carpet squares to the side.
- The group leader stands at the front of the room facing the children.
- The children and behavioral coaches sit in a semi-circle facing the group leader.

Rules: Hot or Cold

- The group leader reads the script below to explain the rules.
- Pick a child to be the *"finding friend,"* the one who looks for the hidden object.
- Pick a child to be the *"helping friend,"* the one who directs the *finding friend* to find the hidden object.
- A behavioral coach will be assigned to assist the *finding friend.*
- The remaining children and behavioral coaches sit and watch until it is their turn to be the *finding friend* or the *helping friend.*
- Instruct the *finding friend* and a behavioral coach to wait outside of the room while the object is hidden.
  - While waiting, the behavioral coach reviews the game rules with the *finding friend.*
  - The behavioral coach remains next to the *finding friend* throughout their turn to ***social coach***.
- The group leader will assist the *helping friend* in hiding the object somewhere in the room.
  - Prior to beginning the lesson, the group leader and behavioral coaches should brainstorm several hiding places.
- The *helping friend* returns to the semi-circle after the object is hidden.
- Call the *finding friend* and the behavioral coach back into the room and instruct them to stand at the front of the room.
- The behavioral coach then ***social coaches*** the *finding friend* to ***ask for help*** from the *helping friend* by asking if they are "*hot or cold*" (i.e., standing close or far away from the hidden object).
- Nearby behavioral coaches sitting in the semi-circle ***social coach*** the *helping friend* to ***give help***.

    - The *helping friend* says "*hot*" if the *finding friend* is standing close to the hidden object or "*cold*" if the *finding friend* is standing far away from the hidden object.
- Repeat ***asking and giving help*** after every few steps until the object is found.
- Once the object is found, ***praise*** the children and continue the game by choosing a new *finding friend.* The previous *finding friend* becomes the next *helping friend.*
- Repeat this cycle until all children have had one turn being the *finding friend* and one turn being the *helping friend.*

Behavioral Rehearsal: Hot or Cold (15 Minutes)

The group leader leads the activity. The behavioral coaches and children sit nearby as the group leader explains the rules.

Group leader: *"Hey friends, now we're going to play a game called 'Hot or Cold.' One friend will be the 'finding friend,' and another friend will be the 'helping friend.' Everybody else will sit nicely and keep cool until it's their turn."*

"The 'finding friend' waits outside while we hide the ____ (small object) (hold up the small object) *somewhere in the room."*

"When the 'finding friend' comes back into the room, they'll ask the 'helping friend' for help in finding the ____ (small object) by saying 'Can you help me? Am I hot or cold?'"

"But friends, there's a secret! We can't (shake your head no) *tell the 'finding friend' where the toy is. The 'helping friend' can only give help by saying 'hot' or 'cold.'"*

(Put the toy down on the floor.)

"So, if our 'finding friend' is close to the toy (take a few steps toward the toy), *we say, 'Hot!' But, if they are far from the toy* (take a few steps away from the toy), *then we say, 'Cold'! So friends, if I'm close to the toy* (take a few steps toward the toy), *what do you say?* (Pause briefly to allow the children to say, *"hot"*). *That's right! And if I'm far from the toy* (take a few steps away from the toy), *what do you say?* (Pause briefly to allow the children to say, *"cold"*). *That's right, friends!"*

"And remember to ask and give help by looking and smiling at your friends. And don't forget to use (pause briefly to prompt the children to say *"names"*)*...NAMES. Okay, _____ (behavioral coach 1) and _____ (behavioral coach 2) go first!"*

Role Play: Hot or Cold

The group leader leads the role play. The two behavioral coaches demonstrate how to play *Hot or Cold.* Behavioral coach 1 is the *finding friend*, and behavioral coach 2 is the *helping friend.* The other behavioral coaches and children sit nearby watching the role play.

Group leader:	(Turn to look at behavioral coach 1.) *"____ (Behavioral coach 1), please stand outside so ____ (behavioral coach 2) can hide the ____ (small object)."*
Behavioral coach 1:	*"Okay, ____ (group leader)."* (Leave the room.)
Behavioral coach 2:	(Hide the small object with help from the group.)
Group leader:	(Loudly call out so that behavioral coach 1 can hear from outside.) *"____ (Behavioral coach 1), the ____ (object) is hidden. Come back in!"*
Behavioral coach 1:	(Enter the room.)
Group leader:	(Turn to look at behavioral coach 1.) *"____ (Behavioral coach 1), ask the helping friend ____ (behavioral coach 2) for help by saying, '____ (behavioral coach 2), can you help me please? Am I hot or cold?'"*
Behavioral coach 1:	(Turn to look and smile at behavioral coach 2.) *"____ (Behavioral coach 2), can you help me? Am I hot or cold?"*
Behavioral coach 2:	(Turn to look and smile at behavioral coach 1.) *"Okay, ____ (behavioral coach 1). You're ____ (hot/cold)."*
Behavioral coach 1:	*"Thanks, ____ (behavioral coach 2)!"* (Take a few steps.) *"____ (Behavioral coach 2), can you help me? Am I hot or cold?"*
Behavioral coach 2:	*"Okay, ____ (behavioral coach 1). You're ____ (hot/cold)."*
Behavioral coach 1:	*"Thanks, ____ (behavioral coach 2)!"* (Take a few steps.)

Repeat these steps several times, demonstrating both *"hot"* and *"cold"* responses until behavioral coach 1 finds the object:

Group leader:	*"Great job asking and giving help, ____ (behavioral coach 1) and ____ (behavioral coach 2)!"* (Turn to look at the group of children and smile.) *"And everyone did a great job keeping cool while you waited! Okay friends, now it's everybody's turn to play Hot or Cold! Are we ready?"*

Behavioral Rehearsal: Hot or Cold

Group leader: *"Our next finding friend is ____ (child) and our next helping friend is ____ (child). ____ (Finding friend), wait outside the room with ____ (behavioral coach)."*

(Outside the room, the behavioral coach reviews the game rules with the *finding friend*, while the *helping friend* hides the object with support from the group leader.)

(Loudly call out so that the *finding friend* and the behavioral coach can hear from outside.) *"____ (Finding friend), the ____ (object) is hidden. Come back in!"*

(Wait for the *finding friend* and the behavioral coach to enter the room.)

"____ (Finding friend), the ____ (object) is hidden. Ask ____ (helping friend) for help by saying, '____ (Helping friend), can you help me? Am I hot or cold?'"

(If needed, ***social coach*** the children to ***give help*** by saying, *"____ (Helping friend), the finding friend asked for help. Remember to help them by saying if they're hot or cold."*)

Behavioral coach: (If needed, ***social coach*** the *finding friend* to ***ask for help*** until the object is found by saying, *"____ (Finding friend), ask ____ (helping friend) for help by saying, '____ (Helping friend), can you help me? Am I hot or cold?'"*)

Group leader: *"Great job asking and giving help, ____ (helping and finding friends). And everyone did a great job keeping cool while you waited! Our next finding friend is ____ (child) and our next helping friend is ____ (previous finding friend)."*

Repeat the sequence above making sure that each child has a turn being the *finding friend* and the *helping friend.*

Behavioral Rehearsal Wrap-Up

Group leader: *"Well friends, great job asking and giving help! Give yourselves a big round of applause!"* (All behavioral coaches clap and cheer and encourage the children to clap as well.)

"Now everyone should come sit in the Listening Circle." (Have children return to the Listening Circle to sit on their carpet squares.)

"Okay friends, you did such a great job asking and giving help by looking at your friend with your (point to your eyes to prompt the children to

say *"eyes")...EYES and smiling with your* (point to your mouth to prompt the children to say *"mouth")...MOUTH when you said, 'Can you help me?' And good job saying, 'okay' when you gave help. And nice job using* (pause briefly to prompt the children to say *"names")...NAMES!"*

"You each earned ____ (number) more stars for asking and giving help! Let's start with ____ (child)."

Award each child the same number of stars by repeating the following with each child:

Group leader: *"Where's ____ (child)?"* (Wait until all the children are looking at the child.)

"____ (Child), how many stars did you earn?" (Pause briefly to allow the child to respond.)

"That's right! Let's all count for ____ (child)! One, two, three... (add stars to the Star Chart as they are counted aloud)*! Everybody clap for ____ (child)!"* (All behavioral coaches clap and cheer and encourage the children to clap as well.)

"Now we're going to play another game with our parents and practice asking and giving help some more!"

Session 12 Continued

Asking and Giving Help

PARENT COACHED PLAY: DYADIC PLAYDATES

Materials Needed

- Games brought by children and parents from home.
- Turn-taking games provided by the treatment team.
- Tables and chairs or carpet squares.
- *Parent Coached Play Cards*.

Room Setup

- If available, organize tables in separate corners of the room with four to six chairs per table.
- If tables are not available, place two carpet squares in separate corners of the room to indicate where the children will sit.

Rules: Dyadic Playdates

- The group leader divides the families into groups of two families each.
  - If there are an odd number of children, pair one child with a behavioral coach. In this case, you will need an additional coach to serve as a behavioral coach for the parent.
- Assign each group to sit at a table or specific play area.
  - Children should sit next to each other.
  - Parents will act as ***social coaches*** by sitting on the other side of their child to minimize interrupting the natural flow of play between the children.
  - One behavioral coach will be assigned to each dyad to provide ***social coaching*** suggestions and feedback to parents.
- Parents will help the children pick the first game to play and ***social coach*** their children to ***keep cool*** if their game was not the first chosen game.
- Rather than helping the children set up the game, parents will ***social coach*** the children to ***ask and give help*** setting up the game with each other.
- Parents should attempt to limit their direct participation during game playing by redirecting and ***social coaching*** the children to ***ask and give help*** to each other as much as possible.
- After approximately nine minutes of play, instruct the parents to prepare the children for the upcoming game swap.
- After approximately one additional minute of play (ten minutes total), instruct the parents to ***social coach*** the children to ***ask and give help*** while cleaning up before swapping games.

- Rather than helping the children set up the game, parents will ***social coach*** the children to ***ask and give help*** setting up the game with each other.
- After approximately nine minutes of play, instruct the parents to prepare the children for clean up.
- After approximately one additional minute of play (ten minutes total), parents will ***social coach*** the children to ***ask and give help*** while cleaning up and then return to the Listening Circle.

Behavioral Coaching: Dyadic Playdates

Behavioral coaches will ***social coach*** parents during dyadic ***playdates*** in the following ways:

- ***Priming***:
  - Begin the play interactions with parents going over the rules for ***asking and giving help*** BEFORE GAME PLAYING.
    - Example: *"Remember to ask for help by looking at your friend with your* (point to your eyes to prompt the child to say *"eyes"*)*...EYES and smiling with your* (point to your mouth to prompt the child to say *"mouth"*)*... MOUTH when you say, 'Can you help me?' And remember to say, 'Okay' when you give help to your friend. And don't forget to use* (pause briefly to prompt the child to say *"names"*)*...NAMES."*
- ***Prompting***:
  - Reminding parents to use the buzzwords to ***prompt*** their child to ***ask and give help*** IN THE MOMENT.
  - Helping parents to identify opportunities to proactively ***prompt*** their child to ***ask and give help.***
    - Example: *"Remember to ask for help."*
    - Example: *"Remember to give help if your friend needs help."*
    - Example: *"What should you say to ask for help?"*
- ***Praising***:
  - Reminding parents to ***praise*** and reinforce their child whenever their child ***asks and gives help*** CORRECTLY.
    - Example: *"Great job asking for help!"*
    - Example: *"Good job looking and smiling when you gave your friend help!"*
    - Example: *"Good job saying, 'Can you help me?'"*
- ***Providing corrective feedback using a praise sandwich***:
  - Reminding parents to ***praise*** their child's ATTEMPTS to ***ask and give help*** and identify what could be done differently next time.
    - Example: *"Good job giving your friend help. Remember to say 'okay' next time, but nice job!"*
    - Example: *"Nice job asking for help. Don't forget to look at me, but good job!"*
    - Example: *"Nice try asking for help. Next time, don't forget to use names, but good try!"*
- Reminding parents to continue to ***social coach*** on previously learned skills:
  - ***Listening and following directions.***
  - ***Meeting and greeting friends.***
  - ***Sharing and giving a turn.***
  - ***Asking for a turn.***
  - ***Keeping cool.***
  - ***Being a good sport.***
  - ***Showing and telling.***
  - ***Don't be bossy.***

- ***Asking a friend to play.***
- ***Joining a game.***
- ***Asking to play something different.***

Parent Coached Play: Dyadic Playdates (20 Minutes)

- Have each child choose a turn-taking game brought from home or provided by the treatment team.
- The group leader sits on the floor at the front of the room.
- The families sit on the floor in a semi-circle facing the group leader.

Group leader: *"Hey friends, we're going to have more playdates and play with the fun games you brought from home. This time, we're going to practice asking and giving help as you play. You can ask for help by looking at your friend with your* (point to your eyes to prompt the children to say *"eyes"*)*...EYES and smiling with your* (point to your mouth to prompt the children to say *"mouth"*)*...MOUTH when you say, 'Can you help me?'"*

"And remember to give help when your friends ask by saying 'okay.' And don't forget to use (pause briefly to prompt the children to say *"names"*)*...NAMES."*

"We'll swap games after a few minutes. Then you'll practice asking and giving help some more. Parents, remember to social coach your children by using your Parent Coached Play Cards. Okay, let's play with our games!"

- Before playing, parents will ***social coach*** their child to ***say "hi"*** to one another ***using names***.
- Rather than helping the children set up the game, parents will ***social coach*** the children to ***ask and give help*** to each other.
- Parents should attempt to limit their direct participation by redirecting and ***social coaching*** the children to ***ask and give help*** to each other as much as possible.
- Parents will also ***social coach*** their children to ***not be bossy, show and tell, ask for a turn***, ***share and take turns, keep cool***, and ***be a good sport*** throughout the game playing.
- After approximately nine minutes of play, instruct the parents to prepare the children for the upcoming game swap by saying, *"Parents, tell your children that we'll be swapping games in one minute."*
- After approximately one additional minute of play (ten minutes total), instruct the parents to swap games by saying, *"Parents, it's time to swap games. Social coach the children to ask and give help by cleaning up before playing the next game."*
- After approximately nine minutes of playing the second game, instruct the parents to prepare the children for clean up by saying, *"Parents, tell your children that we'll be cleaning up in one minute."*
- After approximately one additional minute of play (ten minutes total), ***prompt*** the parents to instruct their children to clean up by saying, *"Parents, it's time to clean up. Let's social coach the children to ask and give help by cleaning up and then say 'bye' to their friend using names before sitting in the Listening Circle."*

- If needed, parents will ***social coach*** their child to ***ask and give help*** to clean up.
- Then parents will ***social coach*** their child to ***say "bye"*** to their friend ***using names.***

Final Wrap-Up (20 minutes)

- The group leader sits on the floor at the front of the room.
- The children sit on the carpet squares in a semi-circle facing the group leader, with parents sitting behind their children.

Group leader: *"Okay friends, you all did a great job playing your games and asking and giving help. When we're asking and giving help, do you think we should LOOK at our friend with our EYES and SMILE with our MOUTH?"* (Pause briefly to allow children to respond *"yes."*)

"That's right, friends! And when we ask for help, do you think we should say, "Can you help me?" and use names?" (Pause briefly to allow children to respond *"yes."*)

"That's right, friends! And when we give our friends help, do you think we should say "okay" and use names?" (Pause briefly to allow children to respond *"yes."*)

"That's right, friends! You all did such a great job asking and giving help today that you each earned ____ (number) more stars! Let's start with ____ (child)."

Award each child the same number of stars by repeating the following with each child:

Group leader: *"Where's _____ (child)?"* (Wait until all the children are looking at the child.)

"_____ (Child), how many stars did you earn?" (Pause briefly to allow the child to respond.)

"That's right! Let's all count for _____ (child)! One, two, three... (add stars to the Star Chart as they are counted aloud)*! Everybody clap for _____ (child)!"* (All behavioral coaches clap and cheer and encourage the children to clap as well.)

"And remember you all earned those stars by asking and giving help! Everyone did a great job, and parents you did an excellent job social coaching! Parents, remember your homework assignments this week are for you and your children to practice asking and giving help and for you to continue practicing all the other things we've learned to be a good friend using the 4 Ps. And don't forget to have a playdate and go to your playgroups."

"Alright little friends, do you want to count our stars?" (Pause briefly to allow the children to respond.)

"Let's all count together and see how many stars we earned today! One, two, three…(count the number of stars for one child)*!"*

"You each earned ____ (total number) stars today! Round of applause for our friends!" (All behavioral coaches should clap and cheer and encourage the families to clap as well.)

"Great job, friends! Don't forget to choose your reward before you leave. See you all next week!"

Session 12 Continued

Asking and Giving Help

PEERS® FOR PRESCHOOLERS: PARENT HANDOUT

Snapshot of the Lesson: Asking and Giving Help

The objective of this lesson is to teach children how to ***ask and give help.*** The steps for ***asking and giving help*** include:

Asking for Help

1. ***Look at your friends with your eyes*** (point to your eyes).
2. ***Smile with your mouth*** (point to your mouth and smile).
3. ***Say, "Can you help me?" using names***.

Giving Help

1. ***Look at your friends with your eyes*** (point to your eyes).
2. ***Smile with your mouth*** (point to your mouth and smile).
3. ***Say "okay" using names***.
4. ***Give help to your friend***.

Parent Social Coaching Strategies for Asking and Giving Help

- **Provide opportunities to practice *asking and giving help* during games and activities that are highly motivating for your child.**
    - ***Prime*** your child that they will be practicing ***asking and giving help*** by going over the rules and steps first.
    - Make the practice more rewarding by pairing it with a highly preferred activity.
    - Do not surprise your child in the middle of playing a highly preferred activity by suggesting that they practice ***asking and giving help***.
        - The rehearsal will distract from the preferred activity and they will be less motivated to practice.
    - Playing the highly preferred activity should be contingent on practicing ***asking and giving help***.

- ***Praise* and relabel natural instances of your child *asking and giving help* using the buzzwords.**
  - Your child will naturally ***ask and give help*** throughout the week.
  - Be on the lookout for these naturally occurring behaviors and ***praise*** them using the buzzwords.
    - Example: *"Great job asking for help to put your shoes on!"*
    - Example: *"Nice job giving me help with the snacks!"*
  - By reframing and labeling their behavior using ***praise***, your child will be more motivated to ***ask and give help*** in the future.

- **Use opportunities that naturally occur throughout the day to have your child practice *asking and giving help.***
  - Examples of opportunities for your child to ***ask and give help***:
    - Setting up and cleaning up games or play activities.
    - Getting dressed, putting on shoes, etc.
    - Preparing snacks and meals.
    - Opening doors for family members.
    - Helping to carry things.
    - Holding their own backpacks.
    - Helping to find items in the grocery store.

- **When practicing *asking and giving help*, keep initial practice opportunities short.**
  - This is likely to help your child feel more successful and less frustrated.
  - Remember to immediately ***praise*** their efforts at ***asking and giving help***.
  - In the context of games and activities, it may also help the children to learn that ***asking and giving help***:
    - Will not take away from being able to play the game or activity.
    - Will make it easier to play the game or activity.
    - Will increase the time spent having fun playing the game or activity.

- **Create opportunities to *ask and give help* by completing most of the steps of a game or fun activity and having your child complete the last one or two steps.**
  - By having your child help in completing the last few steps, they will be reinforced and rewarded for ***asking and giving help***.
  - By pairing ***asking and giving help*** with a reward (e.g., game playing), we create an immediate reinforcement for using the skills with natural reinforcement contingencies.
  - As ***asking and giving help*** becomes easier, parents may want to gradually increase the number of steps completed by their child.

- **Practice *asking and giving help* by having your child take turns with siblings and *playmates.***
  - Consider having your child's sibling or ***playmate*** complete a few steps of some action, then ***social coach*** your child to ***give help*** by completing the remaining steps.
  - Have your child initiate some action and before completing the sequence of steps, ***social coach*** your child to ***ask for help*** from a sibling or ***playmate*** to complete the remaining steps.

    - If your child observes that they are sharing the responsibility of ***helping*** with siblings and ***playmates***, they are less likely to feel frustrated by the practice.

- **During *playdates* and *playgroups*, redirect your child and their *playmates* to *ask and give help* to each other rather than first relying on adult assistance.**
    - ***Playdates*** and ***playgroups*** offer natural social opportunities to ***ask and give help***.
    - Children will often seek help from adults to complete certain tasks during ***playdates*** and ***playgroups.***
    - If the task is not too difficult, consider having your child ***ask and give help*** by saying, *"How about asking your friend for help"* or *"Why don't you help your friend."*
    - The collateral gains of ***social coaching*** your child and their ***playmates*** to ***ask and give help*** during ***playdates*** and ***playgroups*** include:
        - The children assuming an "expert role" during that game or activity.
        - Encouraging and reinforcing more cooperative, reciprocal play interactions.

Homework Assignments

1. **Playdates.**
    - Schedule and have a ***playdate*** with a ***playmate***.
    - Prepare for the ***playdate*** using the ***5 Ws***.
        - ***WHO: Playdates*** should be one-on-one.
        - ***WHAT: Playdates*** should be activity-based.
        - ***WHERE:*** Schedule initial ***playdates*** to take place in your home or somewhere you can provide ***social coaching***.
        - ***WHEN:*** Try to keep initial ***playdates*** to no more than 1–1.5 hours.
        - ***HOW:*** Coordinate how the children will get to and from the ***playdate***.
    - Do a final practice with your child of the games and activities that will be available during the ***playdate***.
    - Gather all the games and activity materials for the ***playdate*** in one area that is VISIBLE and easily accessible to YOU but not the children.
    - Provide ***social coaching*** during the ***playdate*** and assess if this is a good ***playmate*** for your child.

2. **Practice asking and giving help.**
    - Practice having your child ***ask and give help*** this week while providing ***social coaching*** using the ***4 Ps***.
        - ***Priming:*** Review the rules for ***asking and giving help*** with your child BEFORE PRACTICING.
        - ***Prompting:*** Remind your child IN THE MOMENT to ***ask and give help*** whenever the opportunities present.
        - ***Praising: Praise*** your child using the buzzwords whenever they ***ask and give help*** CORRECTLY.
        - ***Providing corrective feedback: Provide corrective feedback*** in the form of a ***praise sandwich*** whenever your child ATTEMPTS to ***ask and give help.***

- Please send us a 30–60-second video of ***social coaching*** your child to ***ask and give help*** to be viewed during homework review.
    - Please include:
        - Skills your child did well.
        - Skills you would like to work on with your child.

3. **Provide *social coaching* on previously learned skills.**
    - Continue providing ***social coaching*** to your child throughout the week using the ***4 Ps.***
    - Previous skills include:
        - ***Listening and following directions.***
        - ***Meeting and greeting friends.***
        - ***Sharing and giving a turn.***
        - ***Asking for a turn.***
        - ***Keeping cool.***
        - ***Being a good sport.***
        - ***Showing and telling.***
        - ***Don't be bossy.***
        - ***Asking a friend to play.***
        - ***Joining a game.***
        - ***Asking to play something different.***

4. **Bring a turn-taking game.**
    - Bring a turn-taking game that your child enjoys playing and can be played with the other children.

Session 12 Continued

Asking and Giving Help

PEERS® FOR PRESCHOOLERS: PARENT COACHED PLAY CARDS

Snapshot of the Lesson: Asking and Giving Help

Asking for Help

1. ***Look at your friends with your eyes*** (point to your eyes).
2. ***Smile with your mouth*** (point to your mouth and smile).
3. ***Say, "Can you help me?" using names***.

Giving Help

1. ***Look at your friends with your eyes*** (point to your eyes).
2. ***Smile with your mouth*** (point to your mouth and smile).
3. ***Say "okay" using names***.
4. ***Give help to your friend***.

Priming BEFORE Game Playing

- Example: *"Remember to ask for help by looking at your friend with your* (point to your eyes to prompt the child to say *"eyes"*)*...EYES and smiling with your* (point to your mouth to prompt the child to say *"mouth"*)*...MOUTH when you say, 'Can you help me?' And remember to say, 'Okay' when you give help to your friend. And don't forget to use* (pause briefly to prompt the child to say *"names"*)*...NAMES."*

Prompting IN THE MOMENT

- Example: *"Remember to ask for help."*
- Example: *"Remember to give help if your friend needs help."*
- Example: *"What should you say to ask for help?"*

Praising for CORRECT Use of Skills

- Example: *"Great job asking for help!"*
- Example: *"Good job looking and smiling when you gave your friend help!"*
- Example: *"Good job saying, 'Can you help me?'"*

Providing Corrective Feedback for ATTEMPTS Using a Praise Sandwich

- Example: *"Good job giving your friend help. Remember to say 'okay' next time, but nice job!"*
- Example: *"Nice job asking for help. Don't forget to look at me, but good job!"*
- Example: *"Nice try asking for help. Next time, don't forget to use names, but good try!"*

- Continue to provide ***social coaching*** on previously learned skills:
  - ***Listening and following directions.***
  - ***Meeting and greeting friends.***
  - ***Sharing and giving a turn.***
  - ***Asking for a turn.***
  - ***Keeping cool.***
  - ***Being a good sport.***
  - ***Showing and telling.***
  - ***Don't be bossy.***
  - ***Asking a friend to play.***
  - ***Joining a game.***
  - ***Asking to play something different.***

Session 12 Continued

Asking and Giving Help

PEERS® FOR PRESCHOOLERS: PARENT HOMEWORK WORKSHEET

Child's Name:	Parent's Name:		Date:	
HOMEWORK ASSIGNMENTS	PRIMING (REVIEWING RULES BEFORE PRACTICE)	PROMPTING (IN THE MOMENT)	PRAISING (USING BUZZWORDS)	PROVIDING CORRECTIVE FEEDBACK (USING A PRAISE SANDWICH)
Asking and giving help				
Practice previous skills: • **Asking to play something different** • **Joining a game** • **Asking a friend to play** • **Don't be bossy** • **Show and tell during play** • **Being a good sport** • **Keeping cool** • **Asking for a turn** • **Sharing and giving turns** • **Meeting and greeting friends** • **Listening and following directions**				

<table>
<tr><td>Child's Name:</td><td colspan="2">Parent's Name:</td><td colspan="2">Date:</td></tr>
<tr><td>HOMEWORK ASSIGNMENTS</td><td>PRIMING (REVIEWING RULES BEFORE PRACTICE)</td><td>PROMPTING (IN THE MOMENT)</td><td>PRAISING (USING BUZZWORDS)</td><td>PROVIDING CORRECTIVE FEEDBACK (USING A PRAISE SANDWICH)</td></tr>
<tr><td>Playdate:
• Plan a playdate using the 5 Ws
• Prime your child before the playdate
• Provide social coaching during the playdate using the 4 Ps</td><td colspan="4"></td></tr>
<tr><td>Bring a turn-taking game</td><td colspan="2">Did you bring a turn-taking game?
YES or NO
(Circle)</td><td colspan="2">Which game did you bring?</td></tr>
</table>

Please fill out this worksheet by describing what you did to complete the homework assignments. Worksheets will be collected during Homework Review at the next session of PEERS® for Preschoolers.

Session 13

Staying in Our Own Space

PARENT SESSION THERAPIST GUIDE

Parent Session Agenda

- Homework Review (40 minutes).
- Didactic Lessons (20 minutes).
- Parent Coached Play (20 minutes).
- Final Wrap-Up (10 minutes).

Materials Needed

- Conference room with a large table and enough chairs for the parent group leader and all parents to sit comfortably around the table.
  - Avoid sitting in a circle without a table as this creates the atmosphere of group therapy.
- Name tags for parents and treatment team.
- *Parent Handouts* (for the current week and the previous week).
- *Parent Homework Worksheets* (for the current week and the previous week).
- *Parent Coached Play Cards* (for the current week and the previous week).
- *Attendance and Homework Compliance Sheets* for parent group leader.
- Pens for note-taking (consider having extra pens for parents who need them).

Homework Review (40 Minutes)

1. **Playdates.**
   - Have parents report on the ***playdate*** and confirm that they planned using the ***5 Ws.***
   - Review what parents did to ***social coach*** their child BEFORE, DURING, and AFTER the ***playdate***.
   - Identify what skills their child did well and what skills they need to work on.
     - Confirm that parents ***praised*** skills that were done well and provided ***priming, prompting,*** and/or ***corrective feedback*** for emerging skills.
   - Have parents assess if this is a good ***playmate*** for their child.
   - Have parents identify who their child might have a ***playdate*** with in the coming week (does not have to be a different ***playmate***).

2. **Practice asking and giving help.**
   - Review the 30–60-second video of ***social coaching*** for ***asking and giving help*** for each family. (For larger groups, you may need to review video recordings in two smaller groups with two different parent group leaders).

DOI: 10.4324/9781003502968-14

  - Have parents identify:
    - Skills their child did well.
    - Skills they would like to work on with their child.
  - Provide ***social coaching*** tips as appropriate for each family.
- If parents did not send a video of ***social coaching***, confirm the following:
  - Parents practiced having their child ***ask and give help*** while providing ***social coaching*** using the ***4 Ps.***
    - ***Priming***: Reviewed the rules for ***asking and giving help*** with their child BEFORE PRACTICING.
    - ***Prompting***: Reminded their child IN THE MOMENT to ***ask and give help*** whenever the opportunity presented.
    - ***Praising***: ***Praised*** their child using the buzzwords whenever they ***asked and gave help*** CORRECTLY.
    - ***Providing corrective feedback***: ***Provided corrective feedback*** in the form of a ***praise sandwich*** whenever their child ATTEMPTED to ***ask and give help***.

3. **Provide *social coaching* on previously learned skills.**
   - Confirm parents continued to provide ***social coaching*** to their child throughout the week using the ***4 Ps*** for previously learned skills:
     - ***Listening and following directions.***
     - ***Meeting and greeting friends.***
     - ***Sharing and giving a turn.***
     - ***Asking for a turn.***
     - ***Keeping cool.***
     - ***Being a good sport.***
     - ***Showing and telling.***
     - ***Don't be bossy.***
     - ***Asking a friend to play.***
     - ***Joining a game.***
     - ***Asking to play something different.***

4. **Bring a turn-taking game.**
   - Confirm the following:
     - Brought a turn-taking game that their child enjoys playing and can be played with the other children. (To avoid distractions, these games should be left with the parents until *Parent Coached Play*.)

Didactic Lessons (20 Minutes)

PEERS® Neuroaffirming Pledge:

- We value neurodiversity, acceptance, and authenticity.
- We honor the diverse ways people experience the world.
- We respect each person's unique perspectives and communication styles.
- We recognize there is no one right way to connect with others.
- If using the strategies taught in PEERS® feels like camouflaging or masking and/or they don't align with your goals or the goals of your family, then you do not have to use them.
- Learning and using the skills taught in PEERS® is a PERSONAL CHOICE.

Didactic Lesson: Staying in Our Own Space

- Distribute *Parent Handouts*.
  - Sections in **bold print** come directly from the *Parent Handout*.
  - Terms that are ***bold and italicized*** are buzzwords and represent important concepts from the didactic lesson.
- Explain, *"For the past several weeks, we have talked about strategies for sustaining play. One important element of successful play interactions includes the use of good body boundaries. Inappropriate body boundaries may lead to peer rejection. The focus of today's child lesson is to help your children maintain appropriate and comfortable body boundaries when playing with playmates and siblings. Before we cover parent coaching strategies for promoting appropriate body boundaries, it will be helpful to review the child lesson to give you some context for thinking about your social coaching."*

Snapshot of the Lesson: Staying in Our Own Space

The objective of this lesson is to teach children how to *stay in their own space.* Steps for *staying in our own space* include:

- ***Don't get too close* (shake your head no).**
  - **If we can touch the person next to us (extend your arm out in front and to the side), then we're *too close* and being a *space hog.***
- ***Stay in our own space* (nod your head yes).**
  - **If we're *too close* and *being a space hog*, then we need to *back up* (lean back) and *stay in our own space.***
  - **If our friends are *too close* and *being a space hog*, then we need to *back up* (lean back), *stay in our own space,* and *not be bossy.***
  - ***Remember to be a "space keeper."***

Parent Social Coaching Strategies for Staying in Our Own Space

- **Parents should provide opportunities to practice *staying in our own space* during games and activities that are highly motivating for your child.**
  - **Your child will be more motivated to practice *staying in their own space* if the rehearsal is paired with a preferred activity.**
  - **Remember to *prime* your child before practicing by saying, *"Now we're going to practice staying in our own space while playing (preferred activity)."***
    - **Then go over the rules for *staying in our own space.***
  - **Example: Playing games with siblings and *playmates.***
    - **When playing games on the floor, you may make continued game play contingent on your child *staying in their own space.***
    - **If your child begins to get *too close* to a sibling or *playmate*, pause the game and *social coach* your child to *stay in their own space.***

- **Once they are demonstrating good body boundaries, *praise* your child and resume the game.**

- **Parents may pretend to be a *playmate* while having your child practice *staying in their own space.***
  - **In the absence of siblings or *playmates* to practice with, you may have the child pretend the parent is a *playmate* while practicing *staying in their own space.***
  - **Since body boundaries are different for parents and their children, be clear that the parent is pretending to be a peer for the sake of practicing.**
  - **Example: In preparation for a *playdate*, have your child pretend that you are their *playmate* and you are having a pretend *playdate* while practicing *staying in your own space.***

- **Practice *staying in our own space* during games and activities that may be more difficult for your child to use appropriate body boundaries.**
  - **Consider playing games or activities on the floor that are usually played while seated at a table.**
    - **Example: Playing a board game on the floor.**
  - **Playing on the floor often leads to poorer use of body boundaries in children, so practicing on the floor may create more opportunities to provide *social coaching* around *staying in our own space.***
  - **When practicing *staying in our own space* on the floor, consider practicing with siblings when possible, or with a parent assuming the role of a child.**
  - **If you have concerns that your child will not be able to *stay in their own space* during games and activities on the floor with real *playmates*, consider structuring activities around a table until your child can more appropriately use body boundaries.**

- **Use opportunities that naturally occur throughout the day to have your child practice *staying in their own space.***
  - **Examples of opportunities for your child to *stay in their own space*:**
    - **Watching television or movies.**
    - **Meal or snack times.**
    - **Waiting in line at the store.**
    - **Waiting for parents to finish a task.**
    - **Playing with games and toys on the floor.**
  - **Because body boundaries with parents and their children are different, be sure to let your child know you are practicing *staying in our own space* as if you were *playmates.***
    - ***Social coaching* your child that they should remain an arm's length away from you may feel rejecting if they don't understand you are pretending to be a *playmate.***

- **If your child does not know what an arm's length away feels like, create fun opportunities to demonstrate this distance.**
  - **Some children have difficulty judging when they are getting *too close* to another person or being a *space hog.***
  - **Creating fun opportunities for your child to learn what an arm's length away feels like will help them better judge this distance in the future.**

- **Example: Create a fun game to practice body boundaries.**
  - **You and your child stand at opposite sides of the room facing each other.**
  - **When you say *"Go!"* you and your child run toward each other while doing something silly.**
  - **Then *social coach* your child to use *stay in their own space* by saying, *"Freeze!"* when you get too close.**
  - **End with praising them for *staying in their own space.***

- **If your child has difficulty judging when they are getting *too close* to another person:**
  - **Consider creating a *verbal prompt* to provide coaching in the moment.**
    - **Example: *"Space check."***
    - **Example: *"Body bubble."***
  - **Consider creating a *nonverbal prompt* to provide coaching in the moment.**
    - **Example: Parent extends their arm.**
  - **Note: It is fine to have your child measure with their arm when learning about body boundaries with you and members of the family but be sure to let them know that we NEVER measure the distance with our arms with *playmates* or other people.**

Parent Coached Play

- Distribute the *Parent Coached Play Cards*.
- Review the examples of the ***4 Ps*** provided on the *Parent Coached Play Card.*
- Remind parents that in a few moments we will be joining the children for *Parent Coached Play* in the context of mock dyadic ***playdates***.
- Parents should keep the *Parent Coached Play Card* in front of them during the dyadic ***playdate*** for recommendations on how to ***social coach*** children on ***staying in our own space.***

Homework Assignments

(Briefly review the homework assignments and troubleshoot any potential problems with parents.)

1. **Playdates.**
   - **Schedule and have a *playdate* with a *playmate.***
   - **Prepare for the *playdate* using the *5 Ws.***
     - ***WHO: Playdates* should be one-on-one.**
     - ***WHAT: Playdates* should be activity-based.**
     - ***WHERE:* Schedule initial *playdates* to take place in your home or somewhere you can provide *social coaching.***
     - ***WHEN:* Try to keep initial *playdates* to no more than 1–1.5 hours.**
     - ***HOW:* Coordinate how the children will get to and from the *playdate.***
   - **Do a final practice with your child of the games and activities that will be available during the *playdate.***
   - **Gather all the games and activity materials for the *playdate* in one area that is VISIBLE and easily accessible to YOU but not the children.**

- **Provide *social coaching* during the *playdate* and assess if this is a good *playmate* for your child.**

2. **Practice staying in your own space.**
   - **DO NOT have your child practice being a *space hog*.**
     - **Notify your child that you are PRETENDING to be a friend who is a *space hog* and have your child practice *staying in their own space* and *being a space keeper.***
   - **Practice having your child *stay in their own space* this week while providing *social coaching* using the *4 Ps.***
     - ***Priming:* Review the rules for *staying in our own space* with your child BEFORE PRACTICING.**
     - ***Prompting:* Remind your child IN THE MOMENT to *stay in their own space* whenever the opportunities present.**
     - ***Praising: Praise* your child using the buzzwords whenever they *stay in their own space* CORRECTLY.**
     - ***Providing corrective feedback: Provide corrective feedback* in the form of a *praise sandwich* whenever your child ATTEMPTS to *stay in their own space.***
   - **Please send us a 30–60-second video of *social coaching* your child to *stay in their own space* to be viewed during homework review.**
     - **Please include:**
       - **Skills your child did well.**
       - **Skills you would like to work on with your child.**

3. **Provide social coaching on previously learned skills.**
   - **Continue providing *social coaching* to your child throughout the week using the *4 Ps.***
   - **Previous skills include:**
     - ***Listening and following directions.***
     - ***Meeting and greeting friends.***
     - ***Sharing and giving a turn.***
     - ***Asking for a turn.***
     - ***Keeping cool.***
     - ***Being a good sport.***
     - ***Showing and telling.***
     - ***Don't be bossy.***
     - ***Asking a friend to play.***
     - ***Joining a game.***
     - ***Asking to play something different.***
     - ***Asking and giving help.***

4. **Bring a turn-taking game that your child enjoys playing and can be played with the other children.**

Session 13 Continued

Staying in Our Own Space

CHILD SESSION THERAPIST GUIDE

Child Session Agenda

- Didactic Lesson: *Staying in Our Own Space* (20 minutes).
- Group Behavioral Rehearsal Activity 1: *Ring Around the Rosie* (15 minutes).
- Break Time (10 minutes).
- Group Behavioral Rehearsal Activity 2: *Simon Says* (15 minutes).
- Parent Coached Play: *Dyadic Playdates* (20 minutes).
- Final Wrap-Up (10 minutes).

Snapshot of the Lesson: Staying in Our Own Space

The objective of this lesson is to teach children how to ***stay in their own space.*** Steps for ***staying in our own space*** include:

- ***Don't get too close*** (shake your head no).
  - If we can touch the person next to us (extend your arm out in front and to the side), then we're ***too close*** and being a ***space hog***.
- ***Stay in our own space*** (nod your head yes).
  - If we're ***too close*** and ***being a space hog***, then we need to ***back up*** (lean back) and ***stay in our own space.***
  - If our friends are ***too close*** and ***being a space hog***, then we need to ***back up*** (lean back), ***stay in our own space,*** and ***not be bossy.***
  - ***Remember to be a "space keeper."***

Materials Needed

- Mouse puppet.
- Frog puppet.
- Several Legos.
- Carpet squares or chairs.
- Making Friends Helper" badge.
- Star chart with names of children.
- Marker for star chart.
- Name tags for families and treatment team.
- Prize bins with prizes.

Preparing for the Lesson

- Use the script below with the group leader using a mouse puppet to play the part of "Marty Mouse."
- A behavioral coach uses a frog puppet to play the part of "Franny Frog."
- An additional behavioral coach assists in behavioral rehearsal and provides encouragement and feedback to the group.
- A child is chosen at the beginning of the lesson as the "Making Friends Helper."
  - The "Making Friends Helper" wears a special badge and is the first child to practice the skill.
- The group leader and the behavioral coach sit on the floor at the front of the room.
- A special colored carpet square (e.g., red) is placed at the front of the room next to the child group leader to be used as the "Good Friend Square."
- For the children, additional carpet squares of the same color (e.g., green) are placed in a semicircle facing the child group leader and the "Good Friend Square."
- Note: If carpet squares are unavailable, the children and behavioral coach may sit on chairs.
- The material in *italics* should be read by the indicated person.
- The material in ***bold and italics*** represents buzzwords and should be emphasized when read.
- The material in CAPITAL LETTERS within the script should be given extra emphasis while the group is encouraged to say the words in unison.

Behavioral Coaching Techniques

Behavioral coaches should use the following coaching techniques described below throughout the lesson and the behavioral rehearsal activities. (Note: ***priming*** occurs during the introduction to the activity.)

- ***Prompting*:**
  - Use the buzzwords to ***prompt*** the children to ***stay in their own space***.
    - Example: *"Remember to stay in your own space."*
    - Example: *"Don't forget to back up if you're too close."*
    - Example: *"Are you being a space hog or a space keeper?"*

- ***Praising*:**
  - Reinforce ***staying in your own space*** by ***praising*** the children.
    - Example: *"Great job being a space keeper!"*
    - Example: *"Great job backing up and not being too close!"*
    - Example: *"Good job staying in your own space!"*

- ***Providing corrective feedback using a praise sandwich:***
  - Reinforce ATTEMPTS to ***stay in your own space*** by ***praising*** the children and identifying what could be done differently next time.
    - Example: *"Nice try staying in your own space. Don't forget to back up next time, but good try!"*
    - Example: *"Good try staying in your own space. Don't get too close next time, but good job!"*
    - Example: *"Good try staying in your own space. Don't be a space hog next time, but nice job!"*

- Behavioral coaches should continue to ***social coach*** on previously learned skills:
  - ***Listening and following directions.***
  - ***Meeting and greeting friends.***
  - ***Sharing and giving a turn.***
  - ***Asking for a turn.***
  - ***Keeping cool.***
  - ***Being a good sport.***
  - ***Showing and telling.***
  - ***Don't be bossy.***
  - ***Asking a friend to play.***
  - ***Joining a game.***
  - ***Asking to play something different.***
  - ***Asking and giving help.***

Didactic Lesson: Staying In Our Own Space (20 minutes)

Have the children sit in a semi-circle on the carpet squares facing the group leader.

Marty Mouse: (Sit at the front of the room and choose a Making Friends Helper.) *"Who wants to be our Making Friends Helper?"*

(Choose from among the children raising their hands and place the "Making Friends Helper" badge on the child. The child stays in their seat for now.)

"Hi friends! I'm Marty Mouse. Squeak, squeak! Today we're going to practice staying in our own space. Staying in our own space is a great way to be nice to our friends!"

"Who should we stay in our own space with? We should stay in our own space with our friends, teachers, brothers, sisters, and people we don't know (shake your head no)*."*

"How do we stay in our own space? We stay in our own space by NOT (shake your head no) *getting too close. If we can touch the person next to us* (extend your arm out in front and to the side)*, then we're too close and being a space hog! When we're too close, then we should back up* (lean back) *and stay in our own space. And when our friend is too close, we should back up* (lean back)*, stay in our own space, and not be bossy. Remember to be a space keeper!"*

"Remember, staying in our own space and NOT (shake your head no) *being a space hog are nice ways to be a good friend! Squeak, squeak!"*

Role Play: Staying In Our Own Space

Marty Mouse and Franny Frog: (Franny Frog plays with the Legos. Marty Mouse sits several feet away.)

Franny Frog: (Turn to look at the group of children.) *"Hey friends! I want to play Legos with my friend Marty Mouse. Do you think I should ask him to play?"* (Nod your head yes and encourage the children to say *"yes."*)

	"That's a great idea! Ribbit, ribbit! Let's do it!" (Turn to look at Marty Mouse and smile.) *"Marty Mouse, do you want to play Legos with me? Ribbit, ribbit!"*
Marty Mouse:	(Turn to look at Franny Frog and smile.) *"Okay, Franny Frog! Squeak, squeak!"*
Franny Frog:	*"Cool! Come here, Marty Mouse!"* (Wave Marty Mouse over with your hand.)
Marty Mouse:	(Turn to look at Franny Frog and smile.) *"Okay, Franny Frog! Squeak, squeak!"*
	(Move over to Franny Frog. Sit so close that you and Franny Frog are shoulder to shoulder.)
Franny Frog:	(Turn to look at Marty Mouse, frown, shake your head, and lean back slightly.)
Marty Mouse:	(Turn to look at the group of children.) *"Hey friends, do you think I'm too close to Franny Frog and being a space hog?"* (Nod your head yes and encourage the children to say *"yes."*)
	"That's right! Squeak, squeak! Do you think I should back up and stay in my own space?" (Nod your head yes and encourage the children to say *"yes."*)
	"That's right! Squeak, squeak! Let's do it!" (***Back up*** until you are an arm's length away from Franny Frog.)
	(Turn to look at the group of children and smile.) *"Hey friends, now do you think I'm doing a good job staying in my own space and being a space keeper?"* (Nod your head yes and encourage the children to say *"yes."*)
	"That's right! Squeak, squeak!"
Marty Mouse and Franny Frog:	(Say *"good job," give a "mouse high-five," and "frog high-five,"* clap, cheer, and encourage the children to clap as well. Franny Frog takes the Legos and sits 2–3 FEET AWAY on the other side of the Good Friend Square (i.e., the Good Friend Square is between Marty Mouse and Franny Frog). ***Social coach*** the children as needed while they ***stay in their own space*** with Franny Frog.)
Marty Mouse:	*"Now let's see _____ (behavioral coach) try! _____ (Behavioral coach), please come sit on the Good Friend Square."*
Behavioral coach:	(Sit on the Good Friend Square.)

Marty Mouse:	*"_____ (Behavioral coach), can you show us how to stay in your own space with Franny Frog?"*
Behavioral coach:	*"Okay, Marty Mouse."*
Marty Mouse:	(Turn to look at the group of children.) *"Remember when we're staying in our own space, we don't get too close* (shake your head no). *If we can touch the person next to us* (extend your arm out in front and to the side), *then we're too close and being a space hog. If we're too close and being a space hog, then we need to back up* (demonstrate leaning back) *and stay in our own space. Remember to be a space keeper!"*
Behavioral coach:	*"Okay, Marty Mouse."*
Franny Frog:	(Play with the Legos. After a few moments, turn to look at the behavioral coach member and smile.) *"_____ (Behavioral coach), do you want to play Legos with me? Ribbit, ribbit!"*
Behavioral coach:	(Turn to look at Franny Frog and smile.) *"Okay, Franny Frog!"*
Franny Frog:	*"Cool! Come here, _____ (behavioral coach)."* (Wave the behavioral coach over with your hand.)
Behavioral coach:	*"Okay, Franny Frog!"* (Leave the Good Friend Square and sit about an arm's length away from Franny Frog.)
Franny Frog and Behavioral coach:	(Play together with the Legos for a few moments while ***showing and telling***.)
Marty Mouse:	*"Great job staying in your own space and being a space keeper, _____ (behavioral coach)! Squeak, squeak!"*
Marty Mouse and Behavioral coach:	(Say *"good job," give a "mouse high-five," and "frog high-five,"* clap, cheers, and encourage the children to clap as well. The behavioral coach leaves the Good Friend Square.)

Behavioral Rehearsal: Staying in Your Own Space

Marty Mouse:	(Turn to look at the group of children.) *"Okay friends! Now let's see our Making Friends Helper _____ try! _____ (Making Friends Helper), come sit on the Good Friend Square and show us how to stay in your own space with Franny Frog."* (The Making Friends Helper should sit on the Good Friend Square.)

(Turn to look at the group of children.) *"Remember when we're staying in our own space, we don't get too close* (shake your head no). *If we can touch the person next to us* (extend your arm out in front and to the side), *then we're too close and being a space hog. If we're too close and being a space hog, then we need to back up* (demonstrate leaning back) *and stay in our own space. Remember to be a space keeper!"*

Franny Frog: (Play with the Legos. After a few moments, turn to look at the Making Friends Helper and smile.)

"_____ (Making Friends Helper), do you want to play Legos with me? Ribbit, ribbit!"

Marty Mouse: (If needed, ***social coach*** the Making Friends Helper to look, smile, say, *"Okay, Franny Frog!"* and leave the Good Friend Square to sit about an arm's length away from Franny Frog.)

(If needed, ***social coach*** the Making Friends Helper to ***back up*** if they are ***too close*** to Franny Frog and being a ***space hog***.)

(If needed, ***social coach*** the Making Friends Helper to begin playing with the Legos with Franny Frog.)

"Great job staying in your own space and being a space keeper, _____ (Making Friends Helper)! Squeak, squeak!"

(Say *"good job," give a "mouse high-five," and "frog high-five,"* clap, cheer, and encourage the children to clap as well.)

"Okay, Making Friends Helper, choose another friend to sit on the Good Friend Square." (If needed, ***social coach*** the Making Friends Helper to choose another child before returning to their seat.)

Repeat the following with each child:

Marty Mouse: (Have each child take turns sitting on the Good Friend Square and practicing ***staying in their own space*** with Franny Frog.)

(Turn to look at the group of children.) *"Okay friends! Now let's see _____ (child) try! _____ (Child), come sit on the Good Friend Square and show us how to stay in our own space with Franny Frog."*

(The child should sit on the Good Friend Square.)

(Turn to look at the group of children.) *"Remember when we're staying in our own space, we don't get too close* (shake your head no). *If we can touch the person next to us* (extend your arm out in front and to the side), *then we're too close and being a space hog. If we're too close and being a space hog, then we need to back up* (demonstrate leaning back) *and stay in our own space. Remember to be a space keeper!"*

Franny Frog: (Play with the Legos. After a few moments, turn to look at the child and smile.)

"_____ (Child), do you want to play Legos with me? Ribbit, ribbit!"

Marty Mouse: (If needed, ***social coach*** the child to look, smile, say, *"Okay, Franny Frog!"* and leave the Good Friend Square to sit about an arm's length away from Franny Frog.)

(If needed, ***social coach*** the child to ***back up*** if they are ***too close*** to Franny Frog and being a ***space hog***.)

(If needed, ***social coach*** the child to begin playing with the Legos with Franny Frog.)

"Great job staying in your own space and being a space keeper, _____ (child)! Squeak, squeak!"

(Say *"good job," give a "mouse high-five," and "frog high-five,"* clap, cheer, and encourage the children to clap as well.)

"Okay, _____ (child), choose another friend to sit on the Good Friend Square." (If needed, ***social coach*** the child to choose another child before returning to their scat.)

Didactic Lesson Wrap-Up

Group leader: *"Well friends, you all did a great job staying in your own space by backing up* (lean back) *if you were too close to Franny Frog! No space hogs here!"*

"You each earned ____ (number) stars for staying in your own space and being a space keeper! Let's start with ____ (child)."

Award each child the same number of stars by repeating the following with each child:

Group leader: *"Where's ____ (child)?"* (Wait until all the children are looking at the child.)

"____ (Child), how many stars did you earn?" (Pause briefly to allow the child to respond.)

"That's right! Let's all count for ____ (child)! One, two, three... (add stars to the Star Chart as they are counted aloud)*! Everybody clap for ____ (Child)!"* (All behavioral coaches clap and cheer and encourage the children to clap as well.)

Session 13 Continued

Ring Around the Rosie

BEHAVIORAL REHEARSAL ACTIVITY 1

Materials Needed

- None.

Room Setup

- Remove or place all carpet squares to the side.
- The group leader sits on the floor in front of the room.
- The children and behavioral coaches sit on the floor in a circle facing the group leader.

Rules: Ring Around the Rosie

- The group leader reads the script below to explain the rules.
- Instruct the children and behavioral coaches to hold hands and walk in a circle as they sing the *Ring Around the Rosie* song:
    - *Ring Around the Rosie* song:
      "Ring around the rosie,
      A pocket full of posies,
      Ashes, ashes,
      We all fall down!"

- The children and behavioral coaches should act out the last line of the song (*"We all fall down!"*) by sitting down on the floor.
- Once familiar with the game, the children will practice ***staying in their own space*** when acting out the last line of the song.
- Each time the children act out the last line of the song and fall down, tell the children to freeze in place before ***social coaching*** the children to ***stay in their own space***.
- To ensure that the children have sufficient opportunities to practice ***staying in their own space***, behavioral coaches will intentionally be ***space hogs*** when acting out the last line of the song.
    - The children will ***back up*** from behavioral coaches that are ***too close***.
- New commands may be introduced in the last line of the song.
    - Before introducing a new command, behavioral coaches demonstrate the new command while the children watch.
    - Examples: Spin around, stand still, kneel down, etc.

Behavioral Rehearsal: Ring Around the Rosie (15 Minutes)

The group leader explains the activity. The behavioral coaches and children sit in a circle nearby as the group leader explains the rules.

Group leader: *"Hey friends, now we're going to play a game called 'Ring Around the Rosie.' Everyone will stand in a circle holding hands. Then you'll walk in a circle singing the 'Ring Around the Rosie' song. The song goes like this: 'Ring around the rosie, a pocket full of posies, ashes, ashes, we all fall down!' And when we say, 'We all fall down,' we'll all fall down and sit on the floor like this* (sit on the floor)*."*

"And every time we fall down, we'll practice staying in our own space. Remember when we're staying in our own space, we don't get too close (shake your head no). *If we can touch the person next to us* (extend your arm out in front and to the side), *then we're too close and being a space hog. If we're too close and being a space hog, then we need to back up* (demonstrate leaning back) *and stay in our own space. And when our friend is too close, we should back up* (lean back), *stay in our own space, and be a space keeper!"*

"Okay, let's have ____ (behavioral coach 1) and ____ (behavioral coach 2) try first!"

Role Play: Ring Around the Rosie

The group leader leads the role play. Behavioral coaches 1 and 2 demonstrate how to play *Ring Around the Rosie* while the other behavioral coaches and children sit in a circle nearly watching the role play.

Group leader: *"Okay ____ (behavioral coach 1) and ____ (behavioral coach 2), let's practice staying in our own space. If you're too close to your friend and being a space hog when you sit down, remember to back up and be a space keeper. Are we ready? All together now."*

Behavioral coaches and children: *"Ring around the rosie, a pocket full of posies, ashes, ashes, we all fall down!"*

Behavioral coaches 1 and 2: (Fall down and sit ***too close*** to one another.)

Group leader: *"____ (Behavioral coach 1) and ____ (behavioral coach 2), look around you. If you're sitting too close to your friend and being a space hog, then you should back up and don't be bossy!"*

Behavioral coaches 1 and 2: (Lean back and move away from one another to be an arm's length away from each other.)

Group leader:	*"____ (Behavioral coach 1) and ____ (behavioral coach 2), great job staying in your own space and being a space keeper! Okay friends, now it's everybody's turn to play."*

Behavioral Rehearsal: Ring Around the Rosie

Group leader:	(Have all the children and behavioral coaches stand up and hold hands in a circle.) *"Are we ready? All together now."*
Behavioral coaches:	(If needed, behavioral coaches instruct the children to sing the *Ring Around the Rosie* song. Once the children are familiar with the game, introduce opportunities to practice ***staying in our own space****.)*
Group leader:	*"Okay friends, now let's practice staying in our own space. If you're too close to your friends when you sit down, remember to back up* (lean back) *and be a space keeper! Are we ready? All together now."*
Behavioral coaches and children:	*"Ring around the rosie, a pocket full of posies, ashes, ashes, we all fall down!"*
Behavioral coaches:	(The children will practice staying in their own space by having the behavioral coaches take turns sitting too close (shoulder to shoulder) to the children when they *"all fall down.")*
Group leader:	*"Okay friends, look around you. If you're being a space hog and are too close to your friends, then you should back up and be a space keeper!"*
Behavioral coaches:	(If needed, ***social coach*** the children to ***stay in their own space*** by having the children back up.)
Group leader:	*"Great job staying in our own space and being a space keeper! Let's keep playing. Are we ready? All together now."*

Repeat the sequence above for a few cycles and then begin to introduce new commands.

Group leader:	*"Okay friends, now make sure to listen and follow directions because we're not going to fall down anymore. We're going to do some other fun things! If I say, 'We all spin around!' what should we do?* (Pause briefly to allow the children to demonstrate spinning around.) *That's right, friends! We should all spin around like this* (spin around)." *"Are we ready? All together now."*
Behavioral coaches and children:	*"Ring around the rosie, a pocket full of posies, ashes, ashes, we all spin around!"*

Group leader:	(After a few moments say, *"FREEZE! (Pause.) And sit!"* and children will practice ***staying in their own space*** by having the behavioral coaches take turns sitting too close (shoulder to shoulder) to the children.)
	"Okay friends, look around you. If you're being a space hog and are too close to your friends, then you should back up and be a space keeper!"
Behavioral coaches:	(If needed, ***social coach*** the children to ***stay in their own space*** by having the children back up.)
Group leader:	*"Great job staying in your own space and being a space keeper! Friends, this time we're going to ____ (command)!* (Demonstrate the command). *Can you all show me how to ____ (command)?"*
	"That's right! Are we ready? All together now."
Behavioral coaches and children:	*"Ring around the rosie, a pocket full of posies, ashes, ashes, we all ____ (command)!"*
Group leader:	(After a few moments say, "*FREEZE!* (Pause.) *And sit!"* and children will practice ***staying in their own space*** by having the behavioral coaches take turns sitting too close (shoulder to shoulder) to the children.)

Table 13.1 Sample Commands

Spin around	Touch the ceiling	Hop on two feet
Crawl like a baby	Gallop like a horse	Fly like a dragon
Walk super slow	Hop on one foot	Slither like a snake
Walk on our knees	Swim like an octopus	Walk backward

Repeat the sequence above, introducing new commands each time until all the children have had multiple opportunities to practice ***staying in their own space***.

Behavioral Rehearsal Wrap-Up

Group leader:	*"Well friends, great job staying in your own space! Give yourselves a big round of applause!"* (All behavioral coaches clap and cheer and encourage the children to clap as well.)
	"Now everyone should come sit in the Listening Circle." (Have children return to the Listening Circle to sit on their carpet squares.)
	"Okay friends, you did such a great job staying in your own space by backing up (lean back) *if you were too close to your friends. And when your friend were too close, you did a good job of backing up* (lean back), *staying in your own space, and being a space keeper. No space hogs here!"*

"You each earned ____ (number) more stars for staying in your own space and being a space keeper! Let's start with ____ (child)."

Award each child the same number of stars by repeating the following with each child:

Group leader: *"Where's _____ (child)?"* (Wait until all the children are looking at the child.)

"_____ (Child), how many stars did you earn?" (Pause briefly to allow the child to respond.)

"That's right! Let's all count for _____ (child)! One, two, three... (add stars to the Star Chart as they are counted aloud)*! Everybody clap for _____ (child)!"* (All behavioral coaches clap and cheer and encourage the children to clap as well.)

Break Time (10 Minutes)

- The puppets may be used to lead the children to and from the bathroom during break time.
- To assist with transitions and limit unstructured time, behavioral coaches may review the lesson with the children while waiting for the remaining children to return from the bathroom.
- You may want to award stars for good behavior after returning from the bathroom.

Session 13 Continued

Simon Says

BEHAVIORAL REHEARSAL ACTIVITY 2

Materials Needed

- None.

Room Setup

- Remove or place all carpet squares to the side.
- The group leader stands at the front of the room facing the children.
- The children and behavioral coaches sit in the play area facing the group leader.

Rules: Simon Says

- The group leader reads the script below to explain the rules.
- All commands begin with *"Simon says…"*
  - The purpose of the game is to practice ***staying in our own space*** rather than to eliminate group members.
- Keep commands simple and fun. Present commands that require some movement.
  - Examples:
    - *"Simon says hop like a kangaroo!"*
    - *"Simon says stomp your feet like a giant!"*
  - The group leader and behavioral coaches may need to model the commands for the children.
- Play two or three rounds to familiarize the children with the game.
- Once the children are familiar with the game, instruct the children to freeze in place before ***social coaching*** them to practice ***staying in their own space*** after each command.

Behavioral Rehearsal: Simon Says (15 Minutes)

The group leader leads the activity. The behavioral coaches and children sit nearby as the group leader explains the rules.

Group leader: *"Hey friends, we're going to play Simon Says! I'm going to tell each of you to do some fun and silly things like 'Simon says fly like a bird' (fly like a bird) or 'Simon says hop like a frog'* (hop like a frog)*."*

"After you fly like a bird or hop like a frog, I'll say 'Simon says FREEZE and sit…and don't be a space hog!'"

"After you freeze, you'll practice staying in your own space. Remember when we're staying in our own space, we don't get too close (shake your head no). *If we can touch the person next to us* (extend your arm out in front and to the side), *then we're too close and being a space hog. If we're too close and being a space hog, then we need to back up* (demonstrate leaning back) *and stay in our own space. And when our friend is too close, we should back up* (lean back), *stay in our own space, and be a space keeper!"*

(Walk over to a nearby behavioral coach member and stand ***too close***.)

"Friends, am I being a space hog and standing too close"? (Pause briefly to allow the children to respond by saying, *"yes."*) *"That's right, friends!"*

"Should I back up and stay in my own space?" (Pause briefly to allow the children to respond by saying, *"yes."*) *"That's right, friends!"*

(Take a step back.)

"Friends, now am I staying in my own space?" (Pause briefly to allow the children to respond by saying, *"yes."*) *"That's right, friends!"*

"Okay, _____ (behavioral coach 1) and _____ (behavioral coach 2) go first!"

Role Play: Simon Says

The group leader presents the commands. The two behavioral coaches demonstrate how to play *Simon Says* while the other behavioral coaches and children sit nearby watching.

Group leader:	*"Okay _____ (behavioral coaches 1 and 2), let's play Simon Says and practice staying in our own space."* *"If you or your friend is standing too and being a space hog when I say 'Simon says freeze!' remember to back up and don't be bossy. Remember to be a space keeper!"* *"Are we ready? _____ (Behavioral coaches 1 and 2), Simon says fly like a bird!"*
Behavioral coaches 1 and 2:	(Fly like birds and get ***too close*** to one another.)
Group leader:	*"Simon says FREEZE and sit...and don't be a space hog!"*
Behavioral coaches 1 and 2:	(Behavioral coaches sit ***too close*** to one another.)

Group leader:	*"_____ (Behavioral coaches 1 and 2), look around you. If you or your friend is standing too and being a space hog, then you should back up and don't be bossy. Remember to be a space keeper!"*
Behavioral coaches 1 and 2:	(Move an arm's length away from one another.)
Group leader:	*"_____ (Behavioral coaches 1 and 2), great job staying in your own space and NOT being space hogs!"* *"Okay friends, now it's everybody's turn to play."*

Behavioral Rehearsal: Simon Says

Group leader:	*"Are we ready? Simon says _____ (command)!" (Allow behavioral coaches and children to follow the command for several moments.)* *"Simon says FREEZE!* (Pause.) *And sit…and don't be a space hog!"*
Behavioral coaches:	(Behavioral coaches randomly sit ***too close*** to the children.)
Group leader:	*"Friends, look around you. If you or your friend is sitting too close and being a space hog, then you should back up and don't be bossy. Remember to be a space keeper!"* (If needed, ***social coach*** the children to ***stay in their own space***. If the children continue to be ***space hogs*** and need additional ***social coaching*** say, *"I still see some space hogs. Who can show us how to be a space keeper? Remember to back up if you're sitting too close to your friends."*) *"I don't see any space hogs! Great job staying in your own space! Let's keep playing!"*

Repeat the sequence above introducing new commands each round and making sure that each child practices ***staying in their own space*** multiple times. Once the children are familiar with the game, introduce opportunities to practice ***staying in your own space*** in which behavioral coaches intentionally sit ***too close*** to the children so children will have to practice ***backing up*** and ***staying in their own space***.

Table 13.2 Examples of Commands

Walk like a robot	Waddle like a penguin	Spin like a top
Peck like a chicken	Gallop like a horse	Wiggle like a worm
Stomp your feet like a giant	Walk backward	Dance
Shake your hips	Crawl like a baby	Move slow like a turtle
Hop like a kangaroo	Give a friend a high-five	Spin like a top
Swim like a shark	Chomp like an alligator	Dig like a dog
Slither like a snake	Act like a monkey	Shake your legs

Behavioral Rehearsal Wrap-Up

Group leader: *"Well friends, great job staying in your own space and being space keepers! Give yourselves a big round of applause!"* (All behavioral coaches clap and cheer and encourage the children to clap as well.)

"Now everyone should come sit in the Listening Circle." (Have children return to the Listening Circle to sit on their carpet squares.)

"Okay friends, you did such a great job staying in your own space by backing up (lean back) *if you or your friends were too close. No space hogs here!"*

"You each earned ____ (number) more stars for staying in your own space! Let's start with _____ (child)."

Award each child the same number of stars by repeating the following with each child:

Group leader: *"Where's ____ (child)?"* (Wait until all the children are looking at the child.)

"____ (Child), how many stars did you earn?" (Pause briefly to allow the child to respond.)

"That's right! Let's all count for ____ (child)! One, two, three... (add stars to the Star Chart as they are counted aloud)*! Everybody clap for ____ (child)!"* (All behavioral coaches clap and cheer and encourage the children to clap as well.)

"Now we're going to play another game with our parents and practice asking and giving help some more!"

Session 13 Continued

Staying in Your Own Space

PARENT COACHED PLAY: DYADIC PLAYDATES

Materials Needed

- Games brought by children and parents from home.
- Turn-taking games provided by the treatment team.
- Tables and chairs or carpet squares.
- *Parent Coached Play Cards*.

Room Setup

- If available, organize tables in separate corners of the room with four to six chairs per table.
- If tables are not available, place two carpet squares in separate corners of the room to indicate where the children will sit.
- The group leader sits on the floor at the front of the room.

Rules: Dyadic Playdates

- The group leader divides the families into groups of two families each.
  - If there are an odd number of children, pair one child with a behavioral coach. In this case, you will need an additional coach to serve as a behavioral coach for the parent.
- Assign each group to sit at a table or specific play area.
- Before the families go to their specified play area, parents will ***social coach*** their children to ***stay in their own space*** when sitting down.
- Once at the play area, parents will hold onto the games until the children are sitting down and ***staying in their own space***.
  - Children should sit next to each other.
  - Parents will act as ***social coaches*** by sitting on the other side of their child to minimize interrupting the natural flow of play between the children.
  - One behavioral coach will be assigned to each dyad to provide ***social coaching*** suggestions and feedback to parents.
- Parents will help the children pick the first game to play and ***social coach*** their children to ***keep cool*** if their game was not the first chosen game.
- Rather than helping the children set up the game, parents will ***social coach*** the children to ***ask and give help*** to each other.
- As the children play their games, parents will continue to ***social coach*** their children to ***stay in their own space*** as needed.

- After approximately nine minutes of play, instruct the parents to prepare the children for the upcoming game swap.
- After approximately one additional minute of play (ten minutes total), instruct the parents to swap games.
- Repeat the cycle with the second game.
- After approximately nine minutes of play, instruct the parents to prepare the children for clean up.
- After approximately one additional minute of play (ten minutes total), parents will ***social coach*** the children to clean up, ***say "bye" using names,*** and return to the Listening Circle.

Behavioral Coaching: Dyadic Playdates

Behavioral coaches will ***social coach*** parents during dyadic ***playdates*** in the following ways:

- ***Priming*:**
  - Begin the play interactions with parents going over the rules for ***staying in our own space*** BEFORE GAME PLAYING.
    - Example: *"Remember when we're staying in our own space, we don't get too close* (shake your head no). *If we can touch the person next to us* (extend your arm out in front and to the side), *then we're too close and being a space hog. If we're too close and being a space hog, then we need to back up* (demonstrate leaning back) *and stay in our own space. Remember to be a space keeper!"*
- ***Prompting*:**
  - Reminding parents to use the buzzwords to ***prompt*** their child to ***stay in their own space*** IN THE MOMENT.
  - Helping parents to identify opportunities to proactively ***prompt*** their child to ***stay in their own space***.
    - Example: *"Remember to stay in your own space."*
    - Example: *"Don't forget to back up if you're too close."*
    - Example: *"Are you being a space hog or a space keeper?"*
- ***Praising*:**
  - Reminding parents to ***praise*** and reinforce their child whenever their child ***stays in their own space*** CORRECTLY.
    - Example: *"Great job being a space keeper!"*
    - Example: *"Great job backing up and not being too close!"*
    - Example: *"Good job staying in your own space!"*
- ***Providing corrective feedback using a praise sandwich*:**
  - Reminding parents to ***praise*** their child's ATTEMPTS to ***stay in their own space*** and identify what could be done differently next time.
    - Example: *"Nice try staying in your own space. Don't forget to back up next time, but good try!"*
    - Example: *"Good try staying in your own space. Don't get too close next time, but good job!"*
    - Example: *"Good try staying in your own space. Don't be a space hog next time, but nice job!"*

- Reminding parents to continue to ***social coach*** on previously learned skills:
    - ***Listening and following directions.***
    - ***Meeting and greeting friends.***
    - ***Sharing and giving a turn.***
    - ***Asking for a turn.***
    - ***Keeping cool.***
    - ***Being a good sport.***
    - ***Showing and telling.***
    - ***Don't be bossy.***
    - ***Asking a friend to play.***
    - ***Joining a game.***
    - ***Asking to play something different.***
    - ***Asking and giving help.***

Parent Coached Play: Dyadic Playdates (20 Minutes)

- Have each child choose a turn-taking game brought from home or provided by the treatment team.
- The group leader sits on the floor at the front of the room.
- The families sit on the floor in a semi-circle facing the group leader.

Group leader: *"Hey friends, we're going to have more playdates and play with the fun games you brought from home. This time, we're going to practice staying in our own space as you play. When you get to your play area, you need to sit down and NOT be a space hog."*

"Remember when we're staying in our own space, we don't get too close (shake your head no). *If we can touch the person next to us* (extend your arm out in front and to the side), *then we're too close and being a space hog. If we're too close and being a space hog, then we need to back up* (demonstrate leaning back) *and stay in our own space. And if our friend is too close, then we need to back up* (demonstrate leaning back), *stay in our own space, and don't be bossy. Remember to be a space keeper!"*

"We'll swap games after a few minutes, and you'll keep practicing staying in your own space. Parents, remember to social coach your children by using your Parent Coached Play Cards. Okay, let's play with our games!"

- Before walking to the play area, instruct the parents to ***social coach*** the children *by saying, "Parents, remember to social coach your children to stay in their own space and to say 'hi' and use names with one another."*
- Rather than helping the children set up the game, parents will ***social coach*** the children to ***ask and give help*** to each other.
- Parents should be monitoring their child's body boundaries during game playing and ***social coaching*** the children to ***stay in their own space***.
- Parents will also ***social coach*** their children to ***not be bossy, show and tell, ask for a turn, share and take turns, keep cool,*** and ***be a good sport*** throughout the game playing.
- After approximately nine minutes of play, instruct the parents to prepare the children for the upcoming game swap by saying, *"Parents, tell your children that we'll be swapping games in one minute."*

- After approximately one additional minute of play (ten minutes total), instruct the parents to swap games by saying, *"Parents, it's time to swap games. Social coach the children to ask and give help by cleaning up before playing the next game."*
- After approximately nine minutes of playing the second game, instruct the parents to prepare the children for clean up by saying, *"Parents, tell your children that we'll be cleaning up in one minute."*
- After approximately one additional minute of play (ten minutes total), ***prompt*** the parents to instruct their children to clean up by saying, *"Parents, it's time to clean up. Let's social coach the children to ask and give help by cleaning up and then say 'bye' to their friend using names before sitting in the Listening Circle."*
- If needed, parents will ***social coach*** their child to ***ask and give help*** to clean up.
- Then parents will ***social coach*** their child to ***say "bye"*** to their friend ***using names.***

Final Wrap-Up (10 minutes)

- The group leader sits on the floor at the front of the room.
- The children sit on the carpet squares in a semi-circle facing the group leader, with parents sitting behind their children.

Group leader: *"Okay friends, you all did a great job playing your games and staying in your own space. When we're staying in our own space, do you think we should back up if we're too close to our friends?"* (Pause briefly to allow children to respond *"yes."*)

"That's right, friends! And if our friends are too close to us, do you think we should back up, stay in our own space, and not be bossy?" (Pause briefly to allow children to respond *"yes."*)

"That's right, friends! You all did such a great job staying in your own space and not being space hogs today that you each earned ____ (number) more stars! Let's start with ____ (child)."

Award each child the same number of stars by repeating the following with each child:

Group leader: *"Where's _____ (child)?"* (Wait until all the children are looking at the child.)

"_____ (Child), how many stars did you earn?" (Pause briefly to allow the child to respond.)

"That's right! Let's all count for _____ (child)! One, two, three... (add stars to the Star Chart as they are counted aloud)*! Everybody clap for _____ (child)!"* (All behavioral coaches clap and cheer and encourage the children to clap as well.)

"And remember you all earned those stars by staying in your own space and being good space keepers! Everyone did a great job, and parents you did an excellent job social coaching! Parents, remember your homework assignments this week are for you and your children to practice staying in your own space and for you to continue practicing all the other things we've learned to be a good friend using the 4 Ps. And don't forget to have a playdate and go to your playgroups."

"Alright little friends, do you want to count our stars?" (Pause briefly to allow the children to respond.)

"Let's all count together and see how many stars we earned today! One, two, three…(count the number of stars for one child)*!"*

"You each earned ____ (total number) stars today! Round of applause for our friends!" (All behavioral coaches should clap and cheer and encourage the families to clap as well.)

"Great job, friends! Don't forget to choose your reward before you leave. See you all next week!"

Session 13 Continued

Staying in Our Own Space

PEERS® FOR PRESCHOOLERS: PARENT HANDOUT

Snapshot of the Lesson: Staying in Our Own Space

The objective of this lesson is to teach children how to ***stay in their own space.*** Steps for ***staying in our own space*** include:

- ***Don't get too close*** (shake your head no).
  - If we can touch the person next to us (extend your arm out in front and to the side), then we're ***too close*** and ***being a space hog***.
- ***Stay in our own space*** (nod your head yes).
  - If we're ***too close*** and ***being a space hog***, then we need to ***back up*** (lean back) and ***stay in our own space.***
  - If our friends are ***too close*** and ***being a space hog***, then we need to ***back up*** (lean back), ***stay in our own space,*** and ***not be bossy.***
  - ***Remember to be a "space keeper."***

Parent Social Coaching Strategies for Staying in Our Own Space

- **Parents should provide opportunities to practice *staying in our own space* during games and activities that are highly motivating for your child.**
  - Your child will be more motivated to practice ***staying in their own space*** if the rehearsal is paired with a preferred activity.
  - Remember to ***prime*** your child before practicing by saying, *"Now we're going to practice staying in our own space while playing (preferred activity)."*
    - Then go over the rules for ***staying in our own space.***
  - Example: Playing games with siblings and ***playmates***.
    - When playing games on the floor, you may make continued game play contingent on your child ***staying in their own space***.
    - If your child begins to get ***too close*** to a sibling or ***playmate***, pause the game and ***social coach*** your child to ***stay in their own space***.
    - Once they are demonstrating good body boundaries, ***praise*** your child and resume the game.

- **Parents may pretend to be a *playmate* while having your child practice *staying in their own space.***
  - In the absence of siblings or ***playmates*** to practice with, you may have the child pretend the parent is a ***playmate*** while practicing ***staying in their own space***.
  - Since body boundaries are different for parents and their children, be clear that the parent is pretending to be a peer for the sake of practicing.
  - Example: In preparation for a ***playdate***, have your child pretend that you are their ***playmate*** and you are having a pretend ***playdate*** while practicing ***staying in your own space***.

- **Practice *staying in our own space* during games and activities that may be more difficult for your child to use appropriate body boundaries.**
  - Consider playing games or activities on the floor that are usually played while seated at a table.
    - Example: Playing a board game on the floor.
  - Playing on the floor often leads to poorer use of body boundaries in children, so practicing on the floor may create more opportunities to provide ***social coaching*** around ***staying in our own space***.
  - When practicing ***staying in our own space*** on the floor, consider practicing with siblings when possible, or with a parent assuming the role of a child.
  - If you have concerns that your child will not be able to ***stay in their own space*** during games and activities on the floor with real ***playmates***, consider structuring activities around a table until your child can more appropriately use body boundaries.

- **Use opportunities that naturally occur throughout the day to have your child practice *staying in their own space.***
  - Examples of opportunities for your child to ***stay in their own space***:
    - Watching television or movies.
    - Meal or snack times.
    - Waiting in line at the store.
    - Waiting for parents to finish a task.
    - Playing with games and toys on the floor.
  - Because body boundaries with parents and their children are different, be sure to let your child know you are practicing ***staying in our own space*** as if you were ***playmates***.
    - ***Social coaching*** your child that they should remain an arm's length away from you may feel rejecting if they don't understand you are pretending to be a ***playmate***.

- **If your child does not know what an arm's length away feels like, create fun opportunities to demonstrate this distance.**
  - Some children have difficulty judging when they are getting ***too close*** to another person or being a ***space hog***.
  - Creating fun opportunities for your child to learn what an arm's length away feels like will help them better judge this distance in the future.
  - Example: Create a fun game to practice body boundaries.
    - You and your child stand at opposite sides of the room facing each other.
    - When you say "*Go!*" you and your child run toward each other while doing something silly.

- Then ***social coach*** your child to use ***stay in their own space*** by saying, *"Freeze!"* when you get ***too close***.
- End with ***praising*** them for ***staying in their own space***.

- **If your child has difficulty judging when they are getting *too close* to another person:**
  - Consider creating a ***verbal prompt*** to provide coaching in the moment.
    - Example: *"Space check."*
    - Example: *"Body bubble."*
  - Consider creating a ***nonverbal prompt*** to provide coaching in the moment.
    - Example: Parent extends their arm.
  - Note: It is fine to have your child measure with their arm when learning about body boundaries with you and members of the family but be sure to let them know that we NEVER measure the distance with our arms with ***playmates*** or other people.

Homework Assignments

1. **Playdates.**
   - Schedule and have a ***playdate*** with a ***playmate***.
   - Prepare for the ***playdate*** using the ***5 Ws***.
     - ***WHO: Playdates*** should be one-on-one.
     - ***WHAT: Playdates*** should be activity-based.
     - ***WHERE:*** Schedule initial ***playdates*** to take place in your home or somewhere you can provide ***social coaching***.
     - ***WHEN:*** Try to keep initial ***playdates*** to no more than 1–1.5 hours.
     - ***HOW:*** Coordinate how the children will get to and from the ***playdate***.
   - Do a final practice with your child of the games and activities that will be available during the ***playdate***.
   - Gather all the games and activity materials for the ***playdate*** in one area that is VISIBLE and easily accessible to YOU but not the children.
   - Provide ***social coaching*** during the ***playdate*** and assess if this is a good ***playmate*** for your child.

2. **Practice staying in your own space.**
   - DO NOT have your child practice being a ***space hog***.
     - Notify your child that you are PRETENDING to be a friend who is a ***space hog*** and have your child practice ***staying in their own space*** and ***being a space keeper.***
   - Practice having your child ***stay in their own space*** this week while providing ***social coaching*** using the ***4 Ps***.
     - ***Priming*:** Review the rules for ***staying in our own space*** with your child BEFORE PRACTICING.
     - ***Prompting*:** Remind your child IN THE MOMENT to ***stay in their own space*** whenever the opportunities present.
     - ***Praising*: *Praise*** your child using the buzzwords whenever they ***stay in their own space*** CORRECTLY.
     - ***Providing corrective feedback*: *Provide corrective feedback*** in the form of a ***praise sandwich*** whenever your child ATTEMPTS to ***stay in their own space.***

- Please send us a 30–60-second video of ***social coaching*** your child to ***stay in their own space*** to be viewed during homework review.
  - Please include:
    - Skills your child did well.
    - Skills you would like to work on with your child.

3. **Provide *social coaching* on previously learned skills.**
   - Continue providing ***social coaching*** to your child throughout the week using the ***4 Ps.***
   - Previous skills include:
     - ***Listening and following directions.***
     - ***Meeting and greeting friends.***
     - ***Sharing and giving a turn.***
     - ***Asking for a turn.***
     - ***Keeping cool.***
     - ***Being a good sport.***
     - ***Showing and telling.***
     - ***Don't be bossy.***
     - ***Asking a friend to play.***
     - ***Joining a game.***
     - ***Asking to play something different.***
     - ***Asking and giving help.***

4. **Bring a turn-taking game.**
   - Bring a turn-taking game that your child enjoys playing and can be played with the other children.

Session 13 Continued

Staying in Our Own Space

PEERS® FOR PRESCHOOLERS: PARENT COACHED PLAY CARD

Snapshot of the Lesson: Staying in Our Own Space

- ***Don't get too close*** (shake your head no).
  - If we can touch the person next to us (extend your arm out in front and to the side), then we're ***too close*** and being a ***space hog***.
- ***Stay in our own space*** (nod your head yes).
  - If we're ***too close*** and ***being a space hog***, then we need to ***back up*** (lean back) and ***stay in our own space.***
  - If our friends are ***too close*** and ***being a space hog***, then we need to ***back up*** (lean back), ***stay in our own space,*** and ***not be bossy.***
  - ***Remember to be a "space keeper."***

Priming BEFORE Game Playing

- *"Remember when we're staying in our own space, we don't get too close* (shake your head no). *If we can touch the person next to us* (extend your arm out in front and to the side), *then we're too close and being a space hog. If we're too close and being a space hog, then we need to back up* (demonstrate leaning back) *and stay in our own space. Remember to be a space keeper!"*

Prompting IN THE MOMENT

- Example: *"Remember to stay in your own space."*
- Example: *"Don't forget to back up if you're too close."*
- Example: *"Are you being a space hog or a space keeper?"*

Praising for CORRECT Use of Skills

- Example: *"Great job being a space keeper!"*
- Example: *"Great job backing up and not being too close!"*
- Example: *"Good job staying in your own space!"*

Providing Corrective Feedback for ATTEMPTS Using a Praise Sandwich

- Example: *"Nice try staying in your own space. Don't forget to back up next time, but good try!"*
- Example: *"Good try staying in your own space. Don't get too close next time, but good job!"*
- Example: *"Good try staying in your own space. Don't be a space hog next time, but nice job!"*

- Continue to provide ***social coaching*** on previously learned skills:
  - ***Listening and following directions.***
  - ***Meeting and greeting friends.***
  - ***Sharing and giving a turn.***
  - ***Asking for a turn.***
  - ***Keeping cool.***
  - ***Being a good sport.***
  - ***Showing and telling.***
  - ***Don't be bossy.***
  - ***Asking a friend to play.***
  - ***Joining a game.***
  - ***Asking to play something different.***
  - ***Asking and giving help.***

Session 13 Continued

Staying in Our Own Space

PEERS® FOR PRESCHOOLERS: PARENT HOMEWORK WORKSHEET

Child's Name:	Parent's Name:		Date:	
HOMEWORK ASSIGNMENTS	PRIMING (REVIEWING RULES BEFORE PRACTICE)	PROMPTING (IN THE MOMENT)	PRAISING (USING BUZZWORDS)	PROVIDING CORRECTIVE FEEDBACK (USING A PRAISE SANDWICH)
Staying in our own space				
Practice previous skills: • **Asking and giving help** • **Asking to play something different** • **Joining a game** • **Asking a friend to play** • **Don't be bossy** • **Show and tell during play** • **Being a good sport** • **Keeping cool** • **Asking for a turn** • **Sharing and giving turns** • **Meeting and greeting friends** • **Listening and following directions**				
Playdate: • **Plan a playdate using the 5 Ws** • **Prime your child before the playdate** • **Provide social coaching during the playdate using the 4 Ps**				

Child's Name:	Parent's Name:		Date:	
HOMEWORK ASSIGNMENTS	PRIMING (REVIEWING RULES BEFORE PRACTICE)	PROMPTING (IN THE MOMENT)	PRAISING (USING BUZZWORDS)	PROVIDING CORRECTIVE FEEDBACK (USING A PRAISE SANDWICH)
Bring a turn-taking game	Did you bring a turn-taking game? YES or NO (Circle)		Which game did you bring?	

Please fill out this worksheet by describing what you did to complete the homework assignments. Worksheets will be collected during Homework Review at the next session of PEERS® for Preschoolers.

Session 14

Using an Inside Voice

PARENT SESSION THERAPIST GUIDE

Announcements

- Graduation is in two weeks!
- Explain post-testing (if applicable).

Parent Session Agenda

- Homework Review (40 minutes).
- Didactic Lessons (20 minutes).
- Parent Coached Play (20 minutes).
- Final Wrap-Up (10 minutes).

Materials Needed

- Conference room with a large table and enough chairs for the parent group leader and all parents to sit comfortably around the table.
  - Avoid sitting in a circle without a table as this creates the atmosphere of group therapy.
- Name tags for parents and treatment team.
- *Parent Handouts* (for the current week and the previous week).
- *Parent Homework Worksheets* (for the current week and the previous week).
- *Parent Coached Play Cards* (for the current week and the previous week).
- *Attendance and Homework Compliance Sheets* for parent group leader.
- Pens for note-taking (consider having extra pens for parents who need them).

Homework Review (40 Minutes)

1. **Playdates.**
   - Have parents report on the ***playdate*** and confirm that they planned using the ***5 Ws.***
   - Review what parents did to ***social coach*** their child BEFORE, DURING, and AFTER the ***playdate***.
   - Identify what skills their child did well and what skills they need to work on.
     - Confirm that parents ***praised*** skills that were done well and provided ***priming, prompting***, and/or ***corrective feedback*** for emerging skills.
   - Have parents assess if this is a good ***playmate*** for their child.
   - Have parents identify who their child might have a ***playdate*** with in the coming week (does not have to be a different ***playmate***).

DOI: 10.4324/9781003502968-15

2. **Practice staying in our own space.**
    - Review the 30–60-second video of ***social coaching*** for ***staying in our own space*** for each family. (For larger groups, you may need to review video recordings in two smaller groups with two different parent group leaders).
        - Have parents identify:
            - Skills their child did well.
            - Skills they would like to work on with their child.
        - Confirm that parents DID NOT have their child practice being a ***space hog***.
            - Parents should have pretended to be a friend who is a ***space hog*** and had their child practice ***staying in their own space*** and ***being a space keeper***.
        - Provide ***social coaching*** tips as appropriate for each family.
    - If parents did not send a video of ***social coaching***, confirm the following:
        - Parents practiced having their child ***stay in their own space*** while providing ***social coaching*** using the ***4 Ps.***
            - ***Priming*****:** Reviewed the rules for ***staying in our own space*** with their child BEFORE PRACTICING.
            - ***Prompting*****:** Reminded their child IN THE MOMENT to ***stay in their own space*** whenever the opportunity presented.
            - ***Praising*****: *Praised*** their child using the buzzwords whenever they ***stayed in their own space*** CORRECTLY.
            - ***Providing corrective feedback*****: *Provided corrective feedback*** in the form of a ***praise sandwich*** whenever their child ATTEMPTED to ***stay in their own space***.

3. **Provide social coaching on previously learned skills.**
    - Confirm parents continued to provide ***social coaching*** to their child throughout the week using the ***4 Ps*** for previously learned skills:
        - ***Listening and following directions.***
        - ***Meeting and greeting friends.***
        - ***Sharing and giving a turn.***
        - ***Asking for a turn.***
        - ***Keeping cool.***
        - ***Being a good sport.***
        - ***Showing and telling.***
        - ***Don't be bossy.***
        - ***Asking a friend to play.***
        - ***Joining a game.***
        - ***Asking to play something different.***
        - ***Asking and giving help.***

4. **Bring a turn-taking game.**
    - Confirm the following:
        - Brought a turn-taking game that their child enjoys playing and can be played with the other children. (To avoid distractions, these games should be left with the parents until *Parent Coached Play*.)

Didactic Lessons (20 Minutes)

PEERS® Neuroaffirming Pledge:

- We value neurodiversity, acceptance, and authenticity.
- We honor the diverse ways people experience the world.
- We respect each person's unique perspectives and communication styles.

- We recognize there is no one right way to connect with others.
- If using the strategies taught in PEERS® feels like camouflaging or masking and/or they don't align with your goals or the goals of your family, then you do not have to use them.
- Learning and using the skills taught in PEERS® is a PERSONAL CHOICE.

Didactic Lesson: Using an Inside Voice

- Distribute *Parent Handouts*.
  - Sections in **bold print** come directly from the *Parent Handout*.
  - Terms that are ***bold and italicized*** are buzzwords and represent important concepts from the didactic lesson.

- Explain, *"The focus of today's child lesson is to help your children use appropriate volume when playing with their friends. Like the previous lesson on staying in our own space, using good volume control is a transferrable skill that applies to many social contexts beyond making and keeping friends. Before we cover parent coaching strategies for promoting appropriate volume use, it will be helpful to review the child lesson to give you some context for thinking about your social coaching."*

> **Snapshot of the Lesson: Using an Inside Voice**
>
> **The objective of this lesson is to teach children how *to use an inside voice.* Rules for *using an inside voice* include:**
>
> - ***Use an inside voice when you're inside*** **(place an index finger in front of your mouth).**
> - ***Don't be a loud talker.***
>   - ***Don't talk too loudly*** **when you're inside.**
> - ***Don't be a quiet talker.***
>   - ***Don't talk too quietly*** **or your friends won't be able to hear you.**

Parent Social Coaching Strategies for Using an Inside Voice

- **Parents should provide opportunities to practice during games and activities that are highly motivating for your child.**
  - **Example: Playing a turn-taking game with your child**
    - **Make turn-taking contingent on your child *using an inside voice.***
    - **If your child begins to talk *too loudly* or *too quietly* to you or their sibling, then pause the game and *social coach* your child to *use an inside voice.***
    - **Once your child is demonstrating appropriate voice volume, resume the game.**

- **During a *playdate*, parents may consider various activities that allow your child and their *playmate* to use different voice volumes.**
  - ***Social coach* your child PRIOR TO STARTING EACH ACTIVITY to use the appropriate voice volume.**

- **Bold text**
    - ***Social coach* your child DURING EACH ACTIVITY to use the appropriate voice volume when necessary.**
    - **Example: Indoor board games and outdoor water play.**
        - **Plan for the children to play a board game indoors and to play with water toys outdoors.**
        - ***Social coach* your child to *use an inside voice* during the board game.**
        - ***Social coach* your child to *use an outside voice* during water play outside.**
            - **An *outside voice* is simply one that is appropriately louder, depending on the context.**

- **Parents should *social coach* your child throughout the week by making your response to your child's requests contingent on your child *using an inside voice.***
    - **Example: Watching a movie.**
        - **If your child is asking you to watch a movie but is either *talking too loudly* or *too quietly*, parents may *social coach* their child by saying one of the following:**
            - ***"We can watch the movie when you ask using an inside voice."***
            - ***"I can't hear you because you're talking too quietly. Try asking me again using an inside voice."***
            - ***"You're talking too loudly. Try again using an inside voice."***
        - **Be sure to *praise* your child when they appropriately adjust their volume.**

- **Parents may consider REFINING your child's skills by *social coaching* your child to *use an inside voice* when using previously learned skills.**
    - **Example: *Asking for a turn.***
        - **If your child does a great job *asking for a turn* but continues to have difficulty looking at their *playmate* and *using an inside voice*, parents may consider focusing on these two specific behaviors when *social coaching.***
            - ***"Remember to look at your friend and use an inside voice when you ask for a turn."***
    - **Remember NOT to focus on too many behaviors at once. This can be overwhelming and frustrating for your child.**
        - **Focus on the larger, main aspects of the skill first before *social coaching* on smaller aspects.**

- **Use opportunities that naturally occur throughout the day to have your child practice *using an inside voice.***
    - **Examples of opportunities for your child to *use an inside voice*:**
        - **Saying *"hi"* and *"bye"* to *playmates* at drop-off and pick-up times.**
        - **Talking to family during meal or snack times.**
        - **Talking with family members in the car.**
        - **Playing with siblings.**

- **Model appropriate and inappropriate voice volume for your child.**
    - **Prepare your child by telling them which voice volume you are demonstrating before you speak by using the following sentence stem:**
        - ***"This is what (______________) sounds like."***
            - **Yelling.**

- **A loud voice.**
- **An *inside voice*.**
- **A whisper.**
- **Silence.**

- **If your child has difficulty judging voice volume, create fun opportunities or games to demonstrate voice volume.**
  - **Example: Voice volume guessing game.**
    - **After you have demonstrated different types of voice volume, have your child guess which voice volume you are using.**
    - **Randomly alternate between yelling, talking loudly, *using an inside voice*, and whispering.**
    - **Use the same sentence stem to have your child guess which voice volume you are using:**
      - ***"Which volume am I speaking at now?"***
    - **Consider having your child practice using different types of voice volume by having you guess which volume they are speaking at.**

- **If your child has difficulty modulating their voice volume, consider creating *verbal or nonverbal* prompts to provide *social coaching* in the moment.**
  - ***Verbal prompts*:**
    - **Example: *"Volume check."***
    - **Example: *"Voice check."***
  - ***Nonverbal prompts*:**
    - **Example: Parent cups their ear (too quiet).**
    - **Example: Parent covers their ear (too loud).**

Parent Coached Play

- Distribute the *Parent Coached Play Cards.*
- Review the examples of the ***4 Ps*** provided on the *Parent Coached Play Card.*
- Remind parents that in a few moments we will be joining the children for *Parent Coached Play* in the context of mock dyadic ***playdates***.
- Parents should keep the *Parent Coached Play Card* in front of them during the dyadic ***playdate*** for recommendations on how to ***social coach*** children on ***using an inside voice.***

Homework Assignments

(Briefly review the homework assignments and troubleshoot any potential problems with parents.)

1. **Playdates.**
   - **Schedule and have a *playdate* with a *playmate*.**
   - **Prepare for the *playdate* using the *5 Ws*.**
     - ***WHO: Playdates* should be one-on-one.**
     - ***WHAT: Playdates* should be activity-based.**

- ◦ ***WHERE:*** **Schedule initial *playdates* to take place in your home or somewhere you can provide *social coaching*.**
- ◦ ***WHEN:*** **Try to keep initial *playdates* to no more than 1–1.5 hours.**
- ◦ ***HOW:*** **Coordinate how the children will get to and from the *playdate*.**

- **Do a final practice with your child of the games and activities that will be available during the *playdate*.**
- **Gather all the games and activity materials for the *playdate* in one area that is VISIBLE and easily accessible to YOU but not the children.**
- **Provide *social coaching* during the *playdate* and assess if this is a good *playmate* for your child.**

2. **Practice using an inside voice.**
   - **DO NOT have your child practice speaking *too loudly* or *too quietly*.**
     - ◦ **Parents may model appropriate and inappropriate voice volume for your child.**
   - **Practice having your child *use an inside voice* this week while providing *social coaching* using the *4 Ps*.**
     - ◦ ***Priming:*** **Review the rules for *using an inside voice* with your child BEFORE PRACTICING.**
     - ◦ ***Prompting:*** **Remind your child IN THE MOMENT to *use an inside voice* whenever the opportunities present.**
     - ◦ ***Praising: Praise*** **your child using the buzzwords whenever they *use an inside voice* CORRECTLY.**
     - ◦ ***Providing corrective feedback: Provide corrective feedback*** **in the form of a *praise sandwich* whenever your child ATTEMPTS to *use an inside voice*.**
   - **Please send us a 30–60-second video of *social coaching* your child to *using an inside voice* to be viewed during homework review.**
     - ◦ **Please include:**
       - ▪ **Skills your child did well.**
       - ▪ **Skills you would like to work on with your child.**

3. **Provide social coaching on previously learned skills.**
   - **Continue providing *social coaching* to your child throughout the week using the *4 Ps*.**
   - **Previous skills include:**
     - ◦ ***Listening and following directions.***
     - ◦ ***Meeting and greeting friends.***
     - ◦ ***Sharing and giving a turn.***
     - ◦ ***Asking for a turn.***
     - ◦ ***Keeping cool.***
     - ◦ ***Being a good sport.***
     - ◦ ***Showing and telling.***
     - ◦ ***Don't be bossy.***
     - ◦ ***Asking a friend to play.***
     - ◦ ***Joining a game.***
     - ◦ ***Asking to play something different.***
     - ◦ ***Asking and giving help.***
     - ◦ ***Staying in our own space.***

4. **Bring a turn-taking game that your child enjoys playing and can be played with the other children.**

Session 14 Continued

Using an Inside Voice

CHILD SESSION THERAPIST GUIDE

Child Session Agenda

- Didactic Lesson: *Using an Inside Voice* (20 minutes).
- Group Behavioral Rehearsal Activity 1: *Duck, Duck, Goose* (15 minutes).
- Break Time (10 minutes).
- Group Behavioral Rehearsal Activity 2: *Sweet Potato Soup* (15 minutes).
- Parent Coached Play: *Dyadic Playdates* (20 minutes).
- Final Wrap-Up (10 minutes).

Snapshot of the Lesson: Using an Inside Voice

The objective of this lesson is to teach children how **to *use an inside voice.*** Rules for ***using an inside voice*** include:

- ***Use an inside voice when you're inside*** (place an index finger in front of your mouth).
- ***Don't be a loud talker.***
    - ***Don't talk too loudly*** when you're inside.
- ***Don't be a quiet talker.***
    - ***Don't talk too quietly*** or your friends won't be able to hear you.

Materials Needed

- Cow puppet.
- Lion puppet.
- Several Legos.
- Carpet squares or chairs.
- "Making Friends Helper" badge.
- Star chart with names of children.
- Marker for star chart.
- Name tags for families and treatment team.
- Prize bins with prizes.

Preparing for the Lesson

- Use the script below with the group leader using a cow puppet to play the part of "Kelly Cow."
- A behavioral coach uses a lion puppet to play the part of "Larry Lion."
- An additional behavioral coach assists in behavioral rehearsal and provides encouragement and feedback to the group.
- A child is chosen at the beginning of the lesson as the "Making Friends Helper."

    - The "Making Friends Helper" wears a special badge and is the first child to practice the skill.
- The group leader and the behavioral coach sit on the floor at the front of the room.
- A special colored carpet square (e.g., red) is placed at the front of the room next to the child group leader to be used as the "Good Friend Square."
- For the children, additional carpet squares of the same color (e.g., green) are placed in a semi-circle facing the child group leader and the "Good Friend Square."
- Note: If carpet squares are unavailable, the children and behavioral coach may sit on chairs.
- The material in *italics* should be read by the indicated person.
- The material in ***bold and italics*** represents buzzwords and should be emphasized when read.
- The material in CAPITAL LETTERS within the script should be given extra emphasis while the group is encouraged to say the words in unison.

Behavioral Coaching Techniques

Behavioral coaches should use the following coaching techniques described below throughout the lesson and the behavioral rehearsal activities. (Note: ***priming*** occurs during the introduction to the activity.)

- ***Prompting***:
    - Use the buzzwords to ***prompt*** the children to ***use an inside voice***.
        - Example: *"Remember to use an inside voice."*
        - Example: *"Remember your friends can't hear you if you talk too quietly."*
        - Example: *"Are you talking too loudly?"*
- ***Praising***:
    - Reinforce ***using an inside voice*** by ***praising*** the children.
        - Example: *"Great job using an inside voice!"*
        - Example: *"Great job not talking too loudly!"*
        - Example: *"Nice job not talking too quietly!"*
- ***Providing corrective feedback using a praise sandwich:***
    - Reinforce ATTEMPTS to ***use an inside voice*** by ***praising*** the children and identifying what could be done differently next time.
        - Example: *"Nice try using an inside voice. Don't forget to talk a little bit louder so your friends can hear you, but good job!"*
        - Example: *"Good try using an inside voice. Remember not to talk too loudly, but nice job!"*
        - Example: *"Nice try using an inside voice. Remember not to talk too quietly, but good job!"*
- Behavioral coaches should continue to ***social coach*** on previously learned skills:
    - ***Listening and following directions.***
    - ***Asking names and using names.***
    - ***Greeting friends.***
    - ***Sharing and giving a turn.***
    - ***Asking for a turn.***
    - ***Keeping cool.***
    - ***Being a good sport.***
    - ***Showing and telling.***
    - ***Don't be bossy.***
    - ***Asking a friend to play.***
    - ***Joining a game.***
    - ***Asking and giving help.***
    - ***Staying in our own space.***

Didactic Lesson: Using an Inside Voice

Have the children sit in a semi-circle on the carpet squares facing the group leader.

Kelly Cow: (Sit at the front of the room and choose a Making Friends Helper.) *"Who wants to be our Making Friends Helper?"*

(Choose from among the children raising their hands and place the "Making Friends Helper" badge on the child. The child stays in their seat for now.)

"Hi friends! I'm Kelly Cow. Moo, moo! Today we're going to practice using an inside voice. Using an inside voice is a great way to be nice to our friends!"

"Who should we use an inside voice with? We should use an inside voice with our FRIENDS, TEACHERS, MOMMIES, DADDIES, BROTHERS AND SISTERS."

"When should we use an inside voice? We should use an inside voice when we're inside, like at school, or a store, or inside our home."

"HOW should we use an inside voice? We should use an inside voice by (increase your volume when saying *"not talking too loudly"*) *not talking too loudly when we're inside* (shake your head no and cover your ears with your hands), *and* (whisper when saying *"not talking too quietly"*) *not talking too quietly or our friends won't be able to hear us. Instead of being a loud talker or a quiet talker, we should use an inside voice when we're inside."*

"Remember, using an inside voice is a nice way to be a good friend! Moo, moo!"

Role Play: Using an Inside Voice

Kelly Cow and Larry Lion: (Larry Lion plays with the Legos. Kelly Cow is nearby, watching Larry Lion play.)

Kelly Cow: (Turn to look at the group of children.) *"Hey friends! My friend Larry Lion is playing with Legos, and I want to play too! Do you think I should ask him to play?"* (Nod your head yes and encourage the children to say *"yes."*)

"That's a great idea! Moo, moo!! Let's do it!" (Turn toward Larry Lion and use LOUD VOLUME.) *"Larry Lion, can I play with you?"*

Larry Lion: (Turn to look at Kelly Cow, make a face, cover your ears, and shake your head no. Resume playing with the Legos.)

Kelly Cow:	(Turn to look at the group of children.) *"Hey friends, I think I hurt Larry Lion's ears! Oh no! Do you think I used an inside voice?"* (Shake your head no and encourage the children to say *"no."*) *"That's right! I talked too loudly. Do you think I should try again?"* (Nod your head yes and encourage the children to say *"yes."*) *"That's a great idea! Moo, moo! Let's do it!"* (Turn toward Larry Lion and speak in a WHISPER.) *"Larry Lion, can I play with you?"*
Larry Lion:	(Continue to play with the Legos without acknowledging Kelly Cow.)
Kelly Cow:	(Turn to look at the group of children.) *"Hey friends, I think Larry Lion couldn't hear me! Oh no! Do you think I talked too quietly?"* (Nod your head yes and encourage the children to say *"yes."*) *"That's right! Do you think I should try again and use an inside voice?"* (Nod your head yes and encourage the children to say *"yes."*) *"That's a great idea! Moo, moo! Let's do it!"* (Turn to look at Larry Lion, smile, and use an ***inside voice*** with a MODERATE VOLUME.) *"Larry Lion, can I play with you?"*
Larry Lion:	(Turn to look at Kelly Cow and smile.) *"Okay, Kelly Cow! Here's some Legos. Grr, Grr!"* (Hand a few Legos to Kelly Cow.)
Kelly Cow:	*"Thanks, Larry Lion! Moo, moo!"*
Larry Lion and Kelly Cow:	(Play Legos together for a few moments while ***showing and telling*** and ***being good sports***.)
Kelly Cow:	(Turn to look at the group of children.) *"Hey friends, did I do a good job using an inside voice?"* (Nod your head yes and encourage the children to say *"yes."*) *"That's right! Moo, moo!"*
Kelly Cow and Larry Lion:	(Say *"good job," give a "cow high-five," and "lion high-five,"* clap, cheer, and encourage the children to clap as well. Larry Lion keeps the Legos and sits on the other side of the Good Friend Square (i.e., the Good Friend Square is between Kelly Cow and Larry Lion). ***Social coach*** the children as needed while they practice ***using an inside voice*** with Larry Lion.)
Kelly Cow:	*"Now let's see _____ (behavioral coach) try! _____ (Behavioral coach), please come sit on the Good Friend Square."*
Behavioral coach:	(Sit on the Good Friend Square.)

Kelly Cow: *"_____ (Behavioral coach), can you show us how to use an inside voice with Larry Lion?"*

Behavioral coach: *"Okay, Kelly Cow."*

Kelly Cow: (Turn to look at the group of children.) *"Remember to* (place an index finger in front of your mouth and lower your volume when saying "*use an inside voice*") *use an inside voice when you ask Larry Lion to play. And don't forget to use* (pause briefly to prompt the children to say *"names"*)*...NAMES."*

Behavioral coach: *"Okay, Kelly Cow."*

Larry Lion: (Begin to play with the Legos.)

Behavioral coach: (Turn to look at Larry Lion, smile, and use an ***inside voice*** with a MODERATE VOLUME.) *"Larry Lion, can I play with you?"*

Larry Lion: (Turn to look at the behavioral coach and smile.) *"Okay, _____(behavioral coach)! Here's some Legos. Grr, Grr!"* (Hand a few Legos to the behavioral coach.)

Larry Lion and Behavioral coach: (Play together for a few moments while ***showing and telling*** and ***being good sports.***)

Kelly Cow: *"Great job using an inside voice, _____ (behavioral coach)! Moo, moo!"*

Kelly Cow and Behavioral coach: (Say *"good job," give a "cow high-five," and "lion high-five,"* clap, cheer, and encourage the children to clap as well. The behavioral coach returns the Legos to Larry Lion and returns to their seat.)

Behavioral Rehearsal: Using an Inside Voice

Kelly Cow: (Turn to look at the group of children.) *"Okay friends! Now let's see our Making Friends Helper _____ try! _____ (Making Friends Helper), come sit on the Good Friend Square and show us how to use an inside voice with Larry Lion."*

(The Making Friends Helper should sit on the Good Friend Square.)

"Remember to (place an index finger in front of your mouth and lower your volume when saying "*use an inside voice*") *use an inside voice when you ask Larry Lion to play. And don't forget to use* (pause briefly to prompt the children to say *"names"*)*...NAMES."*

Larry Lion: (Begin to play with the Legos.)

Kelly Cow: (If needed, ***social coach*** the Making Friends Helper to ***look, smile,*** and ***say, "Larry Lion, can I play with you?" using an inside voice***.)

Larry Lion: *"Okay, _____ (Making Friends Helper)! Here's some Legos. Grr, Grr!"*

(Hand a few Legos to the Making Friends Helper. Play together for a few moments while ***showing and telling*** and ***being good sports***)

Kelly Cow: *"Great job using an inside voice, _____ (Making Friends Helper)! Moo, moo!"*

(Say *"good job," give a "cow high-five," and "lion high-five,"* clap, cheer, and encourage the children to clap as well. The Making Friends Helper should return the Legos to Larry Lion.)

"Okay, Making Friends Helper, choose another friend to sit on the Good Friend Square." (If needed, ***social coach*** the Making Friends Helper to choose another child before returning to their seat.)

Repeat the following with each child:

Kelly Cow: (Have each child take turns sitting on the Good Friend Square and practicing ***using an inside voice*** with Larry Lion.)

(Turn to look at the group of children.) *"Okay friends! Now let's see*

_____ (child) try! _____ (Child), come sit on the Good Friend Square and show us how to use an inside voice with Larry Lion."

(The child should sit on the Good Friend Square.)

"Remember to (place an index finger in front of your mouth and lower your volume when saying "*use an inside voice*") *use an inside voice when you ask Larry Lion to play. And don't forget to use* (pause briefly to prompt the children to say *"names"*)*...NAMES."*

Larry Lion: (Begin to play with the Legos.)

Kelly Cow: (If needed, ***social coach*** the child to ***look, smile,*** and ***say, "Larry Lion, can I play with you?" using an inside voice***.)

Larry Lion: *"Okay, _____ (Child). Here's some Legos. Grr, Grr!"* (Hand a few Legos to the child. Play together for a few moments while ***showing and telling*** and ***being good sports***.)

Kelly Cow: *"Great job using an inside voice, _____ (child)! Moo, moo!"*

(Say *"good job," give a "cow high-five," and "lion high-five,"* clap, cheer, and encourage the children to clap as well. The child should return the Legos to Larry Lion.)

"Okay, ____ (Child), choose another friend to sit on the Good Friend Square." (If needed, ***social coach*** the child to choose another child before returning to their seat.)

After each child has had a turn practicing ***using an inside voice*** with Larry Lion:

Group leader: *"Well friends, you all did a great job using an inside voice by NOT talking too loudly and by NOT talking too quietly today!"*

"You each earned ____ (number) stars for using an inside voice! Let's start with ____ (child)."

Award each child the same number of stars by repeating the following with each child:

Group leader: *"Where's ____ (child)?"* (Wait until all the children are looking at the child.)

"____ (Child), how many stars did you earn?" (Pause briefly to allow the child to respond.)

"That's right! Let's all count for ____ (child)! One, two, three... (add stars to the Star Chart as they are counted aloud)*! Everybody clap for ____ (Child)!"* (All behavioral coaches clap and cheer and encourage the children to clap as well.)

Session 14 Continued

Duck, Duck, Goose

BEHAVIORAL REHEARSAL ACTIVITY 1

Materials Needed

- None.

Room Setup

- Remove or place all carpet squares to the side.
- The group leader sits on the floor in front of the room.
- The children and behavioral coaches sit on the floor in a circle facing the group leader.

Rules: Duck, Duck, Goose

- The group leader reads the script below to explain the rules.
- Choose a child to be a *"farmer."*
- The *farmer* walks around the circle, softly tapping each child on the head while saying, *"duck."*
  - A behavioral coach walks next to the *farmer* to ***social coach*** as needed.
- The *farmer* randomly selects a child by tapping the child's head and saying, *"goose!"*
- The *"goose"* stands up and chases the *farmer* around the circle.
- The *farmer* tries to sit in the *goose's* seat without being tagged.
- To continue the game, the *goose* is the next *farmer* and ***asks*** the current *farmer* ***for a turn***.
  - The purpose of the game is to practice ***asking for a turn*** and ***sharing and giving a turn*** while ***using an inside voice*** rather than to eliminate group members.
- The group leader and behavioral coach ***social coach*** the children to ***use an inside voice*** throughout the game.
  - If the children are ***talking too loudly*** or ***too quietly***, briefly pause the game and ***social coach*** the children to ***use an inside voice***.

Behavioral Rehearsal: Duck, Duck, Goose (15 Minutes)

The group leader explains the activity. The behavioral coaches and children sit in a circle nearby as the group leader explains the rules.

Group leader: *"Hey friends, today we're going to play Duck, Duck, Goose! One friend will be the farmer. The farmer walks around the circle, taps our heads, and says, 'duck, duck..."* (demonstrate by tapping two children on the head while saying *"duck"*) *while using an inside voice."*

"If the farmer taps your head and says, 'goose,' get up and chase the farmer around the circle. The farmer will run around the circle and will try to sit in your seat before being tagged."

"And if we hear friends talking too loudly or too quietly while we play, we're going to say, 'FREEZE' and wait until everyone uses an inside voice."

"If your head was tapped and the farmer says "goose," then you'll be the next farmer and you'll ask for a turn by looking at your friends with your (point to your eyes to prompt children to say *"eyes"*)*...EYES, smiling with your* (point to your mouth to prompt children to say *"mouth"*)*...MOUTH, and saying, 'Can I have a turn please?' while using an inside voice. And don't forget to use* (pause briefly to prompt the children to say *"names"*)*...NAMES."*

"Okay, _____ (behavioral coach 1) and _____ (behavioral coach 2) go first!"

Role Play: Duck, Duck, Goose

The group leader leads the role play. Behavioral coaches 1 and 2 demonstrate how to play *Duck, Duck, Goose*.

Group leader: *"_____ (Behavioral coach 1), you're our first farmer. Are you ready?"*

Behavioral coach 1: (Walk around the circle and softly tap the heads of the behavioral coaches and children. Tap two heads saying *"duck"* while ***using an inside voice*** with MODERATE VOLUME. Then tap two heads saying *"duck"* using LOUD VOLUME.)

Group leader: *"Everyone FREEZE!"*

Behavioral coaches and children: (Freeze in place.)

Group leader: *"Hey friends, did _____ (behavioral coach 1) talk too loudly?*

(Nod your head yes and encourage the children to say *"yes."*)

"That's right, friends! _____ (Behavioral coach 1), remember to use an inside voice."

Behavioral coach 1: *"Okay, _____ (group leader)."*

(Walk around the circle and softly tap the heads of the behavioral coach and children. Tap two heads saying *"duck"* while ***using an inside voice*** with MODERATE VOLUME. Then tap two heads saying *"duck"* using a WHISPER.)

Group leader: *"Everyone FREEZE!"*

Behavioral coaches and children: (Freeze in place.)

Group leader: *"Hey friends, did _____ (behavioral coach 1) talk too quietly?*

(Nod your head yes and encourage the children to say *"yes."*)

"That's right, friends! _____ (Behavioral coach 1), remember to use an inside voice."

Behavioral coach 1: *"Okay, _____ (group leader)."* (Resume playing while ***using an inside voice*** with MODERATE VOLUME.)

Group leader: *"Great job using an inside voice, _____ (behavioral coach 1)!"*

Behavioral coach 1: (Continue to play. Tap behavioral coach 2 on the head to be the first *goose*.) *"Goose!"*

Behavioral coaches 1 and 2: (Run around the circle. Behavioral coach 1 sits down in behavioral coach 2's seat before being tagged.)

Group leader: *"Great job playing! _____ (Behavioral coach 2), ask _____ (behavioral coach 1) for a turn to be the next farmer. Remember to use an inside voice."*

Behavioral coach 2: (Behavioral coach 2 ***asks for a turn*** using LOUD VOLUME.) *"____ (Behavioral coach 1), can I have a turn?"*

Group leader: *"Hey friends, did _____ (behavioral coach 2) talk too loudly?"*

(Nod your head yes and encourage the children to say *"yes."*)

"That's right, friends! _____ (Behavioral coach 2), remember to use an inside voice."

Behavioral coach 2: (Behavioral coach 2 ***asks for a turn*** using a WHISPER.) *"____ (Behavioral coach 1), can I have a turn?"*

Group leader: *"Hey friends, did _____ (behavioral coach 2) talk too quietly?"*

(Nod your head yes and encourage the children to say *"yes."*)

"That's right, friends! _____ (Behavioral coach 2), remember to use an inside voice."

Behavioral coach 2: (Behavioral coach 2 ***asks for a turn using an inside voice*** with MODERATE VOLUME.) *"____ (Behavioral coach 1), can I have a turn?"*

Behavioral coach 1: *"Okay, _____ (behavioral coach 2)."*

Group leader: *"Great job using an inside voice! _____ (Behavioral coach 2), it's your turn to be the next farmer."*

Behavioral coaches 1 and 2: (Play one quick round ***using an inside voice*** with MODERATE VOLUME only.)

Group leader: *"Great job using an inside voice! "Okay friends, now it's everybody's turn to play Duck, Duck, Goose!"*

Behavioral Rehearsal: Using an Inside Voice

Group leader: *"Our next farmer is _____ (child). _____ (Child), remember to use an inside voice when you ask _____ (former farmer) for a turn."*

(If needed, ***social coach*** the children to ***use an inside voice*** when ***asking for a turn*** and when ***sharing and giving a turn***.)

"Great job asking for a turn and using an inside voice, _____ (child)! Let's keep playing. _____ (Child), it's your turn to be the next farmer." Are we ready?"

(If needed, ***social coach*** the child to walk around the circle and softly tap the heads of the behavioral coaches and children ***using an inside voice*** while following the rules for playing *Duck, Duck, Goose*. Whomever the child taps as "*Goose*" will chase the current *farmer* around the circle and become the next *farmer*.)

Continue in the manner described above making sure all the children have equal opportunities to be the *farmer*.

Behavioral Rehearsal Wrap-Up

Group leader: *"Well friends, great job using an inside voice! Give yourselves a big round of applause!"* (All behavioral coaches clap and cheer and encourage the children to clap as well.)

"Okay friends, you did a great job using an inside voice by NOT talking too loudly and by NOT talking too quietly!"

"You each earned ____ (number) more stars for using an inside voice! Let's start with ____ (child)."

Award each child the same number of stars by repeating the following with each child:

Group leader: *"Where's _____ (child)?"* (Wait until all the children are looking at the child.)

"_____ (Child), how many stars did you earn?" (Pause briefly to allow the child to respond.)

"That's right! Let's all count for _____ (child)! One, two, three... (add stars to the Star Chart as they are counted aloud)*! Everybody clap for _____ (child)!"* (All behavioral coaches clap and cheer and encourage the children to clap as well.)

Break Time (10 Minutes)

- The puppets may be used to lead the children to and from the bathroom during break time.
- To assist with transitions and limit unstructured time, behavioral coaches may review the lesson with the children while waiting for the remaining children to return from the bathroom.
- You may want to award stars for good behavior after returning from the bathroom.

Session 14 Continued

Sweet Potato Soup

BEHAVIORAL REHEARSAL ACTIVITY 2

Materials Needed

- Small bucket.

Room Setup

- Remove or place all carpet squares to the side.
- The group leader sits on the floor at the front of the room holding the small bucket.
- The behavioral coaches and children sit on the floor in a circle with the group leader.

Rules: Sweet Potato Soup

- The group leader reads the script below to explain the rules.
- All behavioral coaches and children lightly tap their laps while singing the *Sweet Potato Soup* song:
  - *"Sweet potato, sweet potato, oop, oop, oop! What did ____ (person holding the bucket) put in that soup?"*
- The child or behavioral coach holding the bucket then pretends to place a food item into the bucket while naming it.
  - If needed, behavioral coaches will help the children to think of a food item.
- The child should then practice ***sharing and giving a turn*** by passing the bucket to the person sitting next to them while ***saying "here," using names***, and ***using an inside voice***.
- OPTIONAL: After one round, have the children place other types of objects into the soup.
  - Examples: Insects, toys, favorite snacks, etc.
  - Children may also be allowed to suggest additional objects.
  - Have all children practice using the same category before introducing new categories.
- The group leader and behavioral coaches ***social coach*** the children to ***use an inside voice*** throughout the game.
  - If the children are ***talking too loudly*** or ***too quietly***, briefly pause the game and ***social coach*** the children to ***use an inside voice***.

Behavioral Rehearsal: Sweet Potato Soup (15 Minutes)

The group leader leads the activity. The behavioral coaches and children sit in a circle on the floor with the group leader while the rules are explained.

Group leader: *"Hey friends! Now we're going to play Sweet Potato Soup! We're going to sing a fun song that goes like this, 'Sweet potato, sweet potato, oop, oop, oop! What did ____ (behavioral coach 1)* (point to behavioral coach 1) *put in that soup?'"*

"We're going to use this bucket (hold up the bucket) *to make our yummy soup. When your friends call your name, say what food you want to put in the bucket and then put it in the bucket* (demonstrate placing pretend food in the bucket and stirring)*."*

"You can put in carrots (demonstrate placing pretend food in the bucket) *or potatoes* (demonstrate placing pretend food in the bucket) *or whatever yummy food you like!"*

"Then you'll share and give a turn by giving the bucket to the friend next to you and saying 'here' while using names."

"And remember to use an inside voice by not talking too loudly and by not talking too quietly."

"And remember to listen and follow directions because sometimes we're going to put some silly things like bugs or candy into the soup."

"Okay, _____ (behavioral coach 1) and _____ (behavioral coach 2) will go first!"

Role Play: Sweet Potato Soup

The group leader leads the role play. Two behavioral coaches demonstrate how to play *Sweet Potato Soup*. The two behavioral coaches sit next to each other to one side of the group leader.

Group leader: *"____ (Behavioral coaches 1 and 2), let's play Sweet Potato Soup and practice using an inside voice. _____ (Behavioral coach 1), you'll go first. Are we ready?"*

(Hand the small bucket to behavioral coach 1.)

Behavioral coaches: *"Sweet potato, sweet potato, oop, oop, oop! What did _____ (behavioral coach 1) put in that soup?"*

Behavioral coach 1: (Use LOUD VOLUME.) *"I'm going to put _____ (food) in the soup* (demonstrate placing food in the bucket and stirring)*."*

Group leader: *"Hey friends, did _____ (behavioral coach 1) talk too loudly?*

(Nod your head yes and encourage the children to say *"yes."*)

	"That's right, friends! _____ (Behavioral coach 1), remember to use an inside voice."
Behavioral coach 1:	*"Okay, _____ (group leader)."* (Use a WHISPER.) *"I'm going to put _____ (food) in the soup* (demonstrate placing food in the bucket and stirring)*."*
Group leader:	*"Hey friends, did _____ (behavioral coach 1) talk too quietly?*
	(Nod your head yes and encourage the children to say *"yes."*)
	"That's right, friends! _____ (Behavioral coach 1), remember to use an inside voice."
Behavioral coach 1:	*"Okay, _____ (group leader)."* (***Use an inside voice*** with MODERATE VOLUME.) *"I'm going to put _____ (food) in the soup* (demonstrate placing food in the bucket and stirring)*. So good!"*
Group leader:	*"Great job using an inside voice, _____ (behavioral coach 1)! "Now share and give a turn with _____ (behavioral coach 2) and see what they will put into the soup."*
Behavioral coach 1:	(Look and smile at behavioral coach 2. ***Use an inside voice*** with MODERATE VOLUME.) *"Here, _____ (behavioral coach 2)* (hand the small bucket to behavioral coach 2)*."*
Group leader:	*"Great job using an inside voice and sharing and giving a turn _____ (behavioral coach 1)! Let's keep playing! Are we ready?"*
	"Great job using an inside voice, _____ (behavioral coach 1)! Okay friends, now it's everybody's turn to play Sweet Potato Soup. Are we ready?"

Behavioral Rehearsal: Sweet Potato Soup

Behavioral coaches children:	*"Sweet potato, sweet potato, oop, oop, oop! What did _____ (person holding the bucket) put in that soup?"*

To ***social coach*** the child holding the small bucket to ***use an inside voice***:

Group leader:	*"____ (Child), remember to use an inside voice."*

To ***social coach*** the children in the circle to ***use an inside voice***:

Group leader:	*"I hear lots of loud voices. We can't play until everyone uses an inside voice."*

(If needed, behavioral coaches should ***social coach*** the children to ***use an inside voice***.)

"Great job using an inside voice, _____ (child/children)!"

"Okay friends, let's listen because this time we're going to put ____ (new category) into the soup! Are we ready?"

Table 14.1 Sample Categories

Insects	Favorite snacks	Animals
Candy	Toys	Body parts
Articles of clothing	Things you see at the park	Things you see at the zoo
Things that smell bad	Things that smell good	Things that are furry
Things that are cold	Things that are hot	Anything you want

Behavioral Rehearsal Wrap-Up

Group leader: *"Well friends, great job using an inside voice! Give yourselves a big round of applause!"* (All behavioral coaches clap and cheer and encourage the children to clap as well.)

"Okay friends, you did a great job using an inside voice by NOT talking too loudly and by NOT talking too quietly!"

"You each earned ____ (number) more stars for using an inside voice! Let's start with ____ (child)."

Award each child the same number of stars by repeating the following with each child:

Group leader: *"Where's ____ (child)?"* (Wait until all the children are looking at the child.)

"____ (Child), how many stars did you earn?" (Pause briefly to allow the child to respond.)

"That's right! Let's all count for ____ (child)! One, two, three... (add stars to the Star Chart as they are counted aloud)*! Everybody clap for ____ (child)!"* (All behavioral coaches clap and cheer and encourage the children to clap as well.)

"Now we're going to play another game with our parents and practice using an inside voice some more!"

Session 14 Continued
Using an Inside Voice

PARENT COACHED PLAY: DYADIC PLAYDATES

Materials Needed

- Games brought by children and parents from home.
- Turn-taking games provided by the treatment team.
- Tables and chairs or carpet squares.
- *Parent Coached Play Cards.*

Room Setup

- If available, organize tables in separate corners of the room with four to six chairs per table.
- If tables are not available, place two carpet squares in separate corners of the room to indicate where the children will sit.

Rules: Dyadic Playdates

- The group leader divides the families into groups of two families each.
  - If there are an odd number of children, pair one child with a behavioral coach. In this case, you will need an additional coach to serve as a behavioral coach for the parent.
- Assign each group to sit at a table or specific play area.
- Before the families go to their specified play area, parents will ***social coach*** their children to ***use an inside voice*** when ***greeting*** their friend.
- Once at the play area, parents will hold onto the games until the children practice ***saying "hi" using names***, while ***using an inside voice.***
  - Children should sit next to each other.
  - Parents will ***social coach*** by sitting on the other side of their child in order to minimize interrupting the natural flow of play between the children.
  - If necessary, parents will ***social coach*** the children to ***stay in their own space***.
- Parents will help the children pick the first game to play and ***social coach*** their children to ***keep cool*** if their game was not the first chosen game.
- Rather than helping the children set up the game, parents will ***social coach*** the children to ***ask and give help*** to each other.
- As the children play their games, parents will ***social coach*** their children to ***use an inside voice*** as needed.
- After approximately nine minutes of play, instruct the parents to prepare the children for the upcoming game swap.

- After approximately one additional minute of play (ten minutes total), instruct the parents to swap games.
- Repeat the cycle with the second game.
- After approximately nine minutes of play, instruct the parents to prepare the children for clean up.
- After approximately one additional minute of play (ten minutes total), parents will ***social coach*** the children to clean up, ***say "bye" using names,*** while ***using an inside voice*** before returning to the Listening Circle.

Behavioral Coaching: Dyadic Playdates

Behavioral coaches will ***social coach*** parents during dyadic ***playdates*** in the following ways:

- ***Priming*:**
  - Begin the play interactions with parents going over the rules for ***using an inside voice*** BEFORE GAME PLAYING.
    - Example: *"Remember to use an inside voice* (place an index finger in front of your mouth) *when playing with your friends. Don't be a loud talker when you're inside, and don't be a quiet talker or your friends won't be able to hear you."*
- ***Prompting*:**
  - Reminding parents to use the buzzwords to ***prompt*** their child to ***use an inside voice*** IN THE MOMENT.
  - Helping parents to identify opportunities to proactively ***prompt*** their child to ***use an inside voice***.
    - Example: *"Remember to use an inside voice."*
    - Example: *"Remember to not to talk too loudly."*
    - Example: *"Are you talking too loudly?"*
- ***Praising*:**
  - Reminding parents to ***praise*** and reinforce their child whenever their child ***uses an inside voice*** CORRECTLY.
    - Example: *"Great job using an inside voice!"*
    - Example: *"Great job not talking too quietly!"*
    - Example: *"Nice job not talking too loudly!"*
- ***Providing corrective feedback using a praise sandwich*:**
  - Reminding parents to ***praise*** their child's ATTEMPTS to ***use an inside voice*** and identify what could be done differently next time.
    - Example: *"Nice try using an inside voice. Don't forget to talk a little bit louder so your friends can hear you, but good job!"*
    - Example: *"Good try using an inside voice. Remember not to talk too loudly, but nice job!"*
    - Example: *"Nice try using an inside voice. Remember not to talk too quietly, but good job!"*
- Behavioral coaches will remind parents to continue to ***social coach*** on previously learned skills:
  - ***Listening and following directions.***
  - ***Meeting and greeting friends.***
  - ***Sharing and giving a turn.***
  - ***Asking for a turn.***

- ***Keeping cool.***
- ***Being a good sport.***
- ***Showing and telling.***
- ***Don't be bossy.***
- ***Asking a friend to play.***
- ***Joining a game.***
- ***Asking to play something different.***
- ***Asking and giving help.***
- ***Staying in our own space.***

Parent Coached Play: Dyadic Playdates (20 Minutes)

- Have each child choose a turn-taking game brought from home or provided by the treatment team.
- The group leader sits on the floor at the front of the room.
- The families sit on the floor in a semi-circle facing the group leader.

Group leader: *"Hey friends, we're going to have more playdates and play with the fun games you brought from home. This time, we're going to practice using an inside voice as you play."*

"Remember to use an inside voice when you say 'hi' and 'bye' to your friend and when you ask and give help. And remember NOT to talk too loudly and NOT to talk too quietly when you ask for a turn and share and give a turn."

"We'll swap games after a few minutes, and you'll keep practicing using an inside voice. Parents, remember to social coach your children by using your Parent Coached Play Cards. Okay, let's go play with our games!"

- Before walking to the play area, instruct the parents to ***social coach*** the children *by saying, "Parents, remember to social coach your children to use an inside voice when they say 'hi' and use names with one another."*
- Rather than helping the children set up the game, parents will ***social coach*** the children to ***ask and give help*** to each other while ***using an inside voice***.
- Parents should be monitoring their child's body boundaries during game playing and ***social coaching*** the children to ***stay in their own space***.
- Parents will also ***social coach*** their children to ***not be bossy, show and tell, ask for a turn, share and take turns, keep cool***, and ***be a good sport*** throughout the game playing.
- After approximately nine minutes of play, instruct the parents to prepare the children for the upcoming game swap by saying, *"Parents, tell your children that we'll be swapping games in one minute."*
- After approximately one additional minute of play (ten minutes total), instruct the parents to swap games by saying, *"Parents, it's time to swap games. Social coach the children to ask for a turn and share and give a turn before playing the next game."*
- After approximately nine minutes of playing the second game, instruct the parents to prepare the children for clean up by saying, *"Parents, tell your children that we'll be cleaning up in one minute."*

- After approximately one additional minute of play (ten minutes total), ***prompt*** the parents to instruct their children to clean up by saying, *"Parents, it's time to clean up. Let's social coach the children to listen and follow directions by cleaning up and then say 'bye' to their friend using an inside voice before sitting in the Listening Circle."*
- If needed, parents will ***social coach*** their child to ***listen and follow directions*** to clean up.
- Then parents will ***social coach*** their child to ***say "bye"*** to their friend ***using names*** and ***an inside voice***.

Final Wrap-Up (10 minutes)

- The group leader sits on the floor at the front of the room.
- The children sit on the carpet squares in a semi-circle facing the group leader, with parents sitting behind their children.

Group leader: *"Okay friends, you all did a great job playing your games and using an inside voice. When we're using an inside voice, do you think we should talk too loudly with our friends?"* (Pause briefly to allow children to respond *"no."*)

"That's right, friends! And when we use an inside voice, do you think we should talk too quietly with our friends?" (Pause briefly to allow children to respond *"no."*)

"That's right, friends! You all did such a great job using an inside voice that you each earned ____ (number) more stars! Let's start with ____ (child)."

Award each child the same number of stars by repeating the following with each child:

Group leader: *"Where's _____ (child)?"* (Wait until all the children are looking at the child.)

"_____ (Child), how many stars did you earn?" (Pause briefly to allow the child to respond.)

"That's right! Let's all count for _____ (child)! One, two, three… (add stars to the Star Chart as they are counted aloud)*! Everybody clap for*

_____ (child)!" (All behavioral coaches clap and cheer and encourage the children to clap as well.)

"And remember you all earned those stars by using an inside voice! Everyone did a great job, and parents you did an excellent job social coaching! Parents, remember your homework assignments this week are for you and your children to practice using an inside voice and for you to continue practicing all the other things we've learned to be a good friend using the 4 Ps. And don't forget to have a playdate and go to your playgroups."

"Alright little friends, do you want to count our stars?" (Pause briefly to allow the children to respond.)

"Let's all count together and see how many stars we earned today! One, two, three…(count the number of stars for one child)*!"*

"You each earned ____ (total number) stars today! Round of applause for our friends!" (All behavioral coaches should clap and cheer and encourage the families to clap as well.)

"Great job, friends! Don't forget to choose your reward before you leave. See you all next week!"

Session 14 Continued

Using an Inside Voice

PEERS® FOR PRESCHOOLERS: PARENT HANDOUT

Didactic Lesson: Using an Inside Voice

> **Snapshot of the Lesson: Using an Inside Voice**
>
> The objective of this lesson is to teach children how ***to use an inside voice.*** Rules for ***using an inside voice*** include:
>
> - ***Use an inside voice when you're inside*** (place an index finger in front of your mouth).
> - ***Don't be a loud talker.***
>   - ***Don't talk too loudly*** when you're inside.
> - ***Don't be a quiet talker.***
>   - ***Don't talk too quietly*** or your friends won't be able to hear you.

Parent Social Coaching Strategies for Using an Inside Voice

- **Parents should provide opportunities to practice during games and activities that are highly motivating for your child.**
  - Example: Playing a turn-taking game with your child.
    - Make turn-taking contingent on your child ***using an inside voice***.
    - If your child begins to talk ***too loudly*** or too quietly to you or their sibling, then pause the game and ***social coach*** your child to ***use an inside voice***.
    - Once your child is demonstrating appropriate voice volume, resume the game.
- **During a *playdate*, parents may consider various activities that allow your child and their *playmate* to use different voice volumes.**
  - ***Social coach*** your child PRIOR TO STARTING EACH ACTIVITY to use the appropriate voice volume.
  - ***Social coach*** your child DURING EACH ACTIVITY to use the appropriate voice volume when necessary.
  - Example: Indoor board games and outdoor water play.
    - Plan for the children to play a board game indoors and to play with water toys outdoors.
    - ***Social coach*** your child to ***use an inside voice*** during the board game.

- ***Social coach*** your child to ***use an outside voice*** during water play outside.
  - An ***outside voice*** is simply one that is appropriately louder, depending on the context.

- **Parents should *social coach* your child throughout the week by making your response to your child's requests contingent on your child *using an inside voice.***
  - Example: Watching a movie.
    - If your child is asking you to watch a movie but is either ***talking too loudly*** or ***too quietly***, parents may ***social coach*** their child by saying one of the following:
      - *"We can watch the movie when you ask using an inside voice."*
      - *"I can't hear you because you're talking too quietly. Try asking me again using an inside voice."*
      - *"You're talking too loudly. Try again using an inside voice."*
    - Be sure to ***praise*** your child when they appropriately adjust their volume.

- **Parents may consider REFINING your child's skills by *social coaching* your child to *use an inside voice* when using previously learned skills.**
  - Example: ***Asking for a turn.***
    - If your child does a great job ***asking for a turn*** but continues to have difficulty looking at their ***playmate*** and ***using an inside voice***, parents may consider focusing on these two specific behaviors when ***social coaching***.
      - *"Remember to look at your friend and use an inside voice when you ask for a turn."*
  - Remember NOT to focus on too many behaviors at once. This can be overwhelming and frustrating for your child.
    - Focus on the larger, main aspects of the skill first before ***social coaching*** on smaller aspects.

- **Use opportunities that naturally occur throughout the day to have your child practice *using an inside voice.***
  - Examples of opportunities for your child to ***use an inside voice***:
    - Saying *"hi"* and *"bye"* to ***playmates*** at drop-off and pick-up times.
    - Talking to family during meal or snack times.
    - Talking with family members in the car.
    - Playing with siblings.

- **Model appropriate and inappropriate voice volume for your child.**
  - Prepare your child by telling them which voice volume you are demonstrating before you speak by using the following sentence stem:
    - *"This is what (____________) sounds like."*
      - Yelling.
      - A loud voice.
      - An *inside voice.*
      - A whisper.
      - Silence.

- **If your child has difficulty judging voice volume, create fun opportunities or games to demonstrate voice volume.**

- Example: Voice volume guessing game.
  - After you have demonstrated different types of voice volume, have your child guess which voice volume you are using.
  - Randomly alternate between yelling, talking loudly, ***using an inside voice***, and whispering.
  - Use the same sentence stem to have your child guess which voice volume you are using:
    - *"Which volume am I speaking at now?"*
  - Consider having your child practice using different types of voice volume by having you guess which volume they are speaking at.

- **If your child has difficulty modulating their voice volume, consider creating *verbal or nonverbal prompts* to provide *social coaching* in the moment.**
  - ***Verbal prompts:***
    - Example: *"Volume check."*
    - Example: *"Voice check."*
  - ***Nonverbal prompts:***
    - Example: Parent cups their ear (too quiet).
    - Example: Parent covers their ear (too loud).

Homework Assignments

1. **Playdates.**
   - Schedule and have a ***playdate*** with a ***playmate.***
   - Prepare for the ***playdate*** using the ***5 Ws.***
     - ***WHO: Playdates*** should be one-on-one.
     - ***WHAT: Playdates*** should be activity-based.
     - ***WHERE:*** Schedule initial ***playdates*** to take place in your home or somewhere you can provide ***social coaching.***
     - ***WHEN:*** Try to keep initial ***playdates*** to no more than 1–1.5 hours.
     - ***HOW:*** Coordinate how the children will get to and from the ***playdate***.
   - Do a final practice with your child of the games and activities that will be available during the ***playdate***.
   - Gather all the games and activity materials for the ***playdate*** in one area that is VISIBLE and easily accessible to YOU but not the children.
   - Provide ***social coaching*** during the ***playdate*** and assess if this is a good ***playmate*** for your child.

2. **Practice using an inside voice.**
   - DO NOT have your child practice speaking ***too loudly*** or ***too quietly***.
     - Parents may model appropriate and inappropriate voice volume for your child.
   - Practice having your child ***using an inside voice*** this week while providing ***social coaching*** using the ***4 Ps***.

- ○ ***Priming***: Review the rules for ***using an inside voice*** with your child BEFORE PRACTICING.
- ○ ***Prompting***: Remind your child IN THE MOMENT to ***use an inside voice*** whenever the opportunities present.
- ○ ***Praising***: ***Praise*** your child using the buzzwords whenever they ***use an inside voice*** CORRECTLY.
- ○ ***Providing corrective feedback***: ***Provide corrective feedback*** in the form of a ***praise sandwich*** whenever your child ATTEMPTS to ***use an inside voice.***

- Please send us a 30–60-second video of ***social coaching*** your child to ***use an inside voice*** to be viewed during homework review.
  - Please include:
    - Skills your child did well.
    - Skills you would like to work on with your child.

3. **Provide social coaching on previously learned skills.**
   - Continue providing ***social coaching*** to your child throughout the week using the ***4 Ps.***
   - Previous skills include:
     - ***Listening and following directions.***
     - ***Meeting and greeting friends.***
     - ***Sharing and giving a turn.***
     - ***Asking for a turn.***
     - ***Keeping cool.***
     - ***Being a good sport.***
     - ***Showing and telling.***
     - ***Don't be bossy.***
     - ***Asking a friend to play.***
     - ***Joining a game.***
     - ***Asking to play something different.***
     - ***Asking and giving help.***
     - ***Staying in our space.***

4. **Bring a turn-taking game.**
   - Bring a turn-taking game that your child enjoys playing and can be played with the other children.

Session 14 Continued

Using an Inside Voice

PEERS® FOR PRESCHOOLERS: PARENT COACHED PLAY CARD

Snapshot of the Lesson: Using an Inside Voice

- ***Use an inside voice when you're inside*** (place an index finger in front of your mouth).
- ***Don't be a loud talker.***
  - ***Don't talk too loudly*** when you're inside.
- ***Don't be a quiet talker.***
  - ***Don't talk too quietly*** or your friends won't be able to hear you.

Priming BEFORE Game Playing

- Example: *"Remember to use an inside voice* (place an index finger in front of your mouth) *when playing with your friends. Don't be a loud talker when you're inside, and don't be a quiet talker or your friends won't be able to hear you."*

Prompting IN THE MOMENT

- Example: *"Remember to use an inside voice."*
- Example: *"Remember not to talk too loudly."*
- Example: *"Are you talking too loudly?"*

Praising for CORRECT Use of Skills

- Example: *"Great job using an inside voice!"*
- Example: *"Great job not talking too quietly!"*
- Example: *"Nice job not talking too loudly!"*

Providing Corrective Feedback for ATTEMPTS Using a Praise Sandwich

- Example: *"Nice try using an inside voice. Don't forget to talk a little bit louder so your friends can hear you, but good job!"*
- Example: *"Good try using an inside voice. Remember not to talk too loudly, but nice job!"*
- Example: *"Nice try using an inside voice. Remember not to talk too quietly, but good job!"*

- Continue to provide ***social coaching*** on previously learned skills:
    - ***Listening and following directions.***
    - ***Meeting and greeting friends.***
    - ***Sharing and giving a turn.***
    - ***Asking for a turn.***
    - ***Keeping cool.***
    - ***Being a good sport.***
    - ***Showing and telling.***
    - ***Don't be bossy.***
    - ***Asking a friend to play.***
    - ***Joining a game.***
    - ***Asking to play something different.***
    - ***Asking and giving help.***
    - ***Staying in our space.***

Session 14 Continued

Using an Inside Voice

PEERS® FOR PRESCHOOLERS: PARENT HOMEWORK WORKSHEET

Child's Name:	Parent's Name:		Date:	
HOMEWORK ASSIGNMENTS	PRIMING (REVIEWING RULES BEFORE PRACTICE)	PROMPTING (IN THE MOMENT)	PRAISING (USING BUZZWORDS)	PROVIDING CORRECTIVE FEEDBACK (USING A PRAISE SANDWICH)
Using an inside voice				
Practice previous skills: • **Staying in our own space** • **Asking and giving help** • **Asking to play something different** • **Joining a game** • **Asking a friend to play** • **Don't be bossy** • **Show and tell during play** • **Being a good sport** • **Keeping cool** • **Asking for a turn** • **Sharing and giving turns** • **Meeting and greeting friends** • **Listening and following directions**				

<table>
<tr><td>Child's Name:</td><td colspan="2">Parent's Name:</td><td colspan="2">Date:</td></tr>
<tr><td>HOMEWORK ASSIGNMENTS</td><td>PRIMING (REVIEWING RULES BEFORE PRACTICE)</td><td>PROMPTING (IN THE MOMENT)</td><td>PRAISING (USING BUZZWORDS)</td><td>PROVIDING CORRECTIVE FEEDBACK (USING A PRAISE SANDWICH)</td></tr>
<tr><td>Playdate:
• Plan a playdate using the 5 Ws
• Prime your child before the playdate
• Provide social coaching during the playdate using the 4 Ps</td><td colspan="4"></td></tr>
<tr><td>Bring a turn-taking game</td><td colspan="2">Did you bring a turn-taking game?
YES or NO
(Circle)</td><td colspan="2">Which game did you bring?</td></tr>
</table>

Please fill out this worksheet by describing what you did to complete the homework assignments. Worksheets will be collected during Homework Review at the next session of PEERS® for Preschoolers.

Session 15

Disclosing a Diagnosis or Condition with Others and Final Review (Part 1)

PARENT SESSION THERAPIST GUIDE

Announcements

- Graduation is in one week!
- Explain post-testing (if applicable).

Parent Session Agenda

- Homework Review (40 minutes).
- Didactic Lessons (20 minutes).
- Parent Coached Play (20 minutes).
- Final Wrap-Up (10 minutes).

Materials Needed

- Conference room with a large table and enough chairs for the parent group leader and all parents to sit comfortably around the table.
  - Avoid sitting in a circle without a table as this creates the atmosphere of group therapy.
- Name tags for parents and treatment team.
- *Parent Handout*s (for the current week and the previous week).
- *Parent Homework Worksheets* (for the current week and the previous week).
- *Parent Coached Play Cards* (for the current week and the previous week).
- *Attendance and Homework Compliance Sheets* for parent group leader.
- Pens for note-taking (consider having extra pens for parents who need them).

Homework Review (40 Minutes)

1. **Playdates.**
   - Have parents report on the ***playdate*** and confirm that they planned using the ***5 Ws***.
   - Review what parents did to ***social coach*** their child BEFORE, DURING, and AFTER the ***playdate***.
   - Identify what skills their child did well and what skills they need to work on.
     - Confirm that parents ***praised*** skills that were done well and provided ***priming, prompting***, and/or ***corrective feedback*** for emerging skills.

DOI: 10.4324/9781003502968-16

- Have parents assess if this is a good ***playmate*** for their child.
- Have parents identify who their child might have a ***playdate*** within the coming week (does not have to be a different ***playmate***).

2. **Practice using an inside voice.**
   - Review the 30–60-second video of ***social coaching*** for ***using an inside voice*** for each family. (For larger groups, you may need to review video recordings in two smaller groups with two different parent group leaders).
     - Have parents identify:
       - Skills their child did well.
       - Skills they would like to work on with their child.
     - Confirm that parents DID NOT have their child practice speaking ***too loudly*** or ***too quietly***.
   - Parents may have modeled appropriate and inappropriate voice volume for their child.
     - Provide ***social coaching*** tips as appropriate for each family.
   - If parents did not send a video of ***social coaching***, confirm the following:
     - Parents practiced having their child ***use an inside voice*** while providing ***social coaching*** using the ***4 Ps.***
       - ***Priming***: Reviewed the rules for ***using an inside voice*** with their child BEFORE PRACTICING.
       - ***Prompting***: Reminded their child IN THE MOMENT to ***use an inside voice*** whenever the opportunity presented.
       - ***Praising***: ***Praised*** their child using the buzzwords whenever they ***used an inside voice*** CORRECTLY.
       - ***Providing corrective feedback***: ***Provided corrective feedback*** in the form of a ***praise sandwich*** whenever their child ATTEMPTED to ***use an inside voice***.

3. **Provide social coaching on previously learned skills.**
   - Confirm parents continued to provide ***social coaching*** to their child throughout the week using the ***4 Ps*** for previously learned skills:
     - ***Listening and following directions.***
     - ***Meeting and greeting friends.***
     - ***Shari***ng and giving a turn.
     - Asking for a turn.
     - Keeping cool.
     - Being a good sport.
     - Showing and telling.
     - Don't be bossy.
     - Asking a friend to play.
     - Joining a game.
     - Asking to play something different.
     - Asking and giving help.
     - Staying in our own space.

4. **Bring a turn-taking game.**
   - Confirm the following:
     - Brought a turn-taking game that their child enjoys playing and can be played with the other children. (To avoid distractions, these games should be left with the parents until *Parent Coached Play*.)

Didactic Lessons (20 Minutes)

PEERS® Neuroaffirming Pledge

- We value neurodiversity, acceptance, and authenticity.
- We honor the diverse ways people experience the world.
- We respect each person's unique perspectives and communication styles.
- We recognize there is no one right way to connect with others.
- If using the strategies taught in PEERS® feels like camouflaging or masking and/or they don't align with your goals or the goals of your family, then you do not have to use them.
- Learning and using the skills taught in PEERS® is a PERSONAL CHOICE.

Didactic Lesson: Disclosing a Diagnosis or Condition with Others

- Distribute *Parent Handouts*.
  - Sections in **bold print** come directly from the *Parent Handout*.
  - Terms that are ***bold and italicized*** are buzzwords and represent important concepts from the didactic lesson.

- Explain, *"The focus of today's parent lesson is on disclosing a diagnosis or condition with others. Like all parent lessons, this information is not being shared with your children. However, because part of being a good advocate for yourself may involve disclosing a diagnosis or condition to others, you may want to hold onto this information to share with your child when they are older. The skills taught here might apply to sharing your child's diagnosis or condition with other parents, teachers, family members, or friends. Disclosing a diagnosis or condition is a personal choice that every family needs to make for themselves. Should you choose to share your child's differences with others, it can be helpful to use the following steps to guide the conversation."*

Snapshot of Steps for Disclosing a Diagnosis or Condition with Others

1. **Choose the right time.**
2. **Choose the right person.**
3. **Choose the right context.**
4. **Acknowledge the difference.**
5. **Give an explanation.**
6. **Acknowledge what the difference means for your child.**
7. **Turn a challenge into a strength.**
8. **Make your child's strength an asset to the friendship.**
9. **Be prepared to answer questions.**
10. **Remember friendship is a choice.**

Steps for Disclosing a Diagnosis or Condition with Others

Step 1: Choose the Right Time

- **You may want to avoid disclosing diagnoses or conditions too soon in your acquaintance.**
  - **Consider letting them meet your child and get to know them before disclosing personal details about your child.**
- **You may want to disclose your child's diagnosis or condition sooner if the differences are noticeable.**
  - **Sharing your child's diagnosis or condition when it is visible allows you to influence how others perceive your child by explaining what others see through your own lens.**
- **Reasons for disclosing a diagnosis or condition:**
  - **Some parents share when seeking acceptance from others.**
  - **Other parents share in response to miscommunication and/or when misunderstandings arise.**
  - **Some parents share as they naturally become more comfortable and accepted by others.**
- **Disclosing your child's diagnosis or condition is a personal choice.**
- **You may or may not choose to share your child's diagnosis or condition and that is your family's decision.**

Step 2: Choose the Right Person

- **If you choose to share your child's diagnosis or condition, consider whether it is beneficial that the person knows.**
  - **Good example: Sharing your child's diagnosis with the parent of a preferred *playmate* who may notice that your child's behavior is different.**

Step 3: Choose the Right Context

- **Avoid blurting out your child's diagnosis or condition for no reason.**
- **Wait for the right context to share your child's diagnosis or condition.**
- **Often there is a reason or context for mentioning your child's diagnosis or condition.**

Step 4: Acknowledge the Difference

- **If your child's behavior appears different from other children, chances are others have noticed.**
- **Rather than avoiding talking about these differences, you might avoid any misunderstandings or misinterpretations by acknowledging the differences.**
  - **Good example: You might begin by saying, *"You may have noticed that my child has a tendency to (state the behavior)."***
    - ***"…avoid eye contact."***
    - ***"…talk a lot about certain things."***
    - ***"…ask a lot of personal questions."***

Step 5: Give an Explanation

- **Provide a reason or explanation for why your child behaves in a way that may be seen as different.**
- **People are more likely to understand behaviors that are different if they can be explained in a way that makes sense to them.**
- **If people don't understand why your child does certain things, they are more likely to attribute their behavior to negative interpretations.**
- **People are more likely to be accepting of differences if they understand them.**
  - **Good example: *"My child behaves in this way because they have/are (explain the condition)."***
  - **Good example: *"My child has been diagnosed with (name the condition)."***

Step 6: Acknowledge What the Difference Means for Your Child

- **Explain what having this condition means for your child.**
- **Explain how your child's behavior may affect others around them.**
- **Not everyone will understand what your child's diagnosis or condition means, so you will need to educate them.**
- **Good example: *"That means that when my child (state the behavior), people may think (explain how others perceive them)."***
  - ***"…avoids eye contact, people may think they're not paying attention or they're uninterested."***
  - *"…talks a lot about certain things, people may think they're being willfully annoying."*
  - *"…asks questions that make other people uncomfortable, people may think they're intentionally being rude."*

Step 7: Turn a Challenge into a Strength

- **After you've acknowledged the difference and presented the challenge your child faces in how people perceive them, immediately point out the strengths in your child.**
- **Always change what could be perceived as a negative into something positive.**
- **Good example: *"On the positive side, my child's condition also means that (state the positive characteristics)."***
  - ***"…even though they may look like they're not paying attention, they're actually very focused on what you're saying and are probably more likely to remember what you've said than most people."***
  - *"… they like to talk about things that interest them and are eager to share with others who have similar interests."*
  - *"…even though they may unintentionally ask personal questions, they're really open to feedback and almost never intend to make others uncomfortable."*

Step 8: Make Your Child's Strength an Asset to the Friendship

- **When acknowledging a difference and turning a challenge into a strength, it is useful to make this strength an asset to the friendship.**
- **You might also point out how this strength might be beneficial to the person with whom you are speaking.**
- **Good example: *"I believe (state the positive characteristic) could be a great asset to their friendships."***
    - ***"I believe my child's listening skills could be a great asset to their friendships."***
    - *"I believe my child's enthusiasm for specific interests, like the interests they share with your child, could be a great asset to their friendship."*
    - *"I believe my child's openness to feedback could be a great asset to their friendships."*

Step 9: Be Prepared to Answer Questions

- **Know what your child's diagnosis or condition means and how to briefly explain it.**
    - **Good example: *"Autism is a neurodevelopmental condition that can make social interactions challenging. Autistic people also tend to have specialized interests and repetitive behaviors."***

Step 10: Remember Friendship is a Choice

- ***Friendship is a choice.***
    - ***We don't get to be friends with everyone.***
    - ***Everyone doesn't get to be friends with us.***
- **When it comes to friendships, there are good choices and bad choices.**
- **If you don't like the way a parent reacts to your disclosure, your child doesn't have to be friends with their child.**
- **A person or a parent who doesn't react well to your disclosure may not be a good choice for your child or for you.**

Child Didactic Lesson: Final Review (Part I)

- Explain, *"The focus of today's child lesson will be reviewing and further practicing the skills learned for making and keeping friends. As we go through our final review of the skills learned in PEERS® for Preschoolers this week and next week, consider which skills still need refinement for your child. Next week, we will wrap-up our review and have a graduation ceremony to celebrate everyone's hard work and progress!"*

Snapshot of Previously Learned Lessons: Final Review (Part 1)

The objective of this lesson is to review some of the skills that the children have learned during the program. The skills for this lesson include:

Table 15.1 Previously Learned Skills (Part 1)

ASKING NAMES 1. Look at your friend with your eyes (point to your eyes). 2. Smile with your mouth (point to your mouth and smile). 3. Say, "What's your name?" 4. Say your name ("I'm ____ (Name)."	**USING NAMES** 1. Look at your friend with your eyes (point to your eyes). 2. Smile with your mouth (point to your mouth and smile). 3. Use names when talking to your friend.
GREETING FRIENDS SAYING "HI" 1. Look at your friend with your eyes (point to your eyes). 2. Smile with your mouth (point to your mouth and smile). 3. Wave with your hand (wave your hand). 4. Say "hi" using your friend's name.	**GREETING FRIENDS SAYING "BYE"** 1. Look at your friend with your eyes (point to your eyes). 2. Smile with your mouth (point to your mouth and smile). 3. Wave with your hand (wave your hand). 4. Say "bye" using your friend's name.
SHARING AND GIVING A TURN 1. Look at your friend with your eyes (point to your eyes). 2. Smile with your mouth (point to your mouth and smile). 3. Say "here" using names (demonstrate handing over a toy) when you share and give a turn.	**BEING A GOOD SPORT** 1. Look at your friend with your eyes (point to your eyes). 2. Smile with your mouth (point to your mouth and smile). 3. Say "good job" using names. 4. Give a high-five.
SHOW AND TELL: SHOWING YOUR TOY 1. Look at your friend with your eyes (point to your eyes). 2. Smile with your mouth (point to your mouth and smile). 3. Show your toy to your friend (wave your toy in front of your friend). 4. Tell your friend to look at your toy by saying, "Look at my (cool toy)!" while using names.	**SHOW AND TELL: "WATCH ME"** 1. Look at your friend with your eyes (point to your eyes). 2. Smile with your mouth (point to your mouth and smile). 3. Tell your friend to look at you by saying, "Watch me!" or "Look at me!" while using names. 4. Do something fun with your toy (e.g., fly a toy/plane in the air).
ASKING A FRIEND TO PLAY 1. Look at your friend with your eyes (point to your eyes). 2. Smile with your mouth (point to your mouth and smile). 3. Say, "Do you want to play?" using names. 4. If your friend says yes, think of something fun to play. 5. Say "Let's play _____ (activity/game)!" using names.	**ASKING TO PLAY SOMETHING DIFFERENT** 1. Think of something fun to play (point to your head). 2. Look at your friends with your eyes (point to your eyes). 3. Smile with your mouth (point to your mouth and smile). 4. Ask to play something different using names (e.g., "(Friend), let's play _____!"). If your friend says no: 1. Keep cool and play nicely 2. Look at your friends with your eyes (point to your eyes). 3. Smile with your mouth (point to your mouth and smile). 4. Say "okay" using names. 5. Play nicely with your friends. 6. If you're still upset, then take deep breaths to keep cool (take two slow deep breaths).
USING AN INSIDE VOICE • Use an inside voice when you're inside (place an index finger in front of your mouth). • Don't be a loud talker. • Don't talk too loudly when you're inside. • Don't be a quiet talker. • Don't talk too quietly or your friends won't be able to hear you.	

Parent Coached Play

- Distribute the *Parent Coached Play Cards*.
- Review the examples of the ***4 Ps*** provided on the *Parent Coached Play Card.*
- Remind parents that in a few moments we will be joining the children for *Parent Coached Play* in the context of mock dyadic ***playdates***.
- Parents should keep the *Parent Coached Play Card* in front of them during the dyadic ***playdate*** for recommendations on how to ***social coach*** children on previously learned skills.

Homework Assignments

(Briefly review the homework assignments and troubleshoot any potential problems with parents.)

1. **Playdates.**
   - **Schedule and have a *playdate* with a *playmate.***
   - **Prepare for the *playdate* using the *5 Ws.***
     - ***WHO: Playdates* should be one-on-one.**
     - ***WHAT: Playdates* should be activity-based.**
     - ***WHERE:* Schedule initial *playdates* to take place in your home or somewhere you can provide *social coaching.***
     - ***WHEN:* Try to keep initial *playdates* to no more than 1–1.5 hours.**
     - ***HOW:* Coordinate how the children will get to and from the *playdate.***
   - **Do a final practice with your child of the games and activities that will be available during the *playdate.***
   - **Gather all the games and activity materials for the *playdate* in one area that is VISIBLE and easily accessible to YOU but not the children.**
   - **Provide *social coaching* during the *playdate* and assess if this is a good *playmate* for your child.**

2. **Make a list of previously learned skills that still need refinement.**
   - **Identify which skills your child still needs to improve upon.**
     - **These are the skills you will focus on during your *social coaching* in the coming weeks and months.**
   - **Review the rules and steps for these skills with your child.**
   - **Consider watching the puppet show lessons with your child again (particularly for skills that still need refinement).**
   - **Previously learned skills include:**
     - ***Listening and following directions.***
     - ***Meeting and greeting friends.***
     - ***Sharing and giving a turn.***
     - ***Asking for a turn.***
     - ***Keeping cool.***
     - ***Being a good sport.***
     - ***Showing and telling.***
     - ***Don't be bossy.***
     - ***Asking a friend to play.***
     - ***Joining a game.***
     - ***Asking to play something different.***
     - ***Asking and giving help.***
     - ***Staying in our own space.***
     - ***Using an inside voice.***

3. **Practice a previously learned skill that needs refinement using the 4 Ps.**

- **Practice having your child use a previously learned skill this week while providing *social coaching* using the *4 Ps*.**
  - ***Priming*: Review the rules for the previously learned skill with your child BEFORE PRACTICING.**
  - ***Prompting*: Remind your child IN THE MOMENT to use the previously learned skill whenever the opportunities present.**
  - ***Praising*: *Praise* your child using the buzzwords whenever they use the previously learned skill CORRECTLY.**
  - ***Providing corrective feedback*: *Provide corrective feedback* in the form of a *praise sandwich* whenever your child ATTEMPTS to use the previously learned skill.**
- **Please send us a 30–60-second BOOSTER VIDEO of *social coaching* your child to use the previously learned skill to be viewed during homework review.**

4. **Practice disclosing a diagnosis or condition with others (optional assignment).**
   - **Consider practicing the steps for disclosing a diagnosis or condition with a trusted family member or friend following the steps outlined in the lesson.**
   - **Choosing to disclose a diagnosis or condition with others is a personal choice for each family, so consider discussing this choice (if you have not already).**

Session 15 Continued

Final Review (Part I)

CHILD SESSION THERAPIST GUIDE

Child Session Agenda

- Didactic Lesson: *Final Review (Part I)* (20 minutes).
- Group Behavioral Rehearsal Activity 1: *Red Rover* (15 minutes).
- Break Time (10 minutes).
- Group Behavioral Rehearsal Activity 2: *Swap Draw* (15 minutes).
- Parent Coached Play: *Dyadic Playdates* (20 minutes).
- Final Wrap-Up (10 minutes).

Snapshot of Previously Learned Lessons: Final Review (Part 1)

The objective of this lesson is to review some of the skills that the children have learned during the program. The skills for this lesson include:

Table 15.1 Previously Learned Skills (Part 1)

ASKING NAMES	USING NAMES
1. Look at your friend with your eyes (point to your eyes). 2. Smile with your mouth (point to your mouth and smile). 3. Say, "What's your name?" 4. Say your name ("I'm ____ (Name)."	1. Look at your friend with your eyes (point to your eyes). 2. Smile with your mouth (point to your mouth and smile). 3. Use names when talking to your friend.
GREETING FRIENDS SAYING "HI"	**GREETING FRIENDS SAYING "BYE"**
1. Look at your friend with your eyes (point to your eyes). 2. Smile with your mouth (point to your mouth and smile). 3. Wave with your hand (wave your hand). 4. Say "hi" using your friend's name.	1. Look at your friend with your eyes (point to your eyes). 2. Smile with your mouth (point to your mouth and smile). 3. Wave with your hand (wave your hand). 4. Say "bye" using your friend's name.
SHARING AND GIVING A TURN	**BEING A GOOD SPORT**
1. Look at your friend with your eyes (point to your eyes). 2. Smile with your mouth (point to your mouth and smile). 3. Say "here" using names (demonstrate handing over a toy) when you share and give a turn.	1. Look at your friend with your eyes (point to your eyes). 2. Smile with your mouth (point to your mouth and smile). 3. Say "good job" using names. 4. Give a high-five.

(*Continued*)

Table 15.1 Continued

SHOW AND TELL: SHOWING YOUR TOY	**SHOW AND TELL: "WATCH ME"**
1. Look at your friend with your eyes (point to your eyes). 2. Smile with your mouth (point to your mouth and smile). 3. Show your toy to your friend (wave your toy in front of your friend). 4. Tell your friend to look at your toy by saying, "Look at my (cool toy)!" while using names.	1. Look at your friend with your eyes (point to your eyes). 2. Smile with your mouth (point to your mouth and smile). 3. Tell your friend to look at you by saying, "Watch me!" or "Look at me!" while using names. 4. Do something fun with your toy (e.g., fly a toy/plane in the air).
ASKING A FRIEND TO PLAY 1. Look at your friend with your eyes (point to your eyes). 2. Smile with your mouth (point to your mouth and smile). 3. Say, "Do you want to play?" using names. 4. If your friend says yes, think of something fun to play. 5. Say "Let's play _____ (activity/game)!" using names.	**ASKING TO PLAY SOMETHING DIFFERENT** 1. Think of something fun to play (point to your head). 2. Look at your friends with your eyes (point to your eyes). 3. Smile with your mouth (point to your mouth and smile). 4. Ask to play something different using names (e.g., "(Friend), let's play _____!").
USING AN INSIDE VOICE • Use an inside voice when you're inside (place an index finger in front of your mouth). • Don't be a loud talker. • Don't talk too loudly when you're inside. • Don't be a quiet talker. • Don't talk too quietly or your friends won't be able to hear you.	**If your friend says no:** 1. Keep cool and play nicely 2. Look at your friends with your eyes (point to your eyes). 3. Smile with your mouth (point to your mouth and smile). 4. Say "okay" using names. 5. Play nicely with your friends. 6. If you're still upset, then take deep breaths to keep cool (take two slow deep breaths).

Materials Needed

- Cow puppet.
- Tiger puppet.
- Two toy cars.
- Small book.
- Bucket with building blocks.
- Carpet squares or chairs.
- "Making Friends Helper" badge for EACH CHILD.
- Star chart with names of children.
- Marker for star chart.
- Name tags for families and treatment team.
- Prize bins with prizes.

Preparing for the Lesson

- Use the script below with the group leader using a cow puppet to play the part of "Kelly Cow."
- A behavioral coach uses a tiger puppet to play the part of "Timmy Tiger."
- An additional behavioral coach assists in behavioral rehearsal and provides encouragement and feedback to the group.
- EACH CHILD is chosen at the beginning of the lesson as the "Making Friends Helpers."
    - Each child wears a "Making Friends Helpers" badge and will take turns being among the first to practice the previously learned skills (there are seven skills to rehearse in this lesson).
- The group leader and the behavioral coach sit on the floor at the front of the room.

- A special colored carpet square (e.g., red) is placed at the front of the room next to the child group leader to be used as the "Good Friend Square."
- For the children, additional carpet squares of the same color (e.g., green) are placed in a semi-circle facing the child group leader and the "Good Friend Square."
- Note: If carpet squares are unavailable, the children and behavioral coach may sit on chairs.
- The material in *italics* should be read by the indicated person.
- The material in ***bold and italics*** represents buzzwords and should be emphasized when read.
- The material in CAPITAL LETTERS within the script should be given extra emphasis while the group is encouraged to say the words in unison.

Behavioral Coaching Techniques

Behavioral coaches should use the following coaching techniques described below throughout the lesson and the behavioral rehearsal activities. (Note: ***priming*** occurs during the introduction to the activity.)

- ***Prompting***:
  - Use the buzzwords to ***prompt*** the children to ***be a good friend***.
    - Example: *"Let's remember to use names when you say 'hi.'"*
    - Example: *"Remember to ask a friend to play and think of something fun to play."*
    - Example: *"What can you do with your hand when being a good sport?"*
- ***Praising***:
  - Reinforce ***being a good friend*** by ***praising*** the children.
    - Example: *"Great job telling your friends to 'watch me!'"*
    - Example: *"Great job asking for a turn!"*
    - Example: *"Good job using an inside voice!"*
- ***Providing corrective feedback using a praise sandwich***:
  - Reinforce ATTEMPTS to ***be a good friend*** by ***praising*** the children and identifying what could be done differently next time.
    - Example: *"Good job asking a friend to play. Don't forget to look next time, but nice try!"*
    - Example: *"Good job sharing. Remember to say 'here' next time, but nice try!"*
    - Example: *"Good try showing and telling. Remember to say 'look at me' next time, but good job!"*

Didactic Lesson: Final Review (Part 1)

Kelly Cow: (Sit at the front of the room.) *"Hi friends! I'm Kelly Cow. Moo, moo! Today is a special day because EVERYBODY gets to be a Making Friends Helper! Moo, moo!"* (All behavioral coaches clap and cheer and encourage the children to clap as well.)

(Place a "Making Friends Helper" badge on EACH child. The children stay in their seats for now.)

Kelly Cow: *"Today we're going to have lots of fun playing some of your favorite games and practicing all the different ways to be nice to our friends!"*

"Who should we be nice with? We should be nice with our FRIENDS, TEACHERS, MOMMIES, DADDIES, BROTHERS, AND SISTERS."

"How should we be nice to our friends? We can be nice by using names and saying 'hi' and asking to play something different. We can also be nice by sharing and giving a turn, asking to play, being a good sport, and ALL the other things that we learned together."

"When should we be nice to our friends? We should be nice to our friends ALL the time! Like when we're playing together at the park or eating lunch at school or playing together at home."

"Remember, being nice is a great way to be a good friend! Moo, moo!"

Role Play: Meeting and Greeting Friends

Timmy Tiger: (Quietly reading a book to himself.)

Kelly Cow: (Turn to look at the group of children.) *"Hey friends! I see my new friend reading a book. I want to play with him but I forgot his name. Hmmm...Do you think I should ask his name and then say 'hi' using names?"* (Nod head yes and encourage the children to say *"yes."*)

"That's right, friends! Moo, moo! Let's do it!" (Turn to look at Timmy Tiger and smile.) *"What's your name?"*

Timmy Tiger: (Turn to look at Kelly Cow and smile.) *"Timmy Tiger. Grrr, grrr! What's your name?"*

Kelly Cow: *"Hi, Timmy Tiger* (wave at Timmy Tiger)*! I'm Kelly Cow. Moo, moo!"*

Timmy Tiger: *"Hi, Kelly Cow* (wave at Kelly Cow)*! Grrr, grrr!"*

Kelly Cow: (Turn to look at the group of children.) *"Hey friends, did I do a good job being a good friend by asking and using names?"* (Nod head yes and encourage the children to say *"yes."*)

"That's right! Moo, moo!"

Kelly Cow and Timmy Tiger: (Say *"good job," give a "cow high-five," and "tiger high-five,"* clap, cheer, and encourage the children to clap as well. Timmy Tiger takes the book and sits on the other side of the Good Friend Square (i.e., the Good Friend Square is between Kelly Cow and Timmy Tiger). ***Social coach*** the children as needed while they practice ***asking and using names*** with Timmy Tiger.)

Behavioral Rehearsal: Meeting and Greeting Friends

Kelly Cow: *"Who wants to be the first Making Friends Helper to show us how to ask names and say 'hi' using names?"*

(Choose from among the children raising their hands.)

"_____ (Child), come sit on the Good Friend Square and show us how to ask names and say 'hi' using names with Timmy Tiger."

(The child should sit on the Good Friend Square.)

"Remember to look at Timmy Tiger with your (point to your eyes to prompt the children to say *"eyes"*)*...EYES and smile with your* (point to your mouth and smile to prompt the children to say *"mouth")...MOUTH when you say, 'What's your name?' And when you say 'hi,' don't forget to use* (pause briefly to prompt the children to say *"names"*)*...NAMES."*

Timmy Tiger: (Begin to read the book.)

Kelly Cow: (If needed, ***social coach*** the child to ***look, smile,*** and ***say, "What's your name?"***)

Timmy Tiger: *"Timmy Tiger. Grrr, grrr! What's your name?"*

Kelly Cow: (If needed, ***social coach*** the child to ***look, smile, say their name***, and ***say, "Hi, Timmy Tiger" while waving***.)

Timmy Tiger: *"Hi, _____ (Child)* (wave at the child)*! Grrr, grrr!"*

Kelly Cow: *"Great job asking names and saying 'hi', _____ (child)! Moo, moo!"*

(Say *"good job," give a "cow high-five," and "tiger high-five,"* clap, cheer, and encourage the children to clap as well. If needed, ***social coach*** the child to return to their seat.)

"Who wants to be the next Making Friends Helper to show us how to ask names and say 'hi' using names?"

(Choose from among the children raising their hands.)

"_____ (Child), come sit on the Good Friend Square and show us how to ask names and say 'hi' using names with Timmy Tiger."

(The child should sit on the Good Friend Square.)

"Remember to look at Timmy Tiger with your (point to your eyes to prompt the children to say *"eyes"*)*...EYES and smile with your* (point to your mouth and smile to prompt the children to say *"mouth")...MOUTH when you say,*

'What's your name?' And when you say 'hi,' don't forget to use (pause briefly to prompt the children to say *"names"*)*...NAMES."*

Timmy Tiger: (Begin to read the book.)

Kelly Cow: (If needed, ***social coach*** the child to ***look, smile,*** and ***say, "What's your name?"***)

Timmy Tiger: *"Timmy Tiger. Grrr, grrr! What's your name?"*

Kelly Cow: (If needed, ***social coach*** the child to ***look, smile, say their name,*** and ***say, "Hi, Timmy Tiger" while waving***.)

Timmy Tiger: *"Hi,* _____ (*child*) (wave at the child)***!*** *Grr, grr!"*

Kelly Cow: *"Great job asking names and saying 'hi',* _____ (*child*)*! Moo, moo!"*

(Say *"good job," give a "cow high-five," and "tiger high-five,"* clap, cheer, and encourage the children to clap as well. If needed, ***social coach*** the child to return to their seat.)

Role Play: Using an Inside Voice and Asking a Friend to Play

Kelly Cow: (Place two toy cars nearby but out of reach of Timmy Tiger.)

"Friends, now that I know Timmy Tiger's name, do you think I should use an inside voice and ask my friend to play by thinking of something fun to play?" (Nod head yes and encourage the children to say *"yes."*)

"That's right, friends! Moo, moo! Let's do it!"

Timmy Tiger: (Resume reading the book.)

Kelly Cow: (Turn to look at Timmy Tiger and smile.) *"Timmy Tiger, do you want to play?"*

Timmy Tiger: (Turn to look at Kelly Cow and smile.) *"Sure, Kelly Cow."*

Kelly Cow: *"Timmy Tiger,* (point to the two toy cars) *let's race cars!"*

Timmy Tiger: *"Okay, Kelly Cow! Grrr, grrr!"*

Kelly Cow and Timmy Tiger: (Timmy Tiger puts down the book. They race the toy cars together for a few moments while ***showing and telling*** and ***being good sports***.)

Kelly Cow: *"That was fun, Timmy Tiger! Moo, moo!"*

Timmy Tiger: *"That was so cool, Kelly Cow! Grrr, grrr!*

Kelly Cow: (Turn to look at the group of children.) *"Hey friends, did I do a good job being a good friend by asking my friend to play and using an inside voice?"* (Nod head yes and encourage the children to say *"yes."*)

"That's right! Moo, moo!"

Kelly Cow and Timmy Tiger: (Say *"good job," give a "cow high-five," and "tiger high-five,"* clap, cheer, and encourage the children to clap as well. Timmy Tiger takes the book and sits on the other side of the Good Friend Square (i.e., the Good Friend Square is between Kelly Cow and Timmy Tiger). ***Social coach*** the children as needed while they practice ***asking a friend to play*** and ***using an inside voice*** with Timmy Tiger.)

Behavioral Rehearsal: Using an Inside Voice and Asking a Friend to Play

Kelly Cow: (Place the two toy cars near the Good Friend Square.)

"Who wants to be the first Making Friends Helper to show us how to use an inside voice when asking a friend to play?"

(Choose from among the children raising their hands.)

"_____ (Child), come sit on the Good Friend Square and show us how to use an inside voice when asking your friend Timmy Tiger to play."

(The child should sit on the Good Friend Square.)

"Remember to look at Timmy Tiger with your (point to your eyes to prompt the children to say *"eyes"*)*...EYES and smile with your* (point to your mouth and smile to prompt the children to say *"mouth")...MOUTH when you use an inside voice and say, 'Timmy Tiger, do you want to play?' If Timmy Tiger says yes, then think of something fun to play like racing cars* (point to the toy cars). *And don't forget to use* (pause briefly to prompt the children to say *"names"*)*...NAMES."*

Timmy Tiger: (Resume reading the book.)

Kelly Cow: (If needed, ***social coach*** the child to ***look, smile,*** and ***say, "Timmy Tiger, do you want to play?"*** using an ***inside voice***.)

Timmy Tiger: (Turn to look at the child and smile.) *"Sure, _____ (child). Grrr, grrr!"*

Kelly Cow: (If needed, ***social coach*** the child to ***look, smile,*** and ***say, "Timmy Tiger, let's race cars!"*** using an ***inside voice***.)

Timmy Tiger: *"Okay, _____ (child). Grrr, grrr!"*

(Put down the book. Race the two toy cars with the child for a few moments while ***showing and telling*** and ***being good sports***.)

"That was fun, _____ (child)!"

Kelly Cow: *"Great job using an inside voice and asking a friend to play, _____ (child)! Moo, moo!"*

(Say *"good job," give a "cow high-five," and "tiger high-five,"* clap, cheer, and encourage the children to clap as well. The child should return the toy car to Kelly Cow. Place the two toy cars near the Good Friend Square. If needed, ***social coach*** the child to return to their seat.)

"Who wants to be the next Making Friends Helper to show us how to use an inside voice when asking a friend to play?"

(Choose from among the children raising their hands.)

"_____ (Child), come sit on the Good Friend Square and show us how to use an inside voice when asking your friend Timmy Tiger to play."

(The child should sit on the Good Friend Square.)

"Remember to look at Timmy Tiger with your (point to your eyes to prompt the children to say *"eyes"*)*...EYES and smile with your* (point to your mouth and smile to prompt the children to say *"mouth")...MOUTH when you use an inside voice and say, 'Timmy Tiger, do you want to play?' If Timmy Tiger says yes, then think of something fun to play like racing cars* (point to the toy cars). *And don't forget to use* (pause briefly to prompt the children to say *"names"*)*...NAMES."*

Timmy Tiger: (Resume reading the book.)

Kelly Cow: (If needed, ***social coach*** the child to ***look, smile,*** and ***say, "Timmy Tiger, do you want to play?"*** using an ***inside voice***.)

Timmy Tiger: (Turn to look at the child and smile.) *"Sure, _____ (child). Grrr, grrr!"*

Kelly Cow: (If needed, ***social coach*** the child to ***look, smile,*** and ***say, "Timmy Tiger, let's race cars!"*** using an ***inside voice***.)

Timmy Tiger: *"Okay, _____ (child). Grrr, grrr!"* (Put down the book. Race the two toy cars with the child for a few moments while ***showing and telling*** and ***being good sports***.)

"That was fun, _____ (Child)!"

Kelly Cow: *"Great job using an inside voice and asking a friend to play,* _____ *(child)! Moo, moo!"*

(Say *"good job," give a "cow high-five," and "tiger high-five,"* clap, cheer, and encourage the children to clap as well. The child should return the toy car to Kelly Cow. Place the two toy cars near the Good Friend Square. If needed, ***social coach*** the child to return to their seat.)

Role Play: Showing and Telling and Being a Good Sport

Kelly Cow: (Remove the book as it is no longer needed.) *"Hey friends, I was having so much fun playing with Timmy Tiger. Do you think I should show and tell with Timmy Tiger and be a good sport?"* (Nod head yes and encourage the children to say *"yes."*)

"That's right, friends! Moo, moo! Let's do it!" (Turn to look at Timmy Tiger and smile.) *"Timmy Tiger, watch me* (jump the toy car through the air)*!"*

Timmy Tiger: (Look at Kelly Cow and the toy car and smile.) *"Cool jump, Kelly Cow! Grrr, grrr! Kelly Cow, watch me* (jump the toy car through the air)*!"*

Kelly Cow: *"That's so cool! Good job, Timmy Tiger* (give a high-five to Timmy Tiger)*! Moo, moo!"*

(Turn to look at the group of children.) *"Hey friends, did I do a good job of being a good friend by showing and telling and being a good sport?"* (Nod head yes and encourage the children to say *"yes."*)

"That's right! Moo, moo!"

Kelly Cow and Timmy Tiger: (Say *"good job," give a "cow high-five," and "tiger high-five,"* clap, cheer, and encourage the children to clap as well. Timmy Tiger takes one toy car and sits on the other side of the Good Friend Square (i.e., the Good Friend Square is between Kelly Cow and Timmy Tiger). ***Social coach*** the children as needed while they practice ***showing and telling*** and ***being a good sport*** with Timmy Tiger.)

Behavioral Rehearsal: Showing and Telling and Being a Good Sport

Kelly Cow: *"Who wants to be the first Making Friends Helper to show us how to show and tell and be a good sport?"*

(Choose from among the children raising their hands.)

"_____ (Child), come sit on the Good Friend Square and show us how to show and tell and be a good sport with Timmy Tiger."

(The child should sit on the Good Friend Square.)

"Remember to look at Timmy Tiger with your (point to your eyes to prompt the children to say *"eyes"*)*...EYES and smile with your* (point to your mouth and smile to prompt the children to say *"mouth"*)*...MOUTH when you show* (wave a car in front of the children) *Timmy Tiger your toy and tell Timmy Tiger to 'watch me.'"*

"And remember to be a good sport by saying 'good job' and giving a high-five to Timmy Tiger (give a high-five to Timmy Tiger). *And don't forget to use* (pause briefly to prompt the children to say *"names"*)*...NAMES."*

(Hand a toy car to the child.)

Timmy Tiger: (With the child, begin to play with the toy cars while ***showing and telling*** and ***being a good sport.***)

Kelly Cow: (If needed, ***social coach*** the child to ***look, smile***, jump the toy car through the air, and ***say, "Timmy Tiger, watch me!"***)

Timmy Tiger: *"Cool jump, _____ (child)! Grrr, grrr! _____ (Child), watch me* (jump the toy car through the air)*!"*

Kelly Cow: (If needed, ***social coach*** the child to ***look, smile, say, "Good job, Timmy Tiger!"*** and ***give a high-five*** to Timmy Tiger.)

"Great job showing and telling and being a good sport, _____ (child)! Moo, moo!"

(Say *"good job," give a "cow high-five," and "tiger high-five,"* clap, cheer, and encourage the children to clap as well. The child should return the toy car to Kelly Cow. If needed, ***social coach*** the child to return to their seat.)

"Who wants to be the next Making Friends Helper to show us how to show and tell and be a good sport?"

(Choose from among the children raising their hands.)

"_____ (Child), come sit on the Good Friend Square and show us how to show and tell and be a good sport with Timmy Tiger."

(The child should sit on the Good Friend Square.)

"Remember to look at Timmy Tiger with your (point to your eyes to prompt the children to say *"eyes"*)*...EYES and smile with your* (point to your mouth

	and smile to prompt the children to say *"mouth")...MOUTH when you show* (wave a car in front of the children) *Timmy Tiger your toy and tell Timmy Tiger to 'watch me'."*
	"And remember to be a good sport by saying 'good job' and giving a high-five to Timmy Tiger (give a high-five to Kelly Cow). *And don't forget to use* (pause briefly to prompt the children to say *"names")...NAMES."*
	(Hand a toy car to the child.)
Timmy Tiger:	(With the child, begin to play with the toy cars while ***showing and telling*** and ***being a good sport.***)
Kelly Cow:	(If needed, ***social coach*** the child to ***look, smile,*** jump the toy car through the air, and ***say, "Timmy Tiger, watch me!"***)
Timmy Tiger:	*"Cool jump, _____ (child)! Grrr, grrr! _____ (Child), watch me* (jump the toy car through the air)*!"*
Kelly Cow:	(If needed, ***social coach*** the child to ***look, smile, say, "Good job, Timmy Tiger!"*** and ***give a high-five to Timmy Tiger***.)
	"Great job showing and telling and being a good sport, _____ (child)! Moo, moo!"
	(Say *"good job," give a "cow high-five," and "tiger high-five,"* clap, cheer, and encourage the children to clap as well. The child should return the toy car to Kelly Cow. If needed, ***social coach*** the child to return to their seat.)

Role Play: Asking to Play Something Different and Sharing and Giving a Turn

Kelly Cow:	(Place a small bucket of building blocks nearby but out of reach of Timmy Tiger.) *"Hey friends! I was having fun playing with Timmy Tiger, but I want to play something different. Do you think I should think of something fun to play?"* (Nod head yes and encourage the children to say *"yes."*)
	"That's right, friends! Moo, moo! Maybe we can play with those fun blocks (point to the blocks). *And do you think it's a good idea to share and give a turn with Timmy Tiger?"* (Nod head yes and encourage the children to say *"yes."*)
	"That's right, friends! Moo, moo! Let's do it!"
Timmy Tiger:	(Resumes racing cars for a few moments while commenting to self.)

Kelly Cow:	(Turn to look at Timmy Tiger and smile.) *"Timmy Tiger,* (point to the blocks) *let's play with the blocks!"*
Timmy Tiger:	(Look at Kelly Cow and smile.) *"Okay, Kelly Cow. Grrr, grrr!"*
Kelly Cow and Timmy Tiger:	(Timmy Tiger puts down the toy cars. Begin to SEPARATELY build two towers using the blocks for a few moments.)
Timmy Tiger:	*"Kelly Cow, can I have _____ (a type of block that there is only one of)* (point to the block)*?"*
Kelly Cow:	*"Okay. Here, Timmy Tiger* (hand the block to Timmy Tiger). *Moo, moo!"*
Timmy Tiger:	*"Thanks, Kelly Cow! Grrr, grrr!"*
Kelly Cow and Timmy Tiger:	(Continue to play with the blocks for a few moments while ***showing and telling*** and ***being good sports***.)
Kelly Cow:	(Turn to look at the group of children.) *"Hey friends, did I do a good job of being a good friend by asking to play something different and sharing and giving a turn?"* (Nod head yes and encourage the children to say *"yes."*) *"That's right! Moo, moo!"*
Kelly Cow and Timmy Tiger:	(Say *"good job," give a "cow high-five," and "tiger high-five,"* clap, cheer, and encourage the children to clap as well. Timmy Tiger sits on the other side of the Good Friend Square (i.e., the Good Friend Square is between Kelly Cow and Timmy Tiger). ***Social coach*** the children as needed while they practice ***asking to play something different*** and ***sharing and giving a turn*** with Timmy Tiger.)

Behavioral Rehearsal: Asking to Play Something Different and Sharing and Giving a Turn

Kelly Cow:	(Put the blocks back in the bucket. Place the bucket near the Good Friend Square. Have two cars in hand.) *"Who wants to be the first Making Friends Helper to show us how to ask to play something different and share and give a turn?"* (Choose from among the children raising their hands.) *"_____ (Child), come sit on the Good Friend Square and show us how to ask to play something different and share and give a turn with Timmy Tiger."* (The child should sit on the Good Friend Square.)

"Remember to look at Timmy Tiger with your (point to your eyes to prompt the children to say *"eyes"*)*...EYES and smile with your* (point to your mouth and smile to prompt the children to say *"mouth"*)*...MOUTH when you ask to play something different by thinking of something fun to play like the blocks* (point to the blocks)*."*

"And remember to share and give a turn by saying 'Here, Timmy Tiger.' And don't forget to use (pause briefly to prompt the children to say *"names"*)*...NAMES."*

Timmy Tiger: (Hand one of the toy cars to the child. Play with the toy cars together while ***showing and telling*** and ***being good sports***.)

Kelly Cow: (If needed, ***social coach*** the child to ***look, smile***, and ***say, "Timmy Tiger, let's play with the blocks!"***)

Timmy Tiger: (Look at the child and smile.) *"Okay, _____ (child). Grrr, grrr!"*

Kelly Cow: (If needed, ***social coach*** the child to push the bucket of blocks closer to Timmy Tiger and play with the blocks together.)

Timmy Tiger: *"_____ (Child), can I have _____ (a type of block that there is only one of)* (point to the block)*?"*

Kelly Cow: (If needed, ***social coach*** the child to l***ook, smile, say, "Okay. Here, Timmy Tiger,"*** and ***give*** the block to Timmy Tiger.)

Timmy Tiger: *"Thank you, _____ (child)! Grrr, grrr!"*

Kelly Cow: *"Great job asking to play something different and sharing and giving a turn, _____ (child)! Moo, moo!"*

(Say *"good job," give a "cow high-five," and "tiger high-five,"* clap, cheer, and encourage the children to clap as well. If needed, ***social coach*** the child to return to their seat.)

Timmy Tiger: (Put the blocks back in the bucket. Place the bucket near the Good Friend Square. Timmy Tiger has the two toy cars.)

Kelly Cow: *"Who wants to be the next Making Friends Helper to show us how to play something different and share and give a turn?"*

(Choose from among the children raising their hands.)

"_____ (Child), come sit on the Good Friend Square and show us how to ask to play something different and share and give a turn with Timmy Tiger."

(The child should sit on the Good Friend Square.)

Kelly Cow:	*"Remember to look at Timmy Tiger with your* (point to your eyes to prompt the children to say *"eyes")...EYES and smile with your* (point to your mouth and smile to prompt the children to say *"mouth")...MOUTH when you ask to play something different by thinking of something fun to play like the blocks* (point to the blocks)*."* *"And remember to share and give a turn by saying 'Here, Timmy Tiger.' And don't forget to use* (pause briefly to prompt the children to say *"names")...NAMES."*
Timmy Tiger:	(Hand one of the toy cars to the child. Play with the toy cars together while ***showing and telling*** and ***being good sports***.)
Kelly Cow:	(If needed, ***social coach*** the child to ***look, smile,*** and ***say, "Timmy Tiger, let's play with the blocks!"***)
Timmy Tiger:	(Look at the child and smile.) *"Okay, _____ (child). Grrr, grrr!"*
Kelly Cow:	(If needed, ***social coach*** the child to push the bucket of blocks closer to Timmy Tiger and play with the blocks together.)
Timmy Tiger:	*"_____ (Child), can I have _____ (a type of block that there is only one of)* (point to the block)*?"*
Kelly Cow:	(If needed, ***social coach*** the child to ***look, smile, say, "Okay. Here, Timmy Tiger,"*** and ***give*** the block to Timmy Tiger.)
Timmy Tiger:	*"Thank you, _____ (child)! Grrr, grrr!"*
Kelly Cow:	*"Great job asking to play something different and sharing and giving a turn, _____ (child)! Moo, moo!"* (Say *"good job," give a "cow high-five," and "tiger high-five,"* clap, cheer, and encourage the children to clap as well. If needed, ***social coach*** the child to return to their seat.)

After the last child has returned to their seat:

Group leader:	*"Well friends, you all did a great job practicing some ways you can be nice to your friend!"* *"You each earned ____ (number) stars for being a good friend! Let's start with ____ (child)."*

Award each child the same number of stars by repeating the following with each child:

Group leader: *"Where's ____ (child)?"* (Wait until all the children are looking at the child.)

"____ (Child), how many stars did you earn?" (Pause briefly to allow the child to respond.)

"That's right! Let's all count for ____ (child)! One, two, three... (add stars to the Star Chart as they are counted aloud)*! Everybody clap for ____ (child)!"* (All behavioral coaches clap and cheer and encourage the children to clap as well.)

Session 15 Continued

Red Rover

BEHAVIORAL REHEARSAL ACTIVITY 1

Materials Needed

- None.

Room Setup

- Remove or place all carpet squares to the side.
- The group leader stands at the front of the room facing the children.
- Children and behavioral coach sit in a semi-circle facing the group leader as the rules are explained.

Rules: Red Rover

- The group leader reads the script below to explain the rules.
- Divide the children into two teams.
  - Assign a behavioral coach to each team to act as team leader.
- The two teams should stand approximately 10–15 feet apart and face each other.
  - Intersperse remaining behavioral coaches among the children to ***social coach***.
- Children should hold the hand of the child or behavioral coach next to them to form a chain.
- Throughout the game, help the teams choose which child from the opposing team they want to "call over" (i.e., walk over and join their team) based on various attributes.
  - Examples:
    - *"Call over somebody wearing a blue shirt. Who's wearing a blue shirt?"*
    - *"Call over a friend wearing a hat. Which friend is wearing a hat?"*
    - *"Call over someone with brown hair. Which friend has brown hair?"*
- Before the identified child can walk over, the children on the opposing team should ***ask a friend to play*** by saying, "_______ *(Child), do you want to play Red Rover?"*
- The child should respond to the team by saying, *"yes"* or *"okay."*
- All behavioral coaches and children should then sing the *Red Rover* song:
  - *"Red rover, red rover, let ____ (child from the opposing team) walk over!"*
- As the child leaves their team, they and the team should ***say "bye"*** to each other ***using names***.
- As the child joins the opposing team, they and the team should ***say "hi"*** to each other ***using names***.
- Repeat the cycle EACH time a child is "called over" to the opposing team.

- Once a child is "called over" they will be the new *calling friend.*
- Make sure all children have a turn being "called over" and being the *calling friend.*

Behavioral Rehearsal: Red Rover (15 Minutes)

The group leader leads the activity. The behavioral coaches and children sit nearby as the group leader explains the rules.

Group leader: *"Hey friends, now we're going to play a game called Red Rover! We will have two teams that will take turns calling friends over by singing the Red Rover Song. Each of you will take turns being a 'calling friend.' The calling friend will ask a friend to play from the other team by looking at your friends with your* (point to your eyes to prompt the children to say *"eyes")...EYES and smiling with your* (point to your mouth to prompt the children to say *"mouth"*)... *MOUTH when you say, 'Do you want to play Red Rover?' And don't forget to use...*(pause briefly to prompt the children to say *"names"*)...*NAMES!"*

"And if your friends say yes, then you'll sing the Red Rover song that goes like this: 'Red rover, red rover, let ____ (behavioral coach 1) walk over! Remember to listen because when your name is called, you'll walk over and join the other team."

"And what should we say and do with our hands when a friend JOINS our team?" (Pause briefly to allow the children to say, *"hi friend"* and *"wave our hands."*)

"That's right, friends! And what should we say and do with our hands when a friend LEAVES our team?" (Pause briefly to allow the children to say, *"bye friend"* and *"wave our hands."*)

"That's right, friends! And don't forget to use (pause briefly to prompt the children to say *"names"*)...*NAMES. Okay, let's have ____ (behavioral coach 1), ____ (behavioral coach 2), and ____ (behavioral coach 3) try first!"*

Role Play: Red Rover

The group leader leads the role play. The three behavioral coaches demonstrate how to play *Red Rover*. Behavioral coach 1 is on one team and behavioral coaches 2 and 3 are on the opposing team. The children and other behavioral coaches are interspersed equally across the two groups and stand 10–15 feet apart from each other. Each team holds hands with one another to keep the children from wandering during game playing.

Group leader: *"Okay, let's have ____ (behavioral coach 1)'s team go first. ____ (Behavioral coach 1) will be our first calling friend. ____ (Behavioral coach 1), call over somebody ____ (attribute to describe behavioral coach 2). Who's ____ (attribute to describe behavioral coach 2)?"*

Behavioral coach 1: *"____ (Behavioral coach 2)."*

Group leader: *"Great job, ____ (behavioral coach 1)! Now ask ____ (behavioral coach 2) to play and think of something fun to play like Red Rover."*

Behavioral coach 1: (Turn to look and smile at behavioral coach 2.) *"____ (Behavioral coach 2), do you want to play Red Rover?"*

Behavioral coach 2: (Look and smile at behavioral coach 1.) *"Okay, ____ (behavioral coach 1)."*

Behavioral coach 1 and team: *"Red rover, red rover, let ____ (behavioral coach 2) walk over!"*

Behavioral coach 2: (Look and smile at your team.) *"Bye, friends* (wave your hand)*!"*

Behavioral coach 3 and team: *"Bye, ____ (behavioral coach 2)!"*

Behavioral coach 2: (Walk toward behavioral coach 1's team.) *"Hi, friends* (wave your hand)*!"*

Behavioral coach 1 and team: *"Hi, ____ (behavioral coach 2)!"*

Behavioral coach 2: (Join behavioral coach 1's team.)

Group leader: *"Great job asking your friend to play and great job saying 'hi' and 'bye!' ____ (Behavioral coach 3), now it's your turn to be the calling friend and ask a friend to play. ____ (Behavioral coach 3)'s side, call over somebody ____ (attribute to describe behavioral coach 1). Who's ____ (attribute to describe behavioral coach 1)?"*

Behavioral coach 3: *"____ (Behavioral coach 1)."*

Group leader: *"Great job, ____ (behavioral coach 3)! Now ask ____ (behavioral coach 1) to play and think of something fun to play like Red Rover."*

Behavioral coach 3: (Turn to look and smile at behavioral coach 1.) *"____ (Behavioral coach 1), do you want to play Red Rover?"*

Behavioral coach 1: (Look and smile at behavioral coach 3.) *"Okay, ____ (behavioral coach 3)."*

Behavioral coach 3 and team: *"Red rover, red rover, let ____ (behavioral coach 1) walk over!"*

Behavioral coach 1: (Look and smile at your team.) *"Bye, friends* (wave your hand)*!"*

Behavioral coach 2 and team:	*"Bye, ____ (behavioral coach 1)!"*
Behavioral coach 1:	(Walk toward behavioral coach 3 and team.) *"Hi, friends* (wave your hand)*!"*
Behavioral coach 3 and team:	*"Hi, ____ (behavioral coach 1)!"*
Behavioral coach 1:	(Join behavioral coach 3 and team.)
Group leader:	*"Great job asking your friend to play and great job saying 'hi' and 'bye'! Okay friends, now it's everybody's turn to play Red Rover. Are we ready?"*

Behavioral Rehearsal: Red Rover

Group leader:	*"Okay, let's have ____ (child) be the next calling friend to ask a friend to play. ____ (Child), call over somebody ____ (attribute to describe a child from the opposing team). Who's ____ (attribute to describe a child from the opposing team)?"*
	(If needed, behavioral coaches should ***social coach*** the children to identify the correct child.)
	"Great job, ____ (child)! Now ask ____ (child from the opposing team) to play and think of something fun to play like Red Rover."
	(If needed, behavioral coaches should ***social coach*** the children to ***ask a friend to play*** Red Rover.)
Behavioral coaches and children:	*"Red rover, red rover, let ____ (child from the opposing team) walk over!"*
	(If needed, behavioral coaches should ***social coach*** the children to ***say "hi" and "bye"*** to teammates ***using names***.)
Group leader:	*"Great job asking your friend to play and saying 'hi' and 'bye,' to your friends! Let's keep on playing. Are we ready?"*

Repeat the sequence above until all the children have had at least one turn being the *calling friend* and have had the opportunity to practice ***asking a friend to play*** and ***saying hi and bye using names***.

Behavioral Rehearsal Wrap-Up

Group leader: *"Well friends, great job asking a friend to play and saying 'hi' and 'bye' using names! Give yourselves a big round of applause!"* (All behavioral coaches clap and cheer and encourage the children to clap as well.)

"Now everyone should come sit in the Listening Circle." (Have children return to the Listening Circle to sit on their carpet squares.)

"Okay friends, you did a great job practicing some ways you can be nice to your friends like saying 'hi' and 'bye' and asking a friend to play!"

"You each earned ____ (number) more stars for being good friends! Let's start with ____ (child)."

Award each child the same number of stars by repeating the following with each child:

Group leader: *"Where's _____ (child)?"* (Wait until all the children are looking at the child.)

"_____ (Child), how many stars did you earn?" (Pause briefly to allow the child to respond.)

"That's right! Let's all count for _____ (child)! One, two, three... (add stars to the Star Chart as they are counted aloud)*! Everybody clap for _____ (child)!"* (All behavioral coaches clap and cheer and encourage the children to clap as well.)

Break Time (10 Minutes)

- The puppets may be used to lead the children to and from the bathroom during break time.
- To assist with transitions and limit unstructured time, behavioral coaches may review the lesson with the children while waiting for the remaining children to return from the bathroom.
- You may want to award stars for good behavior after returning from the bathroom.

Session 15 Continued

Swap Draw

BEHAVIORAL REHEARSAL ACTIVITY 2

Materials Needed

- Drawing paper (approximately four to five sheets per group).
- Coloring tools (approximately three to four per group).
  - Examples: washable markers, crayons, colored pencils.
- Tables or hard, flat surfaces to draw on.
  - Chairs (when using tables).

Room Setup

- Organize tables and chairs or drawing surfaces around the room.
- Place sets of paper and coloring tools on the tables or drawing surfaces, providing enough space for children and behavioral coaches to sit around the materials.
- The group leader sits on the floor at the front of the room while explaining the rules.
- The children and behavioral coaches sit on the floor in a semi-circle facing the group leader.

Rules: Swap Draw

- The group leader reads the script below to explain the rules.
- The group leader divides the children into dyads.
  - If there are an odd number of children, pair one child with a behavioral coach.
  - Assign at least one behavioral coach per dyad to ***social coach***.
- Direct each dyad to sit in a circle around a set of materials.
- The behavioral coach will pick one child to be the first "*drawing friend*."
- The other child will be the "*choosing friend*" and will choose a theme for the *drawing friend* to draw.
  - Behavioral coaches may need to help the *choosing friend* identify a theme.
- The behavioral coach places ONE PIECE of paper and the coloring tools in front of the *drawing friend* and instructs the child to begin drawing.
- The *drawing friend* may or may not choose to draw the theme chosen by the *choosing friend.*
- As the children draw, behavioral coaches ***social coach*** the children to ***show and tell*** while ***using an inside voice***.
- After approximately 20 seconds, the behavioral coach prepares the children for the upcoming swap during which the children practice ***being a good sport*** by saying ***'good job!'*** and ***giving high-fives***, then ***asking for a turn*** and ***sharing and giving a turn***.

- After approximately five additional seconds, the behavioral coach instructs the children to swap materials by ***asking for a turn*** and ***sharing and giving a turn***.
- The children continue to draw following the same drawing theme.
- Repeat the cycle every 20–30 seconds.
- After several minutes, behavioral coaches ***social coach*** the children to ***ask to play something different*** and ***share and give a turn*** by allowing the other child to choose a different theme for the next drawing as the new *choosing friend.*
    - The behavioral coach may need to help the *choosing friend* identify something different to draw.
- The *drawing friend* may or may not choose to draw what the *choosing friend* suggests.
- The behavioral coach provides new paper to the children as needed.

Behavioral Rehearsal: Swap Draw (15 Minutes)

The group leader explains the activity. The behavioral coaches and children sit nearby as the group leader explains the rules. The behavioral coaches ***social coach*** the children in dyads to ***not be bossy*** during the game playing.

Group leader: *"Hey friends, now we're going to play Swap Draw. You'll get to draw fun pictures with your friend, like the beach or the jungle or outer space. But only one friend* (hold up one finger) *will draw at a time. If you're drawing, do you think you should show and tell with your friend using an inside voice?"* (Pause briefly to allow the children to say *"yes."*)

"That's right, friends! And when you hear the word 'swap,' you'll practice being a good sport by saying 'good job' and giving a high-five to your friend (demonstrate giving a high-five). *Then you'll practice asking for a turn by saying, 'Can I have a turn please?' Sometimes our friends may ask to play something different like drawing something new. When our friend asks to draw something different do you think we should say 'Okay' and share and give a turn?"* (Pause briefly to allow the children to say *"yes."*)

"That's right, friends! And remember to look at your friend with your (point to your eyes to prompt the children to say *"eyes"*)*...EYES and smile with your* (point to your mouth and smile to prompt the children to say *"mouth")... MOUTH when you're being a good friend. And don't forget to use* (pause briefly to prompt the children to say *"names"*)*...NAMES."*

"Okay, let's play Swap Draw!"

Behavioral Rehearsal: Swap Draw

The children and the behavioral coaches move to their drawing stations.

Behavioral coach: (The behavioral coach places ONE piece of paper and the coloring tools in front of the *drawing friend.*)

"Okay friends, let's practice sharing and giving a turn by letting ____ (child) be the first 'drawing friend' and letting ____ (child) be the first 'choosing friend'." (If needed, ***social coach*** the children to ***share and give a turn***.)

"____ (Child), what should our drawing friend draw first?" (If needed, ***social coach*** the *choosing friend* to choose a theme.)

(If the *drawing friend* chooses to draw something different, help the *choosing friend* practice ***not being bossy*** by saying, *"Our drawing friend wants to draw something different. Let's practice not being bossy and take deep breaths to keep cool."*)

(If the *drawing friend* draws what the *choosing friend* chose, ***praise*** the *drawing friends* by saying, *"Great job sharing and taking turns, _______ (child)."*)

(If needed, ***social coach*** the children to ***show and tell*** and ***use an inside voice*** while drawing. The behavioral coach helps facilitate positive play interactions by asking questions and making comments (e.g., *"What do you think _______ (child) is drawing?"* or *"That's so cool!"*).

Every 10–20 seconds, the behavioral coach instructs the children to swap the drawing materials and the *choosing friend* will become the *drawing friend* and vice versa.

Behavioral coach: *"Friends, in a few seconds we're going to swap the paper and markers and practice asking for a turn and sharing and giving a turn."*

After approximately five additional seconds, have the children swap the drawing materials:

Behavioral coach: *"And...swap! Let's first practice being good sports, by saying 'good job' and giving high-fives."* (If needed, ***social coach*** the children to be ***good sports***.)

"Now we're going to practice sharing and giving a turn by letting ____ (child) be the next 'drawing friend' and letting ____ (child) be the next 'choosing friend'." (Have the children swap the drawing paper and coloring tools.)

"____ (Child), what should our drawing friend draw next?" (If needed, ***social coach*** the *choosing friend* to choose something new to add to the drawing. The behavioral coach helps facilitate positive play interactions by asking questions and making comments (e.g., *"What do you think _______ (child) is drawing?"* or *"That's so cool!"*).

After several minutes, allow the other child to choose a new drawing theme:

Behavioral coach: *"Friends, let's practice sharing and giving a turn by letting ____ (child) choose the next picture we'll draw."* (If needed, ***social coach*** the children to ***be a good sport*** and ***share and give a turn***.)

Repeat the pattern above for the remainder of the playtime. Provide new drawing paper as needed.

Table 15.2 Drawing Theme Examples

House	Outer space	Beach
School	Trains	Underwater world
Park	Forest	Castle
Friends	Jungle	Dinosaurs
Family	Airplanes	Dragons
Cars	Superheroes	Wizards
Animals	Witches	Princesses

Behavioral Rehearsal Wrap-Up

Group leader: *"Well friends, great job being a good friend! Give yourselves a big round of applause!"* (All behavioral coaches clap and cheer and encourage the children to clap as well.)

"Now everyone should come sit in the Listening Circle." (Have children return to the Listening Circle to sit on their carpet squares.)

"Okay friends, you did a great job practicing some ways you can be nice to your friends like sharing and giving a turn, asking for a turn, asking to play something different, using an inside voice, and being a good sport!"

"You each earned ____ (number) more stars for being good friends! Let's start with ____ (Child)."

Award each child the same number of stars by repeating the following with each child:

Group leader: *"Where's ____ (child)?"* (Wait until all the children are looking at the child.)

"____ (Child), how many stars did you earn?" (Pause briefly to allow the child to respond.)

"That's right! Let's all count for ____ (child)! One, two, three… (add stars to the Star Chart as they are counted aloud)*! Everybody clap for ____ (child)!"* (All behavioral coaches clap and cheer and encourage the children to clap as well.)

"Now we're going to play another game with our parents and practice more ways to be a good friend!"

Session 15 Continued

Final Review (Part 1)

PARENT COACHED PLAY: DYADIC PLAYDATES

Materials Needed

- Games brought by children and parents from home.
- Turn-taking games provided by the treatment team.
- Tables and chairs or carpet squares.
- *Parent Coached Play Cards.*

Room Setup

- If available, organize tables in separate corners of the room with four to six chairs per table.
- If tables are not available, place two carpet squares in separate corners of the room to indicate where the children will sit.

Rules: Dyadic Playdates

- The group leader divides the families into groups of two families each.
    - If there are an odd number of children, pair one child with a behavioral coach. In this case, you will need an additional coach to serve as a behavioral coach for the parent.
- Assign each group to sit at a table or specific play area.
- As children sit down, parents will ***social coach*** the children to ***say "hi"*** to one another ***using names*** while ***using an inside voice***.
- Parents will ***social coach*** the children to ***ask a friend to play*** when choosing the first game to play.
- Throughout the game, parents will ***social coach*** the children to ***show and tell, share and give a turn,*** and ***be a good sport*** while ***using an inside voice***.
- After approximately nine minutes of play, instruct the parents to prepare the children for the upcoming game swap.
- After approximately one additional minute of play (ten minutes total), instruct the parents to swap games by having the next child ***ask to play something different.***
- Repeat the cycle with the second game.
- After approximately nine minutes of play, instruct the parents to prepare the children for clean up.

- After approximately one additional minute of play (ten minutes total), parents will ***social coach*** the children to clean up, ***say "bye" using an inside voice*** and return to the Listening Circle.

Behavioral Coaching: Dyadic Playdates

Behavioral coaches will ***social coach*** parents during dyadic ***playdates*** in the following ways:

- ***Priming***:
  - Begin the play interactions with parents going over the rules for ***being a good friend*** BEFORE GAME PLAYING.
    - Example: "*Remember that before you play your games, we want you to practice greeting your friend by using an inside voice when you say 'hi' using your friend's name. Then we're going to practice asking for a turn, showing and telling, and being good sports. And if you or your friend asks to play something different, then we need to share and give a turn.*"
- ***Prompting***:
  - Reminding parents to use the buzzwords to ***prompt*** their child to ***be a good friend***.
  - Helping parents to identify opportunities to proactively ***prompt*** their child to ***be a good friend***.
    - Example: *"Remember to share and give a turn."*
    - Example: *"Remember to think of something fun to play when you ask your friend to play."*
    - Example: *"What should you do if your friend can't hear you?"*
- ***Praising***:
  - Reminding parents to ***praise*** and reinforce their child whenever their child ***is a good friend*** spontaneously or ***prompted***.
    - Example: *"Great job asking for a turn!"*
    - Example: *"Great job asking to play something different!"*
    - Example: *"Good job showing and telling!"*
- ***Providing corrective feedback using a praise sandwich***:
  - Reminding parents to ***praise*** their child's ATTEMPTS to ***be a good friend*** and identify what could be done differently next time.
    - Example: *"Nice try using an inside voice. Remember not to talk too quietly next time, but good job!"*
    - Example: *"Good job showing and telling. Don't forget to use names next time, but nice try!"*
    - Example: *"Good try sharing and giving a turn. Remember to share nicely next time, but nice job!"*
- Reminding parents to continue to ***social coach*** on previously learned skills:
  - ***Listening and following directions.***
  - ***Meeting and greeting friends.***

- ***Sharing and giving a turn.***
- ***Asking for a turn.***
- ***Keeping cool.***
- ***Being a good sport.***
- ***Showing and telling.***
- ***Don't be bossy.***
- ***Asking a friend to play.***
- ***Joining a game.***
- ***Asking to play something different.***
- ***Asking and giving help.***
- ***Staying in our own space.***
- ***Using an inside voice.***

Parent Coached Play: Dyadic Playdates (20 Minutes)

- Have each child choose a turn-taking game brought from home or provided by the treatment team.
- The group leader sits on the floor at the front of the room.
- The families sit on the floor in a semi-circle facing the group leader.

Group leader: *"Hey friends, we're going to have more playdates and play with the fun games you brought from home."*

"When you play with your friends, we want you to practice ALL the different ways to be a good friend."

"If you want to play with your friends, do you think it's a good idea to ask a friend to play?" (Pause briefly to allow the child to say *"yes."*)

"That's right, friends! And do you think you should say 'hi' and 'bye' and use names when you play with your friends?" (Pause briefly to allow the child to say *"yes."*)

"That's right, friends! And when you play, do you think it's a good idea to share and give a turn, show and tell, and be a good sport while using an inside voice?" (Pause briefly to allow the child to say *"yes."*)

"That's right, friends! And don't forget to ask to play something different when it's time to swap games. Okay, let's go play with our games!"

- Before walking to the play area, instruct the parents to ***social coach*** the children to ***say "hi" using names,*** while ***using an inside voice.***
- Parents should have their children choose the first game by practicing ***asking a friend to play***.
- Parents will also ***social coach*** their children to ***show and tell, share and give a turn,*** and ***be a good sport*** throughout the game playing.
- After approximately nine minutes of play, instruct the parents to prepare the children for the upcoming game swap by saying, "*Parents, tell your children that we'll be swapping games in one minute.*"
- After approximately one additional minute of play (ten minutes total), instruct the parents to practice ***asking to play something different*** by swapping games by saying, *"Parents, it's time*

to swap games. Social coach the children to ask to play something different before playing the next game."

- After approximately nine minutes of playing the second game, instruct the parents to prepare the children for clean up by saying, *"Parents, tell your children that we'll be cleaning up in one minute."*
- After approximately one additional minute of play (ten minutes total), ***prompt*** the parents to instruct their children to clean up by saying, *"Parents, it's time to clean up. Let's social coach the children to listen and follow directions by cleaning up and then say 'bye' to their friend using an inside voice before sitting in the Listening Circle."*
- Then parents will ***social coach*** their child to ***say "bye" using names***, while ***using an inside voice.***

Final Wrap-Up (10 minutes)

- The group leader sits on the floor at the front of the room.
- The children sit on the carpet squares in a semi-circle facing the group leader, with parents sitting behind their children.

Group leader: *"Okay friends, you all did a great job playing your games and being a good friend. When we're asking and using names and saying 'hi' and 'bye,' do you think we should look and smile at our friends?"* (Pause briefly to allow the children to say *"yes."*)

"That's right, friends! And when we're sharing and giving a turn, do you think we should say 'here' and share nicely?" (Pause briefly to allow the children to say *"yes."*)

"That's right, friends! And when we're being a good sport and showing and telling, do you think we use an inside voice?" (Pause briefly to allow the children to say *"yes."*)

"That's right, friends! And when we're asking a friend to play or asking to play something different, do you think we should think of something fun to play?" (Pause briefly to allow the children to say *"yes."*)

"That's right, friends! You all did such a great job being a good friend that you each earned ____ (number) more stars! Let's start with ____ (child)."

Award each child the same number of stars by repeating the following with each child:

Group leader: *"Where's _____ (child)?"* (Wait until all the children are looking at the child.)

"_____ (Child), how many stars did you earn?" (Pause briefly to allow the child to respond.)

"That's right! Let's all count for _____ (child)! One, two, three... (add stars to the Star Chart as they are counted aloud)*! Everybody clap for _____ (child)!"* (All behavioral coaches clap and cheer and encourage the children to clap as well.)

"And remember you all earned those stars by being a good friend! Everyone did a great job, and parents you did an excellent job social coaching! Parents, remember your homework assignments this week are for you and your children to practice using all the skills for being a good friend using the 4 Ps. And don't forget to have a playdate and go to your playgroups."

"Alright little friends, do you want to count our stars?" (Pause briefly to allow the children to respond.)

"Let's all count together and see how many stars we earned today! One, two, three...(count the number of stars for one child)*!"*

"You each earned ____ (total number) stars today! Round of applause for our friends!" (All behavioral coaches should clap and cheer and encourage the families to clap as well.)

"Great job, friends! Don't forget to choose your reward before you leave. And remember that next week is graduation and we will be having a very special graduation ceremony. See you all next week for graduation!"

Session 15 Continued

Disclosing a Diagnosis or Condition with Others and Final Review (Part 1)

PEERS® FOR PRESCHOOLERS: PARENT HANDOUT

Snapshot of Steps for Disclosing a Diagnosis or Condition with Others

1. **Choose the right time.**
2. **Choose the right person.**
3. **Choose the right context.**
4. **Acknowledge the difference.**
5. **Give an explanation.**
6. **Acknowledge what the difference means for your child.**
7. **Turn a challenge into a strength.**
8. **Make your child's strength an asset to the friendship.**
9. **Be prepared to answer questions.**
10. **Remember friendship is a choice.**

Steps for Disclosing a Diagnosis or Condition with Others

Step 1: Choose the Right Time

- You may want to avoid disclosing diagnoses or conditions too soon in your acquaintance.
  - Consider letting them meet your child and get to know them before disclosing personal details about your child.
- You may want to disclose your child's diagnosis or condition sooner if the differences are noticeable.
  - Sharing your child's diagnosis or condition when it is visible allows you to influence how others perceive your child by explaining what others see through your own lens.
- Reasons for disclosing a diagnosis or condition:
  - Some parents share when seeking acceptance from others.
  - Other parents share in response to miscommunication and/or when misunderstandings arise.
  - Some parents share as they naturally become more comfortable and accepted by others.
- Disclosing your child's diagnosis or condition is a personal choice.
- You may or may not choose to share your child's diagnosis or condition and that is your family's decision.

Step 2: Choose the Right Person

- If you choose to share your child's diagnosis or condition, consider whether it is beneficial that the person knows.
    - Good example: Sharing your child's diagnosis with the parent of a preferred ***playmate*** who may notice that your child's behavior is different.

Step 3: Choose the Right Context

- Avoid blurting out your child's diagnosis or condition for no reason.
- Wait for the right context to share your child's diagnosis or condition.
- Often there is a reason or context for mentioning your child's diagnosis or condition.

Step 4: Acknowledge the Difference

- If your child's behavior appears different from other children, chances are others have noticed.
- Rather than avoiding talking about these differences, you might avoid any misunderstandings or misinterpretations by acknowledging the differences.
    - Good example: You might begin by saying, *"You may have noticed that my child has a tendency to (state the behavior)."*
        - *"...avoid eye contact."*
        - *"...talk a lot about certain things."*
        - *"...ask a lot of personal questions."*

Step 5: Give an Explanation

- Provide a reason or explanation for why your child behaves in a way that may be seen as different.
- People are more likely to understand behaviors that are different if they can be explained in a way that makes sense to them.
- If people don't understand why your child does certain things, they are more likely to attribute their behavior to negative interpretations.
- People are more likely to be accepting of differences if they understand them.
    - Good example: *"My child behaves in this way because they have/are (explain the condition)."*
    - Good example: *"My child has been diagnosed with (name the condition)."*

Step 6: Acknowledge What the Difference Means for Your Child

- Explain what having this condition means for your child.
- Explain how your child's behavior may affect others around them.
- Not everyone will understand what your child's diagnosis or condition means, so you will need to educate them.
- Good example: *"That means that when my child (state the behavior), people may think (explain how others perceive them)."*
    - *"...avoids eye contact, people may think they're not paying attention or they're uninterested."*

Step 7: Turn a Challenge into a Strength

- After you've acknowledged the difference and presented the challenge your child faces in how people perceive them, immediately point out the strengths in your child.
- Always change what could be perceived as a negative into something positive.
- Good example: *"On the positive side, my child's condition also means that (state the positive characteristics)."*
    - *"...even though they may look like they're not paying attention, they're actually very focused on what you're saying and are probably more likely to remember what you've said than most people."*

Step 8: Make Your Child's Strength an Asset to the Friendship

- When acknowledging a difference and turning a challenge into a strength, it is useful to make this strength an asset to the friendship.
- You might also point out how this strength might be beneficial to the person with whom you are speaking.
- Good example: *"I believe (state the positive characteristic) could be a great asset to their friendships."*
    - *"I believe my child's listening skills could be a great asset to their friendships."*

Step 9: Be Prepared to Answer Questions

- Know what your child's diagnosis or condition means and how to briefly explain it.
    - Good example: *"Autism is a neurodevelopmental condition that can make social interactions challenging. Autistic people also tend to have specialized interests and repetitive behaviors."*

Step 10: Remember Friendship is a Choice

- ***Friendship is a choice.***
    - ***We don't get to be friends with everyone.***
    - ***Everyone doesn't get to be friends with us.***
- When it comes to friendships, there are good choices and bad choices.
- If you don't like the way a parent reacts to your disclosure, your child doesn't have to be friends with their child.
- A person or a parent who doesn't react well to your disclosure may not be a good choice for your child or for you.

Child Didactic Lesson: Final Review (Part I)

Snapshot of Previously Learned Lessons: Final Review (Part 1)

The objective of this lesson is to review some of the skills that the children have learned during the program. The skills for this lesson include:

Table 15.1 Previously Learned Skills (Part 1)

<table>
<tr>
<td>ASKING NAMES

1. Look at your friend with your eyes (point to your eyes).
2. Smile with your mouth (point to your mouth and smile).
3. Say, “What’s your name?”
4. Say your name (“I’m ____ (Name).”</td>
<td>USING NAMES

1. Look at your friend with your eyes (point to your eyes).
2. Smile with your mouth (point to your mouth and smile).
3. Use names when talking to your friend.</td>
</tr>
<tr>
<td>GREETING FRIENDS SAYING “HI”

1. Look at your friend with your eyes (point to your eyes).
2. Smile with your mouth (point to your mouth and smile).
3. Wave with your hand (wave your hand).
4. Say “hi” using your friend’s name.</td>
<td>GREETING FRIENDS SAYING “BYE”

1. Look at your friend with your eyes (point to your eyes).
2. Smile with your mouth (point to your mouth and smile).
3. Wave with your hand (wave your hand).
4. Say “bye” using your friend’s name.</td>
</tr>
<tr>
<td>SHARING AND GIVING A TURN

1. Look at your friend with your eyes (point to your eyes).
2. Smile with your mouth (point to your mouth and smile).
3. Say “here” using names (demonstrate handing over a toy) when you share and give a turn.</td>
<td>BEING A GOOD SPORT

1. Look at your friend with your eyes (point to your eyes).
2. Smile with your mouth (point to your mouth and smile).
3. Say “good job” using names.
4. Give a high-five.</td>
</tr>
<tr>
<td>SHOW AND TELL: SHOWING YOUR TOY

1. Look at your friend with your eyes (point to your eyes).
2. Smile with your mouth (point to your mouth and smile).
3. Show your toy to your friend (wave your toy in front of your friend).
4. Tell your friend to look at your toy by saying, “Look at my (cool toy)!” while using names.</td>
<td>SHOW AND TELL: “WATCH ME”

1. Look at your friend with your eyes (point to your eyes).
2. Smile with your mouth (point to your mouth and smile).
3. Tell your friend to look at you by saying, “Watch me!” or “Look at me!” while using names.
4. Do something fun with your toy (e.g., fly a toy/plane in the air).</td>
</tr>
<tr>
<td>ASKING A FRIEND TO PLAY

1. Look at your friend with your eyes (point to your eyes).
2. Smile with your mouth (point to your mouth and smile).
3. Say, “Do you want to play?” using names.
4. If your friend says yes, think of something fun to play.
5. Say “Let’s play _____ (activity/game)!” using names.</td>
<td rowspan="2">ASKING TO PLAY SOMETHING DIFFERENT

1. Think of something fun to play (point to your head).
2. Look at your friends with your eyes (point to your eyes).
3. Smile with your mouth (point to your mouth and smile).
4. Ask to play something different using names (e.g., “(Friend), let’s play _____!”).

If your friend says no:

1. Keep cool and play nicely
2. Look at your friends with your eyes (point to your eyes).
3. Smile with your mouth (point to your mouth and smile).
4. Say “okay” using names.
5. Play nicely with your friends.
6. If you’re still upset, then take deep breaths to keep cool (take two slow deep breaths).</td>
</tr>
<tr>
<td>USING AN INSIDE VOICE

• Use an inside voice when you’re inside (place an index finger in front of your mouth).
• Don’t be a loud talker.
• Don’t talk too loudly when you’re inside.
• Don’t be a quiet talker.
• Don’t talk too quietly or your friends won’t be able to hear you.</td>
</tr>
</table>

Homework Assignments

1. **Playdates.**
   - Schedule and have a ***playdate*** with a ***playmate.***
   - Prepare for the ***playdate*** using the ***5 Ws.***
     - ***WHO: Playdates*** should be one-on-one.
     - ***WHAT: Playdates*** should be activity-based.
     - ***WHERE:*** Schedule initial ***playdates*** to take place in your home or somewhere you can provide ***social coaching.***
     - ***WHEN:*** Try to keep initial ***playdates*** to no more than 1–1.5 hours.
     - ***HOW:*** Coordinate how the children will get to and from the ***playdate.***
   - Do a final practice with your child of the games and activities that will be available during the ***playdate.***
   - Gather all the games and activity materials for the ***playdate*** in one area that is VISIBLE and easily accessible to YOU but not the children.
   - Provide ***social coaching*** during the ***playdate*** and assess if this is a good ***playmate*** for your child.

2. **Make a list of previously learned skills that still need refinement.**
   - Identify which skills your child still needs to improve upon.
     - These are the skills you will focus on during your ***social coaching*** in the coming weeks and months.
   - Review the rules and steps for these skills with your child.
   - Consider watching the puppet show lessons with your child again (particularly for skills that still need refinement).
   - Previously learned skills include:
     - ***Listening and following directions.***
     - ***Meeting and greeting friends.***
     - ***Sharing and giving a turn.***
     - ***Asking for a turn.***
     - ***Keeping cool.***
     - ***Being a good sport.***
     - ***Showing and telling.***
     - ***Don't be bossy.***
     - ***Asking a friend to play.***
     - ***Joining a game.***
     - ***Asking to play something different.***
     - ***Asking and giving help.***
     - ***Staying in our own space.***
     - ***Using an inside voice.***

3. **Practice a previously learned skill that needs refinement using the 4 Ps.**
   - Practice having your child use a previously learned skill this week while providing ***social coaching*** using the ***4 Ps.***
     - ***Priming*****:** Review the rules for the previously learned skill with your child BEFORE PRACTICING.
     - ***Prompting*****:** Remind your child IN THE MOMENT to use the previously learned skill whenever the opportunities present.
     - ***Praising*****: *Praise*** your child using the buzzwords whenever they use the previously learned skill CORRECTLY.

- ***Providing corrective feedback*****:** ***Provide corrective feedback*** in the form of a ***praise sandwich*** whenever your child ATTEMPTS to use the previously learned skill.
- Please send us a 30–60-second BOOSTER VIDEO of ***social coaching*** your child to use the previously learned skill to be viewed during homework review.

4. Practice disclosing a diagnosis or condition with others (optional assignment).

- Consider practicing the steps for disclosing a diagnosis or condition with a trusted family member or friend following the steps outlined in the lesson.
- Choosing to disclose a diagnosis or condition with others is a personal choice for each family, so consider discussing this choice (if you have not already).

Session 15 Continued

Final Review (Part 1)

PEERS® FOR PRESCHOOLERS: PARENT COACHED PLAY CARD

Snapshot of Previously Learned Lessons: Final Review (Part 1)

Table 15.1 Previously Learned Skills (Part 1)

ASKING NAMES	**USING NAMES**
1. Look at your friend with your eyes (point to your eyes). 2. Smile with your mouth (point to your mouth and smile). 3. Say, "What's your name?" 4. Say your name ("I'm ____ (Name)."	1. Look at your friend with your eyes (point to your eyes). 2. Smile with your mouth (point to your mouth and smile). 3. Use names when talking to your friend.
GREETING FRIENDS SAYING "HI"	**GREETING FRIENDS SAYING "BYE"**
1. Look at your friend with your eyes (point to your eyes). 2. Smile with your mouth (point to your mouth and smile). 3. Wave with your hand (wave your hand). 4. Say "hi" using your friend's name.	1. Look at your friend with your eyes (point to your eyes). 2. Smile with your mouth (point to your mouth and smile). 3. Wave with your hand (wave your hand). 4. Say "bye" using your friend's name.
SHARING AND GIVING A TURN	**BEING A GOOD SPORT**
1. Look at your friend with your eyes (point to your eyes). 2. Smile with your mouth (point to your mouth and smile). 3. Say "here" using names (demonstrate handing over a toy) when you share and give a turn.	1. Look at your friend with your eyes (point to your eyes). 2. Smile with your mouth (point to your mouth and smile). 3. Say "good job" using names. 4. Give a high-five.
SHOW AND TELL: SHOWING YOUR TOY	**SHOW AND TELL: "WATCH ME"**
1. Look at your friend with your eyes (point to your eyes). 2. Smile with your mouth (point to your mouth and smile). 3. Show your toy to your friend (wave your toy in front of your friend). 4. Tell your friend to look at your toy by saying, "Look at my (cool toy)!" while using names.	1. Look at your friend with your eyes (point to your eyes). 2. Smile with your mouth (point to your mouth and smile). 3. Tell your friend to look at you by saying, "Watch me!" or "Look at me!" while using names. 4. Do something fun with your toy (e.g., fly a toy/plane in the air).

<table>
<tr>
<td>ASKING A FRIEND TO PLAY

1. Look at your friend with your eyes (point to your eyes).
2. Smile with your mouth (point to your mouth and smile).
3. Say, "Do you want to play?" using names.
4. If your friend says yes, think of something fun to play.
5. Say "Let's play _____ (activity/game)!" using names.</td>
<td rowspan="2">ASKING TO PLAY SOMETHING DIFFERENT

1. Think of something fun to play (point to your head).
2. Look at your friends with your eyes (point to your eyes).
3. Smile with your mouth (point to your mouth and smile).
4. Ask to play something different using names (e.g., "(Friend), let's play _____!").

If your friend says no:

1. Keep cool and play nicely
2. Look at your friends with your eyes (point to your eyes).
3. Smile with your mouth (point to your mouth and smile).
4. Say "okay" using names.
5. Play nicely with your friends.
6. If you're still upset, then take deep breaths to keep cool (take two slow deep breaths).</td>
</tr>
<tr>
<td>USING AN INSIDE VOICE

• Use an inside voice when you're inside (place an index finger in front of your mouth).
• Don't be a loud talker.
• Don't talk too loudly when you're inside.
• Don't be a quiet talker.
• Don't talk too quietly or your friends won't be able to hear you.</td>
</tr>
</table>

Priming BEFORE Game Playing

- Example: *"Remember that before you play your games, we want you to practice greeting your friend by using an inside voice when you say 'hi' using your friend's name. Then we're going to practice asking for a turn, showing and telling, and being good sports. And if you or your friend asks to play something different, then we need to share and give a turn."*

Prompting IN THE MOMENT

- Example: *"Remember to share and give a turn."*
- Example: *"Remember to think of something fun to play when you ask your friend to play."*
- Example: *"What should you do if your friend can't hear you?"*

Praising for CORRECT Use of Skills

- Example: *"Great job asking for a turn!"*
- Example: *"Great job asking to play something different!"*
- Example: *"Good job showing and telling!"*

Providing Corrective Feedback for ATTEMPTS Using a Praise Sandwich

- Example: *"Nice try using an inside voice. Remember not to talk too quietly next time, but good job!"*
- Example: *"Good job showing and telling. Don't forget to use names next time, but nice try!"*
- Example: *"Good try sharing and giving a turn. Remember to share nicely next time, but nice job!"*

Session 15 Continued

Disclosing a Diagnosis or Condition with Others and Final Review (Part 1)

PEERS® FOR PRESCHOOLERS: PARENT HOMEWORK WORKSHEET

<table>
<tr><td>Child's Name:</td><td colspan="2">Parent's Name:</td><td colspan="2">Date:</td></tr>
<tr><td>HOMEWORK ASSIGNMENTS</td><td>PRIMING (REVIEWING RULES BEFORE PRACTICE)</td><td>PROMPTING (IN THE MOMENT)</td><td>PRAISING (USING BUZZWORDS)</td><td>PROVIDING CORRECTIVE FEEDBACK (USING A PRAISE SANDWICH)</td></tr>
<tr><td colspan="5">Make a list of previously learned skills that still need refinement</td></tr>
<tr><td>Practice a previously learned skill that needs refinement using the 4 Ps:

• Using an inside voice
• Staying in our own space
• Asking and giving help
• Asking to play something different
• Joining a game
• Asking a friend to play
• Don't be bossy
• Show and tell during play
• Being a good sport
• Keeping cool
• Asking for a turn
• Sharing and giving turns
• Meeting and greeting friends
• Listening and following directions</td><td></td><td></td><td></td><td></td></tr>
</table>

Child's Name:	Parent's Name:		Date:	
HOMEWORK ASSIGNMENTS	PRIMING (REVIEWING RULES BEFORE PRACTICE)	PROMPTING (IN THE MOMENT)	PRAISING (USING BUZZWORDS)	PROVIDING CORRECTIVE FEEDBACK (USING A PRAISE SANDWICH)
Playdate: • **Plan a playdate using the 5 Ws** • **Prime your child before the playdate** • **Provide social coaching during the playdate using the 4 Ps**				
Practice disclosing a diagnosis or condition with others (optional)				

Please fill out this worksheet by describing what you did to complete the homework assignments.
Worksheets will be collected during Homework Review at the next session of PEERS® for Preschoolers.

Session 16

Sharing a Diagnosis or Condition with Your Child and Final Review (Part 2)

PARENT SESSION THERAPIST GUIDE

Announcements

- Today is graduation!
  - Per usual, parents will review homework and have a didactic lesson.
  - Children will have a Final Review of previously learned skills (Part 2), followed by two behavioral rehearsal activities to practice skills.
  - There is no Parent Coached Play in this session.
  - We will end the session with a graduation ceremony with parents and children.
- Explain and/or conduct post-testing (if applicable)

Parent Session Agenda

- Homework Review (40 minutes).
- Didactic Lessons (30 minutes).
- Final Wrap-Up and Graduation Ceremony (20 minutes).

Materials Needed

- Conference room with a large table and enough chairs for the parent group leader and all parents to sit comfortably around the table
  - Avoid sitting in a circle without a table as this creates the atmosphere of group therapy.
- Name tags for parents and treatment team.
- *Parent Handouts* (for the current week and the previous week).
- *Parent Homework Worksheets* (for the current week and the previous week).
- *Attendance and Homework Compliance Sheets* for parent group leader.
- Pens for note-taking (consider having extra pens for parents who need them).
- NEW: *Parent Coached Play Cards* (for ALL previous weeks).
- NEW: *Overview of PEERS® for Preschoolers Skills*.

Homework Review (40 Minutes)

1. **Playdates.**
   - Have parents report on the ***playdate*** and confirm that they planned using the ***5 Ws.***

DOI: 10.4324/9781003502968-17

- Review what parents did to ***social coach*** their child BEFORE, DURING, and AFTER the ***playdate***.
- Identify what skills their child did well and what skills they need to work on.
  - Confirm that parents ***praised*** skills that were done well and provided ***priming, prompting,*** and/or ***corrective feedback*** for emerging skills.
- Have parents assess if this is a good ***playmate*** for their child.
- Have parents identify who their child might have a ***playdate*** within the coming week (does not have to be a different ***playmate***).

2. **Make a list of previously learned skills that still need refinement.**
   - Identify which skills their child still needs to improve upon.
   - Confirm that parents reviewed the rules and steps for these skills with their child (including possibly watching the puppet show lessons with their child again).
   - Previously learned skills include:
     - ***Listening and following directions.***
     - ***Meeting and greeting friends.***
     - ***Sharing and giving a turn.***
     - ***Asking for a turn.***
     - ***Keeping cool.***
     - ***Being a good sport.***
     - ***Showing and telling.***
     - ***Don't be bossy.***
     - ***Asking a friend to play.***
     - ***Joining a game.***
     - ***Asking to play something different.***
     - ***Asking and giving help.***
     - ***Staying in our own space.***
     - ***Using an inside voice.***

3. **Practice a previously learned skill that needs refinement using the 4 Ps.**
   - Review the 30–60-second video of ***social coaching*** a previously learned skill for each family. (For larger groups, you may need to review video recordings in two smaller groups with two different parent group leaders).
     - Have parents identify:
       - Skills their child did well.
       - Skills they would like to work on with their child.
     - Provide ***social coaching*** tips as appropriate for each family.
   - If parents did not send a video of ***social coaching***, confirm the following:
     - Parents had their child practice a previously learned skill while providing ***social coaching*** using the ***4 Ps.***
       - ***Priming*****:** Reviewed the rules for a previously learned skill with their child BEFORE PRACTICING.
       - ***Prompting*****:** Reminded their child IN THE MOMENT to use the previously learned skill whenever the opportunity presented.
       - ***Praising*****:** ***Praised*** their child using the buzzwords whenever they used the previously learned skill CORRECTLY.
       - ***Providing corrective feedback*****:** ***Provided corrective feedback*** in the form of a ***praise sandwich*** whenever their child ATTEMPTED to use the previously learned skill.

4. **Practice disclosing a diagnosis or condition with others (OPTIONAL ASSIGNMENT).**
   - Confirm whether the parent practiced disclosing a diagnosis or condition with a trusted family member or friend following the steps outlined in the lesson.

Didactic Lessons (30 Minutes)

PEERS® Neuroaffirming Pledge:

- We value neurodiversity, acceptance, and authenticity.
- We honor the diverse ways people experience the world.
- We respect each person's unique perspectives and communication styles.
- We recognize there is no one right way to connect with others.
- If using the strategies taught in PEERS® feels like camouflaging or masking and/or they don't align with your goals or the goals of your family, then you do not have to use them.
- Learning and using the skills taught in PEERS® is a PERSONAL CHOICE.

Didactic Lesson: Sharing a Diagnosis or Condition with Your Child

- Distribute *Parent Handouts*.
  - Sections in **bold print** come directly from the *Parent Handout*.
  - Terms that are ***bold and italicized*** are buzzwords and represent important concepts from the didactic lesson.

- Explain, *"The focus of today's parent lesson is on sharing a diagnosis or condition with your child. Like the previous lesson on disclosing a diagnosis or condition with others, this information is not being shared with your children. Sharing a diagnosis or condition with your child, and choosing the appropriate time to have this conversation, are personal choices that every family needs to make for themselves. Sharing a diagnosis or a condition is best accomplished when planned and rehearsed. Should you choose to share your child's differences with them now or later, it can be helpful to use the following steps to guide the conversation."*

Snapshot of the Steps for Sharing a Diagnosis or Condition with Your Child

1. **Choose the right time.**
2. **Choose the right context.**
3. **Acknowledge your child's differences.**
4. **Give an explanation.**
5. **Acknowledge what the difference means for your child.**
6. **Normalize the difference.**
7. **Turn your child's difference into a strength.**
8. **Make your child's strength an asset to the family.**
9. **Be prepared to answer questions.**

Steps for Sharing a Diagnosis or Condition with Your Child

Step 1: Choose the Right Time

- **Don't wait to share a diagnosis or condition with your child until there is a problem.**
- **Children with neurodevelopmental disorders appear to have better responses to learning about their diagnoses or conditions earlier in development (before the age of seven).**
- **Consider sharing your child's diagnosis or condition with them sooner if they begin to ask questions.**

Step 2: Choose the Right Context

- **Avoid blurting out your child's diagnosis or condition for no reason.**
- **Wait for the right context to share your child's diagnosis or condition.**
- **There should be a reason for mentioning your child's diagnosis or condition.**

Step 3: Acknowledge Your Child's Difference

- **Begin by acknowledging the difference(s) your child has probably noticed.**
  - **Examples:**
    - **Frequent doctor visits, assessments, and therapy appointments.**
    - **The mention of "autism" or "ADHD" or other diagnostic terms.**
    - **Challenging behaviors.**
    - **Social difficulties.**
    - **Restricted interests.**
    - **Strict adherence to routines.**
    - **Attentional difficulties.**
    - **Sensory issues.**
    - **Hyperactivity.**

Step 4: Give an Explanation

- **Provide an explanation for why your child receives these services or behaves in these ways.**
- **This is the part where you may choose to label your child's differences, diagnosis, or condition.**
  - **Creating a label (or a name) for your child's differences may make it easier to discuss with them in the future.**

Step 5: Acknowledge What the Difference Means for Your Child

- **Explain what having this condition means for your child.**
  - **Examples:**
    - **Frequent doctor visits.**
    - **Assessments.**
    - **Therapy appointments.**

Step 6: Normalize the Difference

- **Normalize your child's differences by explaining that other people have similar differences.**
- **If your child understands that they are not the only person that has these differences, they will feel less "different."**
- **You might also explain that a "difference" doesn't make them "less than."**

Step 7: Turn Your Child's Differences into a Strength

- **After you've acknowledged the difference(s), provided an explanation, and normalized the difference, immediately point out the strengths in your child.**
- **Always change what could be perceived as a challenge into something positive.**
- **You might even describe your child's strengths and talents as "superpowers" so they can more easily relate to what you are saying.**
- **Example: "The good news is that your (condition) also means that (state the positive characteristics)."**
  - **"…you have an amazing memory."**
  - **"…you know a lot about things and like to share with others."**
  - **"…you are very honest and like to tell the truth."**

Step 8: Make Your Child's Strength an Asset to the Family

- **When turning a difference into a strength, it is useful to make this strength an asset to the family.**
- **Good examples:**
  - **"We are so proud of you!"**
  - **"You are such a good helper!"**
  - **"You teach us so many things!"**

Step 9: Be Prepared to Answer Questions

- **Know what your child's diagnosis or condition means and how to explain it to them in words they can understand.**
  - **There are many books and social stories that can help you guide the conversation.**
- **Your child may have questions immediately and/or later.**
- **If you don't know the answer to your child's questions, tell them you don't know but will find the answer.**
  - **You are not expected to know everything.**
  - **It is okay for you to model that you are learning too.**

Didactic Lesson: Tips for Moving Forward

Explain, *"Although this is our final session for PEERS® for Preschoolers, your job as your child's social coach is not over. Our long-term follow-up research shows that the benefits of PEERS® last longer with parent involvement. Here are some helpful tips for moving forward."*

TIP 1: Continue to enroll your child in *playgroups* based on your child's interests.

- ***Playgroups* provide a potential source of friends with *common interests*.**
- **We recommend that your child be enrolled in AT LEAST ONE *PLAYGROUP* at any given time based on their interests.**
- **It is important that your child continue to participate in *playgroups* or other social activities to have a source of potential *playmates*.**
- ***Playgroups* also provide opportunities for your child to practice the skills they learned in PEERS® for Preschoolers with potential *playmates*.**
- **As soon as one *playgroup* is about to come to an end, investigate and enroll your child in other *playgroups*.**
- **Criteria for good *playgroups*:**
    - **Meets regularly (preferably weekly).**
    - **Located close to your home (this may make it easier to have regularly occurring *playdates*).**
    - **Includes accepting children in the same age range and level of support needs as your child.**
    - **Includes informal time so that your child will have opportunities to socialize and play with other children naturally.**
    - **Activities are based on your child's interests, likes, or hobbies.**
    - **Permits some parent involvement for you to *social coach*.**
- **Continue to assess the appropriateness of *playgroups*.**
    - **See which children may be good potential *playmates* for your child.**
    - **Take note of what activities, games, or toys your child and other children are playing with.**
- **Proactively practice or preview games, activities, and toys that may be popular in the *playgroup* but are new for your child.**
- **When appropriate, continue to *social coach* your child in using the skills during the *playgroups*.**
- **Continue to get to know the other parents of potential *playmates* in the *playgroups*.**
    - **Engage in social chitchat with the parents of potential *playmates*.**
    - **Assess your interest in and compatibility with the other parents.**
    - **The goal is to build a foundation for potential *playdates*.**

TIP 2: Continue to have weekly *playdates*.

- **It is essential that your child have regularly occurring *playdates* with friends.**
    - **This is how they will develop stronger friendships.**
    - **We recommend that your child continue to have AT LEAST ONE *PLAYDATE* PER WEEK.**
- **Remember to plan and prepare for *playdates* by using the *5 Ws*:**
    - **WHO will attend the *playdate*.**
        - **This includes the potential *playmate*, their parent, and/or siblings.**
        - **Initial *playdates* should be one-on-one when possible.**
    - **WHAT will the children do during the *playdate*.**

▪ *Playdates* should be activity-based and focused on the *common interests* of your child and their *playmate.*

- **Avoid games and activities that:**
  - **Require significant adult facilitation.**
  - **Entail extensive setup.**
  - **Are difficult for your child to *share and give a turn.***
  - **Are difficult for your child to transition away from.**
- **WHAT will the children do during the *playdate.***
  - **Games and activities should be visible but not accessible to the children.**
  - **Have a variety of structured games and activities available.**
  - **If games or activities lack structure, then create structure.**
- **WHEN will the *playdate* happen.**
  - **Keep it short and sweet at first.**
  - **Try to keep initial play dates to no more than 1–1.5 hours at first.**
- **WHERE will the *playdate* take place.**
  - ***Playdates* in your home may make it easier for you to provide *social coaching.***
- **HOW will the *playdate* happen.**
  - **How will the children get to and from the *playdate.***

TIP 3: Continue to provide *social coaching* on the skills from PEERS® for Preschoolers using the *4 Ps.*

- ***Social coach* your child to use the skills learned in PEERS® to play with their friends during *playgroups, playdates*, and school and/or daycare.**
  - **As your child improves in their use of the skills with less *social coaching*, gradually fade back *social coaching.***
  - **Be sure to periodically provide intermittent *praise* (catch them being good).**
- ***Priming*: Review the rules with your child BEFORE PRACTICING during preferred and highly motivating activities.**
- ***Prompting*: Remind your child IN THE MOMENT to use the skills whenever the opportunities present.**
- ***Praising*: *Praise* your child using the buzzwords whenever they use the skills CORRECTLY.**
- ***Providing corrective feedback*: *Provide corrective feedback* in the form of a *praise sandwich* whenever your child ATTEMPTS to use the skills.**
- **Regularly review the Parent Coached Play Cards.**
  - **These coaching cards can be used to provide support during your *social coaching.***
- **Continued *social coaching* on your part will ensure that your child:**
  - **Will continue to use the skills learned in PEERS® for Preschoolers.**
  - **Will be successful at making and keeping friends.**
- **Be prepared to help your child obtain new social skills as social demands change with development.**
  - **The social skills your child will need to make and keep friends will change as they grow older.**
  - **Major social developmental periods:**

  - **Preschool age.**
  - **Elementary school age.**
  - **Adolescence (middle and high school).**
  - **Adulthood.**

TIP 4: Remember *friendship is a choice.*

- ***Our children don't get to be friends with everyone.***
- ***Everyone doesn't get to be friends with our children.***
- **There are good choices and bad choices when it comes to friendships.**

Table 16.1 Assessing Parent Interest for Playdates

SIGNS OF INTEREST	SIGNS OF DISINTEREST
Making eye contact	Not making eye contact/looking away
Smiling	Not smiling/looking uncomfortable
Turning toward you	Turning away from you
Talking to you/asking questions	Not talking to you/saying very little
Seeming eager to make plans	Acting reluctant/hesitant to make plans
Agreeing about children's mutual interest	Seeming confused/distracted
Agreeing to playdate (even without finalizing)	Sounding busy or unavailable
Exchanging contact information	No exchanging contact information
Agreeing to follow up later	Agreeing to playdate but not following up

  - **It is important to assess the interest of your child's potential *playmates* and respond accordingly.**
  - **It is also important to assess the interest of the *playmate's* parents in having *playdates.***
- **We need to expect that not every *playmate* is going to be a good choice for our child.**
- **We also need to expect that our child is not going to be a good choice for every *playmate.***
- **We cannot force friendships for our children, just as we cannot force friendships for ourselves.**
- ***Friendship is a choice* for all of us!**

TIP 5: Consider embracing neurodiversity.

- **Just as we have shared the PEERS® Neurodiversity Pledge with you at the beginning of each didactic lesson, consider embracing your own ideas about neurodiversity.**
- **These ideas might include:**
  - **Valuing neurodiversity, acceptance, and authenticity.**
  - **Honoring the diverse ways people experience the world.**
  - **Respecting each person's unique perspectives and communication styles.**
  - **Recognizing there is no one right way to connect with others.**
  - **Remembering that if using the strategies taught in PEERS® feels like camouflaging or masking and/or they don't align with your goals or the goals of your family, then you do not have to use them.**
  - **Remembering that learning and using the skills taught in PEERS® is a PERSONAL CHOICE.**

Didactic Lesson: Final Review (Part 2)

Explain, *"The focus of today's child lesson will be continuing to review and further practice the skills learned for making and keeping friends. As we go through our final review of the skills learned in PEERS® for Preschoolers this week, consider which skills still need refinement for your child. After we finish our review of the child lessons, we will join the children for a graduation ceremony and to celebrate everybody's hard work and progress!"* (Note: To allocate time for the graduation ceremony, there is no *Parent Coached Play* in this session.)

Snapshot of Previously Learned Lessons: Final Review (Part 2)

The objective of this lesson is to review some of the skills that the children have learned during the program. The skills for this lesson include:

Table 16.2 Previously Learned Skills (Part 2)

LISTENING AND FOLLOWING DIRECTIONS	ASKING FOR A TURN
1. Listen with your ears (cup your hand behind your ear). 2. Be quiet with your mouth (place your index finger in front of your mouth and say "shhh"). 3. Have calm hands and a calm body (put your hands to your side). 4. Do what you're told to do.	1. Look at your friend with your eyes (point to your eyes). 2. Smile with your mouth (point to your mouth and smile). 3. Say "Can I have a turn please?" using names.
KEEPING COOL	**DON'T BE BOSSY (BE FLEXIBLE)**
1. Look at your friend with your eyes (point to your eyes) 2. Nicely say "okay" using names. 3. Find something else to do. 4. If you're still feeling upset, take deep breaths to keep cool (take two slow deep breaths). a. Smell the flowers (example of breathing in) b. Blow out the candles (example of breathing out)	1. Keep cool. 2. Take deep breaths (demonstrate taking two deep breaths). 3. Nicely say, "Okay." 4. Let your friend have a turn choosing what to do. 5. Keep playing nicely.
ASKING FOR HELP	**GIVING HELP**
1. Look at your friends with your eyes (point to your eyes). 2. Smile with your mouth (point to your mouth and smile). 3. Say, "Can you help me?" using names.	1. Look at your friends with your eyes (point to your eyes). 2. Smile with your mouth (point to your mouth and smile). 3. Say "okay" using names. 4. Give help to your friend.
JOINING A GAME	**STAYING IN OUR OWN SPACE**
1. Watch the game (point to your eyes). 2. Know the rules (point to your head). 3. Move closer (demonstrate moving closer with your body). 4. Look at your friends with your eyes (point to your eyes). 5. Smile with your mouth (point to your mouth and smile). 6. Say, "Can I play?" using names. • If your friends say yes, join the game. • If your friends say no, keep cool and find something else to do.	• Don't get too close (shake your head no) ○ If we can touch the person next to us (extend your arm out in front and to the side), then we're too close and being a space hog. • Stay in our own space (nod your head yes) ○ If we're too close and being a space hog, then we need to back up (lean back) and stay in our own space. ○ Remember to be a space keeper.

Session 16 Continued
Final Review (Part 2) and Graduation

CHILD SESSION THERAPIST GUIDE

Child Session Agenda

- Didactic Lesson: *Final Review (Part 2)* (30 minutes).
  - Note: You have 10 additional minutes for the last didactic lesson.
- Group Behavioral Rehearsal Activity 1: *Ring Around the Rosie* (15 minutes).
- Break Time (10 minutes).
- Group Behavioral Rehearsal Activity 2: *Hot or Cold* (15 minutes).
- Final Wrap-Up and Graduation Ceremony (20 minutes).

Snapshot of Previously Learned Lessons: Final Review (Part 2)

The objective of this lesson is to review some of the skills that the children have learned during the program. The skills for this lesson include:

Table 16.2 Previously Learned Skills (Part 2)

LISTENING AND FOLLOWING DIRECTIONS	ASKING FOR A TURN
1. Listen with your ears (cup your hand behind your ear). 2. Be quiet with your mouth (place your index finger in front of your mouth and say "shhh"). 3. Have calm hands and a calm body (put your hands to your side). 4. Do what you're told to do.	1. Look at your friend with your eyes (point to your eyes). 2. Smile with your mouth (point to your mouth and smile). 3. Say "Can I have a turn please?" using names.
KEEPING COOL	**DON'T BE BOSSY (BE FLEXIBLE)**
1. Look at your friend with your eyes (point to your eyes) 2. Nicely say "okay" using names. 3. Find something else to do. 4. If you're still feeling upset, take deep breaths to keep cool (take two slow deep breaths). a. Smell the flowers (example of breathing in) b. Blow out the candles (example of breathing out)	1. Keep cool. 2. Take deep breaths (demonstrate taking two deep breaths). 3. Nicely say, "Okay." 4. Let your friend have a turn choosing what to do. 5. Keep playing nicely.

<table>
<tr><th>ASKING FOR HELP</th><th>GIVING HELP</th></tr>
<tr><td>1. Look at your friends with your eyes (point to your eyes).
2. Smile with your mouth (point to your mouth and smile).
3. Say, "Can you help me?" using names.</td><td>1. Look at your friends with your eyes (point to your eyes).
2. Smile with your mouth (point to your mouth and smile).
3. Say "okay" using names.
4. Give help to your friend.</td></tr>
<tr><th>JOINING A GAME</th><th>STAYING IN OUR OWN SPACE</th></tr>
<tr><td>1. Watch the game (point to your eyes).
2. Know the rules (point to your head).
3. Move closer (demonstrate moving closer with your body).
4. Look at your friends with your eyes (point to your eyes).
5. Smile with your mouth (point to your mouth and smile).
6. Say, "Can I play?" using names.
• If your friends say yes, join the game.
• If your friends say no, keep cool and find something else to do.</td><td>• Don't get too close (shake your head no)
○ If we can touch the person next to us (extend your arm out in front and to the side), then we're too close and being a space hog.
• Stay in our own space (nod your head yes)
○ If we're too close and being a space hog, then we need to back up (lean back) and stay in our own space.
○ Remember to be a space keeper.</td></tr>
</table>

Materials Needed

- Cow puppet.
- Tiger puppet.
- Mouse puppet.
- Three toy airplanes.
- Bucket with building blocks.
- Hacky sack.
- Carpet squares or chairs.
- "Making Friends Helper" badge for EACH CHILD.
- Star chart with names of children.
- Marker for star chart.
- Name tags for families and treatment team.
- Prize bins with prizes.

Preparing for the Lesson

- Use the script below with the group leader using a cow puppet to play the part of "Kelly Cow."
- A behavioral coach uses a tiger puppet to play the part of "Timmy Tiger."
- A second behavioral coach uses a mouse puppet to play the part of "Marty Mouse."
- An additional behavioral coach assists in behavioral rehearsal and provides encouragement and feedback to the group.
- EACH CHILD is chosen at the beginning of the lesson as the "Making Friends Helpers."
    - Each child wears a "Making Friends Helpers" badge and will take turns being among the first to practice the previously learned skills (there are eight skills to rehearse in this lesson).
- The child group leader and the behavioral coaches sit on the floor at the front of the room.
- A special colored carpet square (e.g., red) is placed at the front of the room next to the child group leader to be used as the "Good Friend Square."
- For the children, additional carpet squares of the same color (e.g., green) are placed in a semi-circle facing the child group leader and the "Good Friend Square."

- Note: If carpet squares are unavailable, the children and behavioral coach may sit on chairs.
- The material in *italics* should be read by the indicated person.
- The material in ***bold and italics*** represents buzzwords and should be emphasized when read.
- The material in CAPITAL LETTERS within the script should be given extra emphasis while the group is encouraged to say the words in unison.

Behavioral Coaching Techniques

Behavioral coaches should use the following coaching techniques described below throughout the lesson and the behavioral rehearsal activities. (Note: ***priming*** occurs during the introduction to the activity.)

- ***Prompting*:**
  - Use the buzzwords to ***prompt*** the children to ***be a good friend***.
    - Example: *"Remember to not be bossy by keeping cool and playing nicely."*
    - Example: *"What can you say if your friend asks for help?"*
    - Example: *"Remember to back up if you're being a space hog."*
- ***Praising*:**
  - Reinforce ***being a good friend*** by ***praising*** the children.
    - Example: *"Great job listening to your friend!"*
    - Example: *"Great job watching and knowing the rules when you joined the game!"*
    - Example: *"Great job keeping cool!"*
- ***Providing corrective feedback using a praise sandwich:***
  - Reinforce ATTEMPTS to ***be a good friend*** by ***praising*** the children and identifying what could be done differently next time.
    - Example: *"Nice try staying in your own space. Don't forget to back up if you're too close next time, but good job!"*
    - Example: *"Good job joining the game. Remember to use your friend's name next time, but nice try!"*
    - Example: *"Nice try keeping cool. Remember to take deep breaths if you're still upset next time, but good job!"*

Didactic Lesson: Final Review (Part 2) (30 minutes)

Kelly Cow: (Sit at the front of the room.) *"Hi friends! I'm Kelly Cow. Moo, moo! Today is our last day to learn how to be a good friend. And on our last day, EVERYBODY gets to be a Making Friends Helper! Moo, moo!"* (All behavioral coaches clap and cheer and encourage the children to clap as well.)

(Place a "Making Friends Helper" badge on EACH child. The children stay in their seats for now.)

"Today we're going to have lots of fun playing some of your favorite games and practicing all the different ways to be nice to our friends!"

"Who should we be nice with? We should be nice with our FRIENDS, TEACHERS, MOMMIES, DADDIES, BROTHERS AND SISTERS."

"How should we be nice to our friends? We can be nice by asking for a turn and keeping cool, asking and giving help, and not being bossy. And we can also be nice by joining a game, staying in our own space, listening and following directions, and all the other things that we learned together."

"When should we be nice to our friends? We should be nice to our friends all the time! Like when we're playing together at the park or eating lunch at school or playing together at home."

"Remember, being nice is a great way to be a good friend! Moo, moo!"

Role Plays: Asking for a Turn and Keeping Cool

Kelly Cow and Timmy Tiger: (Play together with the toy airplanes for a few moments while ***showing and telling*** and ***being good sports***.)

Kelly Cow: (Turn to look at the group of children.) *"Hey friends! I want to play with one of Timmy Tiger's airplanes* (point to one of Timmy Tiger's airplanes). *Do you think I should ask Timmy Tiger for a turn?"* (Nod head yes and encourage the children to say *"yes."*)

"That's right, friends! And friends, if Timmy Tiger says no, should I get upset or should I keep cool?" (Encourage the children to say, "*keep cool*.")

"That's right, friends! Moo, moo! Let's do it!" (Turn to look at Timmy Tiger and smile.) *"Timmy Tiger* (point to one of Timmy Tiger's toy airplanes), *can I have a turn please?"*

Timmy Tiger: (Turn to look at Kelly Cow.) *"Maybe later."*

Kelly Cow: *"Okay, Timmy Tiger."* (Take two ***deep breaths***.)
(Continue to ***play nicely*** with Timmy Tiger while ***showing and telling*** and ***being good sports***.)

"Hey friends, did I do a good job being a good friend by asking for a turn and keeping cool when Timmy Tiger said no?" (Encourage the children to say *"yes."*)

"That's right, friends! Moo moo!"

Kelly Cow and Timmy Tiger: (Say *"good job," give a "cow high-five," and "tiger high-five,"* clap, cheer, and encourage the children to clap as well. Timmy Tiger takes the toy airplanes and sits on the other side of the Good Friend Square (i.e., the Good Friend Square is between Kelly Cow and Timmy Tiger). ***Social coach*** the children as needed while they practice ***asking for a turn*** and ***keeping cool*** with Timmy Tiger.)

Behavioral Rehearsals: Asking for a Turn and Keeping Cool

Kelly Cow: *"Who wants to be the first Making Friends Helper to show us how to ask for a turn and keep cool with Timmy Tiger?"*

(Choose from among the children raising their hands.)

"_____ (Child), come sit on the Good Friend Square."

(The child should sit on the Good Friend Square.)

"Remember to look at Timmy Tiger with your (point to your eyes to prompt the children to say *"eyes"*)*...EYES and smile with your* (point to your mouth and smile to prompt the children to say *"mouth"*)*...MOUTH when you ask for a turn by saying 'Timmy Tiger, can I have a turn please?'"*

"And remember to keep cool by taking deep breaths (take two *deep breaths*) *and saying 'okay' if Timmy Tiger says no. And don't forget to use* (pause briefly to prompt the children to say *"names"*)*...NAMES."*

Timmy Tiger: (Hand a toy airplane to the child and play with the toy airplanes together.)

Kelly Cow: (If needed, ***social coach*** the child to ***look, smile***, and ***say, "Timmy Tiger, can I have a turn please?"***)

Timmy Tiger: *"Maybe later."*

Kelly Cow: (If needed, ***social coach*** the child to ***keep cool*** with Timmy Tiger.)

"Great job asking for a turn and keeping cool, _____ (child)! Moo, moo!"

(Say *"good job," give a "cow high-five," and "tiger high-five,"* clap, cheer, and encourage the children to clap as well. If needed, ***social coach*** the child to return to their seat.)

"Who wants to be the next Making Friends Helper to show us how to ask for a turn and keep cool with Timmy Tiger?"

(Choose from among the children raising their hands.)

	"_____ (Child), come sit on the Good Friend Square."
	(The child should sit on the Good Friend Square.)
	"Remember to look at Timmy Tiger with your (point to your eyes to prompt the children to say *"eyes"*)...*EYES and smile with your* (point to your mouth and smile to prompt the children to say *"mouth"*)...*MOUTH when you ask for a turn by saying 'Timmy Tiger, can I have a turn please?'"*
	"And remember to keep cool by taking deep breaths (take two *deep breaths*) *and saying 'okay' if Timmy Tiger says no. And don't forget to use* (pause briefly to prompt the children to say *"names"*)...*NAMES."*
Timmy Tiger:	(Hand a toy airplane to the child and play with the toy airplanes together.)
Kelly Cow:	(If needed, ***social coach*** the child to ***look, smile,*** and ***say, "Timmy Tiger, can I have a turn please?"***)
Timmy Tiger:	*"Maybe later."*
Kelly Cow:	(If needed, ***social coach*** the child to ***keep cool*** with Timmy Tiger.)
	"Great job asking for a turn and keeping cool, _____ (child)! Moo, moo!"
	(Say *"good job," give a "cow high-five," and "tiger high-five,"* clap, cheer, and encourage the children to clap as well. If needed, ***social coach*** the child to return to their seat. Put the toy airplanes to the side; they are no longer needed.)
	"Okay friends, let's keep playing!"

Role Play: Joining a Game

Marty Mouse and Timmy Tiger:	(Marty Mouse has a hacky sack and joins Timmy Tiger at the front of the room. Begin to play Hot Potato while ***showing and telling*** and ***being good sports***.)
Kelly Cow:	(Turns to look at the group of children.) *"Hey friends, Marty Mouse and Timmy Tiger are playing a fun game together. I wish I could play too. Do you think I should join the game?"* (Nod head yes and encourage the children to say *"yes."*)
	"That's a great idea! Moo, moo! Let's do it!" (Watch Marty Mouse and Timmy Tiger playing Hot Potato for a few moments.)
	(Turn to look at the group of children and smile.) *"Hey friends, I watched the game and I know the rules. They're playing Hot Potato. Now I'm going to ask to play."*

	(Turn to look at Marty Mouse and Timmy Tiger and smile.) *"Marty Mouse and Timmy Tiger, can I play?"*
Marty Mouse and Timmy Tiger:	(Turn to look at Kelly Cow and smile.) *"Okay, Kelly Cow!"*
Kelly Cow:	*"Thanks, Marty Mouse and Timmy Tiger!"*
	(Join Marty Mouse and Timmy Tiger and play Hot Potato for a few moments while ***showing and telling*** and ***being good sports***.)
	(Turn to look at the group of children and smile.) *"Hey friends, did I do a good job being a good friend by joining the game?"* (Nod head yes and encourage the children to say *"yes."*)
	"That's right! Moo, moo!"
Kelly Cow, Marty Mouse, and Timmy Tiger:	(Say *"good job," give a "cow high-five," "tiger high-five,"* and *"mouse high-five,"* clap, cheer, and encourage the children to clap as well. Timmy Tiger takes the hacky sack and sits on the other side of the Good Friend Square (i.e., the Good Friend Square is between Kelly Cow and Timmy Tiger). ***Social coach*** the children as needed while they practice ***joining the game*** with Timmy Tiger and Marty Mouse.)

Behavioral Rehearsal: Joining a Game

Kelly Cow:	*"Who wants to be the first Making Friends Helper to show us how to join the game with Timmy Tiger and Marty Mouse?"*
	(Choose from among the children raising their hands.)
	"_____ (Child), come sit on the Good Friend Square."
	(The child should sit on the Good Friend Square.)
	"Remember to first watch the game (point to your eyes) *and make sure you know the rules* (tap your head with your index finger). *If you know the rules, then you should look at your friends with your* (point to your eyes to prompt the children to say *"eyes"*)...*EYES and smile with your* (point to your mouth to prompt the children to say *"mouth"*)...*MOUTH when you say, 'Marty Mouse and Timmy Tiger, can I play?' And don't forget to use* (pause briefly to prompt the children to say *"names"*)...*NAMES."*
Marty Mouse and Timmy Tiger:	(Begin to play Hot Potato with the hacky sack while ***showing and telling*** and ***being good sports***.)

Kelly Cow: (If needed, ***social coach*** the child to ***watch the game, know the rules***, and then ***look, smile***, and ***say, "Marty Mouse and Timmy Tiger, can I play?"***)

Marty Mouse and Timmy Tiger: (Turn to look at the child and smile.) *"Okay, _____ (child)!"*

Kelly Cow: (If needed, ***social coach*** the child to ***join the game*** and play Hot Potato for a few moments while ***showing and telling*** and ***being good sports***.)

"Great job joining the game, _____ (child)! Moo, moo!"

(Say *"good job," give a "cow high-five," "tiger high-five,"* and *"mouse high-five,"* clap, cheer, and encourage the children to clap as well. If needed, ***social coach*** the child to return to their seat.)

"Who wants to be the next Making Friends Helper to show us how to join the game with Timmy Tiger and Marty Mouse?"

(Choose from among the children raising their hands.)

"_____ (Child), come sit on the Good Friend Square."

(The child should sit on the Good Friend Square.)

"Remember to first watch the game (point to your eyes) *and make sure you know the rules* (tap your head with your index finger). *If you know the rules, then you should look at your friends with your* (point to your eyes to prompt the children to say *"eyes"*)*...EYES and smile with your* (point to your mouth to prompt the children to say *"mouth"*)*...MOUTH when you say, 'Marty Mouse and Timmy Tiger, can I play?' And don't forget to use* (pause briefly to prompt the children to say *"names"*)*...NAMES."*

Marty Mouse and Timmy Tiger: (Begin to play Hot Potato with the hacky sack while ***showing and telling*** and ***being good sports***.)

Kelly Cow: (If needed, ***social coach*** the child to ***watch the game, know the rules,*** and then ***look, smile,*** and ***say, "Marty Mouse and Timmy Tiger, can I play?"***)

Marty Mouse and Timmy Tiger: (Turn to look at the child and smile.) *"Okay, _____ (child)!"*

Kelly Cow: (If needed, ***social coach*** the child to ***join the game*** and play Hot Potato for a few moments while ***showing and telling*** and ***being good sports***.)

"Great job joining the game, _____ (child)! Moo, moo!"

(Say *"good job," give a "cow high-five," "tiger high-five,"* and *"mouse high-five,"* clap, cheer, and encourage the children to clap as well. If needed, ***social coach*** the child to return to their seat. Place the Marty Mouse puppet to the side. The behavioral coach returns to their seat.)

"Okay friends, let's keep playing!"

Role Plays: Staying in Our Own Space and Listening and Following Directions

Kelly Cow and Timmy Tiger: (Build SEPARATE towers using the blocks. A small bucket for cleanup is nearby.)

Timmy Tiger: (Turn to look at Kelly Cow and smile.) *"Kelly Cow, let's put our towers together!"*

Kelly Cow: *"Okay, Timmy Tiger!"* (Lean over to build on Timmy Tiger's tower and be so close that you are touching.)

Timmy Tiger: (Look at Kelly Cow and frown.)

Kelly Cow: (Turn to look at the group of children.) *"Hey friends, do you think I'm too close to Timmy Tiger and being a space hog*?" (Nod head yes and encourage the children to say *"yes."*)

"That's right! Do you think I should back up (lean back) *and stay in my own space?"* (Nod head yes and encourage the children to say *"yes."*)

"That's right, friends! Moo, moo! Let's do it!" (***Back up*** until you are an arm's length away from Timmy Tiger.) *"Did I do a good job staying in my own space and not being a space hog?"* (Nod head yes and encourage the children to say *"yes"*)

"That's right, friends! Let's keep playing!"

Kelly Cow and Timmy Tiger: (Resume building blocks together for a few moments while ***showing and telling*** and ***being good sports***.)

Behavioral coach: *"It's time to clean up!"*

Kelly Cow: *"Hey friends, do you think we should listen and follow directions and clean up?"* (Nod head yes and encourage the children to say *"yes."*)

"That's right! Moo, moo!"

Kelly Cow and Timmy Tiger: (Begin to place the blocks in the small bucket nearby.)

Kelly Cow:	*"Hey friends, did I do a good job being a good friend by staying in my own space and listening and following directions?* (Nod head yes and encourage the children to say *"yes."*)
	"That's right! Moo, moo!"
Kelly Cow and Timmy Tiger:	(Say *"good job," give a "cow high-five," and "tiger high-five,"* clap, cheer, and encourage the children to clap as well. Timmy Tiger sits on the other side of the Good Friend Square (i.e., the Good Friend Square is between Kelly Cow and Timmy Tiger). ***Social coach*** the children as needed while they practice ***staying in their own space*** and ***listening and following directions*** with Timmy Tiger.)

Behavioral Rehearsals: Staying in Our Own Space and Listening and Following Directions

Timmy Tiger:	(Place blocks on the floor near the Good Friend Square. Place the small bucket nearby.)
Kelly Cow:	*"Who wants to be the first Making Friends Helper to show us how to stay in your own space and listen and follow directions with Timmy Tiger?"*
	(Choose from among the children raising their hands.)
	"_____ (Child), come sit on the Good Friend Square."
	(The child should sit on the Good Friend Square.)
	"Remember to back up (lean back) *if you're too close to Timmy Tiger and being a space hog. And don't forget to listen and follow directions."*
Timmy Tiger:	(With the child, begin building with the blocks together while ***showing and telling*** and ***being good sports***. After a few moments, lean over to get a block and be so close to the child that you are touching.)
Kelly Cow:	(If needed, ***social coach*** the child to ***back up*** if Timmy Tiger is ***too close***.)
Timmy Tiger:	(With the child, resume building blocks together for a few moments while ***showing and telling*** and ***being good sports***.)
Behavioral coach:	*"It's time to clean up!"*
Kelly Cow:	(If needed, ***social coach*** the child to ***listen and follow directions*** by placing the blocks in the small bucket.)
	"Great job staying in your own space and listening and following directions, _____ (child)! Moo, moo!"
	(Say *"good job," give a "cow high-five," and "tiger high-five,"* clap, cheer, and encourage the children to clap as well. If needed, ***social coach*** the child to return to their seat.)

Timmy Tiger: (Place blocks on the floor near the Good Friend Square. Place the small bucket nearby.)

Kelly Cow: *"Who wants to be the next Making Friends Helper to show us how to stay in your own space and listen and follow directions with Timmy Tiger?"*

(Choose from among the children raising their hands.)

"_____ (Child), come sit on the Good Friend Square."

(The child should sit on the Good Friend Square.)

"Remember to back up (lean back) *if you're too close to Timmy Tiger and being a space hog. And don't forget to listen and follow directions."*

Timmy Tiger: (With the child, begin building with the blocks together while ***showing and telling*** and ***being good sports***. After a few moments, lean over to get a block and be so close to the child that you are touching.)

Kelly Cow: (If needed, ***social coach*** the child to ***back up*** if Timmy Tiger is ***too close***.)

Timmy Tiger: (With the child, resume building blocks together for a few moments while ***showing and telling*** and ***being good sports***.)

Behavioral coach: *"It's time to clean up!"*

Kelly Cow: (If needed, ***social coach*** the child to ***listen and follow directions*** by placing the blocks in the small bucket.)

"Great job staying in your own space and listening and following directions, _____ (child)! Moo, moo!"

(Say *"good job," give a "cow high-five," and "tiger high-five,"* clap, cheer, and encourage the children to clap as well. If needed, ***social coach*** the child to return to their seat.)

"Let's keep playing!"

Role Plays: Asking and Giving Help and Don't Be Bossy

Kelly Cow and Timmy Tiger: (Resume playing together with the blocks for a few moments while ***showing and telling*** and ***being good sports***.)

Kelly Cow: (Turn to look at the group of children.) *"Hey friends, I want to build a super tall tower. Do you think I should ask and give help with Timmy Tiger so we can build the tower together?"* (Nod head yes and encourage the children to say *"yes."*)

"That's right, friends! And do you think I should NOT (shake your head to indicate no) *be bossy when we're playing together?"* (Encourage the children to say *"yes."*)

"That's right, friends! Moo, moo! Let's do it!" (Turn to look at Timmy Tiger and smile.) *"Timmy Tiger, can you help me build a tower?"*

Timmy Tiger: (Turn to look at Kelly Cow and smile.) *"Okay, Kelly Cow."*

Kelly Cow and Timmy Tiger: (Build a tower together for a few moments while ***showing and telling*** and ***being good sports***.)

Timmy Tiger: (Hold a block upside down and have difficulty putting the block in place. Turn to look at Kelly Cow and smile.) *"Kelly Cow, this block doesn't fit. Can you help me?"*

Kelly Cow: (Turn to look at Timmy Tiger and smile.) *"Okay, Timmy Tiger."* (Help Timmy Tiger by putting the block in place.)

Timmy Tiger: *"Thanks, Kelly Cow!"*

Kelly Cow and Timmy Tiger: (Resume building a tower together for a few moments while ***showing and telling*** and ***being good sports***.)

Kelly Cow: *"Timmy Tiger, let's build a bigger tower like this. I want to make it all red like this!"* (Rearrange several blocks on the tower and make them all red.)

Timmy Tiger: (Look at Kelly Cow and frown.) *"I don't want a red tower."*

Kelly Cow: (Turn to look at the group of children.) *"Hey friends, am I being bossy with Timmy Tiger?"* (Nod head yes and encourage the children to say *"yes."*)

"That's right, friends! And do you think I should NOT (shake your head to indicate no) *be bossy?"* (Encourage the children to say *"yes."*)

"That's right, friends! Instead, I should be flexible! Moo, moo! Let's do it!"

Timmy Tiger: (Look at Kelly Cow and frown.) *"I don't want a red tower."*

Kelly Cow: *"Okay, Timmy Tiger."* (Take two ***deep breaths***. Rearrange the blocks to their original structure.)

"Hey friends, did I do a good job being a good friend by asking and giving help and not (shake your head to indicate no) *being bossy?"* (Encourage the children to say *"yes."*)

"That's right, friends! Moo moo!"

Kelly Cow and Timmy Tiger: (Say *"good job," give a "cow high-five," and "tiger high-five,"* clap, cheer, and encourage the children to clap as well. Disassemble the blocks. Timmy

Tiger sits on the other side of the Good Friend Square (i.e., the Good Friend Square is between Kelly Cow and Timmy Tiger). ***Social coach*** the children as needed while they practice ***asking and giving help*** and ***not being bossy*** with Timmy Tiger.)

Behavioral Rehearsals: Asking and Giving Help and Don't Be Bossy

Kelly Cow: *"Who wants to be the first Making Friends Helper to show us how to ask and give help and not (shake your head to indicate no) be bossy with Timmy Tiger?"*

(Choose from among the children raising their hands.)

"____ (Child), come sit on the Good Friend Square."

(The child should sit on the Good Friend Square.)

"Remember to ask for help by looking at Timmy Tiger with your (point to your eyes to prompt the children to say *"eyes"*)*...EYES and smiling with your* (point to your mouth to prompt the children to say *"mouth"*)*...MOUTH when you say, 'Timmy Tiger, can you help me?' And remember to not* (shake your head to indicate no) *be bossy by keeping cool, nicely saying 'okay,' and letting Timmy Tiger choose what to do. And don't forget to keep playing nicely if Timmy Tiger says no when you try to help or give ideas."*

Timmy Tiger: (Begin to play with the blocks with the child.)

Kelly Cow: (If needed, ***social coach*** the child to ***look, smile,*** and ***say, "Timmy Tiger, can you help me?"***)

Timmy Tiger: *"Okay, _____ (child)."* (Resume playing with the blocks. Hold a block upside down and have difficulty fitting the block on the tower.) *"_____ (Child), this block doesn't fit. Can you help me?"*

Kelly Cow: (If needed, ***social coach*** the child to ***look, smile,*** and ***say, "Okay, Timmy Tiger."***)

Timmy Tiger: *"Thanks, _____ (child)!"* (Resume building a tower together for a few moments. After the child places a few blocks on the tower, remove one of the blocks that they placed to make the tower taller.) *"I don't want a big tower."*

Kelly Cow: (If needed, ***social coach*** the child to ***keep cool***.)

(Turn to look at the child and smile.) *"Great job asking and giving help and not being bossy, _____ (child)! Moo, moo!"*

(Say *"good job," give a "cow high-five," and "tiger high-five,"* clap, cheer, and encourage the children to clap as well. If needed, ***social coach*** the child to return to their seat.)

Timmy Tiger: (Disassemble the blocks.)

Kelly Cow: *"Who wants to be the next Making Friends Helper to show us how to ask and give help and not be bossy with Timmy Tiger?"*

(Choose from among the children raising their hands.)

"____ (Child), come sit on the Good Friend Square."

(The child should sit on the Good Friend Square.)

"Remember to ask for help by looking at Timmy Tiger with your (point to your eyes to prompt the children to say *"eyes"*)*...EYES and smiling with your* (point to your mouth to prompt the children to say *"mouth"*)*...MOUTH when you say, 'Timmy Tiger, can you help me?' And remember to not* (shake your head to indicate no) *be bossy by keeping cool, nicely saying 'okay,' and letting Timmy Tiger choose what to do. And don't forget to keep playing nicely if Timmy Tiger says no when you try to help or give ideas."*

Timmy Tiger: (With the child, begin to play with the blocks.)

Kelly Cow: (If needed, ***social coach*** the child to ***look, smile,*** and ***say, "Timmy Tiger, can you help me?"***)

Timmy Tiger: *"Okay, _____ (child)."* (Resume playing with the blocks. Hold a block upside down and have difficulty fitting the block on the tower.) *"_____ (Child), this block doesn't fit. Can you help me?"*

Kelly Cow: (If needed, ***social coach*** the child to ***look, smile,*** and ***say, "Okay, Timmy Tiger."***)

Timmy Tiger: *"Thanks, _____ (child)!"* (Resume building a tower together for a few moments. After the child places a few blocks on the tower, remove one of the blocks that they placed to make the tower taller.) *"I don't want a big tower."*

Kelly Cow: (If needed, ***social coach*** the child to ***keep cool***.)

(Turn to look at the child and smile.) *"Great job asking and giving help and not being bossy, _____ (child)! Moo, moo!"*

(Say *"good job," give a "cow high-five," and "tiger high-five,"* clap, cheer, and encourage the children to clap as well. If needed, ***social coach*** the child to return to their seat.)

After the last child has returned to their seat:

Group leader: *"Well friends, you all did a great job practicing some ways you can be nice to your friend!"*

"You each earned ____ (number) stars for being a good friend! Let's start with ____ (child)."

Award each child the same number of stars by repeating the following with each child:

Group leader: *"Where's ____ (child)?"* (Wait until all the children are looking at the child.)

"____ (Child), how many stars did you earn?" (Pause briefly to allow the child to respond.)

"That's right! Let's all count for ____ (child)! One, two, three... (add stars to the Star Chart as they are counted aloud)*! Everybody clap for ____ (child)!"* (All behavioral coaches clap and cheer and encourage the children to clap as well.)

Session 16 Continued

Ring Around the Rosie

BEHAVIORAL REHEARSAL ACTIVITY 1

Materials Needed

- None.

Room Setup

- Remove or place all carpet squares to the side.
- The group leader sits on the floor in front of the room.
- The children and behavioral coaches sit on the floor in a semi-circle facing the group leader.

Rules: Ring Around the Rosie

- The group leader reads the script below to explain the rules.
- Pick a child to be the *"joining friend"* to practice ***joining a game***.
  - The *joining friend* stands next to the group leader.
- Instruct the remaining children and behavioral coaches to hold hands and stand in a circle.
- Instruct the children and behavioral coaches to hold hands and walk in a circle as they sing the *Ring Around the Rosie* song:
  - *Ring Around the Rosie* song:
    "Ring around the rosie,
    A pocket full of posies,
    Ashes, ashes,
    We all fall down!"

- The children and behavioral coaches should act out the last line of the song (*"We all fall down!"*) by sitting down on the floor.
- Continue playing, then briefly pause the game to allow the *joining friend* to ***join the game***.
- Once the *joining friend* has joined the circle, resume the game and ***social coach*** the children to ***stay in their own space*** when acting out the last line of the song.
- Each time the children act out the last line of the song, tell them to freeze in place before ***social coaching*** the children to ***stay in their own space***.
- To ensure that the children have sufficient opportunities to practice ***staying in their own space***, behavioral coaches will be ***space hogs*** when acting out the last line of the song.
  - The children will ***back up*** from behavioral coaches that are ***too close***.

- Then resume the game.
- New commands may be introduced in the last line of the song, *"We all ________."*
  - Examples: "*We all spin around,*" "*We all stand still,*" "*We all kneel down,*" etc.
  - Before introducing a new command, the group leader demonstrates the new command with the children and behavioral coaches.
- Repeat this cycle until all children have had at least one turn being the *joining friend.*

Behavioral Rehearsal: Ring Around the Rosie (15 Minutes)

The group leader explains the activity. The behavioral coaches and children sit in a circle nearby as the group leader explains the rules.

Group leader: *"Hey friends, now we're going to play 'Ring Around the Rosie again.' I'll pick one joining friend to stand next to me. Everyone else will stand in a circle holding hands."*

"Then you'll walk in a circle singing the 'Ring Around the Rosie' song. The song goes like this: 'Ring around the rosie, a pocket full of posies, ashes ashes, we all fall down!'"

"And when we say, 'We all fall down,' we'll all fall down and sit on the floor like this (sit on the floor). *And every time we fall down, we'll practice staying in our own space by backing up* (lean back) *if we're too close to the friends next to us and being a space hog."*

"And while we're playing, our joining friend will join the game by first watching the game (point to your eyes) *and knowing the rules* (tap your head with your finger). *If they know the rules, they'll move closer* (demonstrate moving your body closer), *look at their friends with their* (point to your eyes to prompt the children to say *"eyes"*)*...EYES and smile with their* (point to your mouth to prompt the children to say *"mouth"*)*...MOUTH when they say, 'Can I play?' And don't forget to use* (pause briefly to prompt the children to say *"names"*)*...NAMES."*

"And friends, remember to listen and follow directions because we're going to change the way we all fall down. Okay, let's have ____ (behavioral coach 1) and ____ (behavioral coach 2) try first!"

Role Play: Ring Around the Rosie

The group leader leads the role play. Behavioral coaches 1 and 2 demonstrate how to play *Ring Around the Rosie*. Behavioral coach 1 stands in the circle holding hands with the children. Behavioral coach 2 is the first *joining friend* and stands next to the group leader.

Group leader: *"Okay friends, let's play Ring Around the Rosie. ____ (Behavioral coach 2) will be our joining friend and will practice joining the game. ____ (Behavioral coach 2), let's start by watching the game and knowing the rules. Are we ready? All together now."*

Behavioral coach 1 and children: (Hold hands and walk in a circle while singing the song.)

Behavioral coach 2: (Watch the game and know the rules.)

Behavioral coach 1 and children: *"Ring around the rosie, a pocket full of posies, ashes, ashes, we all fall down!"* (Fall down to the floor while acting out the last line of the song.)

Group leader: *"Everybody FREEZE! Let's see what ____ (behavioral coach 2) does next to join the game."*

(Turn to look at behavioral coach 2.) *"____ (Behavioral coach 2), great job watching the game. Do you know the rules?"*

Behavioral coach 2: *"Yes! They're playing 'Ring Around the Rosie.'"*

Group leader: *"Great! Now you can join the game by moving closer, looking at ____ (behavioral coach 1) with your eyes, smiling with your mouth, and saying, '____ (behavioral coach 1), can I play?' If ____ (behavioral coach 1) says yes, then you can join the game."*

Behavioral coach 2: (Move closer while looking and smiling at behavioral coach 1.) *"____ (Behavioral coach 1), can I play please?"*

Behavioral coach 1: *"Okay, ____ (behavioral coach 2)."*

Behavioral coach 2: *"Thanks, ____ (behavioral coach 1)!"*

Behavioral coaches 1 and 2: (Behavioral coach 1 joins the circle. Both behavioral coaches and children play another round of *Ring Around the Rosie*. In acting out the last line, the two behavioral coaches sit ***too close*** to one another.)

Group leader: *"Everybody FREEZE! ____ (Behavioral coach 1) and ____ (behavioral coach 2), look around you. If you're sitting too close to your friend and being a space hog, then you should back up."*

Behavioral coaches 1 and 2: (Lean back and move away from one another in order to be approximately an arm's length away from each other.)

Group leader: *"____ (Behavioral coach 1) and ____ (behavioral coach 2), great job joining the game and staying in your own space!"*

Behavioral Rehearsal: Ring Around the Rosie

Group leader: *"Okay friends, let's keep on playing. Our next joining friend is ____ (child). ____ (Child), come stand next to me and practice joining the game.* (Have the *joining friend* stand next to the group leader outside of the circle.)

"____ (Child), let's start by watching the game and knowing the rules. Are we ready? All together now." (If needed, ***social coach*** the children to sing the *Ring Around the Rosie* song.)

"Okay friends, now it's time for our joining friend to join the game. Let's see how they join the game." (If needed, ***social coach*** the *joining friend* to ***join the game***.)

Behavioral coaches: (If needed, ***social coach*** the children to accept the *joining friends'* requests to ***join the game***.)

Group leader: *"Great job joining the game ____ (child)! Our next joining friend is ____ (child). ____ (Child), come stand next to me and practice joining the game.* (Have the *joining friend* stand next to the group leader.)

"*Okay friends, now make sure to listen and follow directions because we're not going to fall down anymore. We're going to do some other fun things! For example, if I say, 'We all spin around!' we should all spin around like this* (demonstrate spinning around). *Can you me how to spin around?* (Pause briefly to allow the children to demonstrate spinning around.) *That's right, friends!"*

"Are we ready? All together now."

Behavioral coaches and children: *"Ring around the rosie, a pocket full of posies, ashes, ashes, we all spin around!"*

Group leader: (After a few moments say, "*FREEZE!* (Pause.) *And sit!"*)

Behavioral coaches: (Behavioral coaches will be ***space hogs*** when acting out the last line of the song. The children will ***back up*** from behavioral coaches that are ***too close*** to them.)

Group leader: "*Friends, look around you. If you're being a space hog and are too close to your friends, then you should back up!"* (If needed, ***social coach*** the children to ***stay in their own space***.)

"Great job staying in your own space and listening and following directions! Okay friends, this time we're going to ____ (action) (demonstrate the action). *Can you all show me how to ____ (action)?"*

"That's right! Our next joining friend is ____ (child). Are we ready? All together now."

Behavioral coaches: (If needed, instruct the children to sing the *Ring Around the Rosie* song with new commands.)

Group leader: *"Okay friends, now it's time for our joining friend to join the game. Let's see how they join the game."* (If needed, ***social coach*** the child to ***join the game.)***

Behavioral coaches: (If needed, ***social coach*** the children to accept the *joining friends'* requests to ***join the game***.)

Group leader: *"Great job joining the game! Don't forget to stay in your own space when you sit down!"*

Table 16.3 Sample Commands

Spin around	Touch the floor	Touch our toes
Kneel down	Tap our nose	Hop on one foot
Rub our tummies	Tap our heads	Stand on our tip-toes
Stand on one foot	Touch our knees	Swim like an octopus
Hop on two feet	Fly like a bird	Slither like a snake

Repeat the above cycle using new commands after each turn by saying, *"This time we're going ______ (action)!* (Demonstrate the action). *Can you all show me how to ______ (action)?"* Ensure that every child has at least one turn being the *joining friend* and practicing ***joining the game***.

Behavioral Rehearsal Wrap-Up

Group leader: *"Well friends, great job joining the game, staying in your own space, and listening and following directions! Give yourselves a big round of applause!"* (All behavioral coaches clap and cheer and encourage the children to clap as well.)

"Now everyone should come sit in the Listening Circle." (Have children return to the Listening Circle to sit on their carpet squares.)

"Okay friends, you did a great job practicing some ways you can be nice to your friends like joining a game and staying in your own space and listening and following directions!"

"You each earned ____ (number) more stars for being nice to each other and being good friends! Let's start with ____ (child)."

Award each child the same number of stars by repeating the following with each child:

Group leader: *"Where's _____ (child)?"* (Wait until all the children are looking at the child.)

"_____ (Child), how many stars did you earn?" (Pause briefly to allow the child to respond.)

"That's right! Let's all count for _____ (child)! One, two, three... (add stars to the Star Chart as they are counted aloud)*! Everybody clap for _____ (child)!"* (All behavioral coaches clap and cheer and encourage the children to clap as well.)

Break Time (10 Minutes)

- The puppets may be used to lead the children to and from the bathroom during break time.
- To assist with transitions and limit unstructured time, behavioral coaches may review the lesson with the children while waiting for the remaining children to return from the bathroom.
- You may want to award stars for good behavior after returning from the bathroom.

Session 16 Continued

Hot or Cold

BEHAVIORAL REHEARSAL ACTIVITY 2

Materials Needed

- A small object to be hidden.

Room Setup

- Remove or place all carpet squares to the side.
- The group leader stands at the front of the room facing the children.
- The children and behavioral coaches sit in a semi-circle facing the group leader.

Rules: Hot or Cold

- The group leader reads the script below to explain the rules.
- A behavioral coach is chosen to be the *"finding friend,"* the one who looks for the hidden object.
    - Do NOT allow children to be the *finding friend*.
- The children are the *"helping friends"* and direct the *finding friend* to find the hidden object.
- Instruct the *finding friend* to wait outside of the room while the object is hidden.
- Hide the object somewhere in the room with suggestions from the *helping friends*.
    - Prior to beginning the lesson, the group leader and behavioral coaches should brainstorm several hiding places.
- Call the *finding friend* back into the room and instruct them to stand at the front of the room.
- The *finding friend* asks a *helping friend* for help by asking if they are "*hot or cold*" (i.e., standing close or far away from the hidden object) and if they should take steps in a specific manner (forward or back, one or two steps, etc.).
    - Asking ONE *helping friend* at a time ensures that each child gets an opportunity to practice ***not being bossy***.
- Behavioral coaches will ***social coach*** the *helping friend* to ***give help***.
    - The *helping friend* will say "*hot*" if the *finding friend* is standing close to the hidden object or "*cold*" if the *finding friend* is standing far away from the hidden object.
- The *finding friend* randomly chooses to either follow or not follow the *helping friend's* instructions.
- If the *helping friend's* instructions are not followed, then the *helping friend* should practice ***not being bossy***.
- Once the object is found, ***praise*** the children for ***not being bossy*** and for ***giving help*** and continue the game by hiding another object.

Behavioral Rehearsal: Hot or Cold (15 Minutes)

The group leader leads the activity. The behavioral coaches and children sit nearby as the group leader explains the rules.

Group leader: *"Hey friends, now we're going to play Hot or Cold. ____ (Behavioral coach 1) is the 'finding friend' and you will each take turns being the 'helping friends.' The 'finding friend' will wait outside while we hide the ____ (small object)* (hold up the small object) *somewhere in the room."*

"When the 'finding friend' comes back into the room, they will ask the 'helping friend' TWO questions. The first question is if they are hot or cold. The second question is which way they should move, like if they should take one step (take one step) *or two steps* (take two steps) *or move this way* (demonstrate moving to the right) *or move that way* (demonstrate moving to the left)*."*

"But friends, there's a secret! The 'helping friend' can't (shake your head no) *tell the 'finding friend' where the toy is. The 'helping friend' can only say 'hot' or 'cold' and tell the 'finding friend' how or where to move."*

(Put the toy down on the floor.) *"So if our 'finding friend' is close to the toy* (take a few steps toward the toy)*, we say, 'Hot!' But, if they are far from the toy* (take a few steps away from the toy)*, then we say, 'Cold'! So friends, if I'm close to the toy* (take a few steps toward the toy)*, what do you say?* (Pause briefly to allow the children to say, *"hot"*)*. That's right! And if I'm far from the toy* (take a few steps away from the toy)*, what do you say?* (Pause briefly to allow the children to say, *"cold"*)*. That's right, friends!"*

"And friends, sometimes the finding friend may not listen to your ideas. Remember to not (shake your head to indicate no) *be bossy. Instead, you should be flexible by keeping cool, taking deep breaths* (demonstrate taking two ***deep breaths***)*, nicely saying 'okay,' then letting the finding friend have a turn choosing what to do, and keep playing nicely."*

"Okay, _____ (behavioral coach 1) and _____ (behavioral coach 2) will go first!"

Role Play: Hot or Cold

The group leader leads the role play. The two behavioral coaches demonstrate how to play *Hot or Cold*. Behavioral coach 1 is the *finding friend*, and behavioral coach 2 is the *helping friend*. The other behavioral coaches and children sit nearby watching the role play.

Group leader: *"____ (Behavioral coach 1), please stand outside so that we can hide the ____ (small object)."*

Behavioral coach 1: *"Okay, ____ (group leader)."* (Leave the room.)

Group leader: (Hide the small object. Loudly call out so that behavioral coach 1 can hear from outside.) *"____ (Behavioral coach 1), we're ready. Come back in!"*

Behavioral coach 1: (Enter the room.)

Group leader: *"____ (Behavioral coach 1), ask the helping friend ____ (behavioral coach 2) for help by asking if you're hot or cold and how you should move. And ____ (behavioral coach 2) don't forget to give help."*

Behavioral coach 1: *"____ (Behavioral coach 2), can you help me? Am I hot or cold? Should I take one or two steps forward?"*

Behavioral coach 2: *"Okay, ____ (behavioral coach 1). You're ____ (hot/cold). Take two steps* (specify the direction)*."*

Behavioral coach 1: *"Okay, ____ (behavioral coach 2)."* (Take two steps in the specified direction.) *"____ (Behavioral coach 2), can you help me? Am I hot or cold? Should I take big steps or small steps?"*

Behavioral coach 2: *"Okay, ____ (behavioral coach 1). You're ____ (hot/cold). Take small steps."*

Behavioral coach 1: *"No thanks. This time I'll take a big step."* (Take a big step.)

Behavioral coach 2: *"Okay, ____ (behavioral coach 1)."*

Group leader: *"Great job not being bossy, ____ (behavioral coach 2) when ____ (behavioral coach 1) didn't listen to your idea! Let's keep playing. It's your turn ____ (behavioral coach 1)."*

Repeat these steps until the hidden object is found.

Group leader: *"Great job not being bossy and asking and giving help!"* (Turn to look at the group of children and smile.) *"Okay friends, now it's everybody's turn to play Hot or Cold! Are we ready?"*

Behavioral Rehearsal: Hot or Cold

Group leader: *"____ (Behavioral coach 1), please stand outside so that we can hide the ____ (small object)."*

Behavioral coach 1: *"Okay, ____ (group leader)."* (Leave the room.)

Group leader: (Choose a *hiding friend* from among the children and have them hide the small object, then loudly call out so that behavioral coach 1 can hear from outside.) *"____ (Behavioral coach 1), we're ready. Come back in!"*

Behavioral coach 1: (Enter the room.)

Group leader: *"____ (Behavioral coach 1), ask the helping friend ____ (child) for help by asking if you're hot or cold and how you should move. And ____ (child) don't forget to give help and don't be bossy if ____ (behavioral coach 1) doesn't take your help."*

Behavioral coach 1: *"____ (Child), can you help me? Am I hot or cold? Should I take one or two steps and how should I move?"*

Group leader: (***Social coach*** the *helping friend* to ***give help*** as needed.)

Behavioral coach 1: (The behavioral coach will alternate randomly between saying, *"Okay, ____ (child)" and following the instructions,* or saying, *"No thanks. This time I'll ____"* and doing something different.)

Group leader: (When the behavioral coach does not follow the child's instruction say, *"____ (Child), ____ (behavioral coach) didn't listen to your idea. Remember to not be bossy. Instead, you should be flexible by keeping cool, taking deep breaths* (demonstrate taking two ***deep breaths***), *saying 'okay,' then let ____ (behavioral coach) have a turn choosing what to do, and keep playing nicely."*

(If needed, ***social coach*** the child to ***not be bossy***.)

"Great job not being bossy, ____ (child)! Let's keep playing. Now it's ____ (new child) turn to be the helping friend. ____ (Behavioral coach), ask our new helping friend ____ (new child) if you're hot or cold and how you should move."

Repeat the sequence above until the hidden object is found. Continue to play in this manner while finding new hiding places for the hidden object, ensuring that each child has multiple opportunities to practice ***giving help*** and ***not being bossy*** when their instructions are not followed.

Group leader: *"Great job asking and giving help and not being bossy ____ (child)!"* (Turn to look at the group of children and smile.) *"Okay friends, who wants to be our next helping friend?"*

Behavioral Rehearsal Wrap-Up

Group leader: *"Well friends, great job not being bossy and asking and giving help! Give yourselves a big round of applause!"* (All behavioral coaches clap and cheer and encourage the children to clap as well.)

"Now everyone should come sit in the Listening Circle." (Have children return to the Listening Circle to sit on their carpet squares.)

Group leader: *"Okay friends, you did a great job practicing some ways you can be nice to your friends like* ***asking and giving help*** *and* ***not being bossy****!"*

"You each earned ____ (number) more stars for being nice to each other and being good friends! Let's start with ____ (child)."

Award each child the same number of stars by repeating the following with each child:

Group leader: *"Where's ____ (child)?"* (Wait until all the children are looking at the child.)

"____ (Child), how many stars did you earn?" (Pause briefly to allow the child to respond.)

"That's right! Let's all count for ____ (child)! One, two, three... (add stars to the Star Chart as they are counted aloud)*! Everybody clap for ____ (child)!"* (All behavioral coaches clap and cheer and encourage the children to clap as well.)

"Now our parents are going to come in and we're going to count all of our stars and start our Good Friend Graduation Ceremony!"

Session 16 Continued

FINAL WRAP-UP AND GRADUATION CEREMONY

Materials Needed

- Good Friend Awards for EACH child (see example in Appendix F printed on diploma paper and signed by the treatment team).
- Graduation Prizes (optional).
    - Examples: Interactive board games, card games, sports equipment.

Room Setup

- Reposition the carpet squares in a semi-circle.
- The children should sit on the carpet squares, with parents sitting behind their children on the floor facing the group leader.

Final Wrap-Up

Group leader: *"Okay families, let's all come sit in the Listening Circle."* (Have the full attention of the families before continuing.)

"Friends, you all have been doing a great job being good friends!"

"When we're playing with our friends and want to join a game do you think we should listen and follow directions with our friends?" (Pause briefly to allow the children to say *"yes."*)

"That's right, friends! And are asking and giving help, staying in our space, and not being bossy nice ways to play with our friends?" (Pause briefly to allow the children to say *"yes."*)

"That's right, friends! And when we're asking for a turn and our friends say no, do you think we should keep cool?" (Pause briefly to allow the children to say *"yes."*)

"That's right, friends! In a moment we're going to have our graduation ceremony and celebrate all the hard work you've put into being good friends. Before we do that, should we count up all the stars you've earned today?" (Pause briefly to allow the children to say *"yes."*)

"Okay friends, let's all count together and see how many stars we earned today! One, two, three…(count the number of stars for one child)*! ____ (total number of stars)! Round of applause for our friends!"* (All behavioral coaches clap and cheer and encourage the families to clap as well.)

Graduation Ceremony

- The parent and child group leaders and all the behavioral coaches sit at the front of the room with behavioral coaches wearing a puppet on each hand as a final farewell to the children.
- The children and parents sit in the Listening Circle facing the group leaders and behavioral coaches.
- Consider having the children and parents identify each puppet by name as you are beginning to start the graduation ceremony.
- The parent and child group leaders begin by complimenting the families on their hard work.
  - Comment on the progress the group has made.
  - Avoid mentioning specifics about group members.
  - This part of the graduation ceremony should take a couple of minutes.
- The child group leader announces the start of the graduation ceremony.
  - Explain, *"We are now going to have our graduation ceremony for PEERS® for Preschoolers. Who here has graduated before?"* (Allow children to comment and explain what 'graduation' means and where they have graduated from.) *A graduation is a nice way to celebrate finishing something important. Because you are all graduating from PEERS® for Preschoolers today, you will each get a Good Friend Award that looks like this* (show an example of the certificate). *This award is to celebrate all your hard work in being good friends. When you hear your name called, you will come to the front of the room to receive your award. Then everyone will clap and cheer and you will each share high-fives with all our puppet friends!"*
- The child group leader will present the first award by saying, *"Our first Good Friend Award goes to ______ (child)! Please come to the front of the room to collect your award and get high-fives from all our puppet friends."*
  - If the child is too anxious to come to the front of the room alone, the parent may accompany them.
- The child group leader hands the child their Good Friend Award and ***gives a high-five***.
- The child should then ***give a high-five*** to each of the puppets.
- Everyone will continue to clap and cheer.
- The child group leader presents the next award by saying, *"Our next Good Friend Award goes to ______ (child)! Please come to the front of the room to collect your award and get high-fives from all our puppet friends."*
- Call each child individually up to the front of the room and present them with a Good Friend Award.
- When the final Good Friend Award is given:
  - Thank the families for being a part of the program.
  - Make a few final comments about the wonderful progress that has been made.

- Remind the families that just because the group is over, it does not mean that they should stop using the skills they learned in PEERS® for Preschoolers.
- Encourage them to keep practicing what they've learned so that they can continue to make and keep friends.
- Wish them well and encourage them to stay in touch.
- As each child leaves the room, they should choose one graduation prize (optional) and get their reward(s) from the prize boxes.

Session 16 Continued

Sharing a Diagnosis or Condition with Your Child and Final Review (Part 2)

PEERS® FOR PRESCHOOLERS: PARENT HANDOUT

Snapshot of the Steps for Sharing a Diagnosis or Condition with Your Child

1. Choose the right time.
2. Choose the right context.
3. Acknowledge your child's differences.
4. Give an explanation.
5. Acknowledge what the difference means for your child.
6. Normalize the difference.
7. Turn your child's difference into a strength.
8. Make your child's strength an asset to the family.
9. Be prepared to answer questions.

Didactic Lesson: Steps for Sharing a Diagnosis or Condition with Your Child

Step 1: Choose the Right Time

- Don't wait to share a diagnosis or condition with your child until there is a problem.
- Children with neurodevelopmental disorders appear to have better responses to learning about their diagnoses or conditions earlier in development (before the age of seven).
- Consider sharing your child's diagnosis or condition with them sooner if they begin to ask questions.

Step 2: Choose the Right Context

- Avoid blurting out your child's diagnosis or condition for no reason.
- Wait for the right context to share your child's diagnosis or condition.
- There should be a reason for mentioning your child's diagnosis or condition.

Step 3: Acknowledge Your Child's Difference

- Begin by acknowledging the difference(s) your child has probably noticed.
    - Examples:
        - Frequent doctor visits, assessments, and therapy appointments.
        - The mention of "autism" or "ADHD" or other diagnostic terms.
        - Challenging behaviors.
        - Social difficulties.
        - Restricted interests.
        - Strict adherence to routines.
        - Attentional difficulties.
        - Sensory issues.
        - Hyperactivity.

Step 4: Give an Explanation

- Provide an explanation for why your child receives these services or behaves in these ways.
- This is the part where you may choose to label your child's differences, diagnosis, or condition.
    - Creating a label (or a name) for your child's differences may make it easier to discuss with them in the future.

Step 5: Acknowledge What the Difference Means for Your Child

- Explain what having this condition means for your child.
    - Examples:
        - Frequent doctor visits.
        - Assessments.
        - Therapy appointments.

Step 6: Normalize the Difference

- Normalize your child's differences by explaining that other people have similar differences.
- If your child understands that they are not the only person that has these differences, they will feel less "different."
- You might also explain that a "difference" doesn't make them "less than."

Step 7: Turn Your Child's Differences into a Strength

- After you've acknowledged the difference(s), provided an explanation, and normalized the difference, immediately point out the strengths in your child.
- Always change what could be perceived as a challenge into something positive.
- You might even describe your child's strengths and talents as "superpowers" so they can more easily relate to what you are saying.
- Example: "The good news is that your (condition) also means that (state the positive characteristics)."

- "…you have an amazing memory."
- "…you know a lot about things and like to share with others."
- "…you are very honest and like to tell the truth."

Step 8: Make Your Child's Strength an Asset to the Family

- When turning a difference into a strength, it is useful to make this strength an asset to the family.
- Good examples:
  - "We are so proud of you!"
  - "You are such a good helper!"
  - "You teach us so many things!"

Step 9: Be Prepared to Answer Questions

- Know what your child's diagnosis or condition means and how to explain it to them in words they can understand.
  - There are many books and social stories that can help you guide the conversation.
- Your child may have questions immediately and/or later.
- If you don't know the answer to your child's questions, tell them you don't know but will find the answer.
  - You are not expected to know everything.
  - It is okay for you to model that you are learning too.

Didactic Lesson: Tips for Moving Forward

TIP 1: Continue to enroll your child in *playgroups* based on your child's interests.

- ***Playgroups*** provide a potential source of friends with ***common interests***.
- We recommend that your child be enrolled in AT LEAST ONE ***PLAYGROUP*** at any given time based on their interests.
- It is important that your child continue to participate in ***playgroups*** or other social activities to have a source of potential ***playmates***.
- ***Playgroups*** also provide opportunities for your child to practice the skills they learned in PEERS® for Preschoolers with potential ***playmates.***
- As soon as one ***playgroup*** is about to come to an end, investigate and enroll your child in other ***playgroups.***
- Criteria for good ***playgroups***:
  - Meets regularly (preferably weekly).
  - Located close to your home (this may make it easier to have regularly occurring ***playdates***).
  - Includes accepting children in the same age range and level of support needs as your child.
  - Includes informal time so that your child will have opportunities to socialize and play with other children naturally.

- Activities are based on your child's interests, likes, or hobbies.
- Permits some parent involvement for you to ***social coach***.

TIP 2: Continue to have weekly *playdates.*

- It is essential that your child have regularly occurring ***playdates*** with friends.
  - This is how they will develop stronger friendships.
  - We recommend that your child continue to have AT LEAST ONE ***PLAYDATE*** PER WEEK.
- Remember to plan and prepare for ***playdates*** by using the ***5 Ws.***

TIP 3: Continue to provide *social coaching* on the skills from PEERS® for Preschoolers using the *4 Ps.*

- ***Social coach*** your child to use the skills learned in PEERS® to play with their friends during ***playgroups, playdates,*** and school and/or daycare.
  - As your child improves in their use of the skills with less ***social coaching,*** gradually fade back ***social coaching***.
  - Be sure to periodically provide intermittent ***praise*** (catch them being good).
- Regularly review the *Parent Coached Play Cards*.
  - These coaching cards can be used to provide support during your ***social coaching.***
- Continued ***social coaching*** on your part will ensure that your child:
  - Will continue to use the skills learned in PEERS® for Preschoolers.
  - Will be successful at making and keeping friends.
- Be prepared to help your child obtain new social skills as social demands change with development.
  - The social skills your child will need to make and keep friends will change as they grow older.
  - Major social developmental periods:
    - Preschool age.
    - Elementary school age.
    - Adolescence (middle and high school).
    - Adulthood.

TIP 4: Remember *friendship is a choice.*

- ***Our children don't get to be friends with everyone.***
- ***Everyone doesn't get to be friends with our children.***
- There are good choices and bad choices when it comes to friendships.
  - It is important to assess the interest of your child's potential ***playmates*** and respond accordingly.
  - It is also important to assess the interest of the ***playmate's*** parents in having ***playdates***.

TIP 5: Consider embracing neurodiversity.

- Just as we have shared the PEERS® Neurodiversity Pledge with you at the beginning of each didactic lesson, consider embracing your own ideas about neurodiversity.

- These ideas might include:
  - Valuing neurodiversity, acceptance, and authenticity.
  - Honoring the diverse ways people experience the world.
  - Respecting each person's unique perspectives and communication styles.
  - Recognizing there is no one right way to connect with others.
  - Remembering that if using the strategies taught in PEERS® feels like camouflaging or masking and/or they don't align with your goals or the goals of your family, then you do not have to use them.
  - Remembering that learning and using the skills taught in PEERS® is a PERSONAL CHOICE.

Table 16.1 Assessing Parent Interest for Playdates

SIGNS OF INTEREST	SIGNS OF DISINTEREST
Making eye contact	Not making eye contact/looking away
Smiling	Not smiling/looking uncomfortable
Turning toward you	Turning away from you
Talking to you/asking questions	Not talking to you/saying very little
Seeming eager to make plans	Acting reluctant/hesitant to make plans
Agreeing about children's mutual interest	Seeming confused/distracted
Agreeing to playdate (even without finalizing)	Sounding busy or unavailable
Exchanging contact information	No exchanging contact information
Agreeing to follow up later	Agreeing to playdate but not following up

Child Didactic Lesson: Final Review (Part 2)

Snapshot of Previously Learned Lessons: Final Review (Part 2)

Table 16.2 Previously Learned Skills (Part 2)

LISTENING AND FOLLOWING DIRECTIONS	ASKING FOR A TURN
1. Listen with your ears (cup your hand behind your ear). 2. Be quiet with your mouth (place your index finger in front of your mouth and say "shhh"). 3. Have calm hands and a calm body (put your hands to your side). 4. Do what you're told to do.	1. Look at your friend with your eyes (point to your eyes). 2. Smile with your mouth (point to your mouth and smile). 3. Say "Can I have a turn please?" using names.

(*Continued*)

Table 16.2 (Continued)

KEEPING COOL	DON'T BE BOSSY (BE FLEXIBLE)
1. Look at your friend with your eyes (point to your eyes) 2. Nicely say "okay" using names. 3. Find something else to do. 4. If you're still feeling upset, take deep breaths to keep cool (take two slow deep breaths). a. Smell the flowers (example of breathing in) b. Blow out the candles (example of breathing out)	1. Keep cool. 2. Take deep breaths (demonstrate taking two deep breaths). 3. Nicely say, "Okay." 4. Let your friend have a turn choosing what to do. 5. Keep playing nicely.
ASKING FOR HELP	**GIVING HELP**
1. Look at your friends with your eyes (point to your eyes). 2. Smile with your mouth (point to your mouth and smile). 3. Say, "Can you help me?" using names.	1. Look at your friends with your eyes (point to your eyes). 2. Smile with your mouth (point to your mouth and smile). 3. Say "okay" using names. 4. Give help to your friend.
JOINING A GAME	**STAYING IN OUR OWN SPACE**
1. Watch the game (point to your eyes). 2. Know the rules (point to your head). 3. Move closer (demonstrate moving closer with your body). 4. Look at your friends with your eyes (point to your eyes). 5. Smile with your mouth (point to your mouth and smile). 6. Say, "Can I play?" using names. • If your friends say yes, join the game. • If your friends say no, keep cool and find something else to do.	• Don't get too close (shake your head no) ○ If we can touch the person next to us (extend your arm out in front and to the side), then we're too close and being a space hog. • Stay in our own space (nod your head yes) ○ If we're too close and being a space hog, then we need to back up (lean back) and stay in our own space. ○ Remember to be a space keeper.

Reference List

Abidin, R. R. (2012). *Parenting stress index* (4th ed.). Psychological Assessment Resources.

Aldred, C., Green, J., & Adams, C. (2008). A new social communication intervention for children with autism: Pilot randomised controlled treatment study suggesting effectiveness. *Journal of Child Psychology and Psychiatry, 45*(8), 1420–1430. https://doi.org/10.1111/j.1469-7610.2004.00338.x

American Psychiatric Association. (2013). *Diagnostic and statistical manual of mental disorders* (4th ed.). American Psychiatric Association.

Anagnostou, E., Jones, N., Huerta, M., Halladay, A. K., Wang, P., Scahill, L., Horrigan, J. P., Kasari, C., Lord, C., Choi, D., Sullivan, K., & Dawson, G. (2014). Measuring social communication behaviors as a treatment endpoint in individuals with autism spectrum disorder. *Autism, 19*(5), 622–636. https://doi.org/10.1177/1362361314542955

Antezana, L., Albright, J., Scarpa, A., Richey, J. A., Laugeson, E. A., & Factor, R. S. (2022). PEERS® for preschoolers preliminary outcomes and predictors of treatment response. *Journal of Autism and Developmental Disorders, 53*(12), 4671–4684. https://doi.org/10.1007/s10803-022-05724-7

Antezana, L., Factor, R. S., Condy, E. E., Strege, M. V., Scarpa, A., & Richey, J. A. (2018). Gender differences in restricted and repetitive behaviors and interests in youth with autism. *Autism Research, 12*(2), 274–283. https://doi.org/10.1002/aur.2049

Antezana, L., Mosner, M. G., Troiani, V., & Yerys, B. E. (2015). Social-emotional inhibition of return in children with autism spectrum disorder versus typical development. *Journal of Autism and Developmental Disorders, 46*, 1236–1246. https://doi.org/10.1007/s10803-015-2661-9

Antshel, K. M., Polacek, C., McMahon, M., Dygert, K., Spenceley, L., Dygert, L., Miller, L., & Faisal, F. (2011). Comorbid ADHD and anxiety affect social skills group intervention treatment efficacy in children with autism spectrum disorders. *Journal of Developmental and Behavioral Pediatrics, 32*(6), 439–446. https://doi.org/10.1097/DBP.0b013e318222355d

Arnold, D. S., O'Leary, S. G., Wolff, L. S., & Acker, M. M. (1993). The parenting scale: A measure of dysfunctional parenting in discipline situations. *Psychological Assessment, 5*(2), 137–144. https://doi.org/10.1037/1040-3590.5.2.137

Ashbaugh, K., Koegel, R. L., & Koegel, L. K. (2017). Increasing social integration for college students with autism spectrum disorder. *Behavioral Development Bulletin, 22*(1), 183–196. https://doi.org/10.1037/bdb0000057

Azungah, T. (2018). Qualitative research: Deductive and inductive approaches to data analysis. *Qualitative Research Journal, 18*(4), 383–400. https://doi.org/10.1108/QRJ-D-18-00035

Baio, J. (2014, March 28). *Prevalence of autism spectrum disorder among children aged 8 year- Autism and Developmental Disabilities Monitoring Network, 11 sites, United States, 2010.* Centers for Disease Control and Prevention: Morbidity and Mortality Weekly Report. https://stacks.cdc.gov/view/cdc/22182

Baker, J. K., Seltzer, M. M., & Greenberg, J. S. (2011). Longitudinal effects of adaptability on behavior problems and maternal depression in families of adolescents with autism. *Journal of Family Psychology, 25*(4), 601–609. https://doi.org/10.1037/a0024409

Barnhill, G. P. (2001). Social attributions and depression in adolescents with asperger syndrome. *Focus on Autism and Other Developmental Disabilities, 16*(1), 46–53. https://doi.org/10.1177/108835760101600112

Barnhill, G. P. (2007). Outcomes in adults with asperger syndrome. *Focus on Autism and Other Developmental Disabilities, 22*(2), 116–126. https://doi.org/10.1177/10883576070220020301

Baron-Cohen, S., & Wheelwright, S. (2004). The empathy quotient: An investigation of adults with asperger syndrome or high functioning autism, and normal sex differences. *Journal of Autism and Developmental Disorders, 34*(2), 163–175. https://doi.org/10.1023/B:JADD.0000022607.19833.00

Barroso, N. E., Hungerford, G. M., Garcia, D., Graziano, P. A., & Bagner, D. M. (2016). Psychometric properties of the Parenting Stress Index-Short Form (PSI-SF) in a high-risk sample of mothers and their infants. *Psychological Assessment, 28*(10), 1331–1335. https://doi.org/10.1037/pas0000257

Barry, T. D., Klinger, L. G., Lee, J. M., Palardy, N., Gilmore, T., & Bodin, S. D. (2003). Examining the effectiveness of an outpatient clinic-based social skills group for high-functioning children with autism. *Journal of Autism and Developmental Disorders, 33*(6), 685–701. https://doi.org/10.1023/b:jadd.0000006004.86556.e0

Bartley, J. J. (2006). An update on autism: Science, gender, and the law. *Gender Medicine, 3*(2), 73–78. https://doi.org/10.1016/S1550-8579(06)80197-X

Bauminger, N. (2002). The facilitation of social-emotional understanding and social interaction in high-functioning children with autism: Intervention outcomes. *Journal of Autism and Developmental Disorders, 32*(4), 283–298. https://doi.org/10.1023/A:1016378718278

Bauminger, N., & Kasari, C. (2000). Loneliness and friendship in high-functioning children with autism. *Child Development, 71*(2), 447–456. https://doi.org/10.1111/1467-8624.00156

Bauminger, N., Shulman, C., & Agam, G. (2003). Peer interaction and loneliness in high-functioning children with autism. *Journal of Autism and Developmental Disorders, 33*(5), 489–507. https://doi.org/10.1023/A:1025827427901

Bauminger-Zviely, N., & Shefer, A. (2021). Naturalistic evaluation of preschoolers' spontaneous interactions: The Autism Peer Interaction Observation Scale. *Autism, 25*(6), 1520–1535. https://doi.org/10.1177/1362361321989919

Bearss, K., Burrell, T. L., Stewart, L., & Scahill, L. (2015). Parent training in autism spectrum disorder: What's in a name? *Clinical Child and Family Psychology Review, 18*(2), 170–182. https://doi.org/10.1007/s10567-015-0179-5

Bearss, K., Johnson, C., Handen, B., Smith, T., & Scahill, L. (2012). A pilot study of parent training in young children with autism spectrum disorders and disruptive behavior. *Journal of Autism and Developmental Disorders, 43*(4), 829–840. https://doi.org/10.1007/s10803-012-1624-7

Bellini, S., Peters, J. K., Benner, L., & Hopf, A. (2007). A meta-analysis of school-based social skills interventions for children with autism spectrum disorders. *Remedial and Special Education, 28*(3), 153–162. https://doi.org/10.1177/07419325070280030401

Benjamini, Y., & Hochberg, Y. (1995). Controlling the false discovery rate: A practical and powerful approach to multiple testing. *Journal of the Royal Statistical Society: Series B Methodological, 57*(1), 289–300. https://doi.org/10.1111/j.2517-6161.1995.tb02031.x

Benson, P. R. (2015). Longitudinal effects of educational involvement on parent and family functioning among mothers of children with ASD. *Research in Autism Spectrum Disorders, 11*, 42–55. https://doi.org/10.1016/j.rasd.2014.11.011

Blackledge, J. T., & Hayes, S. C. (2006). Using acceptance and commitment training in the support of parents of children diagnosed with autism. *Child & Family Behavior Therapy, 28*(1), 1–18. https://doi.org/10.1300/J019v28n01_01

Bölte, S. (2014). The power of words: Is qualitative research as important as quantitative research in the study of autism? *Autism, 18*(2), 67–68. https://doi.org/10.1177/1362361313517367

Bolton, P., Macdonald, H., Pickles, A., Rios, P., Goode, S., Crowson, M., & Rutter, M. (1994). A case-control family history study of autism. *Journal of Child Psychology and Psychiatry, 35*(5), 877–900. https://doi.org/10.1111/j.1469-7610.1994.tb02300.x

Borckardt, J. J., Nash, M. R., Murphy, M. D., Moore, M., Shaw, D., & O'Neil, P. (2008). Clinical practice as natural laboratory for psychotherapy research. *American Psychologist, 63*(2), 77–95. https://doi.org/10.1037/0003-066X.63.2.77

Bottema-Beutel, K., Kapp, S. K., Lester, J. N., Sasson, N. J., & Hand, B. N. (2020). Avoiding ableist language: Suggestions for autism researchers. *Autism in Adulthood, 3*(1), 18–29. https://doi.org/10.1089/aut.2020.0014

Bottema-Beutel, K., Mullins, T. S., Harvey, M. N., Gustafson, J. R., & Carter, E. W. (2015). Avoiding the "brick wall of awkward": Perspectives of youth with autism spectrum disorder on social-focused intervention practices. *Autism, 20*(2), 196–206. https://doi.org/10.1177/1362361315574888

Bottema-Beutel, K., Park, H., & Kim, S. Y. (2018). Commentary on social skills training curricula for individuals with ASD: Social interaction, authenticity, and stigma. *Journal of Autism and Developmental Disorders, 48*(3), 953–964. https://doi.org/10.1007/s10803-017-3400-1

Boyd, B. A., Hume, K., McBee, M. T., Alessandri, M., Gutierrez, A., Johnson, L., & Odom, S. L. (2014). Comparative efficacy of LEAP, TEACCH and non-model-specific special education programs for preschoolers with autism spectrum disorders. *Journal of Autism and Developmental Disorders, 44*(2), 366–380. https://doi.org/10.1007/s10803-013-1877-9

Bristol, M. M., Gallagher, J. J., & Holt, K. D. (1993). Maternal depressive symptoms in autism: Response to psychoeducational intervention. *Rehabilitation Psychology, 38*(1), 3–10. https://doi.org/10.1037/h0080290

Brookman-Frazee, L., & Koegel, R. L. (2004). Using parent/clinician partnerships in parent education programs for children with autism. *Journal of Positive Behavior Interventions, 6*(4), 195–213. https://doi.org/10.1177/10983007040060040201

Bury, S. M., Jellett, R., Spoor, J. R., & Hedley, D. (2020). "It defines who I am" or "it's something I have": What language do [autistic] Australian adults [on the autism spectrum] prefer? *Journal of Autism and Developmental Disorders, 53*(1), 677–687. https://doi.org/10.1007/s10803-020-04425-3

Camargo, S. P. H., Rispoli, M., Ganz, J., Hong, E. R., Davis, H., & Mason, R. (2014). A review of the quality of behaviorally-based intervention research to improve social interaction skills of children with ASD in inclusive settings. *Journal of Autism and Developmental Disorders*, *44*(9), 2096–2116. https://doi.org/10.1007/s10803-014-2060-7

Caplan, B., Blacher, J., & Eisenhower, A. (2019). Responsive parenting and prospective social skills development in early school-aged children with autism spectrum disorder. *Journal of Autism and Developmental Disorders, 49*(8), 3203–3217. https://doi.org/10.1007/s10803-019-04039-4

Carter, A. S., Davis, N. O., Klin, A., & Volkmar, F. R. (2005). Social development in autism. In F. R. Volkmar, R. Paul, A. Klin, & D. Cohen (Eds.), *Handbook of autism and pervasive developmental disorders: Diagnosis, development, neurobiology, and behavior* (pp. 312–334). John Wiley & Sons. https://doi.org/10.1002/9780470939345

Casagrande, K. A., & Ingersoll, B. R. (2017). Parent-mediated interventions for social communication in young children with ASD. In J. Leaf (Ed.), *Handbook of social skills and autism spectrum disorder* (pp. 285–312). Springer. https://doi.org/10.1007/978-3-319-62995-7_17

Chamberlain, B., Kasari, C., & Rotheram-Fuller, E. (2007). Involvement or isolation? The social networks of children with autism in regular classrooms. *Journal of Autism and Developmental Disorders*, *37*(2), 230–242. https://doi.org/10.1007/s10803-006-0164-4

Chaxiong, P., Burrows, C., Botteron, K. N., Dager, S. R., Estes, A. M., Hazlett, H. C., Schultz, R. T., Zwaigenbaum, L., Piven, J., Wolff, J., Piven, J., Hazlett, H. C., Chappell, C., Shen, M., Swanson, M., Dager, S., Estes, A., Shaw, D., John, T. S., & IBIS Network. (2021). Relations of restricted and repetitive behaviors to social skills in toddlers with autism. *Journal of Autism and Developmental Disorders, 52*, 1423–1434. https://doi.org/10.1007/s10803-021-05014-8

Chen, J. L., Leader, G., Sung, C., & Leahy, M. (2015). Trends in employment for individuals with autism spectrum disorder: A review of the research literature. *Review Journal of Autism and Developmental Disorders, 2*(2), 115–127. https://doi.org/10.1007/s40489-014-0041-6

Chen, J. L., Lin, T-J., Justice, L., & Sawyer, B. (2019). The social networks of children with and without disabilities in early childhood special education classrooms. *Journal of Autism and Developmental Disorders*, *49*(7), 2779–2794. https://doi.org/10.1007/s10803-017-3272-4

Chenausky, K., Norton, A., Tager-Flusberg, H., & Schlaug, G. (2018). Behavioral predictors of improved speech output in minimally verbal children with autism. *Autism Research, 11*(10), 1356–1365. https://doi.org/10.1002/aur.2006

Chevallier, C., Kohls, G., Troiani, V., Brodkin, E. S., & Schultz, R. T. (2012). The social motivation theory of autism. *Trends in Cognitive Sciences, 16*(4), 231–239. https://doi.org/10.1016/j.tics.2012.02.007

Choque Olsson, N., Rautio, D., Asztalos, J., Stoetzer, U., & Bölte, S. (2016). Social skills group training in high-functioning autism: A qualitative responder study. *Autism*, *20*(8), 995–1010. https://doi.org/10.1177/1362361315621885

Chu, P. S., Saucier, D. A., & Hafner, E. (2010). Meta-analysis of the relationships between social support and well-being in children and adolescents. *Journal of Social and Clinical Psychology, 29*(6), 624–645. https://doi.org/10.1521/jscp.2010.29.6.624

Church, C., Alisanski, S., & Amanullah, S. (2000). The social, behavioral, and academic experiences of children with asperger syndrome. *Focus on Autism and Other Developmental Disabilities*, *15*(1), 12–20. https://doi.org/10.1177/108835760001500102

Clements, C. C., Zoltowski, A. R., Yankowitz, L. D., Yerys, B. E., Schultz, R. T., & Herrington, J. D. (2018). Evaluation of the social motivation hypothesis of autism: A systematic review and meta-analysis. *JAMA Psychiatry, 75*(8), 797–808. https://doi.org/10.1001/jamapsychiatry.2018.1100

Coelho, L., Torres, N., Fernandes, C., & Santos, A. J. (2017). Quality of play, social acceptance and reciprocal friendship in preschool children. *European Early Childhood Education Research Journal, 25*(6), 812–823. https://doi.org/10.1080/1350293X.2017.1380879

Condy, E. E., Scarpa, A., & Friedman, B. H. (2017). Respiratory sinus arrhythmia predicts restricted repetitive behavior severity. *Journal of Autism and Developmental Disorders, 47*(9), 2795–2804. https://doi.org/10.1007/s10803-017-3193-2

Condy, E. E., Scarpa, A., & Friedman, B. H. (2019). Restricted repetitive behaviors in autism spectrum disorder: A systematic review from the neurovisceral integration perspective. *Biological Psychology, 148*, Article 107739. https://doi.org/10.1016/j.biopsycho.2019.107739

Conner, C. M., & White, S. W. (2018). Brief report: Feasibility and preliminary efficacy of individual mindfulness therapy for adults with autism spectrum disorder. *Journal of Autism and Developmental Disorders, 48*(1), 290–300. https://doi.org/10.1007/s10803-017-3312-0

Constantino, J. N., & Gruber, C. P. (2012). *Social responsiveness scale* (2nd ed.). Western Psychological Services. https://doi.org/10.1177/0734282913517525

Corona, L. L., Janicki, C., Milgramm, A., & Christodulu, K. V. (2019). Brief report: Reductions in parenting stress in the context of PEERS® – A social skills intervention for adolescents with autism spectrum disorder. *Journal of Autism and Developmental Disorders*, *49*(12), 5073–5077. https://doi.org/10.1007/s10803-019-04201-y

Cox, M. J., & Paley, B. (1997). Families as systems. *Annual Review of Psychology, 48*(1), 243–267. https://doi.org/10.1146/annurev.psych.48.1.243

Crank, J. E., Sandbank, M., Dunham, K., Crowley, S., Bottema- Beutel, K., Feldman, J., & Woynaroski, T. G. (2021). Understanding the effects of naturalistic developmental behavioral interventions: A project AIM meta-analysis. *Autism Research*, *14*(4), 817–834. https://doi.org/10.1002/aur.2471

Cridland, E. K., Jones, S. C., Magee, C. A., & Caputi, P. (2014). Family-focused autism spectrum disorder research: A review of the utility of family systems approaches.*Autism, 18*(3), 213–222. https://doi.org/10.1177/1362361312472261

Davis, N. O., & Carter, A. S. (2008). Parenting stress in mothers and fathers of toddlers with autism spectrum disorders: Associations with child characteristics. *Journal of Autism and Developmental Disorders, 38*(7), 1278–1291. https://doi.org/10.1007/s10803-007-0512-z

Dawson, G. (2008). Early behavioral intervention, brain plasticity, and the prevention of autism spectrum disorder. *Development and Psychopathology, 20*(3), 775–803. https://doi.org/10.1017/S0954579408000370

Dawson, G., Rogers, S., Munson, J., Smith, M., Winter, J., Greenson, J., & Varley, J. (2010). Randomized, controlled trial of an intervention for toddlers with autism: The early start Denver model. *Pediatrics, 125*(1), e17-e23. https://doi.org/10.1542/peds.2009-0958

de Bildt, A., Timmerman, M. E., Mulder, E. J., Nauta, M. H., & Dekker, V. (2014). A randomized controlled study of a social skills training for preadolescent children with autism spectrum disorders: Generalization of skills by training parents and teachers? *BMC Psychiatry*, *14*(1), Article 189. https://doi.org/10.1186/1471-244X-14-189

de Vries, M., & Geurts, H. (2015). Influence of autism traits and executive functioning on quality of life in children with an autism spectrum disorder. *Journal of Autism and Developmental Disorders, 45*(9), 2734–2743. https://doi.org/10.1007/s10803-015-2438-1

DeLucia, E. A., McKenna, M. P., Andrzejewski, T. M., Valentino, K., & McDonnell, C. G. (2022). A pilot study of self-regulation and behavior problems in preschoolers with ASD: Parent broader autism phenotype traits relate to child emotion regulation and inhibitory control. *Journal of Autism and Developmental Disorders, 52*, 4397–4411. https://doi.org/10.1007/s10803-021-05322-z

Denham, S., von Salisch, M., Olthof, T., Kochanoff, A., & Caverly, S. (2002). Emotional and social development in childhood. In P. K. Smith & C. H. Hart (Eds.), *Blackwell handbook of childhood social development* (pp. 307–328). Blackwell.

Dennis, M. L., Neece, C. L., & Fenning, R. M. (2018). Investigating the influence of parenting stress on child behavior problems in children with developmental delay: The role of parent-child relational factors. *Advances in Neurodevelopmental Disorders*, *2*(2), 129–141. https://doi.org/10.1007/s41252-017-0044-2

DeRosier, M. E., Swick, D. C., Davis, N. O., McMillen, J. S., & Matthews, R. (2011). The efficacy of a social skills group intervention for improving social behaviors in children with high functioning autism spectrum disorders. *Journal of Autism and Developmental Disorders, 41*(8), 1033–1043. https://doi.org/10.1007/s10803-010-1128-2

Derguy, C., Michel, G., M'bailara, K., Roux, S., & Bouvard, M. (2015). Assessing needs in parents of children with autism spectrum disorder: A crucial preliminary step to target relevant issues for support programs. *Journal of Intellectual & Developmental Disability*, *40*(2), 156–166. https://doi.org/10.3109/13668250.2015.1023707

DesChamps, T. D., Ibañez, L. V., Edmunds, S. R., Dick, C. C., & Stone, W. L. (2020). Parenting stress in caregivers of young children with ASD concerns prior to a formal diagnosis. *Autism Research*, *13*(1), 82–92. https://doi.org/10.1002/aur.2213

Dichter, G. S. (2018). Motivational impairments in autism may be broader than previously thought. *JAMA Psychiatry, 75*(8), 773–774. https://doi.org/10.1001/jamapsychiatry.2018.1078

Dieleman, L. M., Moyson, T., De Pauw, S. S. W., Prinzie, P., & Soenens, B. (2018). Parents' need-related experiences and behaviors when raising a child with autism spectrum disorder. *Journal of Pediatric Nursing*, *42*, e26–e37. https://doi.org/10.1016/j.pedn.2018.06.005

Dixon, L., Lucksted, A., Stewart, B., Burland, J., Brown, C. H., Postrado, L., & Hoffman, M. (2004). Outcomes of the peer-taught 12-week family-to-family education program for severe mental illness. *Acta Psychiatrica Scandinavica, 109*(3), 207–215. https://doi.org/10.1046/j.0001-690X.2003.00242.x

Duvekot, J., van der Ende, J., Verhulst, F. C., & Greaves-Lord, K. (2018). Examining bidirectional effects between the Autism Spectrum Disorder (ASD) core symptom domains and anxiety in children with ASD. *Journal of Child Psychology and Psychiatry and Allied Disciplines, 59*(3), 277–284. https://doi.org/10.1111/jcpp.12829

Edwards, A. G., Brebner, C. M., McCormack, P. F., & MacDougall, C. J. (2018). From 'parent' to 'expert': How parents of children with autism spectrum disorder make decisions about which intervention approaches to access. *Journal of Autism and Developmental Disorders, 48*, 2122–2138. https://doi.org/10.1007/s10803-018-3473-5

Estes, A., Olson, E., Sullivan, K., Greenson, J., Winter, J., Dawson, G., & Munson, J. (2013). Parenting-related stress and psychological distress in mothers of toddlers with autism spectrum disorders. *Brain & Development, 35*(2), 133–138. https://doi.org/10.1016/j.braindev.2012.10.004

Eyberg, S. M., & Matarazzo, R. G. (1980). Training parents as therapists: A comparison between individual parent-child interaction training and parent group didactic training. *Journal of Clinical Psychology, 36*(2), 492–499. https://doi.org/10.1002/jclp.6120360218

Factor, R. S., Condy, E. E., Farley, J. P., & Scarpa, A. (2016). Brief report: Insistence on sameness, anxiety, and social motivation in children with autism spectrum disorder. *Journal of Autism and Developmental Disorders, 46*(7), 2548–2554. https://doi.org/10.1007/s10803-016-2781-x

Factor, R. S., Moody, C. T., Sung, K. Y., & Laugeson, E. A. (2022). Improving social anxiety and social responsiveness in autism spectrum disorder through PEERS®. *Evidence-based Practice in Child and Adolescent Mental Health, 7*(1), 142–159. https://doi.org/10.1080/23794925.2021.2013138

Factor, R. S., Ollendick, T. H., Cooper, L. D., Dunsmore, J. C., Rea, H. M., & Scarpa, A. (2019). All in the family: A systematic review of the effect of caregiver-administered autism spectrum disorder interventions on family functioning and relationships. *Clinical Child and Family Psychology Review, 22*(4), 433–457. https://doi.org/10.1007/s10567-019-00297-x

Factor, R. S., Rea, H. M., Dahiya, A. V., Albright, J., Ollendick, T. H., Laugeson, E. A., & Scarpa, A. (2022). An initial pilot study examining child social skills, caregiver styles, and family functioning in the PEERS® for preschoolers program for young autistic children and their caregivers. *Research in Developmental Disabilities, 121*, Article 104152. https://doi.org/10.1016/j.ridd.2021.104152

Factor, R. S., Rea, H. M., Laugeson, E. A., & Scarpa, A. (2023). Examining feasibility and outcomes of the PEERS® for preschoolers program. *Journal of Autism and Developmental Disorders, 53*(5), 1821–1833. https://doi.org/10.1007/s10803-022-05502-5

Factor, R. S., Rea, H. M., Dahiya, A. V., Laugeson, E. A., & Scarpa, A. (2023). Pilot study examining caregiver–child and family functioning in PEERS® for preschoolers. *Journal of Child and Family Studies, 32*(6), 1694–1707.

Factor, R. S., Ryan, S. M., Farley, J. P., Ollendick, T. H., & Scarpa, A. (2017). Does the presence of anxiety and ADHD symptoms add to social impairment in children with autism spectrum disorder? *Journal of Autism and Developmental Disorders, 47*(4), 1122–1134. https://doi.org/10.1007/s10803-016-3025-9

Farroni, T., Csibra, G., Simion, F., & Johnson, M. H. (2002). Eye contact detection in humans from birth. *Proceedings of the National Academy of Sciences, 99*(14), 9602–9605. https://doi.org/10.1073/pnas.152159999

Fraire, M. G., & Ollendick, T. H. (2013). Anxiety and oppositional defiant disorder: A transdiagnostic conceptualization. *Clinical Psychology Review, 33*(2), 229–240. https://doi.org/10.1016/j.cpr.2012.11.004

Franchini, M., Glaser, B., Wood de Wilde, H., Gentaz, E., Eliez, S., & Schaer, M. (2017). Social orienting and joint attention in preschoolers with autism spectrum disorders. *PLoS One*, *12*(6), Article e0178859. https://doi.org/10.1371/journal.pone.0178859

Frankel, F. D., Gorospe, C. M., Chang, Y.-C., & Sugar, C. A. (2011). Mothers' reports of play dates and observation of school playground behavior of children having high-functioning autism spectrum disorders: Play dates and school observation. *Journal of Child Psychology and Psychiatry, 52*(5), 571–579. https://doi.org/10.1111/j.1469-7610.2010.02318.x

Frankel, F. D., & Mintz, J. (2008). *Measuring the quality of play dates*. UCLA Parenting and Children's Friendship Program.

Frankel, F. D., & Mintz, J. (2011). Maternal reports of play dates of clinic referred and community children. *Journal of Child and Family Studies, 20*(5), 623–630. https://doi.org/10.1007/s10826-010-9437-9

Frankel, F. D., & Myatt, R. J. (2013). *Children's friendship training*. Routledge.

Frankel, F. D., Myatt, R. J., Sugar, C., Whitham, C., Gorospe, C. M., & Laugeson, E. A. (2010). A randomized controlled study of parent-assisted children's friendship training with children having autism spectrum disorders. *Journal of Autism and Developmental Disorders, 40*(7), 827–842. https://doi.org/10.1007/s10803-009-0932-z

Fritz, C. O., Morris, P. E., & Richler, J. J. (2012). Effect size estimates: Current use, calculations, and interpretation. *Journal of Experimental Psychology: General, 141*(1), 2–18. https://doi.org/10.1037/a0024338

Gabriels, R. L., Agnew, J. A., Pan, Z., Holt, K. D., Reynolds, A., & Laudenslager, M. L. (2013). Elevated repetitive behaviors are associated with lower diurnal salivary cortisol levels in autism spectrum disorder. *Biological Psychology, 93*(2), 262–268. https://doi.org/10.1016/j.biopsycho.2013.02.017

Gantman, A., Kapp, S. K., Orenski, K., & Laugeson, E. A. (2012). Social skills training for young adults with high-functioning autism spectrum disorders: A randomized controlled pilot study. *Journal of Autism and Developmental Disorders, 42*(6), 1094–1103. https://doi.org/10.1007/s10803-011-1350-6

Garbarino, J., Dow-Burger, K., & Ratner, N. B. (2020). Implementation of the program for the education and enrichment of relational skills (PEERS®) social skills intervention in a university-based communication sciences and disorders clinic. *Perspectives of the ASHA Special Interest Groups, 5*(3), 637–645. https://doi.org/10.1044/2020_PERSP-20-00001

Gardner, D. M., Gerdes, A. C., & Weinberger, K. (2019). Examination of a parent-assisted, friendship-building program for adolescents with ADHD. *Journal of Attention Disorders, 23*(4), 363–373. https://doi.org/10.1177/1087054715588188

Gates, J. A., Kang, E., & Lerner, M. D. (2017). Efficacy of group social skills interventions for youth with autism spectrum disorder: A systematic review and meta-analysis. *Clinical Psychology Review, 52*, 164–181. https://doi.org/10.1016/j.cpr.2017.01.006

Gee, D. G., Gabard-Durnam, L., Telzer, E. H., Humphreys, K. L., Goff, B., Shapiro, M., Flannery, J., Lumian, D. S., Fareri, D. S., Caldera, C., & Tottenham, N. (2014). Maternal buffering of human amygdala–prefrontal circuitry during childhood but not adolescence. *Psychological Science, 25*(11), 2067–2078. https://doi.org/10.1177/0956797614550878

Gena, A., Couloura, S., & Kymissis, E. (2005). Modifying the affective behavior of preschoolers with autism using in-vivo or video modeling and reinforcement contingencies. *Journal of Autism and Developmental Disorders, 35*(5), 545–556. https://doi.org/10.1007/s10803-005-0014-9

Gengoux, G. W. (2015). Priming for social activities: Effects on interactions between children with autism and typically developing peers. *Journal of Positive Behavior Interventions*, *17*(3), 181–192. https://doi.org/10.1177/1098300714561862

Gengoux, G. W., Schapp, S., Burton, S., Ardel, C. M., Libove, R. A., Baldi, G., Berquist, K. L., Phillips, J. M., & Hardan, A. Y. (2019). Effects of a parent-implemented developmental reciprocity treatment program for children with autism spectrum disorder. *Autism, 23*(3), 713–725. https://doi.org/10.1177/1362361318775538

Georgiades, S., Tait, P. A., McNicholas, P. D., Duku, E., Zwaigenbaum, L., Smith, I. M., Bennett, T., Elsabbagh, M., Kerns, C. M., Mirenda, P., Ungar, W. J., Vaillancourt, T., Volden, J., Waddell, C., Zaidman-Zait, A., Gentles, S., & Szatmari, P. (2021). Trajectories of symptom severity in children with autism: Variability and turning points through the transition to school. *Journal of Autism and Developmental Disorders, 52*, 392–401. https://doi.org/10.1007/s10803-021-04949-2

Gilmore, R., Ziviani, J., Chatfield, M. D., Goodman, S., & Sakzewski, L. (2022). Social skills group training in adolescents with disabilities: A systematic review. *Research in Developmental Disabilities, 125*, Article 104218. https://doi.org/10.1016/j.ridd.2022.104218

Goh, H. S. E., Roslan, S., Baguri, E. M., Ong, S. Y., & Li, S. Y. (2020). The effects of children's friendship training on social skills and quality of play among children with autism spectrum disorder. *International Journal of Learning, Teaching and Educational Research*, *19*(7), 225–245. http://www.ijlter.net/index.php/ijlter/article/view/295

Goldstein, H., Lackey, K. C., & Schneider, N. J. (2014). A new framework for systematic reviews: Application to social skills interventions for preschoolers with autism. *Exceptional Children, 80*(3), 262–286. https://doi.org/10.1177/0014402914522423

Gotham, K., Bishop, S. L., Hus, V., Huerta, M., Lund, S., Buja, A., Krieger, A., & Lord, C. (2013). Exploring the relationship between anxiety and insistence on sameness in autism spectrum disorders. *Autism Research, 6*(1), 33–41. https://doi.org/10.1002/aur.1263

Granger, S., des Riviéres-Pigeon, C., Sabourin, G., & Forget, J. (2012). Mothers' reports of their involvement in early intensive behavioral intervention. *Topics in Early Special Education, 32*(2), 68–77. https://doi.org/10.1177/0271121410393285

Greenlee, J. L., Stelter, C. R., Piro-Gambetti, B., & Hartley, S. L. (2021). Trajectories of dysregulation in children with autism spectrum disorder. *Journal of Clinical Child and Adolescent Psychology, 50*(6), 858–873. https://doi.org/10.1080/15374416.2021.1907752

Gresham, F. M., & Elliott, S. N. (2008). *Social skills improvement system: Rating scales*. Pearson Assessments.

Gresham, F. M., Elliott, S. N., Vance, M. J., & Cook, C. R. (2011). Comparability of the social skills rating system to the social skills improvement system: Content and psychometric comparisons across elementary and secondary age levels. *School Psychology Quarterly, 26*(1), 27–44. https://doi.org/10.1037/a0022662

Grindle, C. F., Kovshoff, H., Hastings, R. P., & Remington, B. (2009). Parents' experiences of Applied Behaviour Analysis (ABA)-based interventions for children diagnosed with autistic spectrum disorder. *Journal of Autism and Developmental Disorders, 39*, 42–56. https://doi.org/10.1007/s10803-008-0597-z

Grove, R., Hoekstra, R. A., Wierda, M., & Begeer, S. (2018). Special interests and subjective wellbeing in autistic adults. *Autism Research, 11*(5), 766–775. https://doi.org/10.1002/aur.1931

Grzadzinski, R., Di Martino, A., Brady, E., Mairena, M. A., O'Neale, M., Petkova, E., Lord, C., & Castellanos, F. X. (2011). Examining autistic traits in children with ADHD: Does the autism spectrum extend to ADHD? *Journal of Autism and Developmental Disorders, 41*(9), 1178–1191. https://doi.org/10.1007/s10803-010-1135-3

Gulsrud, A. C., Jahromi, L. B., & Kasari, C. (2010). The co-regulation of emotions between mothers and their children with autism. *Journal of Autism and Developmental Disorders, 40*(2), 227–237. https://doi.org/10.1007/s10803-009-0861-x

Gunning, C., Holloway, J., Fee, B., Breathnach, Ó., Bergin, C. M., Greene, I., & Ní Bheoláin, R. (2019). A systematic review of generalization and maintenance outcomes of social skills intervention for preschool children with autism spectrum disorder. *Review Journal of Autism and Developmental Disorders, 6*(2), 172–199. https://doi.org/10.1007/s40489-019-00162-1

Han, G. T., Tomarken, A. J., & Gotham, K. O. (2019). Social and nonsocial reward moderate relation between autism symptoms and loneliness in adults with ASD, depression, and controls. *Autism Research, 12*(6), 884–896. https://doi.org/10.1002/aur.2088

Happé, F., & Frith, U. (2020). Annual research review: Looking back to look forward-changes in the concept of autism and implications for future research. *Journal of Child Psychology and Psychiatry, 61*(3), 218-232. https://doi.org/10.1111/jcpp.13176

Hartley, S. L., & Schultz, H. M. (2015). Support needs of fathers and mothers of children and adolescents with autism spectrum disorder. *Journal of Autism and Developmental Disorders*, *45*(6), 1636–1648. https://doi.org/10.1007/s10803-014-2318-0

Haskett, M. E., Ahern, L. S., Ward, C. S., & Allaire, J. C. (2006). Factor structure and validity of the parenting stress index-short form. *Journal of Clinical Child & Adolescent Psychology, 35*(2), 302–312. https://doi.org/10.1207/s15374424jccp3502_14

Hastings, R., & Brown, T. (2002). Behavior problems of children with autism, parental self-efficacy, and mental health. *American Journal on Mental Retardation, 107*(3), 222–232. https://doi.org/10.1007/s10803-018-3605-y

Hawkins, N. G., Sanson-Fisher, R. W., Shakeshaft, A., D'Este, C., & Green, L. W. (2007). The multiple baseline design for evaluating population-based research. *American Journal of Preventive Medicine, 33*(2), 162–168. https://doi.org/10.1016/j.amepre.2007.03.020

Hayes, S. A., & Watson, S. L. (2013). The impact of parenting stress: A meta-analysis of studies comparing the experience of parenting stress in parents of children with and without autism spectrum disorder. *Journal of Autism and Developmental Disorders, 43*(3), 629–642. https://doi.org/10.1007/s10803-012-1604-y

Higgins, D. J., Bailey, S. R., & Pearce, J. C. (2005). Factors associated with functioning style and coping strategies of families with a child with an autism spectrum disorder. *Autism, 9*(2), 125–137. https://doi.org/10.1177/1362361305051403

Hill, T. L., Gray, S. A. O., Baker, C. N., Boggs, K., Carey, E., Johnson, C., Kamps, J. L., & Varela, E. R. (2017). A pilot study examining the effectiveness of the PEERS® program on social skills and anxiety in adolescents with autism spectrum disorder. *Journal of Developmental and Physical Disabilities, 29*(5), 797–808. https://doi.org/10.1007/s10882-017-9557-x

Horner, R. H., Carr, E. G., Halle, J., McGee, G., Odom, S., & Wolery, M. (2005). The use of single-subject research to identify evidence-based practice in special education. *Exceptional Children, 71*(2), 165–179. https://doi.org/10.1177/001440290507100203

Hollocks, M. J., Charman, T., Baird, G., Lord, C., Pickles, A., & Simonoff, E. (2021). Exploring the impact of adolescent cognitive inflexibility on emotional and behavioural problems experienced by autistic adults. *Autism, 26*(5) 1229–1241. https://doi.org/10.1177/13623613211046160

Huang, C.-Y., Yen, H.-C., Tseng, M.-H., Tung, L.-C., Chen, Y.- D., & Chen, K.-L. (2014). Impacts of autistic behaviors, emotional and behavioral problems on parenting stress in caregivers of children with autism. *Journal of Autism and Developmental Disorders*, *44*(6), 1383–1390. https://doi.org/10.1007/s10803-013-2000-y

Hutchison, L., Feder, M., Abar, B., & Winsler, A. (2016). Relations between parenting stress, parenting style, and child executive functioning for children with ADHD or autism. *Journal of Child and Family Studies, 25*(12), 3644–3656. https://doi.org/10.1007/s10826-016-0518-2

Kallio, H., Pietilä, A.-M., Johnson, M., & Kangasniemi, M. (2016). Systematic methodological review: Developing a framework for a qualitative semi-structured interview guide. *Journal of Advanced Nursing*, *72*(12), 2954–2965. https://doi.org/10.1111/jan.13031

Iadarola, S., Levato, L., Harrison, B., Smith, T., Lecavalier, L., Johnson, C., & Scahill, L. (2018). Teaching parents behavioral strategies for Autism Spectrum Disorder (ASD): Effects on stress, strain, and competence. *Journal of Autism and Developmental Disorders, 48*(4), 1031–1040. https://doi.org/10.1007/s10803-017-3339-2

Iadarola, S., Shih, W., Dean, M., Blanch, E., Harwood, R., Hetherington, S., Mandell, D., Kasari, C., & Smith, T. (2018). Implementing a manualized, classroom transition intervention for students with ASD in under resourced schools. *Behavior Modification, 42*(1), 126–147. https://doi.org/10.1177/0145445517711437

Ichikawa, K., Takahashi, Y., Ando, M., Anme, T., Ishizaki, T., Yamaguchi, H., & Nakayama, T. (2013). TEACCH-based group social skills training for children with high-functioning autism: A pilot randomized controlled trial. *BioPsychoSocial Medicine, 7*, Article 14. https://doi.org/10.1186/1751-0759-7-14

Ingersoll, B., & Gergans, S. (2007). The effect of a parent-implemented imitation intervention on spontaneous imitation skills in young children with autism. *Research in Developmental Disabilities, 28*(2), 163–175. https://doi.org/10.1016/j.ridd.2006.02.004

Ingersoll, B., & Hambrick, D. Z. (2011). The relationship between the broader autism phenotype, child severity, and stress and depression in parents of children with autism spectrum disorders. *Research in Autism Spectrum Disorders, 5*(1), 337–344. https://doi.org/10.1016/j.rasd.2010.04.017

Institute of Education Sciences. (2017). *What works clearinghouse: Procedures handbook, version 4.0.* https://ies.ed.gov/ncee/WWC/Docs/referenceresources/wwc_procedures_handbook_v4.df

Jacobson, N. S., & Truax, P. (1991). Clinical significance: A statistical approach to defining meaningful change in psychotherapy research. *Journal of Consulting and Clinical Psychology, 59*(1), 12–19. https://doi.org/10.1037/0022-006X.59.1.12

Jensen, S. A., & Corralejo, S. M. (2017). Measurement issues: Large effect sizes do not mean most people get better – clinical significance and the importance of individual results. *Child and Adolescent Mental Health, 22*(3), 163–166. https://doi.org/10.1111/camh.12203

Jenson, W. R., Bowen, J., Clark, E., Block, H., Gabrielsen, T., Hood, J., & Springer, B. (2011). *The superheroes social skills program*. Pacific Northwest.

Johnston, C., & Mash, E. J. (1989). A measure of parenting satisfaction and efficacy. *Journal of Clinical Child Psychology, 18*(2), 167–175. https://doi.org/10.1207/s15374424jccp1802_8

Jones, D. R., Morrison, K. E., DeBrabander, K. M., Ackerman, R. A., Pinkham, A. E., & Sasson, N. J. (2021). Greater social interest between autistic and non-autistic conversation partners following autism acceptance training for non-autistic people. *Frontiers in Psychology, 12,* Article 739147. https://doi.org/10.3389/fpsyg.2021.739147

Jones, T. L., & Prinz, R. J. (2005). Potential roles of parental self-efficacy in parent and child adjustment: A review. *Clinical Psychology Review, 25*(3), 341–363. https://doi.org/10.1016/j.cpr.2004.12.004

Kaat, A. J., & Lecavalier, L. (2014). Group-based social skills treatment: A methodological review. *Research in Autism Spectrum Disorders, 8*(1), 15–24. https://doi.org/10.1016/j.rasd.2013.10.007

Kapp, S. K., Steward, R., Crane, L., Elliott, D., Elphick, C., Pellicano, E., & Russell, G. (2019). "People should be allowed to do what they like": Autistic adults' views and experiences of stimming. *Autism, 23*(7), 1782–1792. https://doi.org/10.1177/1362361319 829628

Karst, J. S., & Van Hecke, A. V. (2012). Parent and family impact of autism spectrum disorders: A review and proposed model for intervention evaluation. *Clinical Child and Family Psychology Review, 15*(3), 247–277. https://doi.org/10.1007/s10567-012-0119-6

Karst, J. S., Van Hecke, A. V., Carson, A. M., Stevens, S., Schohl, K., & Dolan, B. (2015). Parent and family outcomes of PEERS®: A social skills intervention for adolescents with autism spectrum disorder. *Journal of Autism and Developmental Disorders, 45*(3), 752–765. https://doi.org/10.1007/s10803-014-2231-6

Kasari, C., Locke, J., Gulsrud, A., & Rotheram-Fuller, E. (2011). Social networks and friendships at school: Comparing children with and without ASD. *Journal of Autism and Developmental Disorders, 41*(5), 533–544. https://doi.org/10.1007/s10803-010-1076-x

Kasari, C., & Sterling, L. (2013). Loneliness and social isolation in children with autism spectrum disorders. In R. J. Coplan & J. C. Bowker (Eds.), *The handbook of solitude* (pp. 409–426). John Wiley. https://doi.org/10.1002/9781118427378.ch23

Kaufman, A. S., & Kaufman, N. L. (2004). *Kaufman brief intelligence test*. John Wiley & Sons.

Kazdin, A. E. (1997). Parent management training: Evidence, outcomes, and issues. *Journal of the American Academy of Child & Adolescent Psychiatry, 36*(10), 1349–1356. https://doi.org/10.1097/00004583-199710000-00016

Kazdin, A. E. (1998). *Research design in clinical psychology* (3rd ed.). Allyn & Bacon.

Kelly, A. B., Garnett, M. S., Attwood, T., & Peterson, C. (2008). Autism spectrum symptomatology in children: The impact of family and peer relationships. *Journal of Abnormal Child Psychology, 36*(7), 1069–1081. https://doi.org/10.1007/s10802-008-9234-8

Kenny, L., Hattersley, C., Molins, B., Buckley, C., Povey, C., & Pellicano, E. (2016). Which terms should be used to describe autism? Perspectives from the UK autism community. *Autism, 20*(4), 442–462. https://doi.org/10.1177/1362361315588200

Kenworthy, L., Black, D. O., Harrison, B., della Rosa, A., & Wallace, G. L. (2009). Are executive control functions related to autism symptoms in high-functioning children? *Child Neuropsychology, 15*(5), 425–440. https://doi.org/10.1080/09297040802646983

Kiami, S. R., & Goodgold, S. (2017). Support needs and coping strategies as predictors of stress level among mothers of children with autism spectrum disorder. *Autism Research and Treatment*, Article e8685950. https://doi.org/10.1155/2017/8685950

Klinger, L. G., Cook, M. L., & Dudley, K. M. (2020). Predictors and moderators of treatment efficacy in children and adolescents with autism spectrum disorder. *Journal of Clinical Child and Adolescent Psychology, 50*(4), 517–524. https://doi.org/10.1080/15374416.2020.1833735

Klinger, L. G., Ence, W., & Meyer, A. (2013). Caregiver-mediated approaches to managing challenging behaviors in children with autism spectrum disorder. *Dialogues in Clinical Neuroscience, 15*(2), 225–233. https://doi.org/10.31887/DCNS.2013.15.2/lklinger

Koegel, L. K., Vernon, T. W., Koegel, R. L., Koegel, B. L., & Paullin, A. W. (2012). Improving social engagement and initiations between children with autism spectrum disorder and their peers in inclusive settings. *Journal of Positive Behavior Interventions, 14*(4), 220–227. https://doi.org/10.1177/1098300712437042

Koegel, R. L., Werner, G. A., Vismara, L. A., & Koegel, L. K. (2005). The effectiveness of contextually supported play date interactions between children with autism and typically developing peers. *Research and Practice for Persons with Severe Disabilities, 30*(2), 93–102. https://doi.org/10.2511/rpsd.30.2.93

Krasny, L., Williams, B. J., Provencal, S., & Ozonoff, S. (2003). Social skills interventions for the autism spectrum: Essential ingredients and a model curriculum. *Child and Adolescent Psychiatric Clinics of North America, 12*(1), 107–122. https://doi.org/10.1016/s1056-4993(02)00051-2

Kratochwill, T. R., & Levin, J. R. (2014). Enhancing the scientific credibility of single-case intervention research: Randomization to the rescue. In T. R. Kratochwill & J. R. Levin (Eds.), *Single-case intervention research: Methodological and statistical advances* (pp. 53–89). American Psychological Association. https://doi.org/10.1037/14376-003

Kroeger, K. A., Schultz, J. R., & Newsom, C. (2007). A comparison of two-group delivered social skills programs for young children with autism. *Journal of Autism and Developmental Disorders, 37*(5), 808–817. https://doi.org/10.1007/s10803-006-0207-x

Kuhn, J., Hickey, E., Lindly, O., Stransky, M., Masaro, M., Patts, G. J., Cabral, H., Crossman, M., Augustyn, M., Feinberg, E., & Broder-Fingert, S. (2023). Parenting stress, child social functioning, and part C early intervention in predominantly low-income families of children with or at high risk for developmental delay from minoritized racial and ethnic groups. *Journal of Early Intervention*, *45*(4), 467–487. https://doi.org/10.1177/10538151231155406

Ladd, G. W., & Hart, C. H. (1992). Creating informal play opportunities: Are parents' and preschoolers' initiations related to children's competence with peers? *Developmental Psychology, 28*(6), 1179–1187. https://doi.org/10.1037/0012-1649.28.6.1179

Lam, S. F., Wong, B. P., Leung, D., Ho, D., & Au-Yeung, P. (2010). How parents perceive and feel about participation in community activities: The comparison between parents of preschoolers with and without autism spectrum disorders. *Autism, 14*(4), 359–377. https://doi.org/10.1177/1362361309346558

Laugeson, E. A. (2017). *PEERS® for young adults social skills training for adults with autism spectrum disorder and other social challenges.* Routledge. https://doi.org/10.4324/9781315297057

Laugeson, E. A., & Frankel, F. (2010). *Social skills for teenagers with developmental and autism spectrum disorder: The PEERS® treatment manual.* Routledge. https://doi.org/10.4324/9780203867686

Laugeson, E. A., Frankel, F., Gantman, A., Dillon, A. R., & Mogil, C. (2012). Evidence-based social skills training for adolescents with autism spectrum disorders: The UCLA PEERS® program. *Journal of Autism and Developmental Disorders, 42*(6), 1025–1036. https://doi.org/10.1007/s10803-011-1339-1

Laugeson, E. A., Frankel, F., Mogil, C., & Dillon, A. R. (2009). Parent-assisted social skills training to improve friendships in teens with autism spectrum disorders. *Journal of Autism and Developmental Disorders, 39*(4), 596–606. https://doi.org/10.1007/s10803-008-0664-5

Laugeson, E. A., Gantman, A., Kapp, S. K., Orenski, K., & Ellingsen, R. (2015). A randomized controlled trial to improve social skills in young adults with autism spectrum disorder: The UCLA PEERS® program. *Journal of Autism and Developmental Disorders, 45*(12), 3978–3989. https://doi.org/10.1007/s10803-015-2504-8

Laugeson, E. A., & Park, M. N. (2014). Using a CBT approach to teach social skills to adolescents with autism spectrum disorder and other social challenges: The PEERS® method. *Journal of Rational-Emotive & Cognitive-Behavior Therapy, 32*(1), 84–97. https://doi.org/10.1007/s10942-014-0181-8

Laugeson, E. A., Park, M. N., Bolton, C., Bolourian, Y., & Sanderson, J. (2016) *A randomized controlled trial of a parent-assisted social skills treatment: The UCLA PEERS® for Preschoolers Program* [Poster presentation]. International Meeting for Autism Research, Baltimore, MD.

Laushey, K. M., & Heflin, L. J. (2000). Enhancing social skills of kindergarten children with autism through the training of multiple peers as tutors. *Journal of Autism and Developmental Disorders, 30*(3), 183–193. https://doi.org/10.1023/A:1005558101038

Leaf, J. B., Leaf, J. A., Milne, C., Taubman, M., Oppenheim-Leaf, M., Torres, N., Townley-Cochran, D., Leaf, R., McEachin, J., & Yoder, P. (2017). An evaluation of a behaviorally based social skills group for individuals diagnosed with autism spectrum disorder. *Journal of Autism and Developmental Disorders, 47*(2), 243–259. https://doi.org/10.1007/s10803-016-2949-4

Lee, S., Odom, S. L., & Loftin, R. (2007). Social engagement with peers and stereotypic behavior of children with autism. *Journal of Positive Behavior Interventions, 9*(2), 67–79. https://doi.org/10.1177/10983007070090020401

Lee, S. J., Gopalan, G., & Harrington, D. (2016). Validation of the parenting stress index–short form with minority caregivers. *Research on Social Work Practice*, *26*(4), 429–440. https://doi.org/10.1177/1049731514554854

Locke, J., Kasari, C., Rotheram-Fuller, E., Kretzmann, M., & Jacobs, J. (2013). Social network changes over the school year among elementary school-aged children with and without an autism spectrum disorder. *School Mental Health*, *5*(1), 38–47. https://doi.org/10.1007/s12310-012-9092-y

Loftin, R. L., Odom, S. L., & Lantz, J. F. (2008). Social interaction and repetitive motor behaviors. *Journal of Autism and Developmental Disorders, 38*(6), 1124–1135. https://doi.org/10.1007/s10803-007-0499-5

Lord, C., & Bishop, S. L. (2010). Autism spectrum disorders: Diagnosis, prevalence, and services for children and families. Social policy report. *Society for Research in Child Development, 24*(2), 1–27.

Lord, C., & MaGill-Evans, J. (1995). Peer interactions of autistic children and adolescents. *Development and Psychopathology, 7*(4), 611–626. https://doi.org/10.1017/S095457940000674X

Lord, C., Rutter, M., DiLavore, P. C., Risi, S., Gotham, K., & Bishop, S. (2012). *Autism diagnostic observation schedule* (2nd ed.). Western Psychological Services. https://doi.org/10.1037/t54175-000

Lord, C., Wagner, A., Rogers, S., Szatmari, P., Aman, M., Charman, T., Dawson, G., Durand, V. M., Grossman, L., Guthrie, D., Harris, S., Kasari, C., Marcus, L., Murphy, S., Odom, S., Pickles, A., Scahill, L., Shaw, E., Siegel, B., & Yoder, P. (2005). Challenges in evaluating psychosocial interventions for autistic spectrum disorders. *Journal of Autism and Developmental Disorders, 35*(6), 695–708. https://doi.org/10.1007/s10803-005-0017-6

Lordo, D. N., Bertolin, M., Sudikoff, E. L., Keith, C., Braddock, B., & Kaufman, D. A. (2017). Parents perceive improvements in socio-emotional functioning in adolescents with ASD following social skills treatment. *Journal of Autism and Developmental Disorders, 47*(1), 203–214. https://doi.org/10.1007/s10803-016-2969-0

Maag, J. W. (2006). Social skills training for students with emotional and behavioral disorders: A review of reviews. *Behavioral Disorders, 32*(1), 4–17. https://doi.org/10.1177/019874290603200104

Mace, F. C., & Nevin, J. A. (2017). Maintenance, generalization, and treatment relapse: A behavioral momentum analysis. *Education and Treatment of Children, 40*(1), 27–42. https://doi.org/10.1353/etc.2017.0001

Maenner, M. J., Shaw, K. A., & Baio, J. (2020). Prevalence of autism spectrum disorder among children aged 8 years-Autism and developmental disabilities monitoring network, 11 sites, United States, 2016. *MMWR Surveillance Summaries, 69*(4), 1–12. https://doi.org/10.15585/mmwr.ss6904a1

Mahoney, G., Powell, A., & Finger, I. (1986). The maternal behavior rating scale. *Topics in Early Childhood Special Education, 6*(2), 44–56. https://doi.org/10.1177/027112148600600205

Mahoney, G., Wiggers, B., & Lash, S. (1996). Using a relationship focused intervention program to enhance father involvement. *Infant-Toddler Intervention, 6*(4), 295-308.

Mandelberg, J., Laugeson, E. A., Cunningham, T. D., Ellingsen, R., Bates, S., & Frankel, F. (2014). Long-term treatment outcomes for parent-assisted social skills training for adolescents with autism spectrum disorders: The UCLA PEERS® program. *Journal of Mental Health Research in Intellectual Disabilities, 7*(1), 45–73. https://doi.org/10.1080/19315864.2012.730600

Marro, B. M., Kang, E., Hauschild, K. M., Normansell, K. M., Abu-Ramadan, T. M., & Lerner, M. D. (2019). Social performance–based interventions promote gains in social knowledge in the absence of explicit training for youth with autism spectrum disorder. *Bulletin of the Menninger Clinic, 83*(3), 301–325. https://doi.org/10.1521/bumc.2019.83.3.301

Marsack, C. N., & Samuel, P. S. (2017). Mediating effects of social support on quality of life for parents of adults with autism. *Journal of Autism and Developmental Disorders, 47*, 2378–2389. https://doi.org/10.1007/s10803-017-3157-6

Matheny, A. P., Wachs, T. D., Ludwig, J. L., & Phillips, K. (1995). Bringing order out of chaos: Psychometric characteristics of the confusion, hubbub, and order scale. *Journal of Applied Developmental Psychology, 16*(3), 429–444. https://doi.org/10.1016/0193-3973(95)90028-4

Matson, J. L., Matson, M. L., & Rivet, T. T. (2007). Social-skills treatments for children with autism spectrum disorders: An overview. *Behavior Modification, 31*(5), 682–707. https://doi.org/10.1177/0145445507301650

Maxwell, C. R., Parish-Morris, J., Hsin, O., Bush, J. C., & Schultz, R. T. (2013). The broad autism phenotype predicts child functioning in autism spectrum disorders. *Journal of Neurodevelopmental Disorders, 5*, 5–25. https://doi.org/10.1186/1866-1955-5-25

Mazefsky, C. A., Pelphrey, K. A., & Dahl, R. E. (2012). The need for a broader approach to emotion regulation research in autism. *Child Development Perspectives, 6*(1), 92–97. https://doi.org/10.1111/j.1750-8606.2011.00229.x

Mazurek, M. O., & Kanne, S. M. (2010). Friendship and internalizing symptoms among children and adolescents with ASD. *Journal of Autism and Developmental Disorders, 40*, 1512–1520. https://doi.org/10.1007/s10803-010-1014-y

McConachie, H., & Diggle, T. (2007). Parent implemented early intervention for young children with autism spectrum disorder: A systematic review. *Journal of Evaluation in Clinical Practice, 13*(1), 120–129. https://doi.org/10.1111/j.1365-2753.2006.00674.x

McConachie, H., Wilson, C., Mason, D., Garland, D., Parr, J. R., Rattazzi, A., Rodgers, J., Skevington, S., Uljarevic, M., & Magiati, I. (2020). What is important in measuring quality of life? Reflections by autistic adults in four countries. *Autism in Adulthood, 2*(1), 4–12. https://doi.org/10.1089/aut.2019.0008

McConnell, S. R. (2002). Interventions to facilitate social interaction for young children with autism: Review of available research and recommendations for educational intervention and future research. *Journal of Autism and Developmental Disorders, 32*(5), 351–372. https://doi.org/10.1023/A:1020537805154

McCrimmon, A., & Rostad, K. (2014). Test review: Autism Diagnostic Observation Schedule (ADOS-2) manual (Part II): Toddler module. *Journal of Psychoeducational Assessment, 32*(1), 88–92. https://doi.org/10.1177/0734282913490916

McVey, A. J., Dolan, B. K., Willar, K. S., Pleiss, S., Karst, J. S., Casnar, C. L., Caiozzo, C., Vogt, E. M., Gordon, N. S., & Van Hecke, A. V. (2016). A replication and extension of the PEERS® for young adults social skills intervention: Examining effects on social skills and social anxiety in young adults with autism spectrum disorder. *Journal of Autism and Developmental Disorders, 46*(12), 3739–3754. https://doi.org/10.1007/s10803-016-2911-5

McVey, A. J., Schiltz, H., Haendel, A., Dolan, B. K., Willar, K. S., Pleiss, S., Karst, J. S., Carson, A. M., Caiozzo, C., Vogt, E., & Van Hecke, A. V. (2017). Brief report: Does gender matter in intervention for ASD? Examining the impact of the PEERS® social skills intervention on social behavior among females with ASD. *Journal of Autism and Developmental Disorders, 47*(7), 2282–2289. https://doi.org/10.1007/s10803-017-3121-5

Meirsschaut, M., Roeyers, H., & Warreyn, P. (2010). Parenting in families with a child with autism spectrum disorder and a typically developing child: Mothers' experiences and cognitions. *Research in Autism Spectrum Disorders, 4*(4), 661–669. https://doi.org/10.1016/j.rasd.2010.01.002

Messinger, D. S., Fogel, A., & Dickson, K. L. (2001). All smiles are positive, but some smiles are more positive than others. *Developmental Psychology, 37*(5), 642–653. https://doi.org/10.1037/0012-1649.37.5.642

Michelson, D., Davenport, C., Dretzke, J., Barlow, J., & Day, C. (2013). Do evidence-based interventions work when tested in the "real world?" A systematic review and meta-analysis of parent management training for the treatment of child disruptive behavior. *Clinical Child and Family Psychology Review, 16*(1), 18–34. https://doi.org/10.1007/s10567-013-0128-0

Midouhas, E., Yogaratnam, A., Flouri, E., & Charman, T. (2013). Psychopathology trajectories of children with autism spectrum disorder: The role of family poverty and parenting. *Journal of the American Academy of Child and Adolescent Psychiatry, 52*(10), 1057–1065. https://doi.org/10.1016/j.jaac.2013.07.011

Milton, D. E. (2012). On the ontological status of autism: The "double empathy problem." *Disability & Society, 27*(6), 883–887. https://doi.org/10.1080/09687599.2012.710008

Minuchin, P. (1985). Families and individual development: Provocations from the field of family therapy. *Child Development, 56*(2), 289–302. https://doi.org/10.2307/1129720

Moody, C. T., & Laugeson, E. A. (2020). Social skills training in autism spectrum disorder across the lifespan. *Child and Adolescent Psychiatric Clinics, 29*(2), 359–371. https://doi.org/10.1016/j.psc.2020.08.006

Moody, C. T., Schiltz, H. K., Ratto, A. B., Gulsrud, A. C., & Laugeson, E. A. (2022). Measurement of social skills treatment outcome in autism: Moving beyond informant report and considering diversity. *International Review of Research in Developmental Disabilities*, *62*, 265–312. https://doi.org/10.1016/bs.irrdd.2022.05.007

Morgan, D. L., & Morgan, R. K. (2008). *Single-case research methods for the behavioral and health sciences*. Sage Publications.

Morse, J. M. (2015). Critical analysis of strategies for determining rigor in qualitative inquiry. *Qualitative Health Research*, *25*(9), 1212–1222. https://doi.org/10.1177/1049732315588501

Mugno, D., Ruta, L., D'Arrigo, V. G., & Mazzone, L. (2007). Impairment of quality of life in parents of children and adolescents with pervasive developmental disorder. *Health and Quality of Life Outcomes, 5*, 1–9. https://doi.org/10.1186/1477-7525-5-22

Mundy, P. (2016). *Autism and joint attention: Developmental, neuroscience, and clinical fundamentals.* Guilford.

Murdock, L. C., Ganz, J., & Crittendon, J. (2013). Use of an iPad play story to increase play dialogue of preschoolers with autism spectrum disorders. *Journal of Autism and Developmental Disorders, 43*(9), 2174–2189. https://doi.org/10.1007/s10803-013-1770-6

Muskett, A., Capriola-Hall, N. N., Radtke, S. R., Factor, R., & Scarpa, A. (2019). Repetitive behaviors in autism spectrum disorder: Associations with depression and anxiety symptoms. *Research in Autism Spectrum Disorders, 68*, Article 101449. https://doi.org/10.1016/j.rasd.2019.101449

Neece, C. L., Green, S. A., & Baker, B. L. (2012). Parenting stress and child behavior problems: A transactional relationship across time. *American Journal on Intellectual and Developmental Disabilities, 117*(1), 48–66. https://doi.org/10.1352/1944-7558-117.1.48

Nelson, C. A., Zeanah, C. H., & Fox, N. A. (2019). How early experience shapes human development: The case of psychosocial deprivation. *Neural Plasticity,* Article 1676285. https://doi.org/10.1155/2019/1676285

Neuhaus, E., Webb, S. J., & Bernier, R. A. (2019). Linking social motivation with social skill: The role of emotion dysregulation in autism spectrum disorder. *Development and Psychopathology, 31*(3), 931–943. https://doi.org/10.1017/S0954579419000361

Nikopoulos, C. K., & Keenan, M. (2007). Using video modeling to teach complex social sequences to children with autism. *Journal of Autism and Developmental Disorders, 37*(4), 678–693. https://doi.org/10.1007/s10803-006-0195-x

Nuske, H. J., Finkel, E., Hedley, D., Parma, V., Tomczuk, L., Pellecchia, M., Herrington, J., Marcus, S. C., Mandell, D. S., & Dissanayake, C. (2019). Heart rate increase predicts challenging behavior episodes in preschoolers with autism. *Stress, 22*(3), 303–311. https://doi.org/10.1080/10253890.2019.1572744

Nuske, H. J., Shih, W. I., Sparapani, N., Baczewski, L., Dimachkie Nunnally, A., Hochheimer, S., Garcia, C., Castellon, F., Levato, L., Fischer, E., Atkinson-Diaz, Z. L., Li, J., Mandell, D. S., & Kasari, C. (2021). Self-regulation predicts companionship in children with autism. *International Journal of Developmental Disabilities, 68*(6), 889–899. https://doi.org/10.1080/20473869.2021.1917109

Oakley, B. F., Tillmann, J., Ahmad, J., Crawley, D., San José Cáceres, A., Holt, R., Charman, T., Banaschewski, T., Buitelaar, J., Simonoff, E., Murphy, D., & Loth, E. (2020). How do core autism traits and associated symptoms relate to quality of life? Findings from the longitudinal European autism project. *Autism, 25*(2), 389–404. https://doi.org/10.1177/1362361320959959

Ong, S. Y., Roslan, S., Ahmad, N. A., Ayub, A. F. M., Ping, C. L., Zaremohzzabieh, Z., & Ahrari, S. (2021). A mixed-methods evaluation of parent-assisted children's friendship training to improve social skills and friendship quality in children with autism in Malaysia. *International Journal of Environmental Research and Public Health, 18*(5), Article 2566. https://doi.org/10.3390/ijerph18052566

Osborne, L. A., McHugh, L., Saunders, J., & Reed, P. (2008). The effect of parenting behaviors on subsequent child behavior problems in autistic spectrum conditions. *Research in Autism Spectrum Disorders, 2*(2), 249–263. https://doi.org/10.1016/j.rasd.2007.06.004

Pacia, C., Holloway, J., Gunning, C., & Lee, H. (2022). A systematic review of family-mediated social communication interventions for young children with autism. *Review Journal of Autism and Developmental Disorders, 9*(2), 208–234. https://doi.org/10.1007/s40489-021-00249-8

Park, M. N., Moulton, E., & Laugeson, E. A. (2022). Parent-assisted social skills training for children with autism spectrum disorder: PEERS® for Preschoolers. *Focus on Autism and Other Developmental Disabilities, 38*(2), 80–89. https://doi.org/10.1177/10883576221110l

Paul, R. (2003). Promoting social communication in high functioning individuals with autistic spectrum disorders. *Child and Adolescent Psychiatric Clinics of North America, 12*(1), 87–106. https://doi.org/10.1016/S1056-4993(02)00047-0

Pickles, A., Le Couteur, A., Leadbitter, K., Salomone, E., Cole-Fletcher, R., Tobin, H., Gammer, I., Lowry, J., Vamvakas, G., Byford, S., Aldred, C., Slonims, V., McConachie, H., Howlin, P., Parr, J. R., Charman, T., & Green, J. (2016). Parent-mediated social communication therapy for young children with autism (PACT): Long-term follow-up of a randomised controlled trial. *The Lancet, 388*(10059), 2501–2509. https://doi.org/10.1016/S0140-6736(16)31229-6

Prinzie, P., Onghena, P., & Helinckx, W. (2007). Reexamining the parenting scale: Reliability, factor structure, and concurrent validity of a scale for assessing the discipline practices of mothers and fathers of elementary-school-aged children. *European Journal of Psychological Assessment, 23*(1), 24–31. https://doi.org/10.1027/1015-5759.23.1.24

Radley, K. C., Ford, W. B., McHugh, M. B., Dadakhodjaeva, K., O'Handley, R. D., Battaglia, A. A., & Lum, J. D. K. (2015). Brief report: Use of superheroes social skills to promote accurate social skill use in children with autism spectrum disorder. *Journal of Autism and Developmental Disorders, 45*(9), 3048–3054. https://doi.org/10.1007/s10803-015-2442-5

Rao, P. A., & Beidel, D. C. (2009). The impact of children with high functioning autism on parental stress, sibling adjustment, and family functioning. *Behavior Modification, 33*(4), 437–451. https://doi.org/10.1177/0145445509336427

Rao, P. A., Beidel, D. C., & Murray, M. J. (2008). Social skills interventions for children with asperger's syndrome or high-functioning autism: A review and recommendations. *Journal of Autism and Developmental Disorders*, *38*(2), 353–361. https://doi.org/10.1007/s10803-007-0402-4

Raulston, T. J., Hansen, S. G., Frantz, R., Machalicek, W., & Bhana, N. (2019). A parent-implemented playdate intervention for young children with autism and their peers. *Journal of Early Intervention, 42*(4), 303–320. https://doi.org/10.1177/1053815119880943

Ray-Subramanian, C. E., & Ellis Weismer, S. (2012). Receptive and expressive language as predictors of restricted and repetitive behaviors in young children with autism spectrum disorders. *Journal of Autism and Developmental Disorders, 42*(10), 2113–2120. https://doi.org/10.1007/s10803-012-1463-6

Rea, H. M., Factor, R. S., Swain, D. M., & Scarpa, A. (2019). The association of the broader autism phenotype with emotion-related behaviors in mothers of children with and without autism spectrum traits. *Journal of Autism and Developmental Disorders, 49*(3), 950–959. https://doi.org/10.1007/s10803-018-3785-5

Reichow, B., Steiner, A. M., & Volkmar, F. (2012). Social skills groups for people aged 6 to 21 with Autism Spectrum Disorders (ASD). *The Cochrane Database of Systematic Reviews*. https://doi.org/10.1002/14651858

Reichow B., & Volkmar F. R. (2010). Social skills interventions for individuals with autism: Evaluation for evidence-based practices within a best evidence synthesis framework. *Journal of Autism and Developmental Disorders*, *40*(2), 149–166. https://doi.org/10.1007/s10803-009-0842-0

Reinke, J. S., & Solheim, C. A. (2015). Online social support experiences of mothers of children with autism spectrum disorder. *Journal of Child and Family Studies*, *24*, 2364–2373. https://doi.org/10.1007/s10826-014-0039-9

Roberts, D., & Pickering, N. (2010). Parent training programme for autism spectrum disorders: An evaluation. *Community Practitioner, 83*(10), 27–30.

Rodriguez, G., Drastal, K., & Hartley, S. L. (2020). Cross-lagged model of bullying victimization and mental health problems in children with autism in middle to older childhood. *Autism, 25*(1), 90–101. https://doi.org/10.1177/1362361320947513

Rogers, S. J. (2000). Interventions that facilitate socialization in children with autism. *Journal of Autism and Developmental Disorders*, *30*(5), 399–409. https://doi.org/10.1023/a:1005543321840

Rogers, S. J., & Dawson, G. (2020). *Early Start Denver Model for young children with autism: Promoting language, learning, and engagement*. Guilford.

Rogers, S. J., Estes, A., Lord, C., Vismara, L., Winter, J., Fitzpatrick, A., Megye, G., & Dawson, G. (2012). Effects of a brief Early Start Denver Model (ESDM)-based parent intervention on toddlers at risk for autism spectrum disorders: A randomized controlled trial. *Journal of the American Academy of Child & Adolescent Psychiatry, 51*(10), 1052–1065. https://doi.org/10.1016/j.jaac.2012.08.003

Rose, V., Paynter, J., Vivanti, G., Keen, D., & Trembath, D. (2020). Predictors of expressive language change for children with autism spectrum disorder receiving AAC-infused comprehensive intervention. *Journal of Autism and Developmental Disorders, 50*(1), 278–291. https://doi.org/10.1007/s10803-019-04251-2

Rotheram-Fuller, E., Kasari, C., Chamberlain, B., & Locke, J. (2010). Social involvement of children with autism spectrum disorders in elementary school classrooms. *Journal of Child Psychology and Psychiatry, 51*(11), 1227–1234. https://doi.org/10.1111/j.1469-7610.2010.02289.x

Ruble, L., McDuffie, A., King, A. S., & Lorenz, D. (2008). Caregiver responsiveness and social interaction behaviors of young children with autism. *Topics in Early Childhood Special Education, 28*(3), 158–170. https://doi.org/10.1177/0271121408323009

Russell, K. M., Frost, K. M., & Ingersoll, B. (2019). The relationship between subtypes of repetitive behaviors and anxiety in children with autism spectrum disorder. *Research in Autism Spectrum Disorders, 62*, 48–54. https://doi.org/10.1016/j.rasd.2019.03.006

Russell, G., Kapp, S. K., Elliott, D., Elphick, C., Gwernan-Jones, R., & Owens, C. (2019). Mapping the autistic advantage from the accounts of adults diagnosed with autism: A qualitative study. *Autism in Adulthood, 1*(2), 124–133. https://doi.org/10.1089/aut.2018.0035

Samson, A. C., Phillips, J. M., Parker, K. J., Shah, S., Gross, J. J., & Hardan, A. Y. (2014). Emotion dysregulation and the core features of autism spectrum disorder. *Journal of Autism and Developmental Disorders, 44*(7), 1766–1772. https://doi.org/10.1007/s10803-013-2022-5

Sasson, N. J., & Touchstone, E. W. (2014). Visual attention to competing social and object images by preschool children with autism spectrum disorder. *Journal of Autism and Developmental Disorders, 44*(3), 584–592. https://doi.org/10.1007/s10803-013-1910-z

Scarpa, A., Swain, D. M., Factor, R. S., Dahiya, A. V., & Bertollo, J. R. (2021). Enhancing flexibility: A biosocial model for resilience to adversity in youth with autism. *Sage Open, 11*(3). https://doi.org/10.1177/21582440211037997

Schertz, H. H., & Odom, S. L. (2006). Promoting joint attention in toddlers with autism: A parent-mediated developmental model. *Journal of Autism and Developmental Disorders, 37*(8), 1562–1575. https://doi.org/10.1007/s10803-006-0290-z

Schieve, L. A., Blumberg, S. J., Rice, C., Visser, S. N., & Boyle, C. (2007). The relationship between autism and parenting stress. *Pediatrics, 119*(Supplement 1), S114–S121. https://doi.org/10.1542/peds.2006-2089Q

Schiltz, H. K., McVey, A. J., Dolan, B. K., Willar, K. S., Pleiss, S., Karst, J. S., & Van Hecke, A. V. (2018). Changes in depressive symptoms among adolescents with ASD completing the PEERS® social skills intervention. *Journal of Autism and Developmental Disorders, 48*(3), 834–843. https://doi.org/10.1007/s10803-017-3396-6

Schiltz, H. K., McVey, A. J., Wozniak, D., Haendel, B., Stanley, A. D., Arias, R., Gordon, A., N., & Van Hecke, A. V. (2021). The role of loneliness as a mediator between autism features and mental health among autistic young adults. *Autism, 25*(2), 545–555. https://doi.org/10.1177/1362361320967789

Schohl, K. A., Van Hecke, A. V., Carson, A. M., Dolan, B., Karst, J., & Stevens, S. (2014). A replication and extension of the PEERS® intervention: Examining effects on social skills and social anxiety in adolescents with autism spectrum disorders. *Journal of Autism and Developmental Disorders, 44*(3), 532–545. https://doi.org/10.1007/s10803-013-1900-1

Schreibman, L., Dawson, G., Stahmer, A. C., Landa, R., Rogers, S. J., McGee, G. G., & McNerney, E. (2015). Naturalistic developmental behavioral interventions: Empirically validated treatments for autism spectrum disorder. *Journal of Autism and Developmental Disorders, 45*(8), 2411–2428. https://doi.org/10.1007/s10803-015-2407-8

Shire, S. Y., Shih, W., Chang, Y. C., Bracaglia, S., Kodjoe, M., & Kasari, C. (2019). Sustained community implementation of JASPER intervention with toddlers with autism. *Journal of Autism and Developmental Disorders, 49*(5), 1863–1875. https://doi.org/10.1007/s10803-018-03875-0

Sigman, M., & Ruskin, E., Arbelle, S., Corona, R., Dissanayake, C., Espinosa, M., Kim, N., Lopez, A., Zierhut, C., Mervis, C. B., & Robinson, B. F. (1999). Continuity and change in the social competence in children with autism, down syndrome, and other developmental delays: A longitudinal study. *Monographs of the Society for Research in Child Development, 64*(1), i–139.

Sivberg, B. (2002). Family system and coping behaviors: A comparison between parents of children with autistic spectrum disorders and parents with non-autistic children. *Autism, 6*(4), 397–409. https://doi.org/10.1177/1362361302006004006

Slaughter, A. M., McNeel, M. M., Storch, E. A., & Mire, S. S. (2020). Where should we go from here? Identified gaps in the literature in psychosocial interventions for youth with autism spectrum disorder and comorbid anxiety. *Children's Health Care, 49*(4), 435–471. https://doi.org/10.1080/02739615.2020.1756818

Sofronoff, K., & Farbotko, M. (2002). The effectiveness of parent management training to increase self-efficacy in parents of children with asperger syndrome. *Autism, 6*(3), 271–286. https://doi.org/10.1177/1362361302006003005

Solomon, M., Goodlin-Jones, B. L., & Anders, T. F. (2004). A social adjustment enhancement intervention for high functioning autism, asperger's syndrome, and pervasive developmental disorder NOS. *Journal of Autism and Developmental Disorders, 34*(6), 649–668. https://doi.org/10.1007/s10803-004-5286-y

South, M., Carr, A. W., Stephenson, K. G., Maisel, M. E., & Cox, J. C. (2017). Symptom overlap on the SRS-2 adult self-report between adults with ASD and adults with high anxiety. *Autism Research, 10*(7), 1215–1220. https://doi.org/10.1002/aur.1764

Sparrow, S. S., Cicchetti, D. V., & Balla, D. A. (2005). *Vineland adaptive behavior scales, 2nd ed.: Survey Form*. American Guidance Service.

Stadnick, N. A., Drahota, A., & Brookman-Frazee, L. (2013). Parent perspectives of an evidence-based intervention for children with autism served in community mental health clinics. *Journal of Child and Family Studies*, *22*(3), 414–422. https://doi.org/10.1007/s10826-012-9594-0

Stahmer, A. C., Brookman-Frazee, L., Rieth, S. R., Stoner, J. T., Feder, J. D., Searcy, K., & Wang, T. (2017). Parent perceptions of an adapted evidence-based practice for toddlers with autism in a community setting. *Autism*, *21*(2), 217–230. https://doi.org/10.1177/1362361316637580

Stahmer, A. C., Rieth, S. R., Dickson, K. S., Feder, J., Burgeson, M., Searcy, K., & Brookman-Frazee, L. (2020). Project ImPACT for toddlers: Pilot outcomes of a community adaptation of an intervention for autism risk. *Autism, 24*(3), 617–632. https://doi.org/10.1177/1362361319878080

Steiner, A. M., & Gengoux, G. W. (2018). Strength-based approaches to working with families of children with ASD. In M. Siller & L. Morgan (Eds.), *Handbook of parent-implemented interventions for very young children with autism* (pp. 155–168). Springer.

Steiner, A. M., Gengoux, G. W., Klin, A., & Chawarska, K. (2013). Pivotal response treatment for infants at-risk for autism spectrum dis- orders: A pilot study. *Journal of Autism and Developmental Disorders, 43*(1), 91–102. https://doi.org/10.1007/s10803-012-1542-8

Strain, P. S., & Schwartz, I. (2001). ABA and the developmental of meaningful social relations for young children with autism. *Focus on Autism and Other Developmental Disorders*, *16*(2), 120–128. https://doi.org/10.1177/108835760101600208

Stratis, E. A., & Lecavalier, L. (2013). Restricted and repetitive behaviors and psychiatric symptoms in youth with autism spectrum disorders. *Research in Autism Spectrum Disorders, 7*(6), 757–766. https://doi.org/10.1016/j.rasd.2013.02.017

The Hanen Centre. (2016). Talkability™ program for parents of verbal children on the autism spectrum. Retrieved April 28, 2022, from http://www.hanen.org/Programs/For-Parents/TalkAbility.aspx

Thompson, L., Lobb, C., Elling, R., Herman, S., Jurkiewicz, T., & Hulleza, C. (1997). Pathways to family empowerment: Effects of family-centered delivery of early intervention services. *Exceptional Children, 64*(1), 99–113. https://doi.org/10.1177/001440299706400107

Tomasello, M. (2001). Perceiving intention and learning words in the second year of life. In M. Bowerman & S. Levinson (Eds.), *Language acquisition and conceptual development* (pp. 133–158). Cambridge University.

Tottenham, N. (2017). The Brain's Emotional Development. *Cerebrum: The Dana Forum on Brain Science*. https://www.ncbi.nlm.nih.gov/pmc/articles/PMC6132040/

Trembath, D., Gurm, M., Scheerer, N. E., Trevisan, D. A., Paynter, J., Bohadana, G., Roberts, J., & Iarocci, G. (2019). Systematic review of factors that may influence the outcomes and generalizability of parent-mediated interventions for young children with autism spectrum disorder. *Autism Research, 12*(9), 1304–1321. https://doi.org/10.1002/aur.2168

Tripathi, I., Estabillo, J. A., Moody, C. T., & Laugeson, E. A. (2022). Long-term treatment outcomes of PEERS® for preschoolers: A parent-mediated social skills training program for children with autism spectrum disorder. *Journal of Autism and Developmental Disorders*, *52*(6), 2610–2626. https://doi.org/10.1007/s10803-021-05147-w

Tripathi, I., Moody, C. T., & Laugeson, E. A. (2024). Parent perspectives on treatment: A mixed methods analysis of PEERS® for preschoolers. *Autism*, *28*(2), 390–402. https://doi.org/10.1177/13623613231172314

Trivette, C. M., Dunst, C. J., & Hamby, D. W. (2010). Influences of family-systems intervention practices on parent-child interactions and child development. *Topics in Early Childhood Special Education, 30*(1), 3–19. https://doi.org/10.1177/0271121410364250

Uljarević, M., Richdale, A. L., Evans, D. W., Cai, R. Y., & Leekam, S. R. (2017). Interrelationship between insistence on sameness, effortful control and anxiety in adolescents and young adults with

Autism Spectrum Disorder (ASD). *Molecular Autism, 8,* Article 36. https://doi.org/10.1186/s13229-017-0158-4

van den Bergh, S. F., Scheeren, A. M., Begeer, S., Koot, H. M., & Geurts, H. M. (2014). Age related differences of executive functioning problems in everyday life of children and adolescents in the autism spectrum. *Journal of Autism and Developmental Disorders, 44*(8), 1959–1971. https://doi.org/10.1007/s10803-014-2071-4

Van Hecke, A. V., Stevens, S., Carson, A. M., Karst, J. S., Dolan, B., Schohl, K., McKindles, R. J., Remmel, R., & Brockman, S. (2015). Measuring the plasticity of social approach: A randomized controlled trial of the effects of the PEERS® intervention on EEG asymmetry in adolescents with autism spectrum disorders. *Journal of Autism and Developmental Disorders, 45*(2), 316–335. https://doi.org/10.1007/s10803-013-1883-y

Van Schalkwyk, G. I., & Dewinter, J. (2020). Qualitative research in the journal of Autism and Developmental Disorders. *Journal of Autism and Developmental Disorders*, *50*(7), 2280–2282. https://doi.org/10.1007/s10803-020-04466-8

van Steensel, F. J. A., Bögels, S. M., & Dirksen, C. D. (2012). Anxiety and quality of life: Clinically anxious children with and without autism spectrum disorders compared. *Journal of Clinical Child & Adolescent Psychology, 41*(6), 731–738. https://doi.org/10.1080/15374416.2012.698725

Vaughn, S., Kim, A., Morris Sloan, C. V., Hughes, M. T., Elbaum, B., & Sridhar, D. (2003). Social skills interventions for young children with disabilities: A synthesis of group design studies. *Remedial and Special Education*, *24*(1), 2–15. https://doi.org/10.1177/074193250302400101

Vivanti, G., Prior, M., Williams, K., & Dissanayake, C. (2014). Predictors of outcomes in autism early intervention: Why don't we know more? *Frontiers in Pediatrics, 2*, Article 58. https://doi.org/10.3389/fped.2014.00058

Wainer, A. L., Hepburn, S., & McMahon Griffith, E. (2017). Remembering parents in parent-mediated early intervention: An approach to examining impact on parents and families. *Autism, 21*(1), 5–17. https://doi.org/10.1177/1362361315622411

Wan, M. W., Green, J., Elsabbagh, M., Johnson, M., Charman, T., & Plummer, F., & Basis Team. (2013). Quality of interaction between at-risk infants and caregiver at 12–15 months is associated with 3- year autism outcome. *Journal of Child Psychology and Psychiatry, 54*(7), 763–771. https://doi.org/10.1111/jcpp.12032

Wang, S. Y., Parrila, R., & Cui, Y. (2013). Meta-analysis of social skills interventions of single-case research for individuals with autism spectrum disorders: Results from three-level HLM. *Journal of Autism and Developmental Disorders, 43*(7), 1701–1716. https://doi.org/10.1007/s10803-012-1726-2

Watkins, L., Kuhn, M., Ledbetter-Cho, K., Gevarter, C., & O'Reilly, M. (2017). Evidence-based social communication interventions for children with autism spectrum disorder. *The Indian Journal of Pediatrics, 84*(1), 68–75. https://doi.org/10.1007/s12098-015-1938-5

Watkins, L., O'Reilly, M., Kuhn, M., Gevarter, C., Lancioni, G. E., Sigafoos, J., & Lang, R. (2015). A review of peer-mediated social interaction interventions for students with autism in inclusive settings. *Journal of Autism and Developmental Disorders, 45*(4), 1070–1083. https://doi.org/10.1007/s10803-014-2264-x

Watson, P. J., & Workman, E. A. (1981). The non-concurrent multiple baseline across-individuals design: An extension of the traditional multiple baseline design. *Journal of Behavior Therapy and Experimental Psychiatry, 12*(3), 257–259. https://doi.org/10.1016/0005-7916(81)90055-0

Wetherby, A. M., Guthrie, W., Woods, J., Schatschneider, C., Holland, R. D., Morgan, L., & Lord, C. (2014). Parent-implemented social intervention for toddlers with autism: An RCT. *Pediatrics*, *134*(6), 1084–1093. https://doi.org/10.1542/peds.2014-0757

White, S. W., Keonig, K., & Scahill, L. (2007). Social skills development in children with autism spectrum disorders: A review of the intervention research. *Journal of Autism and Developmental Disorders, 37*(10), 1858–1868. https://doi.org/10.1007/s10803-006-0320-x

White, S. W., Richey, J. A., Gracanin, D., Coffman, M., Elias, R., LaConte, S., & Ollendick, T. H. (2016). Psychosocial and computer-assisted intervention for college students with autism spectrum disorder: Preliminary support for feasibility. *Education and Training in Autism and Developmental Disabilities, 51*(3), 307–317.

White, S. W., Scarpa, A., Conner, C. M., Maddox, B., & Bonete, S. (2015). Evaluating change in social skills in high-functioning adults with autism spectrum disorder using a laboratory-based observational measure. *Focus on Autism and Other Developmental Disabilities, 30*(1), 3–12. https://doi.org/10.1177/1088357614539836

Whittingham, K., Sofronoff, K., Sheffield, J., & Sanders, M. R. (2009). Stepping stones triple p: An RCT of a parenting program with parents of a child diagnosed with an autism spectrum disorder. *Journal of Abnormal Child Psychology, 37*(4), 469–480. https://doi.org/10.1007/s10802-008-9285-x

Wolstencroft, J., Robinson, L., Srinivasan, R., Kerry, E., Mandy, W., & Skuse, D. (2018). A systematic review of group social skills interventions, and meta-analysis of outcomes, for children with high functioning ASD. *Journal of Autism and Developmental Disorders, 48*(7), 2293–2307. https://doi.org/10.1007/s10803-018-3485-1

Yerys, B. E., Antezana, L., Weinblatt, R., Jankowski, K. F., Strang, J., Vaidya, C. J., Schultz, R. T., Gaillard, W. D., & Kenworthy, L. (2015). Neural correlates of set-shifting in children with autism. *Autism Research, 8*(4), 386–397. https://doi.org/10.1002/aur.1454

Yoder, P., Bottema-Beutel, K., Woynaroski, T., Chandrasekhar, R., & Sandbank, M. (2013). Social communication intervention effects vary by dependent variable type in preschoolers with autism spectrum disorders. *Evidence-Based Communication Assessment and Intervention*, *7*(4), 150–174. https://doi.org/10.1080/17489539.2014.917780

Yoo, H. J., Bahn, G., Cho, I. H., Kim, E. K., Kim, J. H., Min, J. W., Lee, W. H., Seo, J.-S., Jun, S.-S., Bong, G., Cho, S., Shin, M.-S., Kim, B.-N., Kim, J.-W., Park, S., & Laugeson, E. A. (2014). A randomized controlled trial of the Korean version of the PEERS® parent-assisted social skills training program for teens with ASD. *Autism Research, 7*(1), 145–161. https://doi.org/10.1002/aur.1354

Zablotsky, B., Bradshaw, C. P., & Stuart, E. A. (2013). The association between mental health, stress, and coping supports in mothers of children with autism spectrum disorders. *Journal of Autism and Developmental Disorders*, *43*, 1380–1393. https://doi.org/10.1007/s10803-012-1693-7

Zaidman-Zait, A., Mirenda, P., Zumbo, B. D., Georgiades, S., Szatmari, P., Bryson, S., Fombonne, E., Roberts, W., Smith, I., Vaillancourt, T., Volden, J., Waddell, C., Zwaigenbaum, L., Duku, E., & Thompson, A. (2011). Factor analysis of the parenting stress index-short form with parents of young children with autism spectrum disorders. *Autism Research, 4*(5), 336–346. https://doi.org/10.1002/aur.213

Zuckerman, K. E., Sinche, B., Mejia, A., Cobian, M., Becker, T., & Nicolaidis, C. (2014). Latino parents' perspectives on barriers to autism diagnosis. *Academic Pediatrics*, *14*(3), 301–308. https://doi.org/10.1016/j.acap.2013.12.004

Appendix A
Sample PEERS® for Preschoolers Intake Interview Document

DATE OF SERVICE:

CHILD NAME:

CHILD DOB:

PARENT NAME(S):

PRIMARY INFORMANT(S):

HISTORY SUPPLEMENTED BY:

CHIEF COMPLAINT:

HISTORY OF PRESENT CONCERNS:

CHILD DEVELOPMENTAL HISTORY:

CHILD EDUCATIONAL HISTORY:

CHILD PSYCHIATRIC HISTORY:

FAMILY LEGAL HISTORY:

FAMILY PSYCHIATRIC AND MEDICAL HISTORY:

CHILD MEDICAL HISTORY:

CHILD CURRENT MEDICATIONS:

MENTAL STATUS EXAMINATION (CIRCLE AT LEAST ONE PER CATEGORY):

Appearance: No abnormalities noted. Well-groomed. Disheveled. Inappropriate.

Appears: Age-appropriate. Younger than physical age. Older than physical age.

Eye contact: Appropriate. Poorly modulated.

Behavior and Motor Activity: No abnormalities noted. Calm. Hyperactive. Unusual gestures. Mannerisms. Tics. Tremors. Compulsions. Muscle spasms. Psychomotor slowness. Psychomotor agitation.

Speech: No abnormalities noted. Slowed. Decreased. Prolonged speech latency. Soft/hypophonic. Unusual prosody. Loud. Spontaneous. Slurred. Dysarthric. Pressured. Perseverating.

Orientation: Alert. Oriented to time, place, person, situation.

Concentration: Intact. Impaired. Fluctuating.

Attention: Intact. Impaired. Fluctuating.

Intellectual functioning: Average. Below average. Above average.

Judgment: Age-appropriate. Fair. Intact. Impaired (mild, moderate, severe).

Insight: Age-appropriate. Fair. Intact. Impaired (mild, moderate, severe).

DIAGNOSTIC IMPRESSIONS:

ASSESSMENT AND PLAN:

(Clinician Signature) (Date)

CLINICIAN NAME **DATE**
CREDENTIALS

Appendix B
Sample PEERS® for Preschoolers Welcome Letter

WELCOME TO PEERS® FOR PRESCHOOLERS!

- You are confirmed to attend the next cohort of PEERS® for Preschoolers, which is scheduled to start on **[include date]** and will be held from **[include time].**
- Groups typically include **[include number]** families. *PEERS® for Preschoolers* is NOT a friendship matching group and you are not expected to make lasting friendships with other groups members. You are simply there to practice and learn from one another in a supportive and inclusive environment.
- Regular attendance and coming on time are imperative for getting the full benefit of the program. We typically schedule around major holidays. A planned absence sheet and schedule will be distributed during the first session.
- It is important that the **same parent** attend every session consistently. **Other parents are welcome to attend, but we do not permit parents to switch off from week to week**.
- Families will have weekly assignments that require parent involvement (e.g., setting up playdates, finding playgroups), which requires consistency for parent social coaching.
- We ask that you **do not** bring siblings to group sessions.
- The child and parent groups will be led by **[include qualifications of group leaders]**. Other trained therapists and graduate students may assist with the groups under direct supervision.

Skills taught in PEERS® for Preschoolers include:

- Joining playgroups
- Organizing successful playdates
- Listening and following directions
- Meeting and greeting friends
- Sharing and giving turns
- Asking for turns during play
- Keeping cool during play
- Being flexible during play
- Being a good sport
- Maintaining play interactions
- Asking friends to play
- Joining ongoing game play
- Transitioning to new activities
- Asking and giving help
- Maintaining body boundaries
- Managing voice volume

MEETING LOCATION AND PARKING: **[include information]**

CONTACT INFORMATION: **[include contact information].**

Appendix C
Quality of Socialization Questionnaire – Preschool (QSQ-Pre)

We are interested in the number of playdates your child has had in the last month. A play-date is any time that you and your child followed through with a commitment to spend time with a playmate.

- A playdate may be a planned activity like going to the park or playing games.
- A playdate may be organized well in advance or spontaneously the same day.
- A playdate may be with one playmate or a group of playmates (including birthday parties).

1. **How many playdates did you HOST for your child in the last month?** ____________
2. Please list the **first names** of all the playmates who attended playdate(s) HOSTED by you and your child **in the last month**. If you did not HOST a playdate for your child in the last month, leave the section below blank.

Friend's first name ____________________ Friend's first name ____________________
Friend's first name ____________________ Friend's first name ____________________
Friend's first name ____________________ Friend's first name ____________________

3. **How many playdates was your child INVITED to in the last month?** ____________
4. Fill in the **first names** of all the playmates who INVITED your child for playdate(s) **in the last month**. If your child was not INVITED to a playdate in the last month, leave the section below blank.

Friend's first name ____________________ Friend's first name ____________________
Friend's first name ____________________ Friend's first name ____________________
Friend's first name ____________________ Friend's first name ____________________

We are also interested in the number of playgroups your child has attended in the last month. A playgroup is an organized social recreational activity that your child attends with other playmates for the purpose of play.

- A playgroup is a planned social activity with same-aged peers focused on organized play (e.g., sports, arts and crafts, music, dance, games).
- A playgroup is an extracurricular activity that is organized in advance and typically involves an enrollment process.
- Playgroups do not include preschool, kindergarten, or birthday parties.

5. **How many playgroups did your child attend in the last month?** ________________
6. Please list the **names of all the playgroups** your child attended **in the last month**. If your child did attend a playgroup in the last month, leave the section below blank.

Name of playgroup ____________________ Name of playgroup ____________________
Name of playgroup ____________________ Name of playgroup ____________________
Name of playgroup ____________________ Name of playgroup ____________________

Quality of Socialization Questionnaire – Preschool (QSQ-Pre)

Administration and Scoring Key

QSQ-Pre Administration

- The QSQ-Pre is a measure of social engagement with three scales:
  - Social Initiation Scale.
  - Social Reciprocity Scale.
  - Social Engagement Scale.
- The QSQ-Pre should be completed independently by the parent or caregiver.
- The QSQ-Pre takes approximately five minutes to complete.
- The QSQ-Pre may be administered at pre-test, post-test, and follow-up (optional) to track progress in *PEERS® for Preschoolers.*

QSQ-Pre Scoring Key

Social Initiation Scale:

1. The frequency of HOSTED playdates in the last month.
2. The number of different friends the parent and child HOSTED during playdates in the last month.

Social Reciprocity Scale:

3. The frequency of INVITED playdates in the last month.
4. The number of different friends who INVITED the child for a playdate in the last month.

Social Engagement Scale:

5. The frequency of ATTENDANCE at playgroups in the last month.
6. The number of different playgroups ATTENDED by the child in the last month.

Appendix D
PEERS® for Preschoolers Planned Absence Sheet

It is important for you and your child to attend **EVERY SESSION** of PEERS® for Preschoolers to get the full benefit of the program. If you know that you must be absent for a session, please mark which dates you are unable to attend in the table below.

Child's Name: ____________________________________

Session	*Date*	*Planned Absence*
1		
2		
3		
4		
5		
6		
7		
8		
9		
10		
11		
12		
13		
14		
15		
16		

Please return this document to the PEERS® for Preschoolers team by WEEK 2.
Advance information about planned absences will be used to determine if a particular session needs to be rescheduled based on the anticipated number of absences.
If you have any questions, please contact **[insert contact information]**.

Appendix E
PEERS® for Preschoolers Homework Compliance Sheet

Session	*1*	*2*	*3*	*4*	*5*	*6*	*7*	*8*	*9*	*10*	*11*	*12*	*13*	*14*	*15*	*16*
Date																

C = Complete P = Partial I = Incomplete

Child/ Parent	*Present*	*Listen & Follow Directions*	*Meet & Greet Friends*	*Sharing & Giving Turn*	*Ask for a Turn*	*Keeping Cool*	*Good Sport*	*Show & Tell*	*Don't be Bossy*	*Asking a Friend to Play*	*Joining a Game*	*Ask to Play Something Different*	*Asking & Giving Help*	*Body Boundaries*	*Inside Voice*	*Playgroups*	*Playmates & Playdates*
Child: Parent:																	
Child: Parent:																	
Child: Parent:																	
Child: Parent:																	
Child: Parent:																	
Child: Parent:																	
Child: Parent:																	
Child: Parent:																	
Child: Parent:																	
Child: Parent:																	

Appendix F

Sample PEERS® for Preschoolers Graduation Diploma

PEERS® for Preschoolers

Program for the Education and Enrichment of Relational Skills

Certificate of Completion

Presented to

[FIRST AND LAST NAME]

For the successful completion of PEERS® for Preschoolers
[Month, Day, Year]

Index

Made in the USA
Monee, IL
15 September 2026

62978583R10376